# Principles of Critical Care in Obstetrics

Alpesh Gandhi • Narendra Malhotra
Jaideep Malhotra • Nidhi Gupta
Neharika Malhotra Bora
Editors

# Principles of Critical Care in Obstetrics

Volume II

Springer

*Editors*
Alpesh Gandhi
Arihant Women's Hospital
Ahmedabad
Gujarat
India

Narendra Malhotra
Global Rainbow Healthcare
Agra
India

Jaideep Malhotra
Art Rainbow-IVF
Agra
India

Nidhi Gupta
SN Medical College
Obstetrics and Gynecology
Agra
India

Neharika Malhotra Bora
Bharti Vidya Peethmedical College
Pune
India

ISBN 978-81-322-3815-7 ISBN 978-81-322-2686-4 (eBook)
DOI 10.1007/978-81-322-2686-4

Springer New Delhi Heidelberg New York Dordrecht London

Softcover reprint of the hardcover 1st edition 2016


Printed on acid-free paper

Springer (India) Pvt. Ltd. is part of Science+Business Media (www.springer.com)

# Contents

# Part I

# Respiratory Emergencies During Pregnancy

# Bronchial Asthma in Pregnancy

1

Uma Wankhede and Abhijeet Wadate

The majority of women with asthma have normal pregnancies and the risk of complications is small in those with well-controlled asthma.

Asthma is estimated to occur in about 4 % of pregnancies, typically occurring as a pre-existing comorbidity, although some cases of asthma may initially present during pregnancy. The overall management goals of asthma in pregnancy are effective management of symptoms to avoid foetal hypoxia, whilst at the same time minimising any drug-related risks to the foetus [1].

The diagnosis of asthma is based on history, physical examinations and pulmonary function tests. The common symptoms are episodic breathlessness, wheezing cough and chest tightness. Episodic symptoms after incidental allergen exposure, seasonal variability of symptoms and a positive family history of asthma are also helpful diagnostic guides. The most usual physical finding is wheezing on auscultation. Pulmonary function tests like PEFR measurement with the help of a simple tool called peak flow meter can also aid in the diagnosis. The spirometric evaluation of asthma in pregnant patients is similar to that in non-pregnant patients. FVC, forced expiratory volume in 1 s into (FEV1), FEV1/FVC ratio and peak expiratory flow are stable to slightly increased in pregnancy [2].

## Effect of Pregnancy on Asthma

Maternal hyperventilation occurs from increasing concentration of progesterone without a corresponding change in respiratory rate. Pregnancy has variable effects on asthma. About 28 % of pregnant asthmatics improve, 33 % remain unchanged and 35 % deteriorate usually between 24 and 36 weeks of gestation. Asthma symptoms improve during the last 4 weeks (37–40 weeks) [3].

During labour and delivery, only 10 % of asthmatics report symptoms and only half of those require treatment. During postpartum period, the severity of asthma reverts to its pre-pregnancy level. The conclusions of a meta-analysis of 14 studies are in agreement with the commonly quoted generalisation that during pregnancy about one third of asthma patients experience an improvement in their asthma, one third experience a worsening of symptoms and one third remain the same. There is also some evidence that the course of asthma is similar in successive pregnancies.

Studies suggest that 11–18 % of pregnant women with asthma will have at least one emergency department visit for acute asthma, and of these 62 % will require hospitalisation. Severe asthma is more likely to worsen during pregnancy than mild asthma, but some patients with very severe asthma may experience improvement, whilst symptoms may deteriorate in some patients with mild asthma.

U. Wankhede (✉) • A. Wadate
Associate Professor, B.J. Government Medical College, Pune, India
e-mail: drumawankhede@rediffmail.com


A. Gandhi et al. (eds.), *Principles of Critical Care in Obstetrics: Volume II*,
DOI 10.1007/978-81-322-2686-4_1

A systematic review concluded that, if symptoms do worsen, this is most likely in the second and third trimesters, with the peak in the sixth month. In a large cohort study, the most severe symptoms were experienced by patients between the 24th and 36th week of pregnancy. Thereafter symptoms decreased significantly in the last 4 weeks, and 90 % had no asthma symptoms during labour or delivery [4].

Several physiological changes occur during pregnancy that could worsen or improve asthma, but it is not clear which, if any, are important in determining the course of asthma during pregnancy.

Pregnancy can affect the course of asthma and asthma and its treatment can affect pregnancy outcomes.

The following features may improve asthma during pregnancy:

Progesterone-mediated bronchodilatation

- Oestrogen- or progesterone-mediated potentiation of beta-adrenergic bronchodilatation
- Decreased plasma histamine-mediated bronchoconstriction
- Pulmonary effect of increased serum-free cortisol
- Glucocorticosteroid-mediated increased beta-adrenergic responsiveness
- Prostaglandin E-mediated bronchodilatation
- Atrial natriuretic factor-induced bronchodilatation
- Increased half-life or decreased protein binding of endogenous or exogenous bronchodilator

Factors that may worsen asthma during pregnancy:

- Pulmonary refractoriness to cortisol effects because of competitive binding to glucocorticoid receptors by progesterone, aldosterone or deoxycorticosterone
- Prostaglandin F2a-mediated bronchoconstriction
- Decreased functional residual capacity of the lung
- Increased viral or bacterial respiratory infection-triggered asthma [5]
- Increased gastrooesophageal reflux-induced asthma
- Increased stress in pregnancy

Majority of effects are related to changing hormonal level in pregnant woman.

For example, the levels of free cortisol may improve asthma symptoms, whilst this effect may be counterbalanced by the pregnancy-related increase in serum progesterone, aldosterone and deoxycorticosterone.

In asthmatics with improved symptoms during pregnancy, the balance between these hormones may be tipped towards free cortisol, whilst the opposite occurs in those whose symptoms worsen. Improvement in symptoms during the last 4 weeks of pregnancy and the lack of symptoms during labour coincide with the highest level of free cortisol.

## Effect of Asthma on Pregnancy Outcome

In most women asthma has no effect on the outcome of pregnancy. However uncontrolled asthma may lead to increase in preterm birth, low birth weight, neonatal seizure, transient tachypnoea of the newborn and neonatal hypoglycaemia. Uncontrolled asthma can also lead to higher rates of pregnancy-induced hypertension or pre-eclampsia and caesarean section, hyperglycaemia, vaginal haemorrhage and premature rupture of membranes [6].

The risks for preterm delivery and low birth weight were higher in women with more severe asthma necessitating admission. In a large cohort study of women with asthma, there was an association of both mean FEV1 and mean FEV1 <80 % predicted with gestational hypertension, preterm delivery <37 and <32 weeks and low birth weight.

In contrast, if asthma is well controlled throughout pregnancy, there is little or no increased risk of adverse maternal or foetal complications [7]. Pregnancy should therefore be an indication to optimise therapy and maximise lung function in order to reduce the risk of acute asthma attacks and hypoxia.

## Monitoring of Asthmatic Women during Pregnancy

Monitor pregnant women with moderate/severe asthma closely to keep their asthma well controlled. Women should be advised of the importance of maintaining good control of their asthma during pregnancy to avoid problems for both the mother and baby

- Office spirometry at each visit preferably at every 4–6 weeks.
- Peak expiratory flow rate to be measured especially in those who are on medication for asthma.
- Peak flow rate should be taken on admission to labour delivery unit and then every 12 h.
- If asthma symptoms develop, peak flow rates should be measured after treatment to see adequacy of response.
- IV fluids may be necessary to ensure the mother's proper hydration.
- Adequate analgesia will limit the risk of bronchospasm.
- Monitoring of foetus.

Foetus should be monitored with the help of DFMC, USG, NST and biophysical profile regularly.

## Indicator of Good Control of Asthma

- Active without experiencing any asthma symptoms
- Sleeping through the night and not waking due to asthma symptoms
- Attaining her personal best peak flow reading

## Asthma Management during Pregnancy

The management of acute asthma in pregnancy may be affected by concern regarding treatment side effects, but the maternal and foetal risks of uncontrolled asthma are much greater than the risks from using conventional asthma medications for the management of acute asthma.

## Avoidance of Asthma Triggers

Various risk factors which may precipitate asthma should be avoided as under:

1. Avoidance of pollens, moulds, pet dander, house dust mites and cockroaches.
2. Avoidance of substances like paints, chemical fumes, strong odours and environmental pollution.
3. Remove allergy-causing pets or animals at home or workplace.
4. Cessation of smoking – A pregnant women who smokes runs a higher risk of a severe asthma episode. This could also seriously reduce the oxygen supply to the foetus, especially if the blood of the foetus already contains a large amount of carbon monoxide from cigarette smoke.
5. Avoidance of routine skin testing to identify allergens due to potential risk of systemic reaction.
6. Immunotherapy may be safely continued, if already receiving injections, but initiation of immunotherapy is not recommended.

## Principles of Drug Therapy [8–9]

Oxygen should be delivered to maintain saturation of 94–98 % in order to prevent maternal and foetal hypoxia.

Drug therapy should be given as for a non-pregnant patient with acute asthma, including nebulised β2-agonists and early administration of steroid tablets. In severe cases, intravenous β2-agonists and aminophylline can be used as indicated [10].

Continuous foetal monitoring should be performed when asthma is uncontrolled or severe or when foetal assessment on admission is not reassuring. Consideration should be given to early referral to critical care services as impaired ventilatory mechanics in late pregnancy can lower functional residual capacity and may result in earlier oxygen desaturation. Pregnant women may be more difficult to intubate due to anatomical changes especially if they have pre-eclampsia.

Acute severe asthma in pregnancy is an emergency and should be treated vigorously in the hospital.

In general, the medicines used to treat asthma are safe in pregnancy. A large UK population-based case control study found no increased risk of major congenital malformations in children of women receiving asthma treatment in the year before or during pregnancy. The risk of harm to the foetus from severe or chronically under-treated asthma outweighs any small risk from the medications used to control asthma.

Counsel women with asthma regarding the importance and safety of continuing their medication in pregnancy.

Inhaled therapy is better than oral therapy because oral therapy may produce systemic side effects during long-term therapy.

1. Active asthma control to be achieved by making changes in medication during planning of pregnancy, i.e. prior to conception, if possible. Use minimum dose necessary to control symptoms to avoid foetal hypoxia. Dosages should be decreased, if asthma improves during pregnancy. No significant association has been demonstrated between major congenital malformations or adverse perinatal outcome and exposure to inhaled corticosteroids. Inhaled steroids like beclomethasone dipropionate, budesonide and fluticasone help to prevent exacerbations.
2. Inhaled p2-agonist are considered safe. Due to risk of congenital malformation, parenteral epinephrine should be avoided during early stage of pregnancy. Systemic beta-agonist should be avoided near labour as they may inhibit or prolong labour. No significant association has been demonstrated between major congenital malformations or adverse perinatal outcome and exposure to short-acting β2-agonists. Short-acting beta 2-agonists like salbutamol and levosalbutamol and long-acting beta 2-agonists like salmeterol and formoterol are safe in pregnancy.
3. Dosages of theophylline may be adjusted due to changing pharmacokinetics as pregnancy progresses, and it crosses the placenta and may cause jitteriness in the newborn. No significant association has been demonstrated between major congenital malformations or adverse perinatal outcome and exposure to theophylline.
4. If oral steroids are required for asthma control, prednisolone and methylprednisolone are the preferred preparations since they cross the placenta poorly. Try to minimise the dosage and duration of oral corticosteroid and alternate-day dosing be preferred over daily dosing.

There is much published literature showing that steroid tablets are not teratogenic, but there is a slight concern that they may be associated with oral clefts. The association is not definite, and even if it is real, the benefit to the mother and the foetus of steroids for treating a life-threatening disease justifies the use of steroids in pregnancy. Moreover, the various studies of steroid exposure include many patients with conditions other than asthma, and the pattern of steroid use was generally as a regular daily dose rather than as short courses, which is how asthma patients would typically receive oral steroids [11].

Prednisolone is extensively metabolised by placental enzymes so only 10 % reaches to the foetus, making this the oral steroid of choice to treat maternal asthma in pregnancy.

Pregnant women with acute asthma attacks are less likely to be treated with steroid tablets than non-pregnant women. Failure to administer steroid tablets when indicated increases the risk of ongoing asthma attacks and therefore the risk to the mother and her foetus.

Some studies have found an association between steroid tablet use and pregnancy-induced hypertension or pre-eclampsia, preterm labour and foetal growth, but severe asthma may be a confounding variable [12].

Data regarding the safety of leukotriene receptor antagonists (LTRAs) in pregnancy are limited. A case control study with 96 cases exposed to LTRAs found no increased risk of major malformations between women with asthma exposed to LTRA and women with asthma taking only β-agonists.

## Management During Labour

Acute attacks of asthma are very rare in labour due to endogenous steroid production. In women receiving oral steroid, there is a theoretical risk of maternal hypothalamic-pituitary-adrenal axis suppression. Women with asthma may safely use all forms of pain relief in labour but should be asked about any known sensitivity to aspirin or NSAIDS before using these drugs for pain relief.

In some studies there is an association between asthma and an increased caesarean section rate, but this may be due to planned caesarean sections or inductions of labour rather than due to any direct effect of asthma on intrapartum indications. Data suggest that the risk of postpartum asthma attacks is increased in women having caesarean sections. This may relate to the severity of their asthma rather than to the caesarean section or to factors such as postoperative pain with diaphragmatic splinting, hypoventilation and atelectasis. Prostaglandin E2 may safely be used for labour induction.

The following precautions/steps should be undertaken during labour:

1. Advise women that acute asthma is rare in labour.
2. Advise women to continue their usual asthma medications in labour.
3. In the absence of acute severe asthma, reserve caesarean section for the usual obstetric indications.
4. If anaesthesia is required, regional (epidural) blockade is preferred to general anaesthesia
5. PGE2 is safe for induction of labour as it has got some bronchodilator effect.
6. Use prostaglandin F2alpha with extreme caution in women with asthma because of the risk of inducing bronchoconstriction.
7. $MgSO_4$ is a drug of choice for treating preterm labour.
8. Women receiving oral steroid (prednisolone) at a dose exceeding 7.5 mg per day for more than 2 weeks prior to delivery should receive parenteral hydrocortisone 100 mg 6–8 hourly during labour.
9. Oxytocin is safe for labour induction.

## Drug Therapy in Breastfeeding Mothers

The medicines used to treat asthma, including steroid tablets, have been shown to be safe to use in nursing mothers. Less than 1 % of the maternal dose of theophylline is excreted into breast milk. Prednisolone is secreted in breast milk, but milk concentrations of prednisolone are only 5–25 % of those in serum.

Encourage women with asthma to breastfeed.

Use asthma medications as normal during lactation.

## References


1. Blaiss MS. Management of rhinitis and asthma in pregnancy. Ann Allergy Asthma Immunol. 2003;90:16–22.
2. Mawhinnery H, Spector SL. Optimum management of asthma in pregnancy. Drugs. 1986;32:178–87.
3. Schatz M, Harden K, Forsythe A. The course of asthma during pregnancy, post partum and with successive pregnancies: a prospective analysis. J Allergy Clin Immunol. 1988;81:509–17.
4. Gluck JC, Gluck PA. The effects of pregnancy on asthma a prospective study. Ann Allergy. 1976;37:164–8.
5. Chien SJ, Mint ZS. Asthma in pregnancy in menses. In: Weiss EB, Stein M, editors. Bronchial asthma: mechanisms and therapeutics. Boston: Little Brown & Co; 1993.
6. Schatz M. Asthma during pregnancy: a prospective study of 198 pregnancies. Thorax. 1988;43:12–8.
7. Doucette JT, Bracken MB. Possible role of asthma in risk of preterm labour and delivery. Epidemiology. 1993;4:143–50.
8. Demissie K, Breckenridie MB. Infant and maternal outcome in pregnancies of asthmatics women. Am J Respir Crit Care Med. 1998;158:1091–5.
9. Lehrer S, Stone J, Lapinski R. Association between pregnancy induced hypertension and asthma. Am J Obstet Gynecol. 1993;168:1463.
10. Global strategy for asthma management and prevention NHLB/WHO Workshop Report. NIH Publication, 2004.
11. British Thoracic Society; Scottish Intercollegiate Guidelines Network. British guideline for management of asthma. Thorax. 2003;58(S-1):47–50.
12. Nelson-Piercy C. Asthma in pregnancy. Throx. 2001;56:32.

# 2 Acute Respiratory Distress Syndrome (ARDS) in Pregnancy

Revathy Janakiram, Krithika Meenakshi, and J. Madurai

## Definition

ARDS is defined as radiographically documented pulmonary infiltrates with ratio of pulmonary arterial oxygenation to fraction of inspired oxygen ($PaO_2$:$FiO_2$) of less than 200 without evidence of cardiac failure (Mallampalli 2010).

For practical purpose a working diagnosis of ARDS is made if $PaO_2$:$FiO_2$ ratio is <300 along with dyspnoea, tachypnoea, $O_2$ desaturation and radiographic pulmonary infiltrates (Wheels 2007).

ARDS Definition Task Force (2012) describes ARDS in three categories: mild, moderate and severe.

1. Mild – 200 mmHg < $PaO_2/FiO_2$ <300 mmHg
2. Moderate – 100 mmHg < $PaO_2/FiO_2$ <200 mmHg
3. Severe – $PaO_2/FiO_2$ <100 mmHg

Cardiogenic pulmonary oedema and volume overload are important differential diagnoses in pregnancy because pregnant patients have greater predisposition for developing volume overload and peripartum cardiomyopathy (Table 2.1) [1].

## Incidence

Since there is no uniform criteria for diagnosis, the reported incidence is variable from 1/3000 to 1/6000 deliveries. Catanzarite (2001) in his study reported an incidence of 1/6227.

It is associated with a mortality of 45–90 %. If ARDS develops in antepartum, there is corresponding increase in perinatal mortality too.

## Aetiology

ARDS in pregnant women can occur from obstetric or non-obstetric complications (Table 2.2).

The reduced albumin level and resultant reduced plasma oncotic pressure occurring in pregnancy lower the critical pulmonary capillary pressure at which pulmonary oedema develops (Pisani et al. 1989).

**Table 2.1** Diagnostic criteria for ARDS

| |
|---|
| 1. Acute onset of respiratory distress |
| 2. Bilateral pulmonary infiltrates on chest X-ray |
| 3. PAOP <18 mmHg or absence of clinical evidence of left atrial hypertension |
| 4. $PaO_2/FiO_2$ ratio of <200 regardless of PEEP |

R. Janakiram, MD, DGO, MNAMS, FICOG, FICMCH (✉)
Department of Obstetrics and Gynecology, Madurai Medical College, The Dr. MGR Medical University, Chennai, Tamilnadu, India
e-mail: dr.revathyjanakiram@gmail.com

K. Meenakshi, M S OG • J. Madurai
Consultant Gynecologist, Chennai, Tamilnadu, India


A. Gandhi et al. (eds.), *Principles of Critical Care in Obstetrics: Volume II*,
DOI 10.1007/978-81-322-2686-4_2

**Table 2.2** Causes of acute lung injury and respiratory failure in pregnancy

| |
|---|
| Severe sepsis – pyelonephritis, septic abortion, chorioamnionitis, puerperal infection |
| Pre-eclampsia syndrome |
| Pneumonia – bacteria, viral, aspiration |
| Haemorrhage – shock, massive transfusion, TRALI |
| Tocolytic therapy |
| Amniotic fluid embolism, trophoblastic embolism |
| Placental abruption |
| Fetal surgery, drug overdose, pancreatitis, trauma |

From Catanzarite (2001), Sibai (2014)

## Sepsis

The most common cause of ARDS is *sepsis* from pulmonary or extra-pulmonary sources. It accounts for up to 50 % of all cases.

*Chorioamnionitis* is an important cause of pregnancy-specific infectious complication leading to ARDS. They present with fever, fetal tachycardia, uterine tenderness and foul-smelling amniotic fluid. In pregnant patients with ARDS without any clear cause, and without obvious symptoms of chorioamnionitis, diagnostic amniocentesis may be required [4].

Up to 7 % of pregnant women with *pyelonephritis* develop ARDS. Pregnancy-associated dilatation of the ureters, stasis and untreated bacteriuria in pregnancy increase the risk of acute pyelonephritis [2].

Viral/bacterial pneumonia, fungal infection and malaria are other infections linked with ARDS.

## Pre-eclampsia/Eclampsia

In about 3 % of patients with severe pre-eclampsia, ARDS is reported. Mostly 70 % occurs in immediate postpartum period. Elderly, multiparity and pre-existing chronic hypertension are the risk factors. Reduced pulmonary oncotic pressure, altered permeability of pulmonary capillary membranes and increased pulmonary vascular hydrostatic pressure all together contribute to the development of ARDS in pre-eclampsia. Placing pulmonary artery catheter must be individualised. It may help to distinguish fluid overload and cardiogenic pulmonary oedema from ARDS. But its use has not been shown to improve the outcome.

Supplemental oxygenation, mechanical ventilation and judicious use of diuretics are the mainstay in the management.

## Tocolytic-Induced ARDS

β-adrenoreceptor agonists like terbutaline and ritodrine were used previously for tocolysis. When used, in about 10 % of cases, ARDS developed, either during infusion or up to 12 h after discontinuation of the drug. In addition to pregnancy-related cardiovascular changes, factors like medicine-induced increase in heart rate and cardiac output, increased capillary permeability due to infection, myocardial dysfunction as a result of continuous exposure to catecholamines and aggressive volume resuscitation contribute to the development of ARDS.

Multiple gestations, maternal infection and the use of corticosteroids further worsen the condition. Because of such problems, magnesium sulphate is used for tocolysis in place of β-adrenoreceptor agonists.

Management include immediate stopping of the drug, supportive care and diuresis. Most of the time, it resolves within 12 h.

## Aspiration of Gastric Contents

In pregnancy, aspiration of gastric contents is an important cause for ARDS, because of the physiologic and anatomic changes occurring in pregnancy and immediate postpartum. Enlarged pregnant uterus causing increased intra-gastric pressure, decreased tone of the gastro-oesophageal sphincter, reduced gastric motility and emptying, all predispose to aspiration. The well-known Mendelson's syndrome of aspiration of gastric acid during obstetric anaesthesia was published in 1946 [5]. Once witnessed, the diagnosis of aspiration is easy. Otherwise visualisation of gastric contents in the pharynx during laryngoscopy at the time of intubation helps. The higher the volume, the lower the pH of the aspirated material and the more particulate the aspirated material, the worse will be the degree of lung injury. Perioperative aspiration pneumonitis is noticed in 0.11 % of CS and 0.01 % of vaginal deliveries.

## Amniotic Fluid Embolism

Amniotic fluid embolism is another important pregnancy-specific cause of ARDS. It carries very high mortality. The entry of elements from the amniotic fluid into the maternal circulation could trigger the release of pro-inflammatory cytokines. AFE presents classically as acute hypoxic respiratory distress, haemodynamic collapse and DIC. The mortality rate is very high up to 80 %.

ARDS is characterised by three distinct stages:

1. Initial stage of acute exudative phase
2. Fibro-proliferative phase – which begins in 3–4 days and lasts for 21 days
3. Final recovery phase of healing/fibrotic phase

### Acute Exudative Phase

This acute phase is characterised by increased alveolar capillary permeability leading to protein-rich fluid leakage into alveolar spaces causing alveolar damage. The greater the degree of alveolar epithelial damage, the worse is the outcome. Disruption of the balance between pro-inflammatory and anti-inflammatory cytokines plays a major role in the development of ARDS. Formation of platelet thrombi as a result of abnormalities in coagulation system further aggravates lung injury. In many patients the acute phase may resolve completely. In some it progresses to fibro-proliferative phase.

### Fibro-proliferative Phase

Further worsening of lung compliance occurs with the development of pulmonary hypertension. There is histological evidence of interstitial fibrosis with inflammatory changes.

### Final Recovery Phase

Patients who survive recover gradually, with improvement in lung compliance and hypoxaemia. Radiographic changes also resolve completely. After 6–12 months, return of pulmonary function tests to near normal has been shown in the survivors.

## Clinical Presentation

The clinical condition varies depending on the magnitude of insult, patient's ability to compensate it and the stage of the disease.

Initially there is hyperventilation, which is aggravated by pregnancy-induced metabolic acidosis. Further worsening leads to clinical and radiological evidence of pulmonary oedema (Fig. 2.1).

In chest CT, alveolar infiltration, consolidation and atelectasis worst in the dependant portion of the lung may be noticed.

With further progression to acute pulmonary oedema, the patient develops marked dyspnoea, tachypnoea and hypoxaemia.

On clinical examination bilateral crackles, signs of pulmonary oedema, absence of signs of LVF like peripheral oedema, ↑ JVP and absent S3, will be noticed.

Hyperventilation

↓

Pregnancy induced metabolic acidosis

↓

Clinical / radiological e/o pulmonary edema

↓

↓ lung compliance & ↑intra pulmonary blood shunting

↓

Progressive alveolar interstitial edema

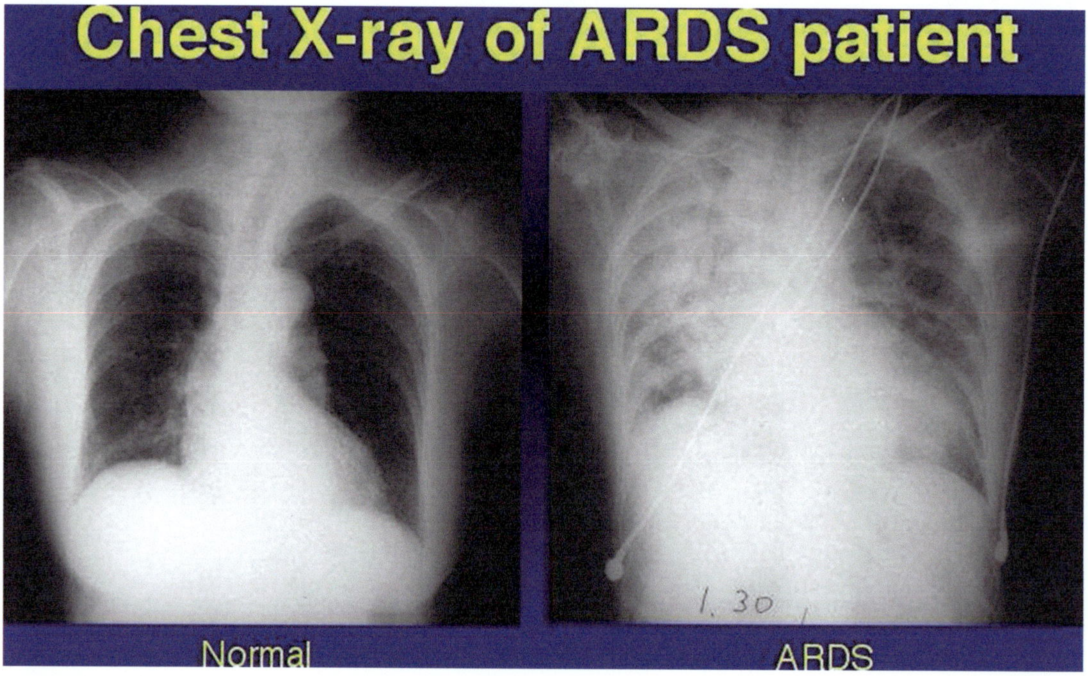


**Fig. 2.1** Bilateral parenchymal and pleural opacification in ARDS without cardiomegaly

When shunting exceeds more than 30 %, it may progress to severe refractory hypoxaemia with metabolic and respiratory acidosis, which can result in myocardial irritability, dysfunction and cardiac arrest.

## Management

ARDS requires emergency management. The mainstay in treatment is supportive therapy to provide adequate oxygenation along with management of the underlying cause, like antimicrobial therapy for sepsis. Trials conducted by the National Heart, Lung, and Blood Institute (2006b) showed that pulmonary artery catheterisation did not improve outcomes. Oxygen delivery can be greatly improved by correcting anaemia. The aim in the management is to attain $PaO_2$ of 60 mmHg, at an inspired $O_2$ content of <50 % and with positive end-expiratory pressure of <15 mmHg.

The management of ARDS in pregnant and non-pregnant women is almost the same. Fetal risk must be taken into consideration. Adequate maternal oxygen saturation is essential for fetal wellbeing. Excessive alkalosis has adverse effect on placental perfusion, whereas maternal acidosis is reasonably tolerated by the fetus.

## Mechanical Ventilation

In early stages, positive-pressure ventilation by face mask may be effective (Roy 2007). In antenatal mothers early intubation helps to maximise the fetal environment. Lower levels of $PaO_2$ should be avoided, because of impairment of placental perfusion (Levinson 1974).

*High-frequency oscillation ventilation* (*HFOP*) is not very effective in ARDS [8].

## Positive End-Expiratory Pressure (PEEP)

This is successful in decreasing the shunt by recruiting the collapsed alveoli. At levels of 5–15 mmHg, it is safe. But at higher levels, impaired venous return leading to decreased uteroplacental perfusion, diminished cardiac output, alveolar overdistension, falling compliance and barotrauma may result [6].

Providing positive-pressure ventilation to pregnant women with ARDS requires endotracheal intubation. Though non-invasive positive-pressure ventilation (NIPPV) has reduced complications, studies evaluating NIPPV in pregnant women with ARDS are not available. A trial of NIPPV in pregnant women may be considered in selected patients, but close monitoring is required because of increased risk of gastric aspiration during pregnancy.

## Ventilator-Induced Lung Injury (VILI)

Mechanical ventilation using large tidal volume and high airway pressure can produce lung injury even in previously normal lungs [3, 7]. In addition to alveolar overdistension, the repetitive opening and closing of surfactant-depleted atelectatic alveoli can itself contribute to VILI. Furthermore it can cause release of pro-inflammatory cytokines which contribute to SIRS leading to multi-organ failure [8]. A lung protective ventilation strategy that aims in avoiding both alveolar overdistension and repetitive opening and closing of atelectatic alveoli helps in reducing the systemic and pulmonary cytokine response [9].

NIH-sponsored ARDS network randomised controlled trial proved the benefit of low tidal volume approach. Comparing 12 ml/kg tidal volume with 6 ml/kg tidal volume in 861 patients, this study showed 22 % risk reduction rate in mortality in the low tidal volume group. This was the first RCT to demonstrate an improvement in mortality.

Unfortunately pregnancy has been an exclusion criterion for RCT. So no trials are available in obstetric patients. The general approach to mechanical ventilation in pregnant patients with ARDS is the same as the general population, to optimise blood gas parameters, while preventing ventilator-induced lung injury. At the same time we have to remember that the degree of respiratory acidosis tolerated by pregnant patients may be lower when compared with the general population. Excessive maternal hyperventilation and hypocapnoea should also be avoided while managing mechanical ventilation in pregnancy, because it is associated with uteroplacental vasoconstriction, diminished uteroplacental blood flow and fetal hypoxia and acidosis [10].

## Extracorporeal Membrane Oxygenation (ECMO)

ECMO has been successfully used in neonatal meconium aspiration. It has been studied in influenza-induced ARDS, by Nair 2011.

## Fetal Oxygenation

Fetal haemoglobin has higher oxygen affinity than adult haemoglobin. Even with severe ARDS and very low $PaO_2$ oxygen, displacement to fetal tissues is favoured.

## Fluid Management

With pre-eclampsia, endothelial activation with leakage causes extravascular albumin loss and fall in serum albumin levels. So in these cases, oncotic pressure becomes 16 mmHg antepartum and 14 mmHg postpartum (Zinaman 1985). Normally the colloid oncotic pressure/wedge pressure gradient exceeds 8 mmHg. When it is less than 4 mmHg, pulmonary oedema develops.

Avoidance of volume overload, together with judicious diuresis and fluid restriction, should be the approach to fluid management.

## Delivery of the Baby

It is controversial whether delivery improves maternal oxygenation (Mallampali 2010).

Many investigators (Chen 2003; Schneider 2003) concluded that delivery does not improve maternal outcome.

Acute pulmonary oedema per se is not an indication for emergency caesarean delivery.

Use of cardio active drugs which might impair utero placental circulation is decided depending on antepartum or post partum period and live or dead fetus.

## Other Therapies

Artificial or replacement surfactant therapy was found to have no benefits (Anzueto 1996).

Inhaled nitric oxide does not change the mortality rates, though there seems to be early improvement (Taylor 2004, Wheeler 2007).

Prolonged methylprednisolone therapy did not seem to reduce mortality rates in the trial by the National Heart, Lung, and Blood Institute (2006a).

## Long-Term Outcomes

No long-term follow-up study is available in pregnant women. In non-pregnant patients in a 5 year follow-up study, Herridge and associates (2011) reported normal lung function, but significant exercise limitation, diminished physical and psychological activity and decreased quality of life. Catanzarite and colleagues reported a mortality of 39 %. The most common cause of death in ARDS in pregnant mothers is multi-organ failure.

### Conclusion

Prompt treatment of the underlying precipitating cause and supportive care in the ICU is essential. Mechanical ventilation and a low tidal volume approach, with care on maternal $PaO_2$ and acid-base status to avoid both excessive hypercarbia and excessive hyperventilation, must be aimed at. Fluid management, haemodynamic support and focus on sepsis management should be considered. The use of nitric oxide, steroids and surfactant needs further study.

A multidisciplinary approach involving maternal-fetal medicine, neonatology, anaesthesiology and intensivist clinician is essential to optimise maternal and fetal outcome.

## References


1. Critical care Obstetrics. – Wiley Blackwell, 5th ed. Chapter 24, Acute Lung Injury and Acute Respiratory distress syndrome in Pregnancy. p. 338–347.
2. Cole DE, Taylor TI, Mc Cullough TM, Schoff CT, Derdak S. Acute respiratory distress syndrome in pregnancy. Crit Care Med. 2005;33:S269–78.
3. Corbridge TC, Wood LD, Crawford G, et al. Adverse effect of large tidal volume. Am Rev Respir Dis. 1990;142:311–5.
4. Lumley J, Wood C. Effect of changes in maternal oxygen & carbon dioxide, tension in the fetus. Clin Anesth. 1974;10:121–37.
5. Petty TL: how we discovered the Acute respiratory distress syndrome. Am J Respir crit care ME. 2001;163:602–3.
6. Mendelson C. The aspiration of stomach contents into lungs during obstetric anesthesia. AM J Obstet Gynecol. 1946;52:191–205.
7. Selected topics in obstetrics and gynecology- 4 Shirish N Daftary, Shyam V Deasi, Chapter 1 – Respiratory disorders in pregnancy. p. 17.
8. Slutsky AS, Trembly LN. Multi organ failure is mechanical ventilation a contributing factor? Am J Respir Crit Care Med. 1998;157:1721–5.
9. Ware LB, Matthay MA. The acute respiratory syndrome. N Engl J Med. 2000;342:1334–49. 180.
10. William's obstetrics. 24th ed. Chapter 47 Critical care and Trauma, Acute Respiratory Distress syndrome. p. 943–946.

# Pregnancy with H1N1 Infection

# 3

J.B. Sharma and Manisha Yadav

## Introduction

The 2009 global pandemic of the novel influenza A (H1N1) virus was characterized by significant clinical variations. The virus has genetic components from human, swine and poultry influenza viruses—a genetic combination that had not been previously identified [1]. The significant mortality related to this viral infection was due to a lack of prior immunity in the population, the virulence of the virus and its transmissibility among humans [2, 3]. Pregnant women are especially at high risk for developing complication with H1N1 influenza A infection. During pregnancy, women are four to five times more prone to develop serious febrile respiratory infection and have increased rate of serious illness and ICU admissions [4]. This is due to the changes in their immune systems to accommodate the developing foetus and adaptations in body as a result of the hormonal and physical changes [5]. Due to these reasons, it is critical that health care providers should know the symptomatology, treatment and prevention of H1N1 infection in pregnancy.

## Influenza Viruses

Influenza viruses are a group of RNA viruses belonging to family Orthomyxoviridae. They are classified into three distinct genera: influenza A, B and C. Influenza A can be further divided into various subtypes depending upon expression pattern of 2 viral genes—haemagglutinin (which mediate viral attachment) and neuraminidase (which mediate viral release). There are 16 types of haemagglutinin and 9 types of neuraminidase variants. So H1N1 implies haemagglutinin1 neuraminidase 1 variant of influenza A. Influenza B and C do not have any subtype. Both influenza A and B cause seasonal viral flu, and dominant strain is included in annual vaccination programme. Influenza C typically causes only mild respiratory illness. In 2009, WHO originally called H1N1 influenza "swine flu" because its genetic appearance is similar to that of viruses that infect pigs in North America. However, further investigation revealed that this new virus is more complex. The new H1N1 virus is a quadruple human reassortant comprising two strains of avian and swine (North American and Eurasian) influenza virus [3, 6, 7].

J.B. Sharma (✉) • M. Yadav
Department of Obstetrics and Gynaecology, All India Institute of Medical Sciences, New Delhi, India
e-mail: jbsharma2000@gmail.com


A. Gandhi et al. (eds.), *Principles of Critical Care in Obstetrics: Volume II*,
DOI 10.1007/978-81-322-2686-4_3

## Epidemiology

The current literature from the recent pandemic and previous outbreaks of H1N1 shows that pregnant women in the second and third trimesters are four times more likely than the general population to be hospitalized, in addition to having a significantly higher mortality rate [4, 5]. Moreover, 8–16 % of all deaths from H1N1 infection in the USA occurred in pregnant women, although this group represented only 1 % of the general population [8]. In Brazil, 156 (9.6 %) of the 1632 total deaths reported during the 2009 pandemic were among pregnant women [9].

## Pathogenesis

The worldwide pandemic of 2009 is the result of infection of influenza A (H1N1 strain) that had not been previously recognized either in pig or in humans. The CDC therefore choose the term *novel H1N1 influenza A infection,* a term that reflects the unique genetic make-up of virus, a genetic reassortment of several swine strain, a human strain and an avian strain. In contrast to genetic drift, which occurs when mutation create antigen variant similar to older strain, while genetic shift (reassortment) lead to a completely new antigen, thereby limiting the capacity of immune system to identify and destroy virus [6, 7]. Seasonal flu and smaller epidemics are due to genetic drift, while genetic shift leads to pandemics. The novel H1N1 virus infection carries various gene segments similar to Spanish flu influenza virus in 1918. Limited immunity contributes to more susceptibility of H1N1 infection. Recent research suggest that swine H1N1 virus replicates more efficiently in human and lead to more severe pathologic lesion in lung, including diffuse alveolar damage.

## Clinical Manifestations

Patients with H1N1 infection typically present with symptoms of acute respiratory illness as sore throat, cough, rhinorrhoea and fever. Other complaints may include headache, fatigue, vomiting and diarrhoea. Their clinical presentation may be complicated by superimposed bacterial infection as pneumonia. Symptoms commonly develop 1 week after the exposure, and patients remain contagious for 8 days [10, 11].

The risk of morbidity with influenza is higher among pregnant women. Pregnancy-related complication of H1N1 influenza virus includes non-reassuring foetal status (most commonly foetal tachycardia) and febrile morbidity. Hyperthermia in early pregnancy leads to neural tube defect and congenital heart disease, and fever during labour and birth is a risk factor for neonatal seizure, neonatal encephalopathy, cerebral palsy and death. Due to H1N1 viral infection, pregnant women may land up in spontaneous abortion, preterm labour and preterm premature rupture of membrane.

## Management of H1N1 Infection in Pregnancy

### Case Identification

*Suspected case*: An individual presenting with acute febrile respiratory illness (fever >38 °C) with the spectrum of disease from influenza-like illness (cough, sore throat, shortness of breath) to pneumonia.

*Probable case*: An individual with an influenza test that is positive for influenza A but is unsubtypable by reagents used to detect seasonal influenza virus infection.

*Confirmed case*: An individual with laboratory confirmed pandemic influenza A(H1N1) 2009 virus infection by one or more of the following tests:

- Real-time (RT) PCR
- Viral culture
- Fourfold rise in pandemic influenza A(H1N1) 2009 virus-specific neutralizing antibodies

### Medical Care

Pregnant mothers should consult a qualified physician (either in government or private sector) immediately if they have above symptoms.

*Pregnant mothers should be admitted to a hospital for specialized care, if they present with features of complicated influenza or progressive disease.*

Features of complicated influenza or progressive disease are:

1. Manifestations of cardiorespiratory distress (e.g. shortness of breath either during physical activity or while resting/dyspnoea, tachypnoea, hypoxia, low blood pressure)
2. Radiological signs of lower respiratory tract disease (e.g. pneumonia)
3. Central nervous system (CNS) involvement (e.g. altered mental status, unconsciousness, drowsiness, recurring or persistent convulsions (seizures), confusion, severe weakness or paralysis)
4. Severe dehydration
5. Persistent high fever and other symptoms beyond 3 days

*A compulsory follow-up visit in 3 days time should be arranged even in the absence of above complications.*

*All pregnant mothers should be admitted to the hospital, if they develop any signs or symptoms of progressive disease or danger signs or if they fail to improve within 72 h of the onset of symptoms.*

## Management in the Hospital

- Provide a disposable/surgical face mask to the patient.
- Ask her to practise hand hygiene and washing often.
- Attending health care providers should also wear face masks properly whenever in contact with infected mother.
- Isolation—care for symptomatic patients should be organized in a separate area of the antenatal ward.
- Consultant or the clinician of the highest rank (Senior Registrar/Registrar/SHO) should be informed immediately on admission.
- Institutions managing pregnant women should request adequate stocks of oseltamivir and consider transferring the patients if they need specialized care only. Most of the pregnant women can be managed if oseltamivir is started early. It is a must to start oseltamivir when H1N1 is suspected without waiting for laboratory confirmation.

## Diagnosis

Clinical specimens to be collected for laboratory diagnosis are respiratory samples. Appropriate laboratory specimens (samples from the upper respiratory tract, including a combination of nasal or nasopharyngeal samples, and a throat swab) should be collected from these patients.

(*Note: If patient has developed pneumonia, swab samples would not be positive and needs bronchial/alveoli aspirates.*)

## Antiviral Therapy

Consultant or his delegate caring for the pregnant mother should start antiviral therapy immediately.

Dose: Oseltamivir 75 mg twice a day for 5 days [12].

In severe cases, higher doses and longer duration of treatment may be considered.

Drug supply: Arrangements should be made to make 24 h availability of antiviral drugs in the hospital and/or obstetric and gynaecological wards.

*The antiviral drug is safe for use even in the first trimester. All pregnant mothers with severe/complicated disease or signs of progression of the disease (or even suspected cases) should be treated with the antiviral oseltamivir. Treatment should be initiated as soon as possible. Treatment with antiviral medications should begin without waiting for collecting specimen or results of diagnostic testing.*

## Supportive Care

The patient should be provided with necessary supportive therapy (adequate nutrition and oral fluids) and medication (e.g. antipyretics, antibiotics where indicated, rehydration. etc.). Oxygen saturation should be monitored by pulse oximetry, whenever possible. Supplemental oxygen should be provided to correct hypoxaemia. Severe cases may need care at an intensive care unit. Therefore, ensure the availability of such facilities beforehand.

*Non-steroidal Anti-inflammatory drugs (NSAIDs) should be avoided.*

Since there is high risk of foetal distress and preterm labour, consider administration of corticosteroids for promotion of foetal lung maturation where applicable.

Organize separate areas for labour and delivery for these women. Provide routine intrapartum and postpartum care. Provide appropriate interventions where indicated for specific complications related to childbirth, the postpartum/postnatal period or the newborn. Tocolytics can be used as for any other obstetric case. However, consider potential harms related to tachycardia, hypotension and other side effects.

Since there is a higher risk of foetal distress, discuss with anaesthesiologist the risks and benefits of vaginal delivery and caesarean delivery. Consider the risks of anaesthesia in a severely ill woman.

*Reduce the length of stay in the postnatal ward to the minimum required by maternal and newborn condition.*

## Newborn Care

- Do not separate the baby from the mother even if the mother has influenza A pandemic (H1N1). Institute rooming-in. (Previously, it is the notion to separate mother (H1N1 positive) from newborn immediately after birth, but according to recent guideline, it is considered that instituting rooming-in and breastfeeding with mother is more beneficial, as it strengthens the immune system of neonate and make less susceptible for viral infection.)
- Mothers should wear a disposable/surgical face mask for next 7 days and practise hand hygiene and handwashing before feeding or handling the baby.
- Support mothers to initiate breastfeeding within 1 h of giving birth and to breastfeed frequently and exclusively on demand. If mother is ill, she should be helped to express her breast milk and feed it to the infant.

  *(Treatment with antivirals to a lactating mother is not a contraindication for breastfeeding.)*
- Newborns of infected mothers should be observed for development of infection.

Newborn infants are unlikely to have typical influenza signs. Influenza or its complications in newborn infants may begin with less typical signs such as apnoea, fever, fast breathing, cyanosis, excessive sleeping, lethargy, feeding poorly and dehydration.

Newborn infants with severe or deteriorating illness and those at risk of more severe or complicated illness should promptly be treated with antiviral drugs.

*Oseltamivir dose for babies: 3 mg/kg twice daily for 5 days* (dosage form in syrup available).

Mothers who are breastfeeding may continue breastfeeding while ill and receiving oseltamivir.

## Discharge Criteria

Pregnant mothers could be discharged after completion of 4 days of treatment if she has clinically recovered. Decision on discharging those with severe disease should be taken by the treating clinicians based on their clinical judgment. Notify the proved positive cases to nearest public health facility.

## Protection Against Infection

1. Pregnant women and women in reproductive age group who have no symptoms of influenza should be educated on early clinical manifestations of pandemic (H1N1) 2009 virus infection (fever along with cough, sore throat, rhinorrhoea, headache, muscle pain and malaise).
2. They should avoid unnecessary travel, crowded public places and public transport as much as possible.
3. They should be advised to stay at home and to practise cough and sneeze etiquette (covering mouth and nose when coughing or sneezing)

or wear a mask (at least a home-made mask) if they have fever and flu-like symptoms.

4. Pregnant women and new mothers should avoid providing care for persons with influenza-like illnesses except for their own newborns.
5. Antenatal clinic visits should be reduced to the minimum required, and women with low-risk pregnancies should be advised to postpone clinic visits in early pregnancy during the outbreak.
6. All preventive measures to avoid transmission of infection should be taken by health care workers when attending to pregnant women.
7. Anyone with respiratory symptoms should not provide care for the pregnant women or the mother and newborn baby.
8. Care for symptomatic pregnant women (with fever and flu-like symptoms) should be organized in a separate area in the clinic or OPD whenever possible.

*Chemoprophylaxis is not recommended during pregnancy.*

## References


1. Machado AA. How to prevent, recognize and diagnose infection with the swine origin influenza A (H1N1) virus in humans. J Bras Pneumol. 2009;35(5):464–9.
2. Picone O, Ami O, Vauloup-Fellous C, Martinez V, Guillet M, Dupont-Bernabé C, et al. Pandemic influenza A H1N1 2009 flu during pregnancy: epidemiology, diagnosis and management. J Gynecol Obstet Biol Reprod. 2009;38(8):615–28.
3. Dawood FS, Jain S, Finelli L, Shaw MW, Lindstrom S, Garten RJ, et al. Emergence of a novel swine-origin influenza A (H1N1) virus in humans. N Engl J Med. 2009;360(25):2605–15.
4. Jamieson DJ, Honein MA, Rasmussen SA, Williams JL, Swerdlow DL, Biggerstaff MS, et al. H1N1 2009 influenza virus infection during pregnancy in the USA. Lancet. 2009;374(9688):451–8.
5. Siston AM, Rasmussen SA, Honein MA, Fry AM, Seib K, Callaghan WM, et al. Pandemic 2009 influenza A(H1N1) virus illness among pregnant women in the United States. JAMA. 2010;303(15):1517–25.
6. Greer LG, Abbassi-Ghanavati M, Sheffield JS, Casey BM. Diagnostic dilemmas in a pregnant woman with influenza A (H1N1) infection. Obstet Gynecol. 2010;115(2 Pt 2):409–12.
7. Shinde V, Bridges CB, Uyeki TM, Shu B, Balish A, Xu X, et al. Triple-reassortant swine influenza A (H1) in humans in the United States, 2005–2009. N Engl J Med. 2009;360(25):2616–25.
8. Jain S, Kamimoto L, Bramley AM, Schmitz AM, Benoit SR, Louie J, et al. Hospitalized patients with 2009 H1N1 influenza in the United States, April-June 2009. N Engl J Med. 2009;361(2):1935–44.
9. Secretariat of Health Surveillance. Epidemiological report pandemic influenza (H1N1) 2009. Year 1. http://portal.saude.gov.br/portal/arquivos/pdf/boletim_influenza_se_47.pdf. Published 2009.
10. Lim ML, Chong CY, Tee WS, Lim WY, Chee JJ. Influenza A/H1N1 (2009) infection in pregnancy – an Asian perspective. BJOG. 2010;117(5):551–6.
11. Louie J, Acosta M, Jamieson D, Honein MA. Severe 2009 H1N1 influenza in pregnant and postpartum women in California. N Engl J Med. 2010;362(1):27–35.
12. Centers for Disease Control and Prevention. Updated interim recommendations for obstetric health care providers related to use of antiviral medications in the treatment and prevention of influenza for the 2009–2010 Season. http://www.cdc.gov/h1n1flu/pregnancy/antiviral_messages.htm. Published 2009.

# Pregnancy with Chicken Pox

4

Prakash K. Mehta

## Introduction

Varicella infection in pregnancy has possibly devastating consequences for both women and their fetus. The overall incidence of varicella in pregnancy ranges from 1 to 5 per 10,000. A relatively benign disease in early childhood, the complications, both fetal and maternal, make it difficult to manage. Several issues are still debated, such as the spectrum and degree of fetal manifestations, the incidence and severity of varicella pneumonia, and the use of antiviral agent [1].

### Skin Lesions in Varicella

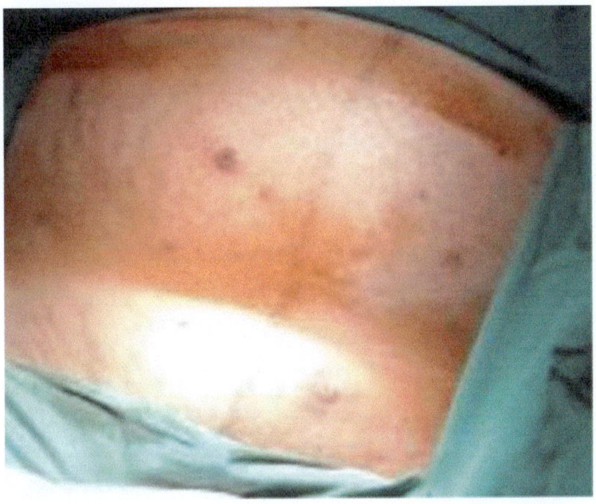

P.K. Mehta
Division of Maternal Fetal Medicine, Bhagwan Mahaveer Jain Hospital, Bangalore, India
e-mail: drprakashmehta@gmail.com

## Virology

Chickenpox (varicella) is caused by a highly contagious DNA herpes virus. Varicella-zoster virus (VZV) is the virus responsible for varicella (chickenpox) and herpes zoster ("shingles"). VZV is a member of the herpes virus family, which includes herpes simplex virus (HSV) types 1 and 2, cytomegalovirus (CMV), Epstein-Barr virus (EBV), and human herpes virus (HHV-6, HHV-7, and HHV-8). Varicella results from primary VZV infection; it is a common childhood illness associated with fever and a generalized pruritic vesicular rash [2].

## Incidence

Chickenpox is an uncommon disease during pregnancy as 93–95 % women of childbearing age are seropositive with virus-specific IgG antibodies. The incidence of varicella is 0.7–3/1000 pregnancies [3].

## Clinical Features

1. Chicken pox is transmitted by respiratory droplets and by direct personal contact with vesicle fluid or indirectly via fomites. It is characterized by fever, malaise, dry cough, and pruritic rash. Varicella-zoster virus (VZV)




A. Gandhi et al. (eds.), *Principles of Critical Care in Obstetrics: Volume II*,
DOI 10.1007/978-81-322-2686-4_4

is 25 times more serious in adults than in children. The incubation period of chickenpox is 10–21 days [3].

2. The primary infection is characterized by fever, malaise, and a pruritic rash. The rash goes through three stages. Initially, it is red and itchy, resembling insect bites, and appears on face, scalp, chest, and back. It then evolves into crops of maculopapules which become vesicular and crust over in next 4–5 days before healing. The vesicular skin lesion is the hallmark of the disease. A total number of 300–400 rashes may appear over the body. The rash may persist for 20 days and begins 48 h after the onset of headache, malaise, and fever. New lesions emerge throughout the first week. The lesions cloud and umbilicate and then crust over. The vesicles usually crust over within 5 days. The vesicles can be easily ruptured and oozes serous fluid. The contact with skin fluid can be another mode of disease transmission [4]. The infection is characterized by the simultaneous development of lesions at various stages; as a result, all three stages of the rash maculopapular, blisters, and scabbed lesions can be present at the same time. The patient is contagious until all of the lesions have crusted [3].
3. Complications include infection of skin lesions, scarring, pneumonia, and, rarely, cerebral edema and death.
4. Diagnosis of chicken pox, either in pregnant or nonpregnant subjects, can be easily performed on the basis of clinical history and clinical classical signs or symptoms. Laboratory workup may not be required. Available laboratory tests include virus/viral antigen detection, virus isolation, and identification or serological diagnosis. These may be useful in atypical cases.

## Pregnancy and Chickenpox

- There is no difference in clinical presentation of chicken pox in pregnancy as compared to the nonpregnant.
- The pregnant woman develops high fever that can last for up to 7 days. The diagnosis of varicella is usually made clinically. The virus may be cultured from vesicular fluid, but this is a cumbersome process. Serologic tests may help document acute infection in confusing cases or indicate immunity. IgM antibody may be detected as soon as 3 days after symptoms appear, and IgG may be detected as early as 7 days after varicella symptoms. Multiple antibody detection assays are available including fluorescent anti-membrane antibody (FAMA), latex agglutination (LA), enzyme-linked immunosorbent assay (ELISA), and complement fixation tests [5].

## Maternal Risks

- Anecdotally, chickenpox infection in pregnancy is more severe than in nonpregnant adults.
- Risks depend on when the infection developed during pregnancy. There could be increased severity of illness in the second half of pregnancy.
- Varicella, the primary infection with varicella-zoster virus in pregnancy, may cause maternal mortality or serious morbidity [6]. The infection can cause pneumonia, hepatitis, and encephalitis. Pneumonia can occur in up to 10 % of pregnant women with chickenpox, and the severity increased in later gestation. Even a healthy pregnant woman is at risk of dying if she develops varicella pneumonia. Mortality rates between 20 and 45 % were reported in the pre-antiviral era but have fallen to 3–14 % with antiviral therapy and improved intensive care [7].
- The chance of preterm labor is increased. Mechanism of the increased prevalence of preterm labor is unknown. It is tempting to speculate on the production of inflammatory mediators due to the viremia as being related to the preterm labor [5].

## Maternal Varicella Pneumonia

Serious life-threatening complications of the infection include pneumonia (up to 20 % of pregnant patients) and encephalitis (up to 1 % of pregnant patients).

Maternal pneumonia complicates about 10–20 % of cases of chickenpox in pregnancy resulting in a higher mortality/morbidity than in nonpregnant adults. Pregnant women with VZV pneumonia should be hospitalized for monitoring and to initiate antiviral therapy because up to 40 % of women may need mechanical ventilation [8]. Mortality in severe cases (those who require mechanical ventilation) in the pre-antiviral era was 20–45 % and is currently estimated to be 3–14 %. Between 1985 and 2002, in the confidential enquiries into maternal deaths in the UK, there were nine indirect and one late maternal death associated with maternal VZV pneumonia [9]. The risk for pneumonia also increases with increasing gestational age. While this has been associated with relative maternal immunosuppression, it still remains unproven and may be purely mechanical with increasing splinting of the diaphragm as the gravid uterus occupies more space.

## Fetal and Neonatal Risks

The transmission rate during maternal viremia has been estimated at approximately 25 %. The consequences for the infant depend on the time of maternal infection [10].

The fetal involvement has been traditionally divided into three forms:

- “Varicella embryopathy”: stemming from maternal disease occurring before 20 weeks of gestation
- Congenital varicella resulting from maternal infection from 20 weeks gestation to term but more commonly close to term
- Neonatal disease occurring when the pregnant patient has active lesions around the time of delivery

The infection rate for fetus has been reported to range from 12 to 30 % [3].

### Infection before 20 Weeks of Pregnancy

- Women who experience chicken pox early in their pregnancy have a very low chance of infecting their unborn baby. The risk appears to be approximately 2 % if the infection occurs before 20 weeks and less than 1 % if it occurs before 13 weeks [11].
- The risk of spontaneous miscarriage is not generally increased if chicken pox occurs in the first trimester.
- Varicella embryopathy was first described by Laforet and Lynch in 1947. The embryopathy includes limb hypoplasia, skin scarring, central nervous system involvement, and other skeletal lesions. Although it is most common before 20 weeks’ gestation, the embryopathy has been reported from infection as late as 26 weeks (0.4 % from conception to 13 weeks and 2.2 % from 13 to 20 weeks) [10].

### Infection before 28 Weeks of Pregnancy

Congenital varicella can result from maternal infection after 20 weeks gestation.

Fetal varicella syndrome occurs in 1–2 % of maternal varicella infection. It is characterized by skin scarring, eye defects, microcephaly, cataract, hypoplasia of limbs, gastrointestinal and urogenital malformations, neurological abnormalities including cerebellar dysplasia (microcephaly, cortical atrophy, mental retardation), and bladder and bowel sphincter dysfunction [11]. Most of these malformations can be seen by ultrasound.

Perhaps the most interesting aspect of congenital varicella is a theory advanced by Higa and co-workers [12]. These authors have postulated that the skin lesions, limb defects, and central nervous system lesions represent zoster infections in utero and that the fetal effects of varicella embryopathy are sequelae of repeated zoster infections in the fetus, including in utero encephalitis. This would explain many of the types of lesions and also the frequent appearance of active vesicles when children are born.

## Between 28 and 36 Weeks of Pregnancy

The late infection is not associated with adverse fetal effect.

It may present as shingles in the first few years of life (reactivation of virus after a primary infection in utero).

## After 36 Weeks to Birth

The baby may become infected and could be born with chickenpox. The timing of maternal infection in relation to delivery determines the risk to the infant – transplacental inoculum vs protective maternal antibody.

## Around the Time of Birth

If varicella manifests in the mother more than 5 days before delivery, there is essentially no risk to the neonate, probably because varicella antibodies have transferred to the fetus [11]. If the mother develops the rash up to 7 days after delivery when cord blood VZV IgG is low [13], the increased peripartum severity is attributed to a large transplacental inoculum of virus in the absence of protective maternal antibody.

Immunoglobulin G (IgG), immunoglobulin M (IgM), and immunoglobulin A (IgA) are produced 2–5 days after the initial infection and reach a maximum after 2–3 weeks. However, maternal varicella infection between 5 days before and 2 days after delivery poses a substantial risk to the neonate. Neonatal varicella is a severe infection that manifests with skin lesions and pneumonia and has a mortality rate of up to 31 %. In the first 10 days of life, up to 50 % of these infants will be affected. The risk of developing severe chicken pox is more if their mother has a rash 4 days before or 2 days after the birth. However, this is extremely rare (1 in 17,000 pregnancies). Furthermore, direct contactor respiratory droplet can lead to infection after birth.

Infection with onset more than 7 days before delivery ensures adequate transplacental passage of specific anti-VZV antibody to protect the infant. Passive immunization of the baby by giving VZIG immediately after delivery prevents or attenuates neonatal varicella and is essential.

Elective delivery should normally be avoided until 5–7 days after the onset of maternal rash to allow for the passive transfer of antibodies from mother to child [13].

Neonatal varicella presents as generalized chicken pox with a fatality rate of 30 %. Congenital varicella is characterized by skin lesions, limb hypoplasia, eye diseases, and neurological defects. About 25 % of infants born with these lesions die during the first months of life.

## Diagnosis of Fetal Infection and Role for Prenatal Invasive Procedures

- Pathogenesis unclear – possibly VZV reactivation in utero. Prenatal diagnosis is by detailed ultrasound examination and detection of VZV DNA by PCR in amniotic fluid.
- No treatment
- *Detailed ultrasound examination:* The findings appear 5 weeks later and include limb deformity, microcephaly, hydrocephalus, soft tissue calcification, and IUGR [14]. The wide spectrum of clinical manifestations in a neonate from maternal varicella included bowel obstruction, urinary tract anomalies, and microtia [15].
- *Fetal magnetic resonance imaging (MRI):* can be useful to identify morphological abnormalities.
- *VZV DNA* can be detected by polymerase chain reaction (PCR) in amniotic fluid [16]. VZV DNA has a high sensitivity but a low specificity for the development of FVS.

- If amniotic fluid is PCR positive for VZV and the ultrasound is normal at 17–21 weeks, the risk of FVS is low.
- If repeat ultrasound is normal at 23–24 weeks, the risk of FVS is remote.
- The risk of FVS is very high if the ultrasound shows features compatible with FVS and the amniotic fluid is positive [16].

## Management During Pregnancy

- General Management
  - Avoid contact with susceptible individual.
  - Symptomatic treatment.
  - The mainstay of treatment for herpes zoster is antiviral medicine [17].
  - Oral antiviral agents (acyclovir, valacyclovir, or famciclovir) have been shown to significantly reduce herpes-related symptoms as well as the duration, intensity, and prevalence of zoster-associated pain when given within 72 h of the first symptom. Acyclovir is the drug that has been most extensively studied in pregnant women and is the agent most commonly used to treat patients with VZV during pregnancy.
  - The dosage form of acyclovir is 800 mg per oral for five times per day for continuous 7 days [17].
  - All HIV and immunocompromised women who are pregnant and are manifesting varicella infection should be admitted to the hospital for intravenous acyclovir IV. The solution contains 25 mg/ml of drug. Each 20 ml vial contains 500 mg of drug. The vial is diluted in 500 ml of fluid and infused slowly every 8 h for 7 days [4].
  - Animal studies have not shown adverse effects from acyclovir on the fetus, and treatment of disseminated herpes simplex in pregnancy in humans has been reported with no apparent fetal damage [18]. Nevertheless, there is still a need for systematic assessment on the risk-benefit of using acyclovir in this scenario. The theoretical risk of teratogenesis persists in the first trimester.
  - Acyclovir appears to be a safe and relatively well-tolerated drug, although it may impair renal function if given to patients who are not adequately hydrated [18].
  - Acyclovir is selectively converted into a monophosphate form by viral thymidine kinase, which is far more effective (3000 times) in phosphorylation than cellular thymidine kinase. Subsequently, the monophosphate form is further phosphorylated into the active triphosphate form, aciclo-GTP, by cellular kinases. Aciclo-GTP is a very potent inhibitor of viral DNA polymerase; it has approximately 100 times higher affinity to viral than cellular polymerase. Its monophosphate form also incorporates into the viral DNA, resulting in chain termination. It has also been shown that the viral enzymes cannot remove aciclo-GMP from the chain, which results in inhibition of further activity of DNA polymerase. Aciclo-GTP is fairly rapidly metabolized within the cell, possibly by cellular phosphatases [18].
  - The low oral bioavailabilities of acyclovir, as well as the emergence of drug-resistant virus strains, have stimulated efforts toward the development of new compounds for the treatment of individuals with VZV infections. Among the new compounds, the oral prodrug form of acyclovir (valacyclovir) and penciclovir (famciclovir) rank among the most promising. Valacyclovir, a category C drug, is a prodrug metabolized to acyclovir. It is an esterified version of acyclovir and has greater oral bioavailability (about 55 %) than acyclovir (10–20 %). It is converted by esterases to the active drug acyclovir, as well as the amino acid valine, via hepatic first-pass metabolism. As with acyclovir itself, all of these drugs are dependent on the virus-encoded thymidine kinase (TK) for their intracellular activation (phosphorylation), and, upon conversion to their triphosphate form, they act as inhibitors/alternative substrate of the viral DNA polymerase. Therefore, cross-resistance to these drugs may be

expected for those virus mutants that are TK deficient and thus resistant to acyclovir [18]. Famciclovir, a category C drug, has not been studied enough in pregnant women.

– Other classes of nucleoside analogues dependent for their phosphorylation on the viral TK that have been used for the treatment of VZV infections include sorivudine, brivudine, fialuridine, fiacitabine, and netivudine. Among oxetanocins, which are partially dependent on viral TK, lobucavir is now under clinical evaluation. Foscarnet, which does not require any previous metabolism to interact with the viral DNA polymerase, is used when TK-deficient varicella virus mutants emerge during acyclovir treatment. IFN-a licensed may be useful for acyclovir-resistant strains [18]

## VZIG: Protection of the Fetus from Infection

- Varicella-zoster immune globulin (VZIG) should be strongly considered for pregnant women without immunity who have been exposed to varicella. Varicella-zoster immune globulin attenuates clinical disease in the mother not necessarily by eradicating viremia but often by lessening it. Given that the large majority of fetuses apparently are not infected even when the mother has a "full" viral load, it is biologically plausible that varicella-zoster immune globulin, which may lessen the viral load to which the fetus is exposed, would lower the fetal infection rate [19].
- All pregnant women who have significant exposure to VZV infection (defined as "living in the same household as a person with active chicken pox or herpes zoster or face-to-face contact with a person with chicken pox or uncovered zoster for at least 5 min"), who have no history of chickenpox, and who are seronegative (or serological testing is not readily available), should be offered VZIG [17].
- VZIG should be administered within 72 h of exposure for maximal effect, although it may provide some benefit up to 96 h after exposure for immunocompromised subjects. US FDA in 2011 has extended administration to up to 10 days. VZIG is ineffective, and should not be given, once clinical illness is established [20].
- VZIG is indicated for the baby if maternal varicella develops up to 7 days before delivery or if the mother develops chicken pox up to 28 days after delivery. If birth occurs within the 7-day period following the onset of the maternal rash or if the mother develops the chickenpox rash within the 7-day period after birth, the neonate should be given VZIG [17]
- The recommended dose is 2 mL for children 0–5 years, 4 mL for children 6–12 years, and 6 mL for adults [17]. Administration is by intramuscular injection, with few adverse effects other than local discomfort reported. This can be lessened if the VZIG is at room temperature when administered. VZIG should never be given intravenously.
- The passive immunization may reduce the risk of fetal infection, but there is no evidence of the prevention of fetal viremia. Passively acquired antibodies may also reduce the severity of neonatal chickenpox.
- Maternal herpes zoster is not an indication for VZIG administration to the baby [17].
- Infants born after 28 weeks' gestation should only be given VZIG if they have had significant exposure and serological tests show the mother to be seronegative.
- All infants born at or before 28 weeks' gestation or born weighing under 1000 g with significant exposure should be given ZIG regardless of the results of serological testing of the mother.

## Quarantine

- A mother and/or her baby with active vesicles should be isolated from other mothers and babies, but an infected mother does not need to be isolated from her own baby.

- The infant should be monitored for signs of infection until 28 days after the onset of maternal infection [17].
- Infants with pneumonitis requiring ventilation must be isolated. Where isolation facilities are unavailable, cases should be transferred to a unit with isolation facilities.
- Quarantine of cases should continue until all lesions have crusted. Aim to discharge all patients requiring quarantine from hospital as soon as possible [17].
- Quarantine of contacts should be from days 7–21 after exposure.
- Although quarantine of cases and those considered to have significant contact is recommended, this should not compromise medical and nursing care of a sick infant [17].

## Primary Prevention

- A previous history of chickenpox infection is 97–99 % predictive of the presence of serum varicella antibodies. Therefore, a reasonable policy is to ask about previous chickenpox/shingles and restrict advice to women who have no history or an uncertain history of previous infection.
- Primary prevention consists of effective vaccination of the mother before conception, while secondary prevention involves the use in susceptible pregnant women of varicella-zoster immune globulin, a specific IgG antibody against varicella-zoster virus, after exposure.
- Women who are seronegative for VZV IgG must be advised to avoid contact with chickenpox and shingles during pregnancy and to immediately inform healthcare workers of a potential exposure.
- Varicella vaccine contains live attenuated virus. Following its introduction, the incidence of primary infection (chickenpox) has fallen by 90 %, and the mortality related to the condition has decreased by two-thirds. Immunity from the vaccine may persist for up to 20 years [21]. Because the effects of the varicella virus on the fetus are unknown, pregnant women should not be vaccinated. Nonpregnant women who are vaccinated should avoid becoming pregnant for 1 month after each injection. For persons without evidence of immunity, having a pregnant household member is not a contraindication for vaccination.
- If a pregnant woman is inadvertently vaccinated or becomes pregnant within 4 weeks after MMR or varicella vaccination, she should be counseled about the theoretical basis of concern for the fetus; however, MMR or varicella vaccination during pregnancy should not be considered a reason to terminate pregnancy [22].

## Delivery and Anesthesia for the Patient with Chickenpox

1. Deciding the timing and route of delivery:
    - Timing and mode of delivery must be individualized.
    - Delivery during the viremic period may be extremely hazardous.
    - The maternal risks are: bleeding, thrombocytopenia, disseminated intravascular coagulopathy, and hepatitis.
    - High risk of varicella of the newborn with significant morbidity and mortality.
    - IV acyclovir is recommended.
    - There is no evidence about the optimum method of anesthesia for women requiring delivery by caesarean section [17].
2. General anesthesia may exacerbate varicella pneumonia.
3. There is theoretical risk of transmitting the virus from skin lesions to the CNS via spinal anesthesia This results in advice that epidural anesthesia may be safer than spinal anesthesia, because the dura is not penetrated.
4. A site free of cutaneous lesions should be chosen for needle placement.

## Prevention and Amelioration of Neonatal Effects

If maternal infection occurs at term:

- If practical delivery should be delayed by 5 days after onset of illness.
- If delivery within 5 days of infection – Give VZIG to neonate.
- If mother develops chickenpox within 2 days of delivery – Give VZIG to neonate.
- VZIG does not prevent neonatal infection but lowers mortality rate.
- Monitor baby for signs of infection for 14–16 days.

If neonatal infection occurs, it should be treated with acyclovir [21].

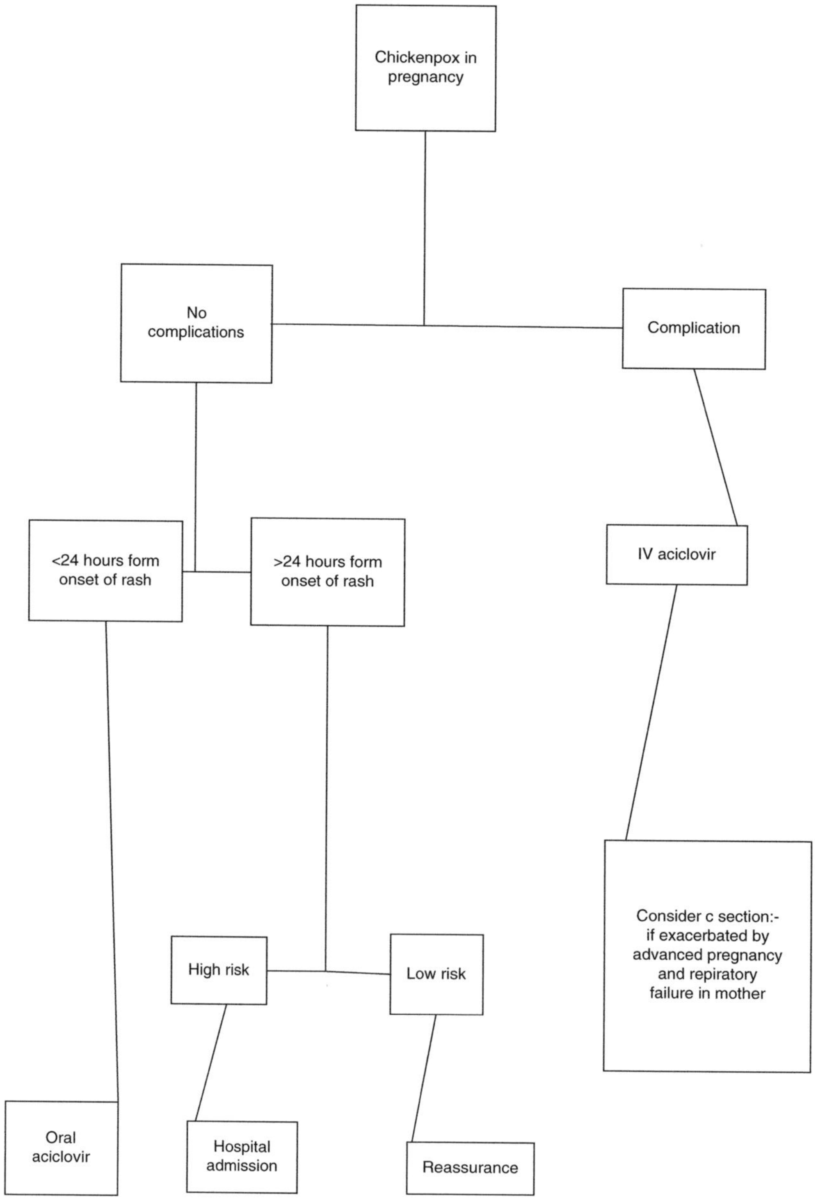

## Breast Feeding

- The chicken pox virus has not been found in breast milk of women with a chicken pox infection [5].
- Breast milk may contain antibodies that can protect baby.
- Prevent baby from coming into direct contact with rash.

## Herpes Zoster and Pregnancy

Following the primary infection, the virus remains dormant in sensory nerve root ganglia but can be reactivated to cause a localized, painful, vesicular erythematous skin rash in a dermatomal distribution known as herpes zoster (HZ) or simply zoster or shingles. Occasionally, chickenpox develops in susceptible mothers after exposure to patients with herpes zoster [2]. This infection is less serious than varicella due to the presence of maternal antibodies; however, it can be very serious in immunocompromised patients. The infection manifests clinically as fever, malaise, and skin rash. The rash is painful and is usually confined to a dermatome. There is no evidence of fetal harm in women who develop herpes zoster. Herpes zoster around the time of delivery is not a risk to the neonate because it is protected by transplacentally acquired maternal antibodies [17].

## Care and Precautions

1. Protection of household contacts/health personnel/newborn/Vaccination/VZIg
2. Healthcare workers:
   (a) A significant exposure in the neonatal unit or on the postnatal ward is defined as: patient sharing the same open ward as a person with chickenpox or zoster.

   Face-to-face contact with a person with chickenpox or zoster for at least 5 min and contact for 1 h or more with person (staff or patient) with chickenpox lesions or who developed lesions up to 48 h later [21].

   (b) All staff who have had significant exposure to an index case and who do not have a history of previous chickenpox infection or of VZV vaccination should have serological tests. If they are VZV antibody negative, they should be removed from clinical duties from days 7–21 after exposure (days 7–28 if they receive ZIG) [23].

   (c) If nonimmune healthcare workers have significant exposure to infection, they should either be:
   - Warned they may develop chickenpox and should be reallocated to minimize patient contact from 8 to 21 days post-contact.
   - Varicella vaccination is recommended for nonimmune healthcare workers. Pregnancy should be avoided for 3 months following vaccination.

**Conclusion**

Both chickenpox and herpes zoster infection are uncommon during pregnancy. The incidence of primary varicella or chickenpox in pregnancy has been estimated to be 1–5 cases per 10,000 pregnancies. Infection with the virus generally confers lifelong immunity. The data currently confirm that vertical transmission risk in the first trimester is extremely low (0–0.4 %) and may be lower for herpes zoster than for chickenpox. The reason for the lower risk in women with zoster may simply be that viremia is uncommon in the immunocompetent individual with zoster compared with chickenpox, thus reducing the risk of placental viral transmission. A pregnant woman who has been exposed to varicella before pregnancy should be reassured that her fetus is safe. A pregnant woman manifesting varicella infection should be counseled about the risk of viral transmission to the fetus and the risks of fetal anomalies. They should also be informed that these risks are very low. Prenatal ultrasound and magnetic resonance imaging have been used to document the extent of tissue damage in fetal varicella syndrome. Neonatal infection may occur in 10–20 % of neonates whose mothers became acutely infected from

5 days before delivery to 2 days after the delivery. Infants become symptomatic 5–10 days postpartum. The clinical picture may vary from skin lesions to systemic illness, pneumonia. For the mother, there could be serious problems including pneumonia which could be fatal. The impact of all the research highlights the need for adequate screening and immunization of women of childbearing age who are susceptible to varicella infection during pregnancy.

## Bibliography


1. Lamont RF, Sobel JD, Carrington D, et al. Varicella-zoster virus (chickenpox) infection in pregnancy. BJOG. 2011;118:1155.
2. Arvin AM. Varicella-zoster virus. In: Fields B, editor. Virology. 3rd ed. New York: Raven; 1995. p. 2547–86.
3. Straus SE, Ostrove JM, Inchauspé G, et al. NIH conference. Varicella-zoster virus infections. Biology, natural history, treatment, and prevention. Ann Intern Med. 1988;108:221.
4. Tunbridge AJ, Breuer J, Jeffery KJ. British Infection Society. Chickenpox in adults – clinical management. J Infect. 2008;57:95–102.
5. Pattanasuttinont S. Maternal chickenpox in peripartum period: a case report and review. J Med Assoc Thai. 2008;91:110–65.
6. Sauerbrei A, Wutzler P. Herpes simplex and varicella-zoster virus infections during pregnancy: current concepts of prevention, diagnosis and therapy. Part 2: varicella-zoster virus infections. Med Microbiol Immunol. 2007;196:95–102.
7. Department of Health. Report of confidential enquiries into maternal deaths in the United Kingdom 1985–87, 1988–90, 1991–93.1994–96. London: HMSO.
8. Cox SM, Cunningham FG, Luby J. Management of varicella pneumonia complicating pregnancy. Am J Perinatol. 1990;7(4):300–1.
9. Harger JH, Ernest JM, Thurnau GR, Moawad A, Momirova V, Landon MB, et al. Risk factors and outcome of varicella-zoster virus pneumonia in pregnant women. J Infect Dis. 2002;185(4):422–7.
10. Paryani SG, Arvin AM. Intrauterine infection with varicella-zoster virus after maternal varicella. N Engl J Med. 1986;314:1542–6.
11. Enders G, Miller E, Cradock-Watson J, et al. Consequences of varicella and herpes zoster in pregnancy: prospective study of 1739 cases. Lancet. 1994;343:1548–51.
12. Higa K, Dan K, Manabe H. Varicella-zoster virus infections during pregnancy: hypothesis concerning the mechanisms of congenital malformations. Obstet Gynecol. 1987;69:214–22.
13. Katz VL, Kuller JA, McMahon MJ, Warren MA, Wells SR. Varicella during pregnancy-maternal and fetal effects. West J Med. 1995;163:446–51.
14. Skibsted L. Abnormal fetal ultrasound findings after maternal chickenpox infection. Ugeskr Laege. 2000;162(18):2546–9.
15. Sauerbrei A, Wutzler P. Neonatal varicella. J Perinatol. 2001;21(8):545–9.
16. Mouly F, Mirlesse V, Meritet J, et al. Prenatal diagnosis of fetal varicella-zoster virus infection with polymerase chain reaction of amniotic fluid in 107 cases. Am J Obstet Gynecol. 1997;177:894–8.
17. Royal College of Obstetricians and Gynaecologists. Green-top guideline no. 13. London: Royal College of Obstetricians and Gynaecologists; 2010. Chickenpox in Pregnancy. p. 1–11.
18. Snoeck R, Andrei G, De Clercq E. Current pharmacological approaches to the therapy of varicella zoster virus infections: a guide to treatment. Drugs. 1999;57(2):187–206.
19. Tan MP, Koren G. Chickenpox in pregnancy: revisited. Reprod Toxicol. 2006;21:410–20.
20. CDC. General recommendations on immunization: recommendations of the Advisory Committee on Immunization Practices (ACIP). MMWR Recomm Rep. 2011;60(2):26–7.
21. Canadian Task Force on Preventive Health Care. New grades for recommendations from the Canadian Task Force on Preventive Health Care. CMAJ. 2003;169:207–8.
22. Marin M, Güris D, Chaves SS, et al. Prevention of varicella: recommendations of the Advisory Committee on Immunization Practices (ACIP). MMWR Recomm Rep. 2007;56:1.
23. Asano Y. Clinicopathologic understanding and control of varicella zoster virus infection. Vaccine. 2008;26:6487–90.

# Part II

# Medical Disorders and Organ System Dysfunctions Requiring Critical Care

# Cardiac Diseases in Pregnancy

5

Hemant Deshpande and Sonali Deshpande

## Introduction

Incidence of heart disease in the population is quite high, and therefore, it is not surprising that many cases of cardiac disease are seen together with pregnancy, and this fact is very true with regard to the Indian setup. Clinically cardiac disease is seen in about 1–4 % pregnancies, but the true incidence of maternal cardiovascular disease is higher because a significant number of such cases go undetected as they are clinically insignificant or were not picked up despite being serious in nature [1]. The absolute number of pregnant women with heart disease is rising because due to increased percentage of antennal care and refinement in the medical and surgical management of congenital and acquired heart defects so greater proportion of such women reaching to child-bearing age. The pregnancy may affect the well-being of both mother and fetus by imposing a grave haemodynamic burden and hence aggravating the pre-existing heart disease. Whatever the lesion, it is certain that close clinical attention and preparedness to avoid acute events and to manage them successfully are the right clinical approaches for these patients to ensure the best maternal and fetal outcome.

H. Deshpande (✉)
Department of Obst. Gynaecology, Dr D. Y. Patil Medical College, Pune, Maharashtra, India
e-mail: drhemantdeshpande@gmail.com

S. Deshpande
Department of Obst. Gynaecology, Government Medical College, Aurangabad, Maharashtra, India

## Haemodynamic Alterations in Normal Pregnancy

**Antepartum Changes** The growing fetus demands a nearly tenfold increase in uterine blood flow from 2 % of cardiac output in non-pregnant state to 17 % cardiac output at term. This requires immense alteration in maternal haemodynamic beginning as early as 5 weeks of gestation. Plasma volume increases by 45 % and red cell mass increases by 20–30 %. This discrepancy leads to haemodilution and the physiological anaemia of pregnancy [2].

**Table 5.1** Cardiac disease in pregnancy (CARPREG) risk score

| |
|---|
| *One point for each:* |
| History of prior cardiac event or arrhythmias |
| New York Heart Association functional classification > II or cyanosis |
| Left heart obstruction (mitral valve area <2 $cm^2$, aortic valve area <1.5 $cm^2$ or left ventricular outflow tract gradient >30 mmHg) |
| Left ventricular ejection fraction <0.40 |
| *Chance of cardiac complication:* |
| 0 points = 5 %<br>1 point = 27 %<br>≥2 points = 75 % |

Developed by Siu et al. (2001) [6]


A. Gandhi et al. (eds.), *Principles of Critical Care in Obstetrics: Volume II*,
DOI 10.1007/978-81-322-2686-4_5

Increase in heart rate and stroke volume lead to a 30–50 % increase in cardiac output during pregnancy. Stroke volume begins to increase at 5 weeks of gestation, peaks at approximately 31 weeks of gestation, and then gradually declines until term. At approximately 32 weeks of gestation, the maximal heart rate of 15–20 beats/min above nonpregnant values is achieved and remains stable until delivery. The relative tachycardia counteracts the declining stroke volume; cardiac output declines only a small amount during the last 6 weeks of pregnancy [2].

Systemic vascular resistance decreases by approximately 20 % with the greatest decrease at 16–24 weeks. This parallels the decrease of arterial blood pressure in the second trimester with gradual increase at term [2].

**Intrapartum Changes** Cardiac output increases even further during labour by 12–31 % during the first stage and up to 49 % during the second stage. Part of the increase is due to pain causing increased sympathetic stimulation, tachycardia, increased blood pressure, and increased myocardial oxygen consumption, and the rest is due to autotransfusion from uterine to systemic circulation with each contraction.

During the second stage of labour with maternal pushing efforts, the Valsalva manoeuvre produces even wider fluctuations in maternal haemodynamics. During the straining period, increased intrathoracic pressure results in decreased venous return to the heart, whereas systemic vascular resistance increases and mean arterial pressure remains constant or slightly elevated. Initially, there is a transient reflex bradycardia; after a few seconds, sympathetic stimulation occurs to decrease preload and increase afterload. After the strain is completed, a rapid increase in venous return causes increase in stroke volume and markedly increased blood pressure, which are again associated with reflex bradycardia.

**Postpartum Changes** Immediately after delivery, relief of vena cava compression by the gravid uterus and autotransfusion of uteroplacental blood cause cardiac output to increase even further for a brief period. Within 1 h of delivery, cardiac output returns to third trimester values. The postpartum period is characterised by mobilisation of extravascular fluid and diuresis.

| Parameter | Percentage of change | |
|---|---|---|
| Cardiac output | 40–50 % | Increase |
| Stroke volume | 30 % | Increase |
| Heart rate | 15–25 % | Increase |
| Intravascular volume | 45 % | Increase |
| Systemic vascular resistance | 20 % | Decrease |
| Systolic BP | | Minimal |
| Diastolic BP | 20 % | Decrease at mid-pregnancy<br>Pre-pregnant values at term |
| CVP | | Unchanged |
| $O_2$ consumption | 30–40 % | Increase |

**Diagnosis and Evaluation of Heart Disease** Many women with heart disease would have been diagnosed and treated before pregnancy. Alternatively, heart disease may be diagnosed for the first time during pregnancy owing to symptoms precipitated by increased cardiac demands, or the patient might have tolerated heart disease well throughout the pregnancy and present during labour or postpartum period with acute symptoms for the first time, a not so unrare fact in India.

The classic symptoms of cardiac disease are palpitation, shortness of breath with exertion, and chest pain. Because these symptoms also may accompany normal pregnancy, a careful history and meticulous examination is needed to determine whether the symptoms are of particular concern in a patient with other reasons to suspect underlying cardiac disease.

A systolic murmur is present in 80 % of pregnant women, most likely due to the increased flow volume in the aorta and pulmonary artery. Any diastolic murmur and any systolic murmur that is loud (grade 3 or higher) or radiates to the carotids should be considered pathologic. Careful evaluation of jugular venous pulse, for peripheral cyanosis or clubbing and pulmonary crackles, is needed in women with suspected cardiac disease. The preferred next step evaluation includes transthoracic echocardiography but may not be available in an acute cardiac event. A chest X-ray is useful if CCF is suspected; dilated cardiac shadow with congestion in lungs with or without plural effusion may be seen. ECG may be helpful to suggest underlying heart disease, but both of these simple tests have limitation during pregnancy due to alteration in cardiac position due to gravid uterus late in pregnancy.

Ischaemic heart disease presenting for the first time during pregnancy is very challenging to diagnose. Heartburn due to GERD/oral iron intake and shortness of breath are not uncommon during pregnancy, and not only these but mild ECG changes may be normal findings during pregnancy besides elevated CPK-MB during pregnancy. Positive TROP-*T* test and change in cardiac enzyme (falling levels) will help to diagnose it retrogradely.

## General Care

Deterioration in cardiac status during pregnancy is frequently insidious. Early registration and frequent and regular visits are a must. Attention is given to the HR, weight gain, and oxygen saturation. The physiological changes of pregnancy are usually continuous and offer adequate time for maternal compensation. Intercurrent events superimposed on pregnancy in the context of maternal heart disease are usually responsible for acute decompensation. The most common events are febrile episodes. Patients should be instructed to report to the hospital in case of fever, upper respiratory tract infection, and burning micturition. Iron and folic acid supplementation may decrease cardiac work.

First trimester dating scan would not only help in knowing exact EDD but also in monitoring growth of fetus in subsequent scan; detailed malformation scan would help if patient conceived on cardiac medication including fetal heart echocardiography specifically if mother is having congenital cardiac lesion.

Intrauterine growth restriction may be either due to ongoing medication or due to compromised oxygenation of fetus; Doppler studies may help in deciding pregnancy termination and mode of delivery.

Standard care in labour and delivery:

1. Accurate diagnosis
2. Close monitoring of maternal and fetal well-being
3. Mode of delivery based on obstetric indications
4. Prophylactic antibiotic when at risk for endocarditis, valvular heart disease, prosthetic heart valves, structured congenital heart diseases, previous infective endocarditis, and hypertrophic cardiomyopathy
5. Maintenance of haemodynamic stability
6. Avoidance of pain – epidural analgesia
7. Avoidance of maternal pushing efforts – instrumental delivery
8. Avoidance of maternal blood loss – active management of third stage of labour
9. Early volume management postpartum – often careful but aggressive diuresis [3]

## Cardiac Lesions and the Associated Maternal Cardiac Risks during Pregnancy

**Maternal mortality associated with heart disease in pregnancy**

| | |
|---|---|
| *Group 1: mortality <1 %* | |
| | Atrial septal defect<br>Ventricular septal defect; PDA<br>Pulmonary/tricuspid disease<br>Tetralogy of Fallot, corrected; bioprosthetic valve<br>Mitral stenosis, NYHA classes I and II |
| *Group 2: mortality 5–15 %* | |
| *2A*<br>*2B* | Mitral stenosis NYHA classes III–IV; aortic stenosis<br>Coarctation of aorta, without valvular involvement<br>Uncorrected tetralogy of Fallot<br>Previous myocardial infarction<br>Marfan syndrome with normal aorta<br>Mitral stenosis with atrial fibrillation<br>Artificial valve |
| *Group 3: mortality 25–50 %* | |
| | Primary pulmonary hypertension or Eisenmenger's syndrome<br>Coarctation of aorta, with valvular involvement<br>Marfan syndrome with aortic involvement |

## NYHA (New York Heart Association) Functional Classification [4]

1. Class I (mild) – no limitation of physical activity. Ordinary physical activity does not cause undue fatigue, palpitation, or dyspnoea.
2. Class II (mild) – slight limitation of physical activity. Comfortable at rest but ordinary physical activity results in symptoms.
3. Class III (moderate) – marked limitation of physical activity, comfortable at rest, but less than normal activity cause symptoms.
4. Class IV (severe) – unable to carry out any physical activity without discomfort. Symptoms of cardiac insufficiency at rest.

Medical termination of pregnancy is to be advised to patients specifically with high risk of cardiac lesion, in view of increased mortality in such cases, but even low-risk patients can complicate in such an outcome.

## Carpreg Score, Hamilton, and Thompson

Bad prognostic criteria will help in guiding outcome during this pregnancy (Table 5.1).

## Valvular Disease

**Mitral Stenosis** Mitral stenosis is the most common cardiac disease occurring mostly as a consequence of rheumatic heart disease. Risk of maternal complications in MS is strongly associated with the severity of MS, NYHA functional class, previous history of pulmonary oedema, and embolic phenomena. Complications include pulmonary oedema, right ventricular failure, and atrial arrhythmias with risk of embolisation. Pregnancy is detrimental to cardiac function in mitral stenosis for several reasons. Expanded blood volume can increase the risk of pulmonary congestion and oedema. The physiological tachycardia of pregnancy decreases filling time which leads to elevated left arterial pressure that causes pulmonary oedema and decreased forward flow that causes hypotension, fatigue, and syncope.

The severity of mitral stenosis is classified based on the valve area: a valve area of >1.5 $cm^2$ is mild, 1.1–1.5 $cm^2$ is moderate and <1 $cm^2$ is severe. Treatment of mitral stenosis in patients who have a history of RHD includes daily prophylactic penicillin, gentle diuresis to prevent pulmonary oedema without decreasing placental function and ß-blockers as needed to prevent tachycardia. Atrial fibrillation can be treated with cardioversion; digoxin or ß-blockers may be used for rate control. Patients with atrial fibrillation should be anticoagulated to prevent systemic embolism. The most common surgical treatment of mitral stenosis is percutaneous balloon mitral valvotomy. This procedure should be preferably performed before conception but in women with critical mitral stenosis may be formed during second trimester of pregnancy with less fetal risk. [2]

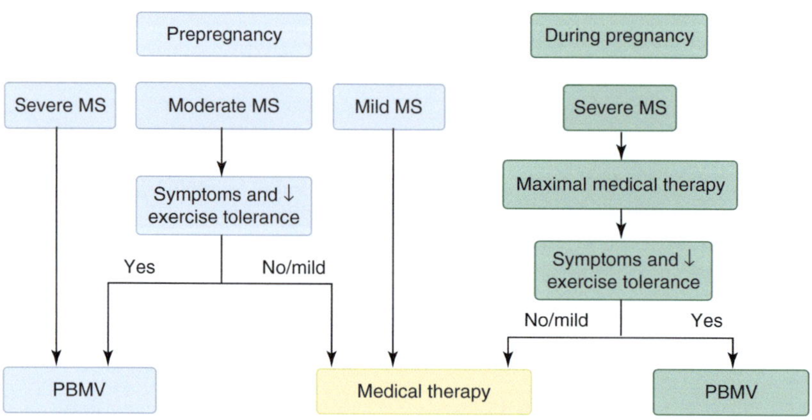

**Aortic Stenosis** Most common cause of AS in young women is a congenital bicuspid valve. RHD is a less common cause. The severity of AS can be described by average valve area or peak pressure gradient across the valve. Severe AS is defined as a peak gradient greater than 50 mmHg. Patients having severe AS have difficulty in achieving the increased cardiac output as their stroke volume is fixed by the obstructed valve, so heart rate is the key determinant of cardiac output. Bradycardia causes decreased cardiac output and hypotension; however, excessive tachycardia decreases excessive ventricular filling time and again causes decreased cardiac output and the risk for myocardial ischaemia. Women with severe AS are advised to undergo operative procedure before planning for pregnancy. Sudden death and irreversible heart failure are the most common causes of maternal death.

Management of mild to moderate AS during pregnancy is conservative. For women with severe symptomatic AS, balloon valvuloplasty has been reported during pregnancy without complications. This procedure is *contraindicated* in presence of significant aortic regurgitation. Concomitant AR is found most often in patients who have congenital bicuspid aortic valves; these valves do not open or close properly. Open valve replacement is also an option for patients who have decompensation during pregnancy but is associated with more fetal mortality. During labour, epidural anaesthesia may be used continuously with generous fluid hydration to prevent hypotension and reflex tachycardia. Assisted vaginal delivery is useful to curtail second stage of labour. Because of the acute decrease in preload that is associated with PPH, women should be managed aggressively to prevent postpartum collapse [2].

**Pulmonary Stenosis** – Isolated pulmonary stenosis is a rare clinical entity, but it seems to be well tolerated in pregnancy. PS in association with congenital heart disease has much worse prognosis. The prognosis in these cases depends on the degree of obstruction to the flow that is assessed by peak-to-peak velocity gradient across the valve. Gradient more than >50 mmHg is severe PS and consideration should be given to balloon valvuloplasty [2].

**Mitral Regurgitation** – MR in pregnant women is most commonly due to mitral valve prolapse. The haemodynamic changes are beneficial to patients because a state of increased volume and decreased systemic vascular resistance promotes forward flow across the regurgitant valve. Pregnancy is well tolerated. Patients having pulmonary congestion can be treated with diuretics. Vasodilators such as hydralazine are beneficial for women who have associated systemic hypertension. Severe MR can lead to marked left arterial dilatation and consequent atrial fibrillation. Epidural anaesthesia can be used safely with intravenous hydration. All patients of mitral regurgitation should receive infective endocarditis prophylaxis regardless of mode of delivery. Rheumatic mitral regurgitation patients should continue penicillin prophylaxis. Patients of MS who undergo PBMV may develop acute MR leading to rapid rise of LA pressure and present flash pulmonary oedema. Pregnancy is *contraindicated* in such patients [2].

**Mitral Valve Prolapse (MVP)** It is the most common maternal cardiac condition seen in women of child-bearing age. This is a benign condition characterised by a redundant valve that prolapses into the ventricle during systole. MVP also can be secondary and associated with ASD, endocarditis and MS [2].

**Aortic Regurgitation** Causes of AR include a dilated aortic annulus, a bicuspid aortic valve and previous endocarditis. Similarly to MR, pregnancy is uncomplicated. Symptomatic patients can be treated by diuretics and vasodilators. LVF is sometimes reported near term. Epidural analgesia can be administered safely [2].

## Non-valvular Congenital Heart Disease

**Conditions with a Left to Right Shunt** Generally left to right shunts are well tolerated in pregnancy. Patients are at high risk for stroke from paradoxical embolisation across the shunt.

Left to right shunt may be due to a ventricular septal defect (VSD), atrial septal defect (ASD) or patent ductus arteriosus.

Small shunts do not usually cause problems.

Moderate shunts may increase if SVR increases due to pain and catecholamine release. If there is a large drop in SVR (e.g. following spinal block), then the shunt may reverse in direction and may result in hypoxia.

Large shunts (most likely from a VSD) can result in pulmonary hypertension.

Infective endocarditis prophylaxis is indicated in all patients with VENTRICULAR septal defects and PDA [5].

**Tetralogy of Fallot (ToF)** Most common cyanotic congenital heart lesion.

Large VSD, right ventricular outflow tract obstruction, right ventricular hypertrophy and overriding aorta.

Risks dependent on the status of the repair.

Pregnancy is often well tolerated in those with repaired ToF, but women should have their right ventricle fully assessed; deaths have occurred in recent years from arrhythmias secondary to unrecognised right heart failure [5].

**Coarctation of the Aorta** Pregnancy in women with coarctation of the aorta is a challenge for the obstetrician. In most cases, narrowing of the aorta occurs distal to the left subclavian artery, resulting in isolated hypertension in the right arm. Determining the arm-leg blood pressure gradient, which is abnormal when greater than 20 mmHg, assesses the severity of lesion. Due to high maternal morbidity and mortality reported during pregnancy, pre-pregnancy counselling should be insisted, although most women presenting with coarctation will have had a previous repair.

Problems during labour and delivery are unlikely if successfully repaired; however late hypertension, re-coarctation and aneurysm formation at the site of previous repair may occur. All women with previous repairs should be closely monitored throughout pregnancy by echocardiography and regular BP measurement (measure BP in both arms since left subclavian may have been used as part of previous repair).

If present with un-repaired coarctation (native coarctation), risks to both mother and fetus are high due to hypertension refractory to medical treatment.

Regional anaesthesia or analgesia must be carefully titrated with close monitoring of BP and drugs to maintain SVR (phenylephrine, metaraminol).

In severe cases women are at risk of aortic rupture, dissection and left ventricular failure due to fluctuations in blood pressure that occur during second stage of labour. That is why caesarean section is preferred in such cases. They need prophylaxis for bacterial endocarditis at the time of delivery [5].

## Pulmonary Hypertension (PH) and Eisenmenger's Syndrome

There is a very high risk of maternal mortality with PH, and termination of pregnancy is often recommended.

There is increased pulmonary vascular resistance resulting in an increased workload placed on the right heart.

PH may be primary or secondary.

Primary pulmonary hypertension is characterised by an increase in the thickness of the pulmonary arterioles. On M/E typical onion skin configuration of vessels is seen due to intimal fibrosis and fibroelastosis.

The causes of secondary PH include: cardiac and respiratory conditions (chronic obstructive or parenchymal conditions, cystic fibrosis, obstructive sleep apnoea, thoracic cage abnormalities), venous thromboembolism, vasculitis, hyperviscosity syndrome, infection, portal hypertension, cirrhosis and drugs (oral contraceptive, crotalaria teas, appetite suppressants)

PH is poorly tolerated due to insufficient adaptation of the right heart to the increased cardiac output and poor compliance of the pulmonary vasculature.

Symptoms of right ventricular decompensation are: shortness of breath, fatigue, chronic cough, haemoptysis and syncope.

Signs include: tachycardia, cyanosis, right ventricular heave, elevated JVP and hepatomegaly.

Death occurs from irreversible right ventricular failure and arrhythmias.

Therapies targeted at pulmonary arterial vasodilatation may be useful during pregnancy (e.g. prostaglandin analogues including iloprost).

Timing of delivery is dependent on the impact of PH on the mother as pregnancy progresses.

If possible, aim to deliver at 32–34 weeks.

Increases in pulmonary vascular resistance (PVR) must be prevented by avoiding rises in $PaCO_2$, falls in $PaO_2$ and pH, hypothermia, high ventilatory pressures and sympathetic agents.

Right ventricular preload, left ventricular afterload and right ventricular contractility must be maintained.

Vaginal delivery is probably the safest mode of delivery with a low-dose epidural to reduce pain, stress and haemodynamic fluctuations while maximising oxygen consumption. Avoid pushing in second stage due to the reduction in venous return and right heart preload that results.

Elective caesarean is sometimes performed especially when delivery is preterm. Regional anaesthesia may be appropriate, but single-shot spinals should be avoided due to the inability of the right ventricle to respond to hypotension.

Pulmonary arterial pressure may rise significantly during intubation if general anaesthesia is provided. Measures to obtund the pressor response to laryngoscopy should be used. (See later.)

Oxytocin should be used cautiously after delivery.

Women should be monitored closely after delivery since most deaths occur 2–9 days postpartum. Observation for at least 72 h on a high dependency unit should be provided [5].

## Eisenmenger's Syndrome

Eisenmenger's syndrome is pulmonary hypertension developing after a long-standing left to right shunt, which induces vascular remodelling and leads to increased pulmonary vascular resistance which meets or exceeds systemic resistance.

The shunt flow depends on the PVR/SVR ratio.

After Eisenmenger's pathophysiology is established, pulmonary hypertension is permanent and surgical correction is unhelpful.

Hypovolaemia will lead to shunt reversal, reduced cardiac output and increased cyanosis.

Mortality in pregnancy and delivery is very high due to right ventricular failure [5].

## Cardiac Disease Developing in Pregnancy

**Cardiomyopathy** – Peripartum cardiomyopathy is defined as onset of cardiac failure with no identifiable cause in the last month of pregnancy or within 5 months after delivery, in the absence of pre-existing heart disease.

The incidence is 1:1500–1:4000 live births.

Risk factors include previous peripartum cardiomyopathy, hypertension, pre-eclampsia, obesity, diabetes, Afro-Caribbean origin, increased parity, older maternal age and multiple gestations.

The aetiology remains unclear but includes viral myocarditis, abnormal immune response to pregnancy or terbutaline tocolytic therapy.

Diagnosis is difficult as many symptoms are similar to those you would expect in the last trimester (peripheral oedema, fatigue and shortness of breath).

Suspected cases should be investigated by echocardiography as there are strict echo criteria for diagnosis (1) which includes ejection fraction <45 % or M-mode fractional shortening less than 30 % or both and (2) end-diastolic dimension >2.7 cm/m$^2$.

Treatment is supportive with medical stabilisation. As most cases present late in pregnancy, delivery of the fetus may significantly improve symptoms.

Vaginal delivery may be best with low-dose epidural and close monitoring of BP and fluid status.

Patients should be monitored on a high dependency unit or cardiac care unit post delivery.

Medical treatment includes salt restriction, diuretics, vasodilators, digoxin for arrhythmias and inotropy and anticoagulation due to the high risk of thromboembolism.

Mortality ranges from 18 to 56 % and often occurs several months after delivery. In severe cases patients will be referred for heart transplantation after delivery.

Idiopathic dilated cardiomyopathy can also develop which is similar to the above but does not fit the diagnostic criteria and has a worse long-term outcome.

Pre-existing *hypertrophic cardiomyopathy* is generally well tolerated, and most undergo successful vaginal delivery.

Cardiac function depends on preload and afterload, so if using regional anaesthesia it must be carefully titrated with invasive blood pressure monitoring.

Pre-existing *dilated cardiomyopathy* may decompensate in pregnancy. Women with severe LV impairment secondary to dilated cardiomyopathy may be counselled against pregnancy due to the high risk of mortality [5].

## Ischaemic Heart Disease and Myocardial Infarction

This is now the leading cause of cardiac maternal mortality in the UK.

In the last confidential enquiry of maternal deaths, all women who died from ischaemic heart disease had identifiable risk factors including:

Obesity
Advanced maternal age
Higher parity
Pre-existing hypertension
Smoking
Family history of cardiac disease
Type 2 diabetes mellitus

Previously undiagnosed ischaemic heart disease (IHD) usually manifests itself in the 3rd trimester, during labour or post delivery at a time when maternal stress and cardiac demand are at their greatest. Most commonly it presents with chest pain, ischaemic changes on the ECG and elevated troponin but may sometimes present atypically with abdominal or epigastric pain. Any woman with chest pain suspicious of ischaemia, particularly in those with risk factors, should have an ECG.

Coronary angiography may be indicated in women with IHD to treat coronary artery occlusion and coronary artery dissection by stenting and angioplasty.

In the event of myocardial infarction, primary percutaneous transluminal coronary angioplasty (PTCA) should be performed. If PTCA is not available, thrombolysis should not be withheld in the pregnant or postpartum woman as the risk of bleeding is less than the risk of no treatment.

Beware the use of uterotonics. Ergometrine causes coronary artery vasospasm and should be avoided if there is a history of IHD [5].

## Aortic Dissection

It is associated with hypertension due to preeclampsia or coarctation of the aorta and connective tissue disorders including Marfan and Ehlers-Danlos syndrome.

Pregnancy-related aortic dissection accounts for 50 % of all aortic dissections in women under 40 years of age.

Maternal mortality may be as high as 25 %.

It usually occurs in late pregnancy or post delivery.

It presents with severe chest pain, interscapular pain, end-organ ischaemia or acute MI.

Investigations include chest CT, MRI or transoesophageal echocardiogram (TOE).

Management varies depending on the gestation of the fetus.

If it presents before 28 weeks, then surgical repair with fetus in situ is recommended as without surgery mortality may reach 80 %.

Cardiopulmonary bypass is associated with congenital malformations in the first trimester but is safer in the second and third trimester.

After 32 weeks of delivery by caesarean section followed by corrective surgery.

Between 28 and 32 weeks of gestation, unless there is severe cardiovascular instability, medical management is provided to allow the fetus to mature.

Goals of anaesthetic management are: maintenance of cardiovascular stability with regional anaesthesia and labetalol infusion for control of BP.

For caesarean section under GA, the hypertensive response to laryngoscopy must be avoided [5].

## Management of Women with Transplanted Heart

Pregnancy is generally well tolerated if cardiac function is good.

There are problems due to the side effects of the immunosuppressant drugs.

Spontaneous vaginal delivery is the best management option.

## General Approaches to Management of Pregnant Women with Cardiac Disease

### Monitoring

Basic monitoring for mothers with heart disease during labour and delivery and in the immediate postpartum period includes: blood pressure, pulse oximetry and continuous 3-lead ECG.

Invasive blood pressure monitoring is very useful in higher risk cases and can be easily managed on labour ward with appropriate anaesthetic input.

There is debate over the use of central venous pressure (CVP) and pulmonary artery catheter (PAC) monitoring. These interventions are not without risk and benefits may sometimes be limited.

Long lines placed in the antecubital fossa can be used to measure CVP and infuse vasoactive drugs and may be a safer approach to central venous cannulation.

### Delivery

For most cardiac conditions, a normal vaginal delivery with good analgesia is the safest mode of delivery for the mother because of less blood loss and less rapid haemodynamic changes than caesarean section.

Consultant-led delivery in a hospital used to dealing with cardiac disease with a high dependency area that can provide invasive monitoring is essential.

Stress on the mother and her cardiovascular system must be minimised while maintaining placental and fetal circulation.

Effective pain relief results in less tachycardia and catecholamine release. It also reduces the haemodynamic effects of pushing.

Limited pushing in second stage, i.e. assisted second stage, may reduce cardiovascular instability.

Low-dose epidural anaesthesia sited early in labour for effective pain control and reduced catecholamine release is highly beneficial in most cases.

If caesarean section is required due to obstetric indications or decompensation of the underlying disease, then this can be done with either general or regional anaesthesia.

If general anaesthesia is planned, measures to suppress the pressor response to laryngoscopy must be provided, e.g. alfentanil 10–20 mcg/kg [5].

If regional anaesthesia is planned, single-shot spinals are best avoided. Alternative options include: careful titration of an epidural and combined spinal-epidural or incremental spinal anaesthesia (via spinal catheter).

There are many factors that influence the decision whether to proceed with regional or general anaesthesia and these include:

Requirement for other procedures which may demand general anaesthesia, e.g. DC cardioversion, post-delivery cardiac surgery, high inspired oxygen concentration (pulmonary hypertension), postoperative ventilation and prolonged or complex surgery following previous surgery

Risk of reducing SVR with regional anaesthesia (left-sided stenotic lesion and those with shunts) versus impairment of cardiac contractility with general anaesthesia
Impact of anticoagulation; risks of withholding it and risk of epidural haematoma
Risk of maternal or fetal death and how the mother feels about this
Airway abnormalities
Anaesthetic preference
Patient preference

## Prophylactic Antibiotics to Prevent Endocarditis

American Heart Association (2007) guidelines and the UK National Institute for Health and Care Excellence (NICE) 2008 guidelines do *not* recommend administration of antibiotics solely to prevent endocarditis in patients who undergo a gynaecological or obstetric procedure since there is no beneficial evidence of this practice.

Patients requiring antibiotic coverage: prosthetic heart valves, previous infective endocarditis, hypertrophic cardiomyopathy, valvular heart disease with stenosis or regurgitation and structural CHD (uncomplicated ASD, fully corrected VSD and PDA)

High-risk patients: ampicillin 2.0 g IM/IV + gentamicin 1.5 mg/kg within 30 min of starting procedures. Six hours later ampicillin 1.0 g IM/IV or amoxicillin 1.0 g po. In patients allergic to penicillin, vancomycin 1.0 g over 1–2 h with gentamicin is recommended.

Moderate-risk patients: amoxicillin 2.0 g po 1 h before procedure or ampicillin 2.0 g IM/IV within 30 min of starting the procedure. In patients allergic to penicillin, vancomycin 1.0 g over 1–2 h within 30 min of starting the procedure is recommended [4].

## Anticoagulation

Warfarin is teratogenic and not recommended during the first trimester of pregnancy. It is avoided in the third trimester since it crosses the placenta and can cause fetal haemorrhage. It also precludes regional anaesthesia, and its effects may be difficult to rapidly reverse in an emergency.

In patients receiving warfarin, the INR should be maintained between 2.0 and 3.0 with the lowest possible dose and low-dose aspirin should be added. If labour begins during treatment with warfarin, *caesarean section* should be performed.

Low-molecular-weight heparin (LMWH) can be used instead of warfarin throughout the whole of pregnancy. Regional anaesthesia can be performed provided adequate time has elapsed since the last dose of LMWH.

For women receiving prophylactic LMWH, regional anaesthesia or removal of epidural catheter can be performed 12 h after last dose of LMWH. After insertion of epidural or spinal, a dose can be given 4 h later.

In women receiving therapeutic doses of LMWH, 24 h should elapse after the last dose of LMWH before regional anaesthesia or removal of epidural catheter. After insertion of epidural/spinal, a dose can be given 4 h later [5].

## Uterine Atony

Many oxytocics have severe consequences for those with cardiac disease, but withholding them can lead to haemorrhage. A balanced individualised approach is best.

Oxytocin can cause profound tachycardia, vasodilatation and hypotension when administered as an IV bolus, so administer the bolus as an infusion (e.g. 5 units in 20 ml over 5–10 min). If at particular risk of cardiovascular effects (e.g. severe aortic stenosis), then it may be best omitted. A low-dose infusion with 10 units per hour can be used post delivery with careful monitoring.

Ergometrine causes pulmonary vasoconstriction and hypertension, so avoid in most cardiac cases especially pulmonary hypertension.

Prostaglandin F2$\alpha$ (carboprost) can cause severe bronchospasm, hypertension, cardiovascular collapse and pulmonary oedema making it unsuitable in most cases.

- Uterine massage can be used to provide temporary relief but may require adequate analgesia.

Other surgical options in the event of refractory uterine atony include: an intrauterine balloon that can be left in 1–2 days after caesarean section or vaginal delivery, uterine compression sutures (e.g. B-Lynch suture), internal iliac balloon catheterization/ligation and hysterectomy [5].

## Contraceptive Advice

Barrier contraceptive is best suited but it has a high failure rate with atypical uses. IUDs and hormonal contraceptive belong in class C of WHO where risk outweighs its usage in heart disease patients. Early completion of family as all heart diseases progress with age and permanent contraception is better approach. Tubectomy in women would involve anaesthesia-related risk, so vasectomy in men is the safest approach.

## Summary

Women at low risk in pregnancy are those who have few or no symptoms and good ventricular function without haemodynamically compromising or potentially life-threatening arrhythmias. They lack severe left ventricular inflow or outflow obstruction, do not have significant pulmonary or systematic hypertension and do not need to take anticoagulants.

After full cardiac assessment, low-risk patients can be managed locally while maintaining potential links with the obstetric cardiac centre should any question or problem arise.

Patients at higher risk need to be managed within or from the cardiac centre, and the highest risk patients will need admission for about 20 weeks.

The mode and time of delivery should be discussed and decisions made well in advance. Vaginal delivery is usually advised. Exceptions are patients with dilated Marfan aortic roots or aortic dissections, uncorrected coarctation, pulmonary vascular disease (including Eisenmenger's syndrome) and/or cyanosis and patients with mechanical valve prostheses in order to minimise the period of heparin withdrawal. Epidural anaesthesia is favoured, but vasodilatation should be avoided in patients with cyanosis or when stroke output is compromised. Adequate fluid volume loading is important but should not be overdone in patients with left ventricular obstruction or severe hypertrophic cardiomyopathy. Invasive monitoring is rarely justified by its inherent risks.

Antibiotic prophylaxis is discretionary for anticipated normal delivery. The risk of endocarditis has been shown to be very low and the benefits have not been proved, but cover is logical and wise for surgical deliveries, for patients with intracardiac prostheses of any sort and for patients who have had previous endocarditis.

In patients with pulmonary hypertension postpartum week and be conducted in the CCU for high-risk patients with continuous pulse oximetry as this is their period of highest risk when an increase.

## References


1. Ray P, Murphy GJ, Shutt LE. Recognition and management of maternal cardiac disease in pregnancy. Br J Anaesth. 2004;93:428–39.
2. Dob DP, Yentis SM. Practical management of the parturient with congenital heart disease. Int J Obstet Anaesth. 2006;15:137–44.
3. Confidential Enquiry into Maternal and Child Health (CEMACH). Saving Mothers' Lives: Reviewing Maternal Deaths to Make Motherhood Safer 2003–2005. The Seventh Report on Confidential Enquiries into Maternal Deaths in the United Kingdom. London: CEMACH; 2007.
4. Joubert IA, Dyer RA. Anaesthesia for the pregnant patient with acquired valvular heart disease. Update Anaesth. 2005;19:1–2.
5. Wilson W et al. Prevention of infective endocarditis. Guidelines from the American Heart Association. Circulation. 2007;16:1736.
6. Klein LL, Galan HL. Cardiac disease in pregnancy. Obstet Gynecol Clin N Am. 2004;31:429–59.

# 6 Acute Renal Failure (Acute Kidney Injury) in Pregnancy

Gita Arjun and M. Sivalingam

## Introduction

Acute renal failure (ARF or acute kidney injury [AKI]) in pregnancy is characterized by a rapid decrease in the glomerular filtration rate (GFR) over a matter of minutes or days. It may result from many of the same causes that occur in nonpregnant women. However, there are specific conditions in pregnancy that may precipitate ARF [1]. Understanding the causes of renal functional deterioration in pregnancy is important in arriving at a rational differential diagnosis and initiating appropriate treatment. In pregnancy, development of ARF is a major clinical challenge because it affects both mother and fetus. Management options, therefore, need to take both maternal and fetal well-being into consideration. Prevention, early recognition, and appropriate therapeutic decisions are imperative in improving maternal and perinatal outcomes. ARF in pregnancy is a complex entity, requiring a multidisciplinary approach with the nephrologist playing an important role.

G. Arjun, FACOG (✉)
Department of Obstetrics and Gynaecology,
E V Kalyani Medical Foundation,
3 Second Street, R K Salai, Chennai 600004, India
e-mail: gitarjun@gmail.com

M. Sivalingam, MRCP (UK), FRCP (Lon)
Department of Medicine, Sundaram Medical
Foundation, Dr. Rangarajan Memorial Hospital,
Shanthi Colony, 4th Avenue, Anna Nagar West,
Chennai 600 040, India
e-mail: drmsivalingam@gmail.com


A. Gandhi et al. (eds.), *Principles of Critical Care in Obstetrics: Volume II*,
DOI 10.1007/978-81-322-2686-4_6

## Incidence

Though the incidence of pregnancy-related ARF has dropped in developed countries (reported incidence of 1–2.8 %) [1, 2], it continues to be as high as 9–25 % in developing countries like India [3–6].

## General Causes of Acute Renal Failure

Acute tubular necrosis (ATN) resulting from infection, glomerulonephritis related to lupus, or drug toxicity may induce ARF in both nonpregnant and pregnant patients [7].

## Causes of Acute Renal Failure Unique to Pregnancy

ARF is associated with two distinct periods in pregnancy: the first trimester and the third trimester [8]. Postpartum ARF resulting from hemorrhage and sepsis also contributes to its incidence.

### Causes in the First Trimester

In the first trimester, the causes of ARF are usually prerenal (Table 6.1). The commonest causes are the following:

- Hyperemesis gravidarum
- Septic abortion

## Hyperemesis Gravidarum

The ARF in hyperemesis is prerenal and results from severe volume depletion. The reduction in renal perfusion is recognized by the rise in blood urea nitrogen, out of proportion to the serum creatinine [1]. Adequate fluid replacement should be instituted to correct the acid-base and electrolyte abnormalities. The hyperemesis should be addressed with a multipronged approach with antiemetics playing an important part in its management.

## Septic Abortion

Septic abortion still plays a major role in the development of ARF in developing countries like India. In India, the incidence of ARF due to postabortal complications has dropped from 59.7 % [9] in the 1970s to 20 % [6] at present. This is a direct result of the legalization of abortion and a decrease in the incidence of sepsis.

**Table 6.1** Common causes of acute renal failure in pregnancy

| | | |
|---|---|---|
| Prerenal | First trimester | Hyperemesis gravidarum |
| | | Septic abortion |
| | Third trimester | Hemorrhage |
| | | Placental abruption |
| | Postpartum | Postpartum hemorrhage |
| Intrarenal | Third trimester | Preeclampsia |
| | | HELLP syndrome |
| | | Acute fatty liver of pregnancy |
| | | Thrombotic microangiopathy |
| Postrenal | Any trimester | Obstruction (nephrolithiasis) |

As opposed to Western countries, the incidence of bilateral renal cortical necrosis (BRCN) following septic abortion is very high in India and has been reported to occur in 14.28–28.57 % of cases [4, 6, 10]. Bilateral renal cortical necrosis may lead to chronic kidney disease (CKD).

## Causes in the Third Trimester

The causes of ARF in the third trimester can be divided into prerenal and intrarenal (Table 6.1).

### Prerenal Causes

- Hemorrhage (Placental abruption)

### Intrarenal Causes

- Preeclampsia
- Hemolysis, elevated liver enzymes, and low platelet count (HELLP) syndrome
- Acute fatty liver of pregnancy
- Thrombotic microangiopathies

The four most common causes of ARF in late pregnancy and the postpartum period are the following:

- Preeclampsia
- HELLP syndrome
- Acute fatty liver of pregnancy
- Thrombotic microangiopathy

## Preeclampsia

Preeclampsia is the most common form of high blood pressure (BP) that complicates pregnancy. It is the association of new-onset hypertension (≥140/90 mm of Hg) that develops after 20 weeks of gestation, with new-onset proteinuria [11].

When a woman presents with hypertension with no proteinuria, there are other criteria that may lead to classifying her as having preeclampsia [11]. These criteria are the following:

- Thrombocytopenia (platelet count less than 100,000/μl)
- Impaired liver function (elevated blood levels of liver transaminases to twice the normal concentration)
- The new development of renal insufficiency (elevated serum creatinine greater than 1.1 mg/dL or a doubling of serum creatinine in the absence of other renal disease)
- Pulmonary edema
- New-onset cerebral or visual disturbances

Preeclampsia is classified as *non-severe* or *severe*. Signs that point to severe preeclampsia are the following [12]:

- Blood pressure ≥160/110 mmHg
- Significant proteinuria
- Multiorgan involvement

Non-severe preeclampsia is not associated with ARF. Renal failure is unusual even with severe cases (1–5 %) [13]. Severe preeclampsia may be associated with a mild degree of azotemia, due in part to reduced permeability of the glomerular capillary wall [6].

Seventy percent of patients with preeclampsia develop glomeruloendotheliosis which persists in the immediate postpartum period. However, these changes reverse completely in the majority of patients.

The changes in preeclampsia that may lead to acute renal failure in preeclampsia are listed in Table 6.2.

Pregnancy complications superimposed on preeclampsia may precipitate ARF. These complications are the following:

**Table 6.2** Causes of ARF in preeclampsia

| | |
|---|---|
| Primary changes | Glomeruloendotheliosis |
| | Decrease in GFR |
| | Decrease in renal plasma flow |
| Secondary effects | Intravascular volume depletion |
| | Vasoconstriction |
| | Activation of inflammatory cascade |
| | Activation of coagulation cascade |

- Significant bleeding with hemodynamic instability
- Marked disseminated intravascular coagulation (DIC)
- HELLP syndrome (*h*emolysis, *e*levated *l*iver enzymes, and *l*ow *p*latelets) [14]
- Placental abruption which may occur with severe preeclampsia

## HELLP Syndrome

HELLP is a syndrome characterized by *h*emolysis, *e*levated *l*iver enzymes, and *l*ow *p*latelet count. Though it is associated with severe preeclampsia, 15–20 % of women with HELLP syndrome do not have hypertension or proteinuria [15]. Unlike preeclampsia, it is more common in multiparous women.

In the HELLP syndrome, hepatic involvement and hemolysis are more severe than in preeclampsia. Infarction and hemorrhage are more pronounced and rupture of liver hematoma is more common.

ARF occurs in 7–36 % of women with the HELLP syndrome [15, 16]. As in severe preeclampsia, ARF may be a result of direct renal injury or as a consequence of abruption.

The ARF that develops as a consequence of the HELLP syndrome can necessitate dialysis in the acute phase in approximately 10–46 % of pregnant women [17]. However, even women requiring dialysis demonstrate a complete recovery of kidney function [18]. Though the maternal mortality following ARF in the HELLP syndrome is low (1 %), perinatal mortality rate is higher, ranging between 7 and 34 % [15, 19, 20]. Perinatal mortality is more common in early-onset disease, which tends to be more severe [15].

## Acute Fatty Liver of Pregnancy

Acute fatty liver of pregnancy (AFLP) is associated with fatty infiltration of hepatocytes without inflammation or necrosis. The disease is caused by an autosomal recessive genetic error. An excessive fetal fatty acid accumulation is released into the maternal circulation. The resulting increased load of long-chain fatty acids is deposited in liver tissue and leads to impaired hepatic function.

Though a rare complication of pregnancy, it is an obstetric emergency which can lead to fulminant hepatic failure. AFLP is associated with acute renal failure in up to 60 % of cases [21–23]. There is decreased renal perfusion or acute tubular necrosis.

In the early stages, it may be difficult to differentiate AFLP from severe preeclampsia and/or HELLP syndrome [24]. The diagnosis should be suspected when preeclampsia is associated with [7]:

- Hypoglycemia
- Hypofibrinogenemia
- Liver function test abnormalities with hyperbilirubinemia
- Prolonged partial thromboplastin time (PTT) in the absence of abruptio placentae

Most severely affected women will have complete recovery of liver and kidney function after delivery. However, AFLP is associated with substantial maternal and perinatal morbidity and mortality [25].

## Thrombotic Microangiopathies

Thrombotic microangiopathies are a combination of thrombocytopenia and microangiopathic anemia. They are rare and affect 1 in 25,000 pregnancies. They are characterized by the presence of fibrin and/or platelet thrombi in the microcirculation of multiple organs [26]. It might be difficult to differentiate severe preeclampsia from thrombotic microangiopathies because of the similar clinical and histologic characteristics [7]. A history of preceding hypertension and proteinuria favors a diagnosis of preeclampsia.

Thrombotic microangiopathies can be divided into two distinct entities depending on which organ is more affected and the timing of onset:

1. *Thrombotic thrombocytopenic purpura (TTP)*:
   (a) Neurologic abnormalities are dominant and kidney injury is minimal.
   (b) Diagnosed predominantly in the second and third trimesters.
2. *Hemolytic-uremic syndrome (HUS)*:
   (a) Renal failure is profound.
   (b) Diagnosed primarily in the postpartum period.

In actual practice the distinction may be difficult since the clinical manifestations of these two conditions may overlap.

TTP is identified by the presence of fever, thrombocytopenia (usually severe), microangiopathic hemolytic anemia, mild renal failure (creatinine <1.4 mg/dL), and neurologic symptoms like disorientation, ataxia, headache, focal changes, seizures, or aphasia [27]. The clinical features of HUS are similar, but neurological involvement is rare while renal involvement is profound.

*A disintegrin and metalloproteinase with thrombospondin motifs 13* (ADAMTS-13) is also known as *von Willebrand factor-cleaving protease* (VWFCP). An enzyme produced by liver stellate cells, endothelial cells, and platelets, it is responsible for cleaving large von Willebrand factor multimers. When ADAMTS-13 is deficient (defined by ADAMT-13 activity of <10 %), these large multimers continue to circulate, leading to platelet aggregation and red cell fragmentation. This enzymatic deficiency can be congenital (rare), but is mostly acquired due to autoantibodies [28].

The differentiating features of severe preeclampsia, HELLP syndrome, acute fatty liver of pregnancy, thrombotic thrombocytopenic purpura, and hemolytic-uremic syndrome are listed in Table 6.3.

## Uterine Hemorrhage and ARF

Acute renal failure is especially common in pregnancy complicated by:

- Placental abruption
- Disseminated intravascular coagulation
- Postpartum hemorrhage

**Table 6.3** Severe preeclampsia, HELLP syndrome, acute fatty liver of pregnancy, TTP, and HUS: differentiating features

| | Severe preeclampsia | HELLP | AFLP | TTP | HUS |
|---|---|---|---|---|---|
| Onset of symptoms | 3rd trimester | 3rd trimester | 3rd trimester | 2nd or 3rd trimester | Postpartum |
| Hypertension | 100 % | 80 % | 25–50 % | Occasionally | + |
| Acute renal failure | Mild | Mild/moderate | Moderate | Mild/moderate | Severe |
| Thrombocytopenia | +/– | + | – | ++ | ++ |
| Hemolytic anemia | – | – | –/+ | ++ | + |
| Increased PTT | –/+ | –/+ | + | – | – |
| Increased liver transaminase | –/+ | + | ++ | – | – |
| ADAMTS-13 activity <10 % | – | – | – | ++ | + |
| Renal outcome | Good | Good | Good | Poor | Poor |

*AFLP* acute fatty liver of pregnancy, *HELLP* hemolysis, elevated liver enzymes, and low platelet count, *TTP* thrombotic thrombocytopenic purpura, *HUS* hemolytic-uremic syndrome

Massive hemorrhage is implicated as a cause of ARF in pregnancy. If there is associated severe preeclampsia or HELLP syndrome, the renal consequences of hemorrhage are worsened [29]. Hemorrhage will exacerbate the hypovolemic state already associated with severe preeclampsia and precipitate the development and progression of acute tubular necrosis (ATN).

If acute hemorrhage, and the resultant hypovolemia, is not treated adequately and immediately, transient acute tubular necrosis may result. ATN is potentially reversible and with supportive therapy, the damage can be minimal. Since pregnancy is associated with heightened inflammation and is a prothrombotic state, without immediate intervention, the ATN can progress rapidly to bilateral renal cortical necrosis (BRCN). This almost always leads to permanent and irreversible renal damage. Twenty percent of cases of acute renal failure of obstetric origin progress to BRCN [10].

Diagnosis of ATN:

- Urinary sodium >25 mEq/L.
- Urine exam shows tubular cell debris and brown granular (pigmented) casts.
- Oliguria (50 % of cases).

Diagnosis of BRCN:

- Anuria persisting for >1 week
- CT with contrast or selective renal angiography (imaging not essential)
  - Delayed filling
  - Poor arborization of the interlobar arteries
  - Absent or nonhomogeneous filling at the level of the cortex
- Renal biopsy

## Management of ARF in Pregnancy

Treatment of acute kidney injury in pregnancy poses special challenges, as there are risks to both the mother and the fetus. Management is best provided by a multidisciplinary team that involves obstetricians, nephrologists, neonatologists, and other specialists as needed.

The key issues in the management of ARF in pregnancy include:

- Correction of hypovolemia when present
- Prevention of further injury
- Initiation of renal replacement therapy (dialysis) when indicated
- Treatment of underlying cause
- The delivery of a baby and the placenta as promptly as possible

It would be prudent to discontinue and avoid nephrotoxic drugs as well as to treat any associated infection such as urinary tract infection [30]. Commonly used nephrotoxic drugs include nonsteroidal anti-inflammatory drugs (NSAIDs) and aminoglycoside antibiotics such as amikacin and gentamicin. Patients who are hypovolemic would require intravenous fluids to restore and maintain renal as well as uroplacental perfusion. Although rarely undertaken in pregnancy, it would also be important to avoid radiocontrast studies in patients with ARF.

## Complications of ARF in Pregnancy

Complications of ARF in pregnancy are similar to other patient groups and include:

- Hypertension
- Electrolyte abnormalities
  - Hyperkalemia
  - Hypocalcemia
- Metabolic acidosis
- Anemia
- Volume overload

### Hypertension

Hypertension is common in patients with ARF, and there is no consensus about the blood pressure level at which antihypertensives should be started in pregnancy [12, 31, 32]. NICE guidelines [33] recommend starting treatment when the blood pressure is ≥150/100 mm of Hg. *Labetalol* is the initial drug of choice. The target blood pressure to be achieved is a systolic of <150 mm of Hg and a diastolic blood pressure between 80 and 100 mm of Hg.

Other antihypertensives such as methyldopa, hydralazine, and nifedipine can also be used safely in pregnancy. Hydralazine is often used intravenously in pregnant women who present with severe hypertension due to preeclampsia [34]. However, a meta-analysis of randomized controlled trials for the treatment of moderate to severe hypertension in pregnancy was not in favor of using hydralazine as its use was associated with a higher incidence of maternal side effects including hypotension, placental abruption, and oliguria [35]. Methyldopa should also be switched to an alternative antihypertensive in the postnatal period as it increases the risk of postnatal depression [36]. Other commonly used antihypertensives such as angiotensin-converting enzyme (ACE) inhibitors and angiotensin II receptor blockers (ARB) should be avoided in pregnancy.

### Hyperkalemia

Hyperkalemia can be treated with either insulin and dextrose or cation exchange resin although persistent and severe hyperkalemia would be an indication for renal replacement therapy [37]. Care should be taken to avoid hypoglycemia when treating hyperkalemia with insulin and dextrose, given the risks to the mother as well as the fetus.

### Metabolic Acidosis

Mild acidosis is common in pregnancy and sodium bicarbonate can be used to correct worsening metabolic acidosis [38].

### Anemia

Anemia is also common in ARF and can be managed with blood transfusion which, however, may exacerbate hyperkalemia and volume overload in patients with renal failure [39]. Human recombinant erythropoietin (EPO) has been used safely in pregnancy, but higher doses may be required to achieve the desired target hemoglobin [40].

## Renal Replacement Therapy (RRT) or Dialysis

The indications for renal replacement therapy (RRT) or dialysis are similar to other patients with ARF and are listed in Table 6.4.

No specific guidelines exist to steer RRT in pregnant women. However, relying on experience with RRT in nonpregnant women alone fails to take account the impact of the physiological changes that often accompany pregnancy [41].

**Table 6.4** Indications for renal replacement therapy

| |
|---|
| 1. Electrolyte imbalance |
| 2. Metabolic acidosis |
| 3. Volume overload |
| 4. Symptomatic uremia (pericarditis, neuropathy, mental status changes) |

Glomerular filtration rate increases by about 50 % in pregnancy as a result of increased renal plasma flow [42]. These changes occur early and persist till term, resulting in a fall in serum creatinine by about 20–30 % during pregnancy, compared to pre-pregnancy values [43]. Given this, standard dose of RRT used in nonpregnant patients may not be adequate in the setting of ARF in pregnancy.

Available evidence in women with end-stage renal disease (ESRD) suggests that intensified dialysis regimens are associated with improved maternal and fetal outcomes [44, 45]. A large registry study done in Belgium also suggested that increasing dialysis time was more likely to be associated with successful pregnancy, although premature deliveries were common in ESRD patients [46]. Similar findings were recently reported in a comparative analysis of a Canadian and US cohort of pregnant hemodialysis patients [47].

It is recommended that dialysis be started early in pregnant women with ARF [48] when:

- GFR is ≤20 ml per minute.
- Serum creatinine is between 3.5 and 5 mg/dl.

## Options for RRT

The options for RRT in ARF include:

- Intermittent hemodialysis
- Peritoneal dialysis (PD)
- Continuous hemofiltration (CRRT)
- Slow low efficiency dialysis (SLED)

### Hemodialysis

Daily intermittent dialysis is advised, aiming for >20 h of dialysis per week to keep pre-dialysis blood urea nitrogen (BUN) levels to <40 mg/dL or blood urea levels to <60 mg/dL [37, 44, 48]. Frequent dialysis is critical as this:

- Lowers ultrafiltration volume per session
- Minimizes the risk of intra-dialytic hypotension thus reducing:
  – The risk of fetal hypoperfusion
  – Significant metabolic shifts

When calculating dry weight, it is important to take account of the normal weight gain of 0.3–0.5 kg per week in the second and third trimesters. As pregnancy is associated with respiratory alkalosis with metabolic compensation, dialysate bicarbonate should be lowered to keep serum bicarbonate in the low pregnancy range of 18–20 mmol/L. Additional folate supplements are recommended for these patients, as there is increased removal of water-soluble vitamins, in particular folate, with frequent dialysis [51]. Both heparin and low molecular weight heparin are safe in pregnancy as they do not cross the placental barrier and can be used for anticoagulation during dialysis [48]. Frequent dialysis may lead to hypokalemia and hypophosphatemia, and levels of electrolytes should be checked after dialysis and replaced as required. In addition, some patients also require nutritional supplements.

Although there are no randomized studies showing benefit for any particular modality, hemodialysis is preferred over PD because:

- It is more efficient.
- It might be difficult to insert a PD catheter in pregnancy [49].
- The gravid uterus may limit the volume of fluid used in each exchange.
- PD is associated with the potential risk of peritonitis [50].

Despite these limitations, PD may be the only option in rural areas in developing countries. Patients who are critically ill with hemodynamic instability and/ or multi-organ failure would benefit from continuous hemofiltration (CRRT). However, this is expensive and not widely available, particularly in developing countries. Hybrid therapies such as slow low efficiency dialysis (SLED) would be an

**Table 6.5** Dialysis in pregnancy: specific concerns

| Variable | Concerns in pregnancy |
|---|---|
| Hemodynamics | Avoid hypotension, volume changes, and fluid fluctuations |
| Pre-dialysis serum BUN | Maintain < 40 mg/dL |
| Serum bicarbonate levels | Pregnancy is associated with respiratory alkalosis and metabolic compensation. Dialysate bicarbonate should be lowered to keep serum bicarbonate in the low pregnancy range |
| Folate supplements and vitamins | Increased supplementation required since serum folate and other water-soluble vitamins are removed by dialysis |
| Anemia | Therapeutic dosage of erythropoietin (if required) is higher in pregnancy |
| Serum calcium, potassium, and phosphates | Watch out for hypercalcemia, hypokalemia, and hypophosphatemia |
| Uterine contractions | Watch for preterm contractions and preterm labor associated with dialysis |
| Maternal weight gain | When calculating dry weight, it is important to take account of the normal weight gain of 0.3–0.5 kg/week in the second and third trimesters |

alternative option where CRRT is not available. Available evidence suggests that SLED provides comparable hemodynamic stability to continuous renal replacement therapy (CRRT) in nonpregnant ARF patients and so would be appropriate when CRRT is not available [52].

Table 6.5 lists the important considerations specific to dialysis in pregnancy.

## Management Based on Underlying Disorder

### Hyperemesis Gravidarum

Patients with ARF in the first trimester of pregnancy due to hyperemesis gravidarum usually respond to adequate volume replacement with normal saline with or without potassium supplements and antiemetics. Although uncommon, some patients with severe ARF due to hyperemesis may require dialysis [53].

### Septic Abortion

In patients with ARF due to septic abortion, treatment includes broad-spectrum antibiotics and evacuation of uterine contents. Some patients with septic abortion develop acute cortical necrosis and require renal replacement therapy.

### Preeclampsia and HELLP Syndrome

Preeclampsia is a progressive, multisystemic disease process, as mentioned earlier. To date, the most effective treatment strategy is delivery of the fetus and placenta. Therefore, in the case of preeclampsia-related ARF, delivery is indicated. The mode of delivery (vaginal vs. cesarean) is based on the clinical situation.

When the gestational age is 34 weeks or more, delivery should be immediate. When the gestational age is less than 34 weeks, the use of glucocorticoids is indicated to accelerate fetal pulmonary maturity.

Prompt delivery is also indicated when life-threatening maternal complications are present such as severe hypertension refractory to treatment, pulmonary edema, acute kidney injury, hepatic rupture, and eclampsia (Table 6.6). Induction of labor does not seem to increase neonatal morbidity but is rarely successful in patients with severe preeclampsia who present at <28 weeks [54].

The principles of management of ARF precipitated by preeclampsia and its complications are supportive and, depending on the clinical scenario, include [55]:

- Replacement of blood products
- Maintenance of intravascular volume
- Renal replacement therapy

**Table 6.6** Indications for immediate delivery

| |
|---|
| 1. Severe hypertension refractory to treatment |
| 2. Pulmonary edema |
| 3. Acute kidney injury |
| 4. Hepatic rupture |
| 5. Eclampsia |

The major causes of maternal mortality are cerebrovascular accidents and pulmonary edema. Therefore, the control of blood pressure and postpartum fluid management are vital in patients with preeclampsia [56, 57].

Excessive fluid administration in patients with severe preeclampsia can lead to pulmonary edema particularly in the postpartum period, and so it is important to monitor patients closely and limit the intravenous fluids [58]. Acute pulmonary edema may lead to mortality in pregnant women. In the absence of ongoing fluid loss, it would be advisable to limit the fluid to <80 ml per hour. Fluid challenges should be avoided. The presence of features of pulmonary edema would be an indication for using intravenous diuretics such as furosemide. Nitroglycerin (NTG) infusion may be used and would also be effective in lowering blood pressure in these patients. Patients who are oliguric and do not respond to the above measures need to be considered for renal replacement therapy. Management of fluid administration in severe preeclampsia is summarized in Table 6.7.

Magnesium sulfate is the mainstay of treatment for eclampsia [59]. As the kidneys excrete magnesium sulfate, dosing should be adjusted in patients with renal failure to avoid magnesium toxicity. Hypermagnesemia can lead to respiratory depression and weak or absent deep tendon reflexes. Patients with renal failure need to be monitored intensively for signs of magnesium toxicity. Calcium gluconate and diuretics can be used to reverse the effects of hypermagnesemia.

## Acute Fatty Liver of Pregnancy (AFLP)

As in preeclampsia/HELLP syndrome, patients with AFLP require urgent delivery once the mother is stabilized and most patients improve afterwards. The major issues are hypoglycemia and coagulopathy. Hypoglycemia requires continuous dextrose infusion, and coagulopathy is corrected with blood products such as FFP, cryoprecipitate, and platelets as required. Though recovery tends to be prolonged, most patients recover renal function after delivery with supportive measures. RRT is rarely indicated [55].

**Table 6.7** Management of fluid administration in severe preeclampsia

| | |
|---|---|
| Fluid replacement | Restricted to <80 ml/h |
| Fluid challenges | To be avoided |
| In the presence of pulmonary edema | Furosemide |
| | Nitroglycerin infusion |
| In the presence of persistent oliguria | Renal replacement therapy |

## Bilateral Renal Cortical Necrosis (BRCN)

Most patients with BRCN require dialysis and treatment is supportive. No specific treatment has been shown to be effective for BRCN. Some patients have partial recovery of renal function, and few remain free of dialysis for up to 12 years [60].

## Thrombotic Microangiopathies

Acute renal failure occurs in two thirds of these patients [61]. Plasmapheresis is the standard treatment of choice for TTP/HUS and can reduce the mortality from 90 to 10–20 % [62]. Corticosteroids have also been used as an adjunctive treatment for ADAMTS-13 deficiency-related thrombotic microangiopathy, but there has been no definitive evidence of efficiency of steroids in this setting [63]. In the presence of high titer autoantibodics, plasmapheresis or FFP may fail to induce or maintain remission [64]. Rituximab, a B cell depleting antibody, has been used as a second-line option in these patients, but its use in pregnancy has potential for fetal toxicity. Rituximab undergoes an active transplacental transport through Fc receptors during the third trimester of pregnancy leading to fetal accumulation [63]. However, rituximab is cleared within 3–4 months postpartum from the newborn circulation [65]. A retrospective review of women treated with rituximab during pregnancy for conditions such as lymphomas and autoimmune disorders reported that 60 % managed live births with only 2.2 % congenital abnormalities [66]. Less than 10 % of the neonates had evidence of B cell depletion. Although the short-term outcome data seems good, long-term prospective studies are needed to assess the impact of rituximab on the immune system of neonates.

About 80 % of those with pregnancy-associated HUS fail to recover renal function despite plasmapheresis and FFP infusions, and most of these patients have complement abnormalities [28]. Eculizumab, a monoclonal humanized IgG, is a potent inhibitor of complement activation. It inhibits the cleavage of C5 and so prevents the generation of C5a and C5b and thus blocks the common terminal activation step of all three-complement pathways [67]. Several case reports have been published which show the effectiveness of eculizumab both in HUS and atypical HUS and affecting native and transplant kidneys [68, 69]. In addition, the efficacy of eculizumab does not seem to be affected by the presence or absence of complement gene mutations. There have been reports of using eculizumab in pregnant women with paroxysmal nocturnal hemoglobinuria (PNH) with no reported safety issues for the fetus [70]. However, it is out of reach for most patients in developing countries as it costs almost half a million dollars per patient per year.

## Fetal Considerations

Pregnancy-related acute renal failure is associated with adverse perinatal outcomes. Most of the problems arise due to altered uteroplacental hemodynamics. There is also an increased risk of preterm labor with the use of dialysis. Attention must be paid to the volume status, adverse fetal effects of maternal medication, and maternal solute load [55]. Frequent fetal assessment using non-stress testing and biophysical profile is indicated. In women with hemodynamic instability, the monitoring is intensified since the fetus is at grave risk in those situations. However, maternal stability must be ensured before intervention is applied for fetal benefit. Steroids for fetal lung maturity should be administered if delivery is expected between 28 and 34 weeks.

### Conclusion

Acute renal failure has different incidence, etiology, and consequences in pregnant women in developing countries as compared to those in developed countries. Septic abortion and puerperal sepsis still play a large etiological role in developing countries. Less than 1 in 10,000–15,000 pregnancies needed RRT in the developed world [71] as compared to 60 % of women with pregnancy-related ARF in a developing nation [72]. Peritoneal dialysis and intermittent hemodialysis still continue to be the more cost-effective and affordable RRT modalities in developing countries.

## References

1. Krane NK. Acute renal failure in pregnancy. Arch Intern Med. 1988;148(11):2347.
2. Stratta P, Besso L, Canavese C, Grill A, Todros T, Benedetto C, et al. Is pregnancy-related acute renal failure a disappearing clinical entity? Ren Fail. 1996;18:575–84.
3. Prakash J, Kumar H, Sinha DK, Kedalaya PG, Pandey LK, Srivastava PK, et al. Acute renal failure in pregnancy in a developing country: twenty years of experience. Ren Fail. 2006;28:309–13.
4. Prakash J, Tripathi K, Pandey LK, Sahai S, Usha, Srivastava PK. Spectrum of renal cortical necrosis in acute renal failure in eastern India. Postgrad Med J. 1995;71:208–10.
5. Kumar KS, Krishna CR, Siva Kumar V. Pregnancy related acute renal failure. J Obstet Gynecol India. 2006;56:308–10.
6. Goplani KR, Shah PR, Gera DN, et al. Pregnancy-related acute renal failure: a single-center experience. Indian J Nephrol. 2008;18(1):17–21.
7. August P, George JN. Acute kidney injury (acute renal failure) in pregnancy. Lockwood CJ, Palevsky PM, editors. In: UpToDate. Waltham: UpToDate; 2014. Accessed 14 Nov 2014.
8. Machado S, Figueiredo N, Borges A, et al. Acute kidney injury in pregnancy: a clinical challenge. J Nephrol. 2012;25(01):21–30.
9. Chugh KS, Singhal PC, Sharma BK. ARF of obstetric origin. J Obstet Gynecol. 1976;108:253–61.
10. Prakash J, Tripathi K, Pandey LK, Gadela SR, Usha. Renal cortical necrosis in pregnancy related acute renal failure. J Indian Med Assoc. 1996;94:227–9.
11. Report of the ACOG Task Force on Hypertension in Pregnancy. Obstet Gynecol. 2013;122(5).
12. Leeman L, Fontaine P. Hypertensive disorders of pregnancy. Am Fam Physician. 2008;78(1):93–100.
13. Lafayette RA, Druzin M, Sibley R, et al. Nature of glomerular dysfunction in pre-eclampsia. Kidney Int. 1998;54:1240.
14. Sibai BM, Ramadan MK. Acute renal failure in pregnancies complicated by hemolysis, elevated liver enzymes, and low platelets. Am J Obstet Gynecol. 1993;168:1682.
15. Picinni P, Gallo G. Diagnosis and management of HELLP syndrome. In: Ronco C, Bellomo R, Kellum J, editors. Critical care nephrology. 2nd ed. Philadelphia: Saunders; 2009. p. 337–40.

16. Baxter JK, Weinstein L. HELLP syndrome: the state of the art. Obstet Gynecol Surv. 2004;59(12):838–45.
17. Haram K, Svendsen E, Abildgaard U. The HELLP syndrome: clinical issues and management: a Review. BMC Pregnancy Childbirth. 2009;9(1):8. 65.
18. Drakeley AJ, Le Roux PA, Anthony J, Penny J. Acute renal failure complicating severe preeclampsia requiring admission to an obstetric intensive care unit. Am J Obstet Gynecol. 2002;186(2):253–6.
19. Gul A, Aslan H, Cebeci A, Polat I, Ulusoy S, Ceylan Y. Maternal and fetal outcomes in HELLP syndrome complicated with acute renal failure. Ren Fail. 2004;26(5):557–62.
20. Sibai BM. Diagnosis, controversies, and management of the syndrome of hemolysis, elevated liver enzymes, and low platelet count. Obstet Gynecol. 2004;103(5 Pt 1):981–91.
21. Castro MA, Fassett MJ, Reynolds TB, et al. Reversible peripartum liver failure: a new perspective on the diagnosis, treatment, and cause of acute fatty liver of pregnancy, based on 28 consecutive cases. Am J Obstet Gynecol. 1999;181:389.
22. Santana L, Hernández Medina E, O'Shanahan G, Sánchez-Palacios M. Acute renal failure in acute fatty liver of pregnancy: apropos of a case. Nefrologia. 2005;25(4):453–4.
23. Koroshi A, Babameto A. Acute renal failure during acute fatty liver of pregnancy. Nephrol Dial Transplant. 2002;17(6):1110–2.
24. Guntupalli SR, Steingrub J. Hepatic disease and pregnancy: an overview of diagnosis and management. Crit Care Med. 2005;33(10 Suppl):S332–9.
25. Nelson DB, Yost NP, Cunningham FG. Acute fatty liver of pregnancy: clinical outcomes and expected duration of recovery. Am J Obstet Gynecol. 2013;209:456.e1.
26. Fakhouri F, Frémeaux-Bacchi V. Does hemolytic uremic syndrome differ from thrombotic thrombocytopenic purpura? Nat Clin Pract Nephrol. 2007;3(12):679–87.
27. George J. The thrombotic thrombocytopenic purpura and hemolytic uremic syndrome: evaluation, management and long-term outcomes experience of the Oklahoma TTP-HUS registry, 1989–2007. Kidney Int. 2009;112:S52–4.
28. Fakhouri F, Roumenina L, Provot F, et al. Pregnancy-associated hemolytic uremic syndrome revisited in the era of complement gene mutations. J Am Soc Nephrol. 2010;21(5):859–67.
29. Drakely AJ, Le Roux PA, Anthony J, Penny J. Acute renal failure complicating severe preeclampsia requiring admission to an obstetric intensive care unit. Am J Obstet Gynecol. 2002;186:253–6.
30. Prakash J, Niwas SS, Parekh A, et al. Acute kidney injury in late pregnancy in developing countries. Ren Fail. 2010;32(3):309–13.
31. Kellum JA, Lameire N. Diagnosis, evaluation, and management of acute kidney injury: a KDIGO summary (Part 1). Crit Care. 2013;17:204.
32. Podymow T, August P. Update on the use of antihypertensive drugs in pregnancy. Hypertension. 2008; 51:960–9.
33. Visintin C, Mugglestone MA, Almerie MQ, Nherera LM, James D, Walkinshaw S. Management of hypertensive disorders during pregnancy: summary of NICE guidance. BMJ. 2010;341:c2207.
34. Vidaeff AC, Carroll MA, Ramin SM. Acute hypertensive emergencies in pregnancy. Crit Care Med. 2005;33:S307–12.
35. Magee LA, Cham C, Waterman EJ, Ohlsson A, von Dadelszen P. Hydralazine for treatment of severe hypertension in pregnancy: meta-analysis. BMJ. 2003;327:955–60.
36. Chandiramani M, Shennan A. Hypertensive disorders of pregnancy: a UK-based perspective. Curr Opin Obstet Gynecol. 2008;20:96–101.
37. Machado S, Figueiredo N, Borges A, et al. Acute kidney injury in pregnancy: a clinical challenge. J Nephrol. 2012;25:19–30.
38. Acharya A, Santos J, Linde B, Anis K. Acute kidney injury in pregnancy-current status. Adv Chronic Kidney Dis. 2013;20:215–22.
39. Tanhehco YC, Berns JS. Red blood cell transfusion risks in patients with end-stage renal disease. Semin Dial. 2012;25:539–44.
40. Jungers P, Chauveau D. Pregnancy in renal disease. Kidney Int. 1997;52:871–85.
41. Barraclough K, Leone E, Chiu A. Renal replacement therapy for acute kidney injury in pregnancy. Nephrol Dial Transplant. 2007;22:2395–7.
42. Davison JM, Dunlop W. Renal hemodynamics and tubular function normal human pregnancy. Kidney Int. 1980;18:152–61.
43. Sturgiss SN, Dunlop W, Davison JM. Renal haemodynamics and tubular function in human pregnancy. Baillieres Clin Obstet Gynaecol. 1994;8:209–34.
44. Bagon JA, Vernaeve H, De Muylder X, Lafontaine JJ, Martens J, Van Roost G. Pregnancy and dialysis. Am J Kidney Dis. 1998;31:756–65.
45. Gangji AS, Windrim R, Gandhi S, Silverman JA, Chan CT. Successful pregnancy with nocturnal hemodialysis. Am J Kidney Dis. 2004;44:912–6.
46. Okundaye I, Abrinko P, Hou S. Registry of pregnancy in dialysis patients. Am J Kidney Dis. 1998;31:766–73.
47. Hladunewich MA, Hou S, Odutayo A, et al. Intensive hemodialysis associates with improved pregnancy outcomes: a Canadian and United States cohort comparison. J Am Soc Nephrol. 2014;25:1103–9.
48. Krane NK, Hamrahian M. Pregnancy: kidney diseases and hypertension. Am J Kidney Dis. 2007;49: 336–45.
49. Davenport A. Peritoneal dialysis in acute kidney injury. Perit Dial Int. 2008;28:423–4; author reply 424.
50. Briones-Garduno JC, Diaz de Leon-Ponce MA, Rodriguez-Roldan M, Briones-Vega CG, Torres-Perez J. Peritoneal dialysis in obstetric patients. Cir Cir. 2006;74:15–20.
51. Hou S. Modification of dialysis regimens for pregnancy. Int J Artif Organs. 2002;25:823–6.
52. Fieghen HE, Friedrich JO, Burns KE, et al. The hemodynamic tolerability and feasibility of sustained low

efficiency dialysis in the management of critically ill patients with acute kidney injury. BMC Nephrol. 2010;11:32.
53. Hill JB, Yost NP, Wendel GDJ. Acute renal failure in association with severe hyperemesis gravidarum. Obstet Gynecol. 2002;100:1119–21.
54. Blackwell SC, Redman ME, Tomlinson M, et al. Labor induction for the preterm severe pre-eclamptic patient: is it worth the effort? J Matern Fetal Med. 2001;10:305–11.
55. Gammill HS, Jeyabalan A. Acute renal failure in pregnancy. Crit Care Med. 2005;33(10 Suppl):S372–84.
56. Bushnell C, Chireau M. Preeclampsia and stroke: risks during and after pregnancy. Stroke Res Treat. 2011;2011:858134.
57. Dennis AT, Solnordal CB. Acute pulmonary oedema in pregnant women. Anaesthesia. 2012;67:646–59.
58. Churchill D, Duley L, Thornton JG, Jones L. Interventionist versus expectant care for severe pre-eclampsia between 24 and 34 weeks' gestation. Cochrane Database Syst Rev. 2013;(7):CD003106.
59. Group TETC. Which anticonvulsant for women with eclampsia? Evidence from the Collaborative Eclampsia Trial. Lancet. 1995;345:1455–63.
60. Chugh KS, Jha V, Sakhuja V, Joshi K. Acute renal cortical necrosis–a study of 113 patients. Ren Fail. 1994;16:37–47.
61. Esplin MSM, Branch DW. Diagnosis and management of thrombotic microangiopathies during pregnancy. Clin Obstet Gynecol Ambul Gynecol. 1999;42:360–7.
62. Rock G, Shumak KH, Buskard MA, et al. Comparison of plasma exchange with plasma infusion in the treatment of thrombotic thrombocytopenic purpura. Canadian Apheresis Study Group. N Engl J Med. 1991; 325:393–7.
63. Fakhouri F, Vercel C, Fremeaux-Bacchi V. Obstetric nephrology: AKI and thrombotic microangiopathies in pregnancy. Clin J Am Soc Nephrol. 2012;7: 2100–6.
64. Kremer Hovinga JA, Vesely SK, Terrell DR, Lammle B, George JN. Survival and relapse in patients with thrombotic thrombocytopenic purpura. Blood. 2010;115:1500–11; quiz 1662.
65. Gall B, Yee A, Berry B, et al. Rituximab for management of refractory pregnancy-associated immune thrombocytopenic purpura. J Obstet Gynaecol Can. 2010;32:1167–71.
66. Chakravarty EF, Murray ER, Kelman A, Farmer P. Pregnancy outcomes after maternal exposure to rituximab. Blood. 2011;117:1499–506.
67. Kaplan M. Eculizumab (Alexion). Curr Opin Investig Drugs. 2002;3:1017–23.
68. Mache CJ, Acham-Roschitz B, Fremeaux-Bacchi V, et al. Complement inhibitor eculizumab in atypical hemolytic uremic syndrome. Clin J Am Soc Nephrol. 2009;4:1312–6.
69. Legendre CM, Licht C, Muus P, et al. Terminal complement inhibitor eculizumab in atypical hemolytic-uremic syndrome. N Engl J Med. 2013;368: 2169–81.
70. Kelly R, Arnold L, Richards S, et al. The management of pregnancy in paroxysmal nocturnal haemoglobinuria on long term eculizumab. Br J Haematol. 2010;149:446–50.
71. Clark SL. Handbook of critical care obstetrics. Boston: Blackwell Scientific Publications; 1994.
72. Najar MS, Shah AR, Wani IA, et al. Pregnancy related acute kidney injury: a single center experience from the Kashmir Valley. Indian J Nephrol. 2008;18(4): 159–61.

# Acute Fatty Liver of Pregnancy

# 7

Asha Reddy

## Introduction

AFLP is an uncommon but potentially fatal complication that occurs in the third trimester or early postpartum period [1–3]. Sheehan first described it as an "acute yellow atrophy of the liver" in 1940. AFLP is characterized by microvesicular fatty infiltration of hepatocytes without any inflammation or necrosis. It has an incidence of approximately one in 7000–15,000 pregnancies. In the past, maternal and perinatal mortality were reported to be as high as 75–85 %. With prompt diagnosis and treatment, the current maternal and perinatal mortality have greatly decreased. The exact pathogenesis is undetermined. Supportive care and expeditious delivery remain the best treatment [1–3]. This article provides a brief review of AFLP, including etiology, pathophysiology, clinical presentations, diagnosis, and management.

## Etiopathogenesis

Studies suggest that AFLP may be a consequence of mitochondrial dysfunction. Association of AFLP with long-chain 3-hydroxyacyl-CoA dehydrogenase (LCHAD) deficiency, a genetic, autosomal recessive, inborn error of metabolism in the fetus, is well recognized. Mitochondrial fatty acid beta-oxidation consists of a series of enzymatic reactions and generates energy from free fatty acids (FFA) for essential organs when the glycogen stores are depleted. Deficiency of LCHAD results in accumulation of medium- and long-chain fatty acids has been identified in some women with AFLP [1, 4–6].

The most common mutation in the LCHAD gene occurs in the alpha-unit of the trifunctional protein gene (1528G $\rightarrow$ C), which alters amino acid 474 from glutamic acid to glutamine (E474Q). This mutation is associated with approximately 65–90 % of the LCHAD-deficient patients. It is hypothesized because the mutation is recessive; under normal physiological conditions, the mother does not have abnormal fatty acid oxidation. However, when both parents are heterozygous for this abnormality and the fetus acquires both of these mutations, the fetus is unable to oxidize the long-chain fatty acids. The unmetabolized FFA return to the maternal circulation, which strains maternal hepatic activity leading to AFLP. Delivery of the fetus eliminates the strain on the maternal liver and explains eventual postpartum normalization fatty acid oxidation.

Some studies have not been able to confirm the association between AFLP and LCHAD deficiency. There are a number of mutations leading to LCHAD deficiency and only specific genetic defects will lead to an increased risk of AFLP. It is also possible that there are several mutations in the LCHAD gene which are currently unknown.

A. Reddy
Consultant Reproductive Endocrinologist, Obstetrician and Gynecologist Primary Medicare Centre, Bengaluru, India
e-mail: ashadeepc@yahoo.com


A. Gandhi et al. (eds.), *Principles of Critical Care in Obstetrics: Volume II*,
DOI 10.1007/978-81-322-2686-4_7

In AFLP, there is a progressive lipid accumulation within the hepatocytes. Normal hepatic fat content is approximately 5 %. In AFLP, hepatic fat content can range from 13 to 19 %. Progressive lipid accumulation along with ammonia production by the hepatocytes leads to coagulopathy and hypoglycemia secondary to evolving hepatic failure. The liver in AFLP is usually small, soft, and yellow, due to hepatocytolysis and hepatocyte atrophy. The kidney, pancreas, brain, and bone marrow may also demonstrate microvesicular fat infiltration.

## Risk Factors

Deficiency of the enzyme LCHAD seems to predispose women to AFLP.

Other known risk factors for AFLP are:

1. Primigravidas.
2. Pre-eclampsia.
3. Male fetus.
4. Multiple gestation. [There is no causal relationship identified between these potential risk factors and AFLP as yet, although hypothesis is that multiple gestations may place women at increased risk for AFLP because there is an increased production of fatty acid metabolites by more than one fetus.]
5. Drugs have also been proposed to be associated with AFLP and there is a report of association between acetylsalicylic acid and AFLP. Nonsteroidal anti-inflammatory drugs, including salicylates, inhibit trifunctional protein and thereby mitochondrial long-chain fatty acid oxidation in mitochondria, leading to AFLP in a heterozygous (LCHAD mutation) mother with a homozygous fetus.

Ethnicity does not seem to be associated with AFLP.

## Clinical Presentation

1. Most women who are diagnosed with AFLP are in the third trimester of pregnancy and the mean gestational age is 35–36 weeks, with a range of 28–40 weeks. Isolated case reports of AFLP have shown that it can occur as early as 22 weeks and as late as the immediate postpartum period.
2. Clinical findings in AFLP vary because it may occur with different degrees of clinical severity and in conjunction with other third trimester symptoms, making early diagnosis of AFLP difficult.
3. Patients often present with nonspecific symptoms such as anorexia, nausea, vomiting, malaise, fatigue, headache, and abdominal pain.
4. Fever and jaundice are very common and occur in more than 70 % of patients with AFLP. Tenderness in the right upper quadrant or midepigastric area may be present. The liver is usually small and nonpalpable.
5. In severe cases, there is multisystem involvement including acute renal failure, encephalopathy, gastrointestinal bleeding, pancreatitis, and coagulopathy.
6. Some may also have pre-eclampsia as well, with edema and hypertension. It is believed that the hemolysis, elevated liver enzymes, and low platelets (HELLP) syndrome, pre-eclampsia, thrombotic thrombocytopenia purpura, and AFLP may all be a spectrum of the same illness.
7. Transient diabetes insipidus may also occur but is very rare (Table 7.1).

**Table 7.1** Common features of AFLP [3–5, 7, 8]

| Common signs and symptoms of AFLP | |
|---|---|
| Common signs and symptoms | (%) |
| Nausea, vomiting, jaundice | 70 |
| Abdominal pain | 60–70 |
| Nervous system (altered sensorium, confusion, disorientation, psychosis, restlessness, seizures, coma) | 60–80 |
| Disseminated intravascular coagulation | 55–80 |
| Gastrointestinal bleeding | 20–60 |
| Acute renal failure | 50 |
| Oliguria | 40–60 |
| Tachycardia | 50 |
| Late-onset pyrexia | 50 |

A. *Lab findings in AFLP* [4–9]

1. *Hematology*

| | |
|---|---|
| Hemoglobin | Normal (unless hemorrhage/hemolysis) |
| Hematocrit | Normal (unless hemorrhage/hemolysis) |
| White blood cells | Mildly elevated |
| Platelets | Normal to mild decrease |

2. *Liver function*

| | |
|---|---|
| Aspartate aminotransferase | Moderate to marked elevation |
| Alanine aminotransferase | Moderate to marked elevation |
| Gamma-glutamyltransferase | Mild elevation |
| Alkaline phosphatase | Moderate to marked elevation |
| Lactate dehydrogenase | Normal and then mild decrease |
| Bilirubin, total | Moderate to marked elevation |
| Bilirubin, direct | Moderate to marked elevation |
| Ammonia | Mild elevation |
| Lactate | Mild elevation |
| Glucose | Moderate-marked decrease |
| Cholesterol | Mild decrease |
| Triglycerides | Mild decrease |

3. *Coagulation tests*

| | |
|---|---|
| International normalized ratio | Moderately to markedly elevated |
| Prothrombin time | Mildly elevated |
| Partial thromboplastin time | Mildly elevated |
| Fibrinogen | Moderately to markedly decreased |
| Fibrin split products | Present |
| Antithrombin III | Moderately to markedly decreased |

4. *Renal*

| | |
|---|---|
| Uric acid | Moderately to markedly elevated |
| Blood urea nitrogen | Mildly elevated |
| Creatinine | Moderately to markedly elevated |

B. *Imaging*: Ultrasound and computed tomography may show fatty infiltration of the liver; however, the findings are not sensitive or specific enough to make a definitive diagnosis of AFLP. False-negative results are common.

C. *Histopathology*: Liver biopsy is usually not necessary for diagnosis. History, clinical findings, and lab and imaging results are sufficient to make the diagnosis in most cases. Liver biopsy should not be performed to confirm a diagnosis of AFLP or to distinguish AFLP from severe pre-eclampsia, because management of both conditions are the same. Liver biopsy may be justified rarely in cases when liver function does not return to normal postpartum. Histologically, microvesicular steatosis with sparing of zone 1 is the characteristic feature. There may be patchy hepatocellular necrosis. Widespread necrosis or inflammation is absent.

## Diagnosis

1. Diagnosis of AFLP is challenging because the initial clinical presentation may be nonspecific.
2. Among other causes of pathological hepatic dysfunction, acute fatty liver of pregnancy (AFLP) is uncommon compared to pre-eclampsia and HELLP syndrome.
3. History, clinical features, and biochemical abnormalities may mimic acute viral hepatitis, pre-eclampsia, HELLP syndrome, obstetric cholestasis, or other causes of hepatic dysfunction.
4. AFLP is uncommon. Therefore, the best approach to any pregnant women with liver dysfunction is to quickly rule out other, more likely causes.

## Differentiating AFLP from Other Causes of Pathological Hepatic Dysfunction in Pregnancy [3–9]

1. Pre-eclampsia and eclampsia:
   (a) Onset: 2nd or 3rd trimester.
   (b) Incidence: 5–10 %.

   (c) Features: Nausea, vomiting, epigastric pain, edema, hypertension, mental status changes, and jaundice (late feature).
   (d) Labs: ALT <500 U/L, proteinuria, and DIC (7 %).
   (e) Maternal complications: Hypertensive crisis, renal impairment, hepatic rupture/infarct, and neurological (seizures, cerebrovascular accidents).
   (f) Fetal complications: Abruption and prematurity; IUGR and perinatal morbidity and mortality.
   (g) One of the most common multiorgan diseases of late pregnancy.
   (h) Women with AFLP can also have pre-eclampsia; however women with pre-eclampsia alone do not usually have jaundice or hypoglycemia which are characteristic of AFLP.
   (i) AFLP often presents more acutely whereas pre-eclampsia develops over several days or weeks.
   (j) Pre-eclampsia rarely presents with severe coagulopathy.
2. HELLP syndrome:
   (a) Onset: 3rd trimester
   (b) Incidence: 0.10 % (4–12 % of women with pre-eclampsia)
   (c) Features: Symptoms of pre-eclampsia (hypertension, headache, blurred vision), epigastric or right upper quadrant pain, nausea, vomiting, hematuria, and jaundice (late feature)
   (d) Labs: Hemolysis, ALT <500 U/L, platelets <100 × 109/L, elevated LDH, and DIC (20–40 %)
   (e) Maternal complications: Seizures; acute renal failure; hepatic rupture, hematoma, or infarct; and high mortality (1–3 %)
   (f) Fetal complications: Abruption and prematurity; IUGR and perinatal morbidity and mortality
3. Obstetric cholestasis:
   (a) Onset: 2nd or 3rd trimester.
   (b) Incidence : 0.1–0.2 %.
   (c) Features: Intense pruritus, jaundice (20–60 %, occurs about 1–4 weeks after onset of pruritus), and steatorrhea.
   (d) Labs: ALT <500 U/L, markedly elevated ALP and GGT, and increased bile acids; bilirubin (<103 μmol/L).
   (e) Maternal complications: Predisposed to cholestasis on subsequent pregnancies.
   (f) Fetal complications: Still birth, prematurity, and fetal mortality (3.5 %).
   (g) OC may cause jaundice; however, it is predominantly characterized by intense pruritus and elevated alkaline phosphatase.
   (h) OC is not associated with abdominal pain, nausea, vomiting, liver failure, or DIC.
4. Viral hepatitis:
   (a) Onset: Any trimester.
   (b) Incidence: Same as general population.
   (c) Features: Nausea, vomiting, and fever. Signs of pre-eclampsia are absent in viral hepatitis.
   (d) Labs: Serum transaminases are much higher (often more than 1000 U/L). Bilirubin is high. Viral serology tests will be positive. Uric acid levels are rarely elevated in fulminant hepatitis.
   (e) Maternal complications: Increased mortality with hepatitis E.
5. Drug-induced hepatitis:
   (a) Onset: Any trimester
   (b) Incidence: Variable
   (c) Features: Nausea, vomiting, pruritis, and jaundice (in cholestatic hepatitis)
   (d) Labs: Variable
   (e) Maternal and fetal complications: Variable
6. Acute fatty liver of pregnancy:
   (a) Onset: 3rd trimester (rarely during 2nd)
   (b) Incidence: 0.01 %
   (c) Features: Malaise, upper abdominal pain, nausea, vomiting, jaundice (very very common), and encephalopathy (late feature)
   (d) Labs: ALT <500 U/L, hyperbilirubinemia, hypoglycemia, and elevated ammonia, leukocytosis, and DIC (>75 %) – thrombocytopenia, prolonged PT, and hypofibrinogenemia
   (e) Maternal complications: Acute renal failure, encephalopathy, ascites, sepsis, wound seroma, pancreatitis, and increased mortality

(f) Fetal complications: Increased mortality from asphyxia, prematurity, IUGR, and LCHAD deficiency

## Management [3–12]

(a) *Maternal Stabilization*
1. Early diagnosis, prompt delivery, and intensive supportive care are the cornerstones in the management of AFLP.
2. Lab findings in AFLP frequently do not reflect the magnitude of the condition. High level of suspicion, with low threshold for inpatient admission to monitor, is important. If at high risk for multisystem organ failure and death, admission to the intensive care unit is recommended.
3. Maternal stabilization should be achieved before delivery, which includes airway management, treatment of hypertension, correction of hypoglycemia, and electrolyte and coagulation abnormalities.
4. Careful maintenance of intravenous fluids and blood products and frequent assessment of maternal vital signs and mental status are all crucial.
5. Frequent fetal assessment is necessary.
6. Multidisciplinary care involving different specialties such as intensive care, gastroenterology, and perinatology is essential.

(b) *Delivery of the Fetus*
7. Once the mother is stabilized, delivery of the fetus is the next step.
8. Vaginal birth is probably the best approach if tolerated; however, caesarean birth is often performed because of rapidly deteriorating maternal-fetal status.

(c) *Postpartum Management*
1. During the postpartum recovery period, continued hemodynamic monitoring is necessary because of high risk of bleeding due to coagulopathy.
2. Transfusion of fluids and blood products may be needed.
3. Patients are also at risk of hypoglycemia and glucose infusion may be needed.
4. Potential complications of AFLP usually develop after the onset of hepatic and renal dysfunction. The development of pseudocysts with secondary infections or hemorrhagic pancreatitis with resultant retroperitoneal bleeding can be difficult to control, especially when patient has coagulopathy. Serial screening of serum lipase and amylase for several days after the onset of hepatic dysfunction is necessary.
5. Imaging studies such as computed tomography or magnetic resonance imaging may be useful in assessing the development of pseudocysts or hemorrhagic pancreatitis.
6. The safety and effect of plasma exchange with continuous renal replacement therapy for AFLP need evaluation.
7. Liver transplantation has rarely been performed for AFLP. Orthotopic liver transplantation should be considered for those women with fulminant hepatic failure/multisystem failure, irreversible liver failure despite delivery and aggressive supportive care, hepatic encephalopathy, severe metabolic acidosis, or worsening coagulopathy or those with liver rupture complicated by hepatic necrosis as indicated by computed tomography.

## Outcomes [3–12]

### Maternal Outcomes

1. Mortality from AFLP is around 18 %.
2. Deaths are usually secondary to sepsis, renal failure, circulatory collapse, pancreatitis, or gastrointestinal bleeding.
3. Among survivors, liver function tests may show continued deterioration for up to 1 week postpartum but then slowly recover. On CT the liver volume initially decreases and recovers eventually in the postpartum.
4. Resolution of the disease is indicated by the improvement of hepatic function. Liver enzymes, ammonia, and coagulation studies will begin to normalize and will be followed

by a decrease in serum creatinine, as long as there is no permanent renal damage.
5. Full clinical recovery usually occurs in several weeks with no long-term sequelae, although histological changes in the liver may persist for months.

## Recurrence of AFLP

1. AFLP can recur in subsequent pregnancies.
2. The theoretical recurrence risk in subsequent pregnancies is 25 % with a mother carrying a homozygous mutant or compound heterozygous fetuses; it is uncommon and only a few cases have been documented. However, this may be an underestimation, because many women may refrain from having further pregnancies after the first occurrence.
3. Affected women should be counseled. If necessary the neonate and the mother should be tested for LCHAD deficiency.
4. If the patient decides to be pregnant again, she should be closely monitored for any early signs of acute fatty liver.
5. Women should be counseled about the risk of recurrence and regularly monitored during the next pregnancy, even if the search for gene mutation is negative.

## Fetal Outcomes

1. Previously, the neonatal mortality rate had been as high as 85 %. Over the recent times, with prompt recognition and treatment, the mortality rate has dramatically decreased to approximately 20 %.
2. Though perinatal survival rate has improved, evidence of fetal compromise is not uncommon and can be present even in a clinically stable mother.
3. Close fetal surveillance and neonatal care are essential.
4. Cause for increased fetal distress and neonatal death in the absence of maternal clinical decompensation is not very clear. However, this could be due to premature delivery.
5. Maternal metabolic acidosis secondary to impaired lactate clearance affects fetal acid-base status. Prompt correction of maternal metabolic acidosis is essential to the fetal well-being.

## LCHAD Deficiency in Infants

1. Accumulation of the toxic metabolites in the mitochondria causes degeneration and fatty infiltration of muscle fibers affecting both skeletal and cardiac muscles. Lipid depositions within the hepatocytes lead to impaired bilirubin metabolism and progressive jaundice.
2. Inherited LCHAD deficiency may not be recognizable right away and usually presents in the neonatal period or in early childhood, frequently after a period of fasting or viral illness. At the time of diagnosis, infants frequently have severe liver failure, severe cardiomyopathy, and hypoketotic hypoglycemic encephalopathy which may be difficult to reverse. LCHAD deficiency can be suddenly lethal.
3. Molecular testing for this deficiency should be performed in infants as well as in affected mothers and fathers. Although there are a number of mutations for LCHAD deficiency, testing only for E474Q might be sufficient because fetuses of affected mothers almost always have the E474Q mutation on at least one allele.
4. A diet low in long-chain fatty acids and supplemented with medium-chain triglycerides is recommended. Dietary therapy may improve long-term prognosis, although it does not prevent irreversible ophthalmological changes such as fundal pigmentation.

**Conclusion**

1. AFLP is an uncommon, life-threatening disorder developing in the third trimester of pregnancy or early postpartum period.
2. Early diagnosis sometimes can be difficult because AFLP shares features with other common disorders such as pre-eclampsia, viral hepatitis, or cholestasis of pregnancy.

3. Careful history, physical examination, and laboratory and imaging results are often sufficient to make the diagnosis. Liver biopsy is rarely indicated.
4. Prompt delivery of the infant and intensive supportive care remain as the mainstay treatment for AFLP.

## References


1. Ko H, Yoshida EM. Acute fatty liver of pregnancy. Can J Gastroenterol. 2006;20(1):25–30.
2. Castro MA, Fassett MJ, Reynolds TB, Shaw KJ, Goodwin TM. Reversible peripartum liver failure: a new perspective on the diagnosis, treatment, and cause of acute fatty liver of pregnancy, based on 28 consecutive cases. Am J Obstet Gynecol. 1999;181(2):389–95.
3. Treem WR, Shoup ME, Hale DE, Bennett MJ, Rinaldo P, Millington DS, Stanley CA, Riely CA, Hyams JS. Acute fatty liver of pregnancy, hemolysis, elevated liver enzymes, and low platelets syndrome, and long chain 3-hydroxyacyl-coenzyme A dehydrogenase deficiency. Am J Gastroenterol. 1996;91(11):2293–300.
4. Paul S, Sepehr GJ, Allison HV. Abnormal liver function tests in the third trimester: a diagnostic dilemma. Acute fatty liver of pregnancy. Gastroenterology. 2014;146(4):910.
5. Mjahed K, Charra B, Hamoudi D, Noun M, Barrou L. Acute fatty liver of pregnancy. Arch Gynecol Obstet. 2006;274(6):349–53.
6. Loganathan G, Eapen CE, Chandy RG, Jasper P, Mathai M, Seshadri L, Ramakrishna B, Jana AK, John G, Chandy GM. Acute fatty liver of pregnancy: a report of two cases. Natl Med J India. 2002;15(6): 336–8.
7. Sheehan HL. The pathology of acute yellow atrophy and delayed chloroform poisoning. J Obstet Gynaecol Br Emp. 1940;47:49–62.
8. Usta IM, Barton JR, Amon EA, Gonzalez A, Sibai BM. Acute fatty liver of pregnancy: an experience in the diagnosis and management of fourteen cases. Am J Obstet Gynecol. 1994;171(5):1342–7.
9. Papafragkakis H, Singhal S, Anand S. Acute fatty liver of pregnancy. South Med J. 2013;106(10): 588–93.
10. Nelson DB, Yost NP, Cunningham FG. Acute fatty liver of pregnancy: clinical outcomes and expected duration of recovery. Am J Obstet Gynecol. 2013;209(5):456.
11. Goel A, Jamwal KD, Ramachandran A, Balasubramanian KA, Eapen CE. Pregnancy-related liver disorders. J Clin Exp Hepatol. 2014;4(2): 151–62.
12. Yu CB, Chen JJ, Du WB, Chen P, Huang JR, Chen YM, Cao HC, Li LJ. Effects of plasma exchange combined with continuous renal replacement therapy on acute fatty liver of pregnancy. Hepatobiliary Pancreat Dis Int. 2014;13(2):179–83.

# 8 Fulminant Hepatitis

Suchitra N. Pandit and Deepali P. Kale

## Introduction

Acute viral hepatitis (AVH) continues to be a public health problem in India despite improving sanitation, health awareness, and socioeconomic conditions. India is hyperendemic for hepatitis A and E [8].

Hepatitis E virus (HEV), a member of the genus *Hepevirus* in the family *Hepeviridae* [10], is a major cause of enterically transmitted non-A non-B hepatitis in many developing countries with large epidemics already being reported in Asia, Africa, and Latin America [13]. High mortality rates have been reported for HEV-related infection during pregnancy [8, 9].

## Definition

Fulminant hepatitis or acute liver failure is defined as development of hepatic encephalopathy within 4 weeks of acute hepatitis in a patient without pre existing liver disease [1].

Acute viral hepatitis (AVH) is an infection predominantly involving the liver. Hepatitis virus A, B, C, D, E, and G are the causative agents [5].

Acute viral hepatitis is defined usually by acute self-limited disease and a serum aspartate aminotransferase elevation of at least fivefold or clinical jaundice or both (Table 8.1).

Hepatic encephalopathy usually sets in fulminant hepatic failure in all classifications and has transition from a severe condition to a deadly disease. The interval between the onset of symptoms or jaundice and the appearance of encephalopathy enables grouping of patients with similar etiologies, clinical characteristics, and prognosis. Liver disorders in pregnancy encompass a wide spectrum, but FH is the condition which has the most alarming and devastating course.

Acute liver failure is a broad term that encompasses both fulminant hepatic failure and subfulminant hepatic failure (or late-onset hepatic failure). Fulminant hepatic failure is generally used to describe the development of encephalopathy within 8 weeks of the onset of symptoms in a patient with a previously healthy liver. Subfulminant hepatic failure is reserved for patients with liver disease for up to 26 weeks before the development of hepatic encephalopathy.

S.N. Pandit, MD, DGO, DNB, FRCOG, B. Pharm (✉)
Department of Obstetrics and Gynecology,
Kokilaben Dhirubhai Ambani Hospital
and Research Centre, Mumbai, India
e-mail: snpandit.president@gmail.com

D.P. Kale, DNB, DGO(MUHS), FCPS, FMAS
Department of Obstetrics and Gynecology,
Nowrosjee Wadia Maternity Hospital and Seth
G.S Medical College, Mumbai, India


A. Gandhi et al. (eds.), *Principles of Critical Care in Obstetrics: Volume II*,
DOI 10.1007/978-81-322-2686-4_8

**Table 8.1** Different classifications of fulminant hepatic failure

| Trey and Davidson [1] | England [10] | France [13] | International Association for the Study of the Liver 15 Acute liver failure (occurrence of HE within 4 weeks after onset of symptoms) [11] |
|---|---|---|---|
| Fulminant hepatic failure: development of HE within 8 weeks of onset of symptoms | Acute liver failure (includes only patients with encephalopathy) | Acute hepatic failure: a rapidly developing impairment of liver function | *Subclassification*<br>Acute liver failure, hyperacute: within 10 days<br>Acute liver failure, fulminant: 10–30 days<br>Acute liver failure, not otherwise specified |
| | *Subclassification* depending on the interval between jaundice and HE | Severe acute hepatic failure: prothrombin time or factor V concentration below 50 % of normal with or without HE | *Subacute liver failure* (development of ascites and/or HE from 5 to 24 weeks after onset of symptoms)<br>*Subclassification* by etiology<br>Hepatitis A–E<br>Other viruses |
| | Hyperacute liver failure: 0–7 days | *Subclassification*<br>Fulminant hepatic failure: HE within 2 weeks of onset of jaundice | |
| | Acute liver failure: 8–28 days | *Subfulminant hepatic failure*: HE between 3 and 12 weeks of onset of jaundice | |
| | Subacute liver failure: 29–72 days | | |
| | Late-onset acute liver failure: 56–182 days | | |

## Etiology

The most common etiology implicated in FH is viral hepatitis. The viruses have different geographic distribution. Thus, hepatitis B virus (HBV) is a common cause of FHF in the Far East, and hepatitis E virus (HEV) is relevant in India [14].

Studies carried out in India, Iran, Africa, and the Middle East have found the incidence of fulminant hepatitis to be higher in pregnancy [3, 4].

Occurrence of FHF within the larger number of patients with viral hepatitis, however, is rare (0.2–0.4 % for hepatitis A, 1–4 % for hepatitis B) [15]. Pregnant women infected by HEV seem to have a special propensity for developing FHF.

## Epidemiology

Hepatitis E virus infection is highly endemic in certain countries. It causes frequent waterborne outbreaks and around 50 % of all cases of acute viral hepatitis in many countries and is contributed by factors like rapid urbanization, with limited access to safe drinking water and food and proper sanitation, which subsequently augments the risk of these infections. Thus, hepatitis viruses have a significant disease burden in the Southeast Asia Region, in the form of both acute and chronic hepatitis, with approximately 500,000 deaths annually in the region. Available data from the region on rates of infection with hepatitis viruses, rates of clinical disease caused by these viruses, and the associated morbidity and mortality are limited and may not reflect the true picture. Also the data available on the social and economic impact, expenditure on medical care, etc., of these infections in the region is not available [12].

Hepatitis E is caused by infection with the hepatitis E virus (HEV), a non-enveloped, positive-sense, single-stranded RNA virus [16–18], with four genotypes, 1, 2, 3, and 4. Each HEV genotype appears to have a specific geographic distribution. Genotype 1 HEV has been isolated from human cases of epidemic and sporadic hepatitis E in parts of Asia and Africa, where the disease is highly endemic. Outbreaks of HEV infection of up to several hundred to several thousand persons have been reported frequently in the Indian subcontinent, China, Southeast and Central Asia, the Middle East, and northern and western parts of Africa [2, 19].

Hepatitis E outbreaks are characteristically associated with a high disease attack rate among pregnant women. Further, affected pregnant women are more prone to develop fulminant hepatitis [19–23]. Hepatitis E outbreaks are characteristically associated with a high disease attack rate among pregnant women. Further, the affected pregnant women are more likely to develop fulminant hepatitis (15–22 %) or to have a fatal outcome. Fulminant hepatitis E infection has been reported among 40.3 % of pregnant women who were coinfected with chronic hepatitis B [24–26].

Hepatitis E during pregnancy is also associated with prematurity, low birth weight, and an increased risk of perinatal mortality [22].

**Hepatitis E** Self-limiting – the overall mortality rate in FHF is 1–3 %; in pregnant women the rate is 15–25 %.

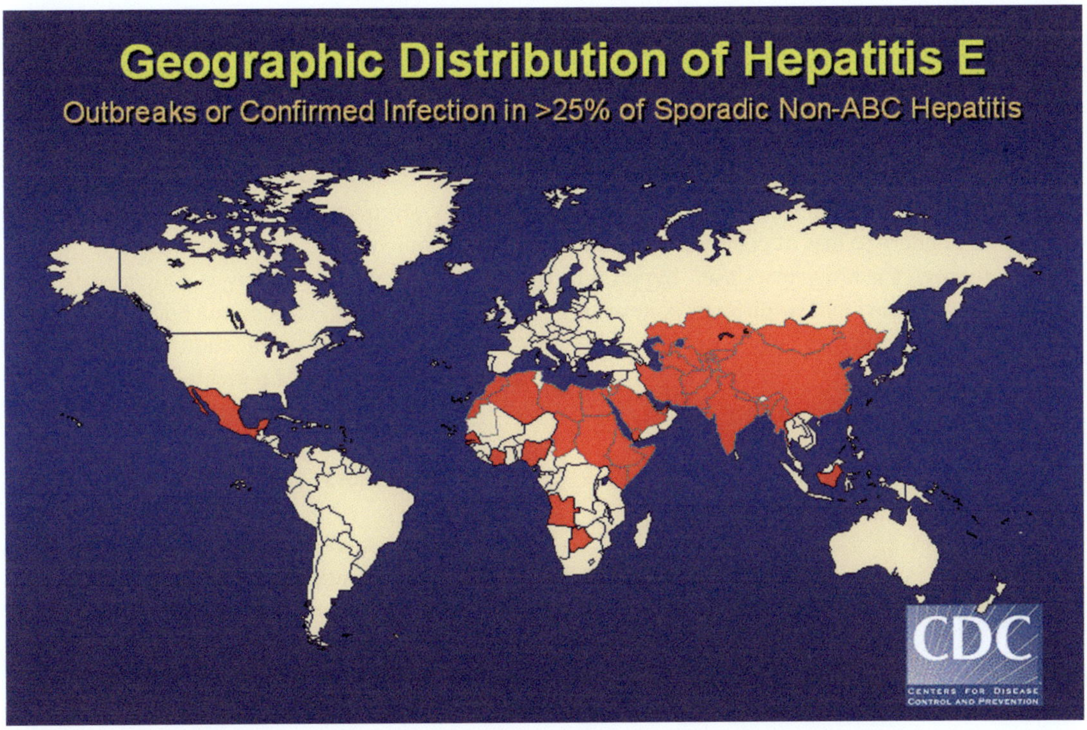

## Pathology

### Encephalopathy

Hepatic encephalopathy is a reversible neuropsychiatric dysfunction associated with acute or chronic liver failure preceded by agitation, hyperkinesis, and delusions with rapid progression to coma.

| Grade I | Grade II - | Grade III - | Grade IV - |
|---|---|---|---|
| Diagnosis in retrospect, mild personality changes, fine tremor | Mild obtundation, drowsiness, lethargy, tremor ++, asterixis | Stupor, somnolence, arousal to voice, tremor if cooperative, hyperreflexia | Coma, response to pain (A) or no response (B), posturing |

Grades of encephalopathy

*Precipitating factors include* gastrointestinal bleeding, SBP, sepsis, drugs, dietary protein load, alkalosis, diuretics, dehydration, constipation, and azotemia.

### Cerebral Edema

Cerebral edema is detected in 75 % of grade IV encephalopathy and is the leading cause of death. It occurs secondary to loss of cell membranes and BBB integrity. Cushing response, hypertonia, posturing, and brain stem respiratory patterns are late signs.

### Coagulopathy

- Decreased II, V, VII, IX, and X
- Decreased PLT
- FFP are of no value in absence of bleeding

### Renal and CV

- Distributive hemodynamic
- Hypotension, decreased SVR
- Hepatorenal syndrome

### Oxygen Transport and Delivery

- Severe peripheral shunting may result from peripheral PLT plugs, interstitial edema, and abnormal vasomotor tone – diminished $O_2$ extraction.

### Metabolic Changes

- Hypoglycemia is common (defective gluconeogenesis, decreased glycogen stores); dextrose 10 % may be required.
- Hypokalemia.
- Hyponatremia.
- Hypophosphatemia.

### Infections

Risks – decreased level of consciousness, immunocompromise (diminished opsonic activity, PMN function, phagocytosis, impaired CMI, humoral immunity). Portosystemic collaterals allow bacteria to bypass the hepatic reticuloendothelial system. Bacteremia and fungemia are common. Patients with GPC (*S. aureus* and epidermidis, strep) and GNR infection do not benefit from prophylactic ATB but empiric broad-spectrum antibiotic therapy is indicated if there are signs of sepsis. Pneumonia and UTI were the most common signs of infection; bacteremia was documented in 26 % of patients.

### Pathologenesis

The mechanism of severe liver injury in pregnant women with hepatitis E is not known.

### Immunological Factors

The immunological changes during pregnancy are of such nature that they help the rejection of the fetal allograft by suppressing T-cell-mediated immunity. The cellular immunity clearly alters the ratio of Th1/Th2 cell with definite increase in Th1 than Th2 which is the reverse occurring in normal pregnancy. This increase in Th2 is required for the survival of the fetus and thus explains the higher fetal morbidity observed in fulminant hepatitis. When HEV infection occurs, a cytotoxic immune response (Th1) is likely to be elicited in the Th2-biased pregnant women. Fulminant hepatic failure is always associated with high HEV load. For that a strong Th1 response is required. If this elevated Th1 immune response remains insufficient to fight with such a high HEV load, there is a possibility that Th1 response goes on increasing, but in the due process, the cytotoxic immune response may result in reduced fetal protection and eventually fetal demise. Opinions differ over the maternal and fetal outcome of pregnancies associated with viral hepatitis. Poor prenatal care and maternal nutrition appear to have contributed significantly to the increased severity of infection.

**Hormonal Factors** Viral replication is promoted in pregnancy due to the high levels of steroid hormones. The direct inhibition on hepatic cells predispose to hepatic dysfunction/failure when exposed to infectious pathogens [27]. Steroid hormones are immunosuppressive [28] Figs. 8.1, 8.2 and 8.3.

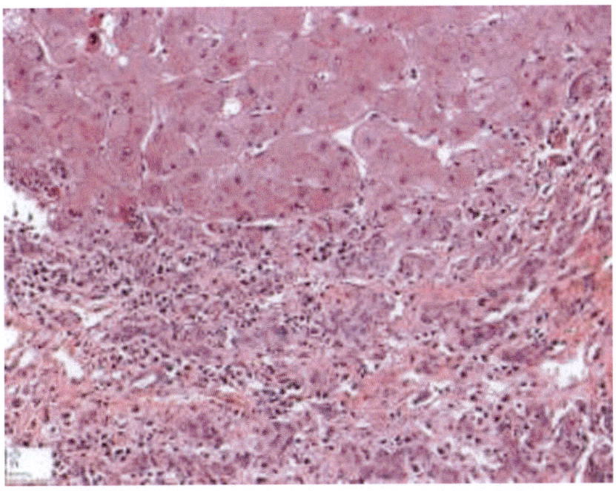

**Fig. 8.1** FHF

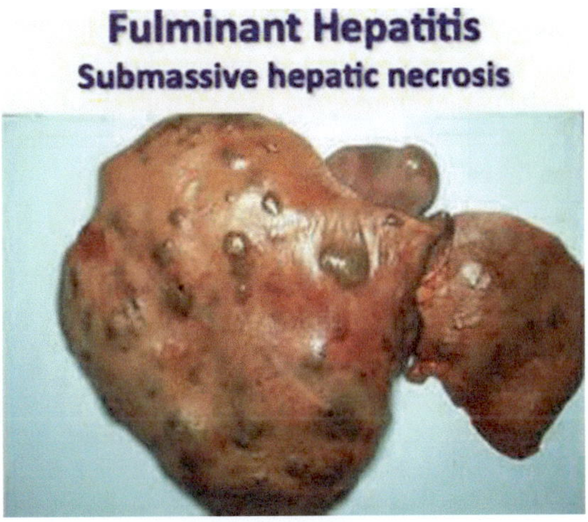


**Fig. 8.2** Submassive hepatic necrosis,3 FHF

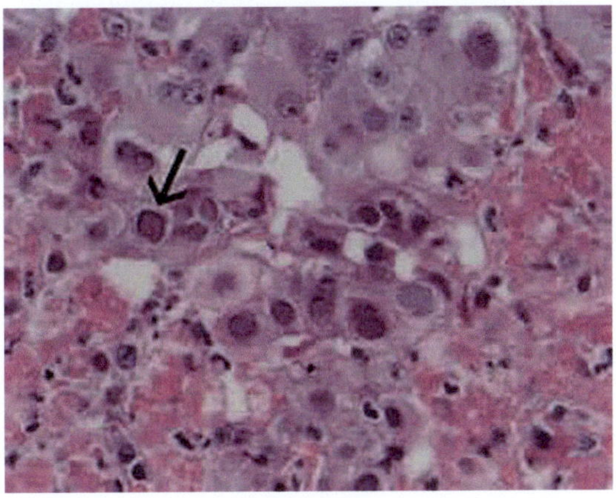

**Fig. 8.3** Pathogenesis of severe hepatic injury in hepatitis E

#### Management of Fulminant Hepatitis

The management of fulminant hepatic failure demands the availability of a critical care setup and the involvement of critical care specialists. In normal pregnancy the liver is difficult to palpate due to the enlarged uterine size and also the signs of liver pathology like telangiectasia and palmar erythema may be observed in 60 % of normal pregnancies, the hormone estrogen being the cause for the same.

The fulminant hepatic failure needs to be differentiated from acute fatty liver of pregnancy associated with preeclampsia-HELLP syndrome, hepatic hemorrhage, rupture, and hepatic infarction, infections – herpes simplex virus and hepatitis. The mortality rate for pregnant women with hepatitis E is 20 %. Serology helps to identify these viral infections as cause of hepatic decompensation.

## A Critically Ill Obstetric Patient: Management in Indian Scenario

It is now realized that maternal critical care is the least discussed area of obstetrics. Auditing data on maternal mortality has shown the cause in many cases to be suboptimal care. The concept of high dependency unit and intensive care unit is to be differentiated from the critical care [6].

This term was first defined in Comprehensive Critical Care and subsequently updated in 2009 [6].

The levels of support:

| | |
|---|---|
| Level 0 | Patients whose needs can be met through normal ward care<br>Low-risk patient |
| Level 1 | Patients at risk of their condition deteriorating and needing a higher level of observation or those recently relocated from higher levels of care (oxytocin infusion, mild preeclampsia on antihypertensive) |
| Level 2 | Patients requiring invasive monitoring/ intervention that includes support for a single failing organ system (excluding advanced respiratory support)<br>*Neurological support*<br>Magnesium infusion to control seizures (not prophylaxis)<br>Intracranial pressure monitoring<br>Hepatic support<br>Management of acute fulminant hepatic failure, e.g., from HELLP syndrome or acute fatty liver, such that transplantation is being considered<br>Patient requiring basic respiratory support and basic and advance cardiac support |
| Level 3 | Patients requiring advanced respiratory support (mechanical ventilation) alone or basic respiratory support along with support of at least one additional organ into the single entity of "critical care." Maternal critical care, high dependency care, and high-risk maternity care are not interchangeable, the term critical care having a more precise definition<br>Advanced respiratory support, two or more organs requiring support |

The levels of support

This approach has proven useful as it has facilitated some aspects of critical illness management especially some aspects of level 2 care.

Maternal critical care has to be distinguished from "high-risk" obstetrics because fetal issues are excluded and maternal risk factors or obstetric complications that require closer observations or intervention, but not support of an organ system, are also outside the term [6].

We should identify physicians, anesthetists, midwife, and establishments in different zones which deal with critically ill obstetric patients. The availability of a standard intensive care unit managed by a qualified intensivist is essential. The management of critically ill obstetric patients should be done aggressively as there are two lives involved. Practitioners should be encouraged to acquire experience in the subject of maternal-fetal medicine as in some western countries. Pregnant women should be motivated to report for regular antenatal care and educate them to report early in times of illness.

Defining the level of critical care required by the mother will be dependent on the number of organs requiring support and the type of support required as determined by the Intensive Care Society's "Level of Care" document [6]. This term was first defined in Comprehensive Critical Care and subsequently updated in 2009.

## Prevention and Control of HEV Infection

The primary route of transmission for HEV is by fecal-oral route through contamination of drinking water supplies and possibly food. The virus is shed in the feces of infected individuals during the late incubation period (beginning a few days before the onset of illness). In the phase of clinical illness it reaches the various surface water sources, such as rivers, ponds, superficial wells, canals, etc., leading to disease outbreaks. Such contamination is particularly common during periods of heavy rains and flooding. Also, reduction of water flow during summer may increase the concentration of fecal contaminants in rivulets and streams, increasing the risk of epidemics. In urban areas, contamination of piped water supply systems with intermittent supply has been reported to occur where the pipes pass through soil contaminated with human feces or sewage. This occurs due to the sewage getting sucked into the pipes during the periods of low water pressure in pipes.

Prevention of HEV infection depends primarily on improving overall hygiene and sanitation, including proper sewage disposal, and ensuring safe drinking water supplies. Boiling and chlorination of water appear to inactivate the HEV and may be used during outbreaks of hepatitis E, if safety of water used for drinking purposes is uncertain or cannot be ensured. It may be useful to target the preventive measures at persons who have a particularly high risk of developing severe disease such as pregnant women or persons with preexisting chronic liver disease. Two recombinant subunit vaccines been developed and have shown promising results in clinical trials, in terms of good immunogenicity and short-term protective efficacy. However, no data are yet available on long-term protection or efficacy when the vaccine is administered after exposure, as is the case in outbreak settings. One of these vaccines has not been commercially developed. The other vaccine is approved for use in China, but not in any other country. The exact public health role of this vaccine remains unclear at this time, and further data are needed to determine the population groups and settings, in which it may be useful [12].

## Management of Complications

**Hepatic Encephalopathy** The treatment of infections and other precipitant factors should be instituted. The use of lactulose in fulminant hepatic failure should be with caution because of the risk of hypernatremia and functional ileus. Assessment of mental state although very important for assessing prognosis, sedation, and intubation may be required in advanced stages of encephalopathy.

### Cerebral Edema

Cerebral edema and intracranial hypertension may develop rapidly in patients with deep encephalopathy. An arterial ammonia level higher than 200 g/dL in stage III and IV encephalopathy is a strong predictor of brain herniation [29]. Intracranial pressure should be maintained below 15 mmHg and cerebral perfusion pressure over 50 mmHg. Monitoring of jugular bulb oxygen saturation with a reversed jugular venous catheter can also guide interventions to avoid intracranial hypertension. Decreased saturations (<55 %) indicate cerebral ischemia, and high saturations (<85 %) indicate either decreased metabolic demands of the brain or cerebral hyperemia, more commonly the latter. It is recommended to maintain the patient's head at a 20° angle to improve jugular venous outflow. In episodes of intracranial hypertension, a bolus of 0.5–1 g/kg of mannitol can be administered intravenously and repeated until plasma osmolarity reaches 310 mOsm/L. Patients with oliguria and renal failure may require hemodialysis to avoid hyperosmolarity. Hyperventilation produces cerebral vasoconstriction and reduces cerebral blood flow, but the effect is usually transient. New therapies like mild hypothermia reduced intracranial pressure and cerebral blood flow and improved cerebral perfusion pressure both in patients with FHF [30]. Indomethacin also reduced cerebral blood flow and prevented brain edema in experimental models, and it has been used in isolated cases in humans, with encouraging results [31]. In a recent controlled clinical trial, a prophylactic infusion of phenytoin decreased the incidence of subclinical seizure activity and appeared to prevent brain edema [32].

## Management of Liver Failure

### Liver Transplantation

Liver transplantation is the only measure that can radically influence the course of fulminant hepatic failure. However, the cost factor limits its utility as a management option in the Indian scenario. Also it is a high-risk procedure with considerable morbidity and represents a commitment to indefinite immunosuppression.

Moreover, patients transplanted for fulminant hepatic failure have a worse outcome than those transplanted for other causes in most series, in part because of their poor clinical condition at the time of the procedure.

Early identification of which patients would die if orthotopic liver transplant were not performed is thus a very important objective.

Liver transplantation is the definitive treatment in liver failure. In selected patients for whom no allograft is immediately available, consider support with a bioartificial liver, till a suitable donor liver is found. However, no controlled study has shown long-term benefit.

Bioartificial liver-assist device, hepatocyte transplantation, and auxiliary liver transplantation are other therapeutic options to mention. This is a short-term measure that only leads to survival if the liver spontaneously recovers or is replaced.

Nonbiologic extracorporeal liver support systems, such as hemodialysis, hemofiltration, charcoal hemoperfusion, plasmapheresis, and exchange transfusions, permit temporary liver support until a suitable donor liver is found. However, no controlled study has shown long-term benefit.

## Conclusion

Fulminant hepatic failure in pregnancy is caused by HEV. This infection in pregnancy leads to poor maternal and fetal outcome. Affected patients show Th1 bias in terms of higher IL-12/IL-10 ratio. Thus, this shift of Th2 increase, which is a characteristic of normal pregnancy, in the HEV-infected pregnant women is suggestive of the role of immunological shift during hepatitis E-related fulminant hepatic failure in pregnancy. This immune alteration in turn leads to reduced fetal protection which is probably due to higher activity of NK cells, leading to fetal death. Viral load is comparatively higher in fulminant hepatic failure as compared to acute viral hepatitis and also higher in patients with fetal mortality in both these conditions, suggesting its role with the disease severity.

Rapid urbanization, overpopulated cities, and lack of access to clean water and sanitation, inadequate financial and manpower resource allocation, and public spending on programs for surveillance are some of the hindrances to the prevention and control of hepatitis E which is the major cause of FHF in the pregnant population [12].

Good intensive care is critical for patient survival. Orthotopic liver transplantation (OLT) remains a definitive therapeutic option. Involvement of critical care physician and shifting the patient to critical care unit is the central plan of management of fulminant hepatic failure. In the Indian scenario, the rural as well as urban population should be encouraged to seek for antenatal care and early identification of viral hepatitis E so that subsequent maternal morbidity and mortality can be attenuated.

## References

1. Trey C, Davidson CS. The management of fulminant hepatic failure. Prog Liver Dis. 1970;3:282–98; Trey C, Davidson LS. The management of FHF. In: Popper H, Schafnner F, editors. Progress in liver disease. New York: Grune & Stration; 1970. p. 282–98.
2. Bhatia V, Singhal A, Panda SK, Acharya SK. A 20-year single-centre experience with acute liver failure during pregnancy: is the prognosis really worse? Hepatology. 2008;48:1577–85. PubMed PMID: 18925633.
3. Kamat SK. Prognosis of infective hepatitis in pregnant women. In: Vakil BJ, Shah SG, editors. Hepatitis. Bombay: Adoni Printers & Publishers; 1975. p. 50–3.
4. Borhanmanesh F, Haghighi P, Hekmat K, Rezaizadeh K, Ghavani AG. Viral hepatitis during pregnancy: severity and effect on gestation. Gastroentrology. 1973;64:304–12.
5. Aggarwal R, Krawczynski K, Hepatitis E. An overview and recent advances in clinical and laboratory research. J Gastroenterol Hepatol. 2000;15(1):9–20.
6. Levels of critical care for adult patients. Standards and guidelines. ICS: London. 2009. www.ics.ac.uk/intensive_care_professional/standards_and_guidelines/levels_of_critical_care_for_adult_patients.
7. McCashland TM, Shaw BW, Tape E. The American experience with transplantation for acute liver failure. Semin Liver Dis. 1996;16:427–33.
8. Khuroo MS, Teli MR, Skidmore S, Sofi MA, Khuroo MI. Incidence and severity of viral hepatitis in pregnancy. Am J Med. 1981;70:252–5.
9. Nayak NC, Panda SK, Datta R, Zuckerman AJ, Guha DK, Madanagopalan N, et al. Aetiology and outcome of acute viral hepatitis in pregnancy. J Gastroenterol Hepatol. 1989;4:345–52.

10. O'Grady JG, Schalm SW, Williams R. Acute liver failure: redefining the syndromes. Lancet. 1993; 342:273–5.
11. Tandon BN, Bernauau J, O'Grady J, et al. Recommendations of the International Association for the Study of the Liver Subcommittee non nomenclature of acute and subacute liver failure. J Gastroenterol Hepatol. 1999;14:403–4. 2000;15:9–20.
12. Regional strategy for prevention and control of viral hepatitis. WHO Regional office for South East Asia.
13. Bernuau J, Rueff B, Benhamou JP. Fulminant and subfulminant liver failure: definitions and causes. Semin Liver Dis. 1986;6:97–106.
14. Acharya SK, Dasarathy S, Kumer TL, et al. Fulminant hepatitis in a tropical population: clinical course, cause, and early predictors of outcome. Hepatology. 1996;23:1448–55.
15. Hoofnagle JH, Carithers RL, Shapiro C, Ascher N. Fulminant hepatic failure: summary of a workshop. Hepatology. 1995;21:240–52.
16. Lu L, Li C, Hagedorn CH. Phylogenetic analysis of global hepatitis E virus sequences: genetic diversity, subtypes and zoonosis. Rev Med Virol. 2006; 16:5–36.
17. Huang CC, Nguyen D, Fernandez J, et al. Molecular cloning and sequencing of the Mexico isolate of hepatitis E virus (HEV). Virology. 1992;191:550–8.
18. Van Cuyck-Gandre H, Zhang HY, Tsarev SA, et al. Characterization of hepatitis E virus (HEV) from Algeria and Chad by partial genome sequence. J Med Virol. 1997;53:340–7.
19. Pal R, Aggarwal R, Naik SR, Das V, Das S, Naik S. Immunological alterations in pregnant women with acute hepatitis E. J Gastroenterol Hepatol. 2005;20:1094–101.
20. Navaneethan U, Al Mohajer M, Shata MT. Hepatitis E and pregnancy: understanding the pathogenesis. Liver Int. 2008;28:1190–9.
21. Kar P, Jilani N, Husain SA, et al. Does hepatitis E viral load and genotypes influence the final. Outcome of acute liver failure during pregnancy? Am J Gastroenterology. 2008;103:495–501.
22. Mamun-Al-Mahtab, Rahman S, Khan M, Karim F. HEV infection as an aetiologic factor for acute hepatitis: experience from a tertiary hospital in Bangladesh. J Health Popul Nutr. 2009;27(1):14–19.
23. Ippagunta SK, Naik S, Sharma B, Aggarwal R. Presence of hepatitis E virus in sewage in Northern India: frequency and seasonal pattern. J Med Virol. 2007;79:1827–31.
24. Husain MM, Srivastava R, Akondy R, Aggarwal R, Jameel S, Naik S. Evidence of hepatitis E virus exposure among seronegative healthy residents of an endemic Area. Intervirology. 2011;54(3):139–43.
25. Shrestha MP, Scott RM, Joshi DM, et al. Safety and efficacy of a recombinant hepatitis E vaccine. N Engl J Med. 2007;356:895–903.
26. Zhang J, Liu CB, Li RC, et al. Randomized-controlled phase II clinical trial of a bacterially expressed recombinant hepatitis E vaccine. Vaccine. 2009;27: 1869–74.
27. McGovern BH, Ditelberg JS, Jeremy S, et al. Hepatic Steatosis is associated with fibrosis, nucleoside analogue use, and hepatitis C virus genotype 3 infection in HIV-seropositive patients. Clin Infect Dis. 2006;43:365–72.
28. Mellor AM, Munn DH. Tryptophan catabolism and T-cell tolerance: immunosuppression by starvation? Immunol Today. 1999;20:469–73.
29. Clemmesen JO, Larsen FS, Kondrup J, et al. Cerebral herniation in patients with acute liver failure is correlated with arterial ammonia concentration. Hepatology. 1999;29:648–53.
30. Jalan R, Damink SW, Deutz NE, et al. Moderate hypothermia for uncontrolled intracranial hypertension in acute liver failure. Lancet. 1999;354:1164–8. This study shows the efficacy of hypothermia to reduce cerebral blood flow, restore cerebral blood flow autoregulation, and control intracranial hypertension in the clinical setting. It also confirms previous.
31. Clemmesen JO, Hansen BA, Larsen FS. Indomethacin normalizes intracranial pressure in acute liver failure: a twenty three-year-old woman treated with indomethacin. Hepatology. 1997;26:1423–5.
32. Ellis AJ, Wendon JA, Williams R. Subclinical seizure activity and prophylactic phenytoin infusion in acute liver failure: a controlled clinical trial. Hepatology. 2000;32:536–41.

# Acute Pancreatitis in Pregnancy

# 9

Sunita Ghike and Madhuri Gawande

## Introduction

Acute pancreatitis is defined as inflammation of pancreas involving peripancreatic tissue. AP (acute pancreatitis) during pregnancy is rare but a serious condition when associated with pregnancy. The incidence varies between 1 in 1000 and 1 in 12,000 pregnancies. Acute pancreatitis is usually prevalent in advanced gestational age occurring more commonly in the second and third trimester or in early postpartum period [1–3]. Although rare, AP can occur in the first trimester and always be distinguished with hyperemesis gravidarum [4]. The spectrum of AP in pregnancy ranges from mild to severe pancreatitis. The severe pancreatitis can be associated with necrosis, abscess, pseudocyst, and multiple organ failure [5]. Older review of AP in pregnancy reported high maternal and fetal mortality in preendoscopic era. It was always associated with greater concerns as it deals with two lives. Diagnostic studies such as endoscopic ultrasound, magnetic resonance cholangiopancreatography and endoscopic retrograde cholangiopancreatography, and therapeutic modalities that include endoscopic sphincterotomy, biliary stenting, common bile duct (CBD) stone extraction, and laparoscopic cholecystectomy are major milestones in gastroenterology. When properly managed, AP in pregnancy does not carry poor prognosis as in the past [4].

## Pathophysiology

The most common causes of AP in pregnancy are gallstones (65–100 %), alcohol abuse, and hypertriglyceridemia [6]. Above all the commonest cause is biliary which is caused by gallstones or sludge. The incidence by gallstones varies with ethnicity. It is lesser in Asians and Africans than in Native Americans. The rare causes are hyperparathyroidism, connective tissue diseases, abdominal injuries, and iatrogenesis caused by medications (diuretics, antihypertensives) [3, 4]. Pregnancy does not primarily predispose the pregnant woman to pancreatitis, but it does increase the risk of cholelithiasis and biliary sludge [3, 5].

S. Ghike (✉) • M. Gawande
Department of OBGY, NKP Salve Institute of Medical Sciences and Lata Mangeshkar Hospital, Nagpur, Maharashtra, India
e-mail: sunita_dr@yahoo.co.in; madhuri.vaidya@rediffmail.com


A. Gandhi et al. (eds.), *Principles of Critical Care in Obstetrics: Volume II*,
DOI 10.1007/978-81-322-2686-4_9

## Why in Pregnancy There Is Increased Risk of Cholelithiasis or Biliary Sludge?

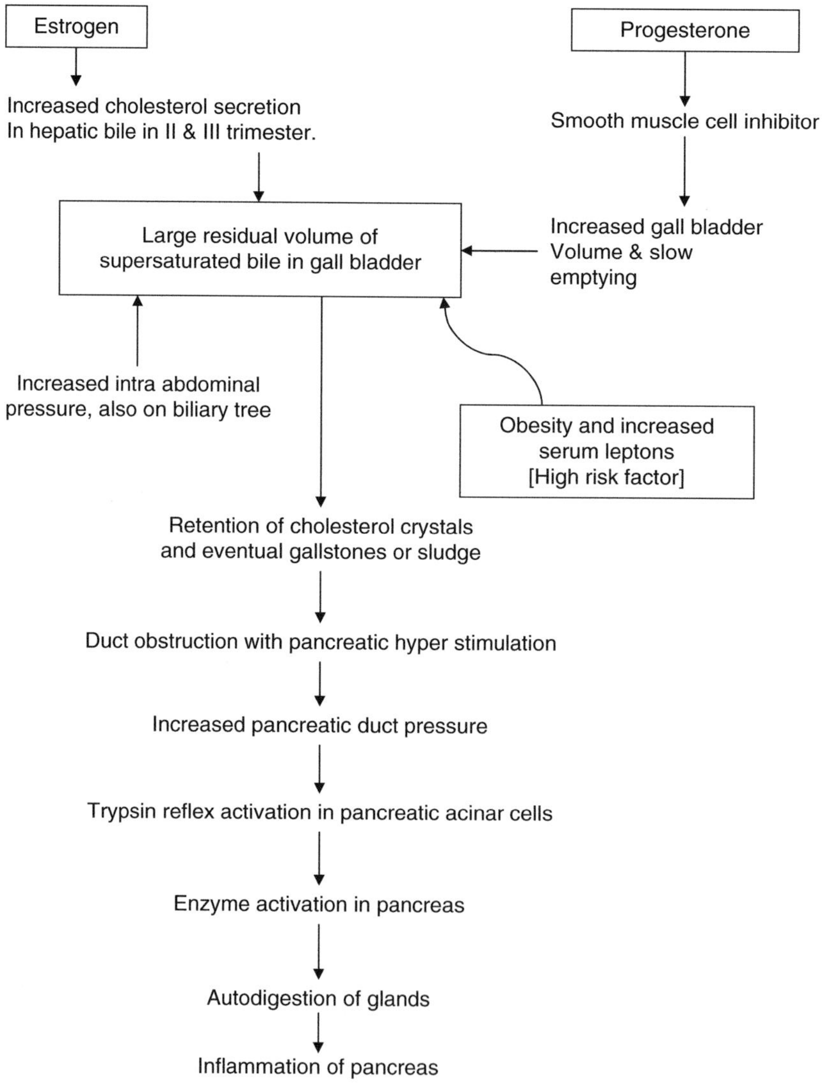


## Symptomatology

Acute pancreatitis in pregnancy presents in a similar way as during nonpregnant status. However, it is difficult to diagnose in pregnancy due to similarity to many acute abdominal illnesses. The signs and symptoms of gallbladder disease usually precede pancreatitis such as colicky abdominal pain radiating to right flank, scapula, and shoulder. It is rapid in onset with maximum intensity in 10–20 min. These are typical symptoms of gallbladder disease. Also, there can be anorexia, nausea, vomiting, dyspepsia, low-grade fever, and fatty food intolerance [1, 3].

## Physical Examination

In moderate to severe disease, patient appears acutely ill lying with limbs flexed (fetal position). There might be fever, tachycardia, dyspnea, and low blood pressure due to loss of fluid in the third space. On abdominal examination, there might be tenderness guarding and rigidity and sluggish or absent bowel sounds. The altered acid-base balance can lead to fetal hypoxia. Severe and sustained hypoxemia can lead to fetal demise [3, 4].

## Diagnosis of Acute Pancreatitis

AP is usually diagnosed by symptomatology, laboratory investigations, and imaging.

1. *Laboratory diagnosis*:
   (i) Serum amylase and lipase (increased by threefold).
   Amylase starts rising within 6–12 h of onset of disease and remains elevated for 3–5 days. But it is nonspecific. Serum lipase starts rising within an hour and remains high for a longer time than amylase. Lipase is more specific to amylase [5, 7].
   (ii) S. amylase to s. creatinine clearance ratio may be helpful in pregnancy (ratio >5 % suggests acute pancreatitis) [7].
   (iii) Increase in serum aminotransferase levels (more than threefold rise) is a very suggestive biochemical marker of biliary pancreatitis [4, 5].
   (iv) Any changes in liver enzymes and bilirubin should suggest biliary etiology [5].
2 *Imaging techniques*:
   (i) Abdominal ultrasound: It is safe in pregnancy and detects dilated pancreatic duct, pseudocysts, and focal accumulation more than 2–3 cm. It can also detect gallbladder stones, but insensitive for detection of stone or sludge in CBD.
   (ii) EUS (endoscopic ultrasound): It can detect stones in CBD even <2 mm or sludge. It has high positive predictive value. It can be done under mild sedation and is safe in pregnancy. EUS is appropriate prior to therapeutic ERCP.
   (iii) MRCP (magnetic resonance cholangiopancreatography): It can be used if USG is inconclusive. There is paucity of data regarding safety of MRCP in the first trimester.
   (iv) RCP (endoscopic retrograde cholangiopancreatography): It has lost its value because of risk of radiation. ERCP should only be used in selected cases of CBD stones or sludge. In cases of severe acute biliary pancreatitis, ERCP within 24 h is recommended to decompress CBD, removal of gallstones, and subsequent papillotomy. ERCP should be done by experienced endoscopist and radiologist with confirmed diagnosis. The fetus should be shielded all the time during procedure to minimize exposure [5].

## Management

Management of AP depends on four questions:

(i) Does the patient have AP (diagnosis)?
(ii) If having AP, what is predicted severity?
(iii) Is there biliary etiology?
(iv) What is the trimester of pregnancy?

**Conventional Treatment** Mainly, it includes fluid restoration, analgesics, antiemetics, monitoring of vital signs, and estimation of fetal heart rate. Oxygen is given whenever it is required.

**Nutrition** Enteral nutrition by nasojejunal feeding is better than TPN (total parenteral nutrition) in patients with severe AP. Keeping patient nil by mouth might increase the risk of infection. Enteral nutrition is physiological, helps the gut flora maintain the gut mucosal immunity, and reduces translocation of bacteria, while simultaneously avoiding all the risks of TPN [5].

**Antibiotics** There is a lot of controversy regarding the use of antibiotics in AP. It might be protective against non-pancreatic infections. Antibiotics which are safe in pregnancy can be administered. The therapy should be modified to reflect the organisms recovered in blood cultures and the clinical status of the patient [5].

Mild pancreatitis usually resolves in 7 days. Among all, 10 % of patients have severe course, and they are best managed in the intensive care unit. In severe pancreatitis, hypovolemia is common due to loss of fluid in the third space. It can lead to organ hypoperfusion to the tissue resulting in multiple organ failure [8]. Hence, patients of severe AP are to be managed in the intensive care unit with meticulous hydration therapy.

## Management of Underlying Cause

### Management of Gallstones

Surgical management is best for patients who failed to respond to conservative management. For surgical management, major decision is for:

(a) Choice of procedure
(b) Timing and approach of cholecystectomy

The factors which influence surgical decision are trimester of pregnancy, presence or absence of CBD dilatation, cholangitis, and severity of AP. Cholecystectomy can be performed in all trimesters but preferably in the second trimester. Studies show that both laparotomy and laparoscopy have similar results. But morbidity is less with laparoscopic cholecystectomy [3, 5]. Guidelines by the Society of American Gastrointestinal and Endoscopic Surgeons for laparoscopy in pregnancy (2011) are:

(i) Open technique for insertion of trochar
(ii) Avoidance of high intraperitoneal pressure
(iii) Left lateral position of patient to prevent aortocaval compression
(iv) Use of electrocautery cautiously and away from uterus

Early cholecystectomy needs to be performed in mild acute biliary pancreatitis. In severe acute biliary pancreatitis and in cholangitis, this procedure should be done within 4–6 weeks. Meanwhile, ERCP with sphincterotomy with fetal shielding and clearance of CBD stones is indicated [5, 9]. Some advocate biliary stent placement rather than performing sphincterotomy and stone extraction and therefore eliminating complications that accompany sphincterotomy. However, stenting carries risks of stent occlusion and cholangitis and the need for a second procedure. The sterile necrosis of pancreas is treated with antibiotics and necrosectomy [5].

**Hyperlipidemic Pancreatitis** Hypertriglycerid emia is the second most common cause of AP, when the serum triglyceride is >1000 mg/dL. In the third trimester of pregnancy, there is a threefold rise in serum triglyceride levels. This is thought to be due to estrogen-induced increases in triglyceride synthesis and very low-density lipoprotein secretion. Hypertriglyceridemia may be more severe in persons with familial hyperlipidemia, predisposing them to develop pancreatitis. Treatment of hyperlipidemic AP is mostly supportive [5].

## Algorithm: Diagnosis and Management of Acute Pancreatitis in Pregnancy

*Clinical features*: acute pain in abdomen, nausea, dyspepsia, fever, dyspnea

*Laboratory investigations*: threefold increase in lipase and amylase

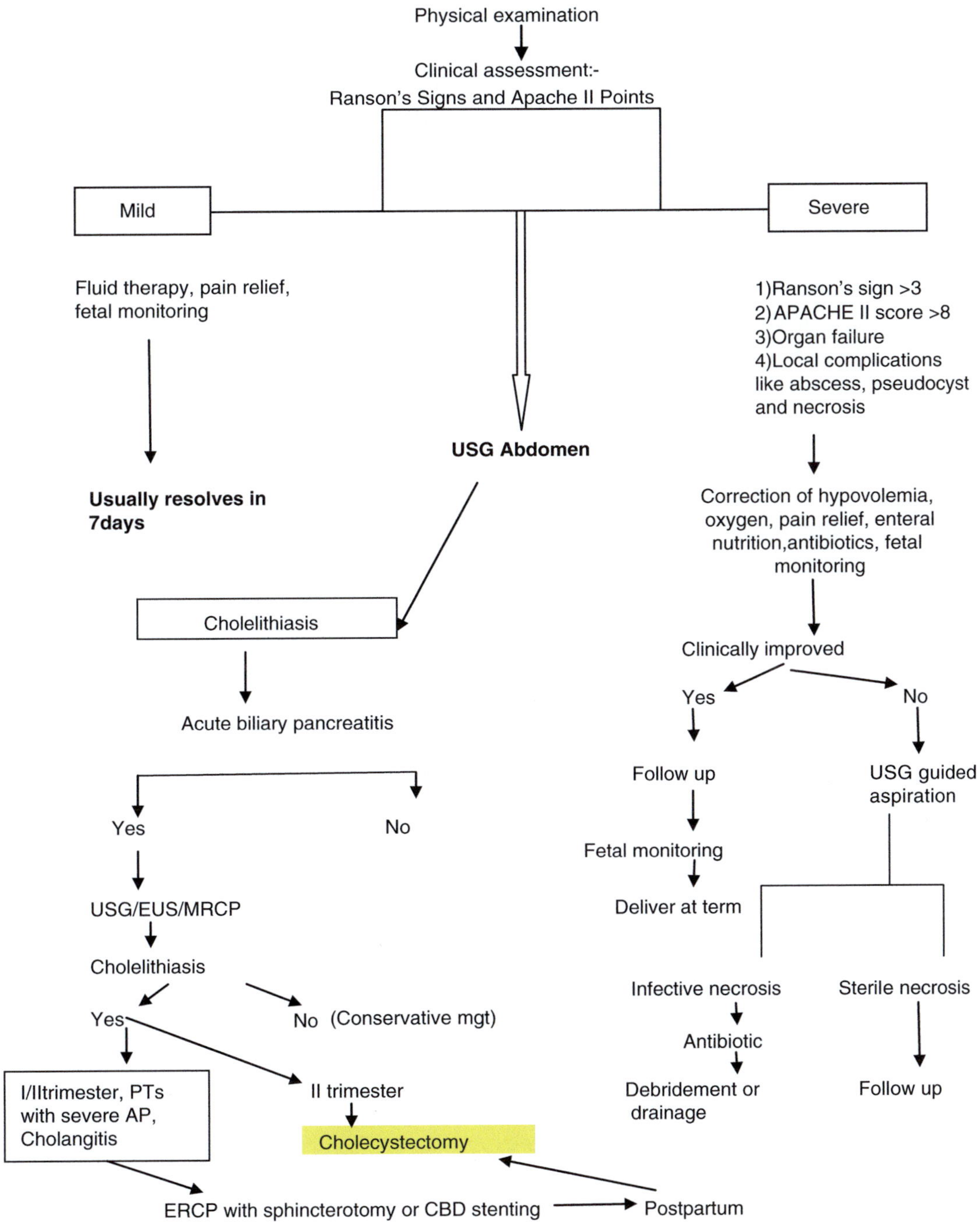
Physical examination
Clinical assessment:-
Ranson's Signs and Apache II Points
Mild
Severe
Fluid therapy, pain relief, fetal monitoring
Usually resolves in 7days
USG Abdomen
1)Ranson's sign >3
2)APACHE II score >8
3)Organ failure
4)Local complications like abscess, pseudocyst and necrosis
Correction of hypovolemia, oxygen, pain relief, enteral nutrition,antibiotics, fetal monitoring
Clinically improved
Yes
No
Follow up
Fetal monitoring
Deliver at term
USG guided aspiration
Infective necrosis
Antibiotic
Debridement or drainage
Sterile necrosis
Follow up
Cholelithiasis
Acute biliary pancreatitis
Yes
No
USG/EUS/MRCP
Cholelithiasis
Yes
No (Conservative mgt)
I/IItrimester, PTs with severe AP, Cholangitis
II trimester
Cholecystectomy
ERCP with sphincterotomy or CBD stenting
Postpartum

## Prognosis

Mild acute pancreatitis when managed conservatively has excellent prognosis. In olden days, severe cases of acute pancreatitis were associated with high maternal and perinatal mortality. In 1973, Wilkinson et al. noted 30 % maternal and 60 % fetal mortality in cases of severe AP [10]. The mechanism of fetal demise includes placental abruption and profound metabolite disturbance leading to acidemia. But over the decades, perinatal morbidity and mortality have reduced due to improvement in neonatal intensive and supportive care. In 2005, Sunil Kumar et al. reported eight patients of acute pancreatitis in pregnancy over the span of 2 years. Out of 83 who underwent laparoscopic cholecystectomy, five were treated conservatively. All patients recovered well and delivered at term with good neonatal outcome [4].

In other study by Talukdar and Vege (2009), the perinatal death rate was <17 % and was similar for maternal mortality in India [11]. The outcome of pregnant patients with AP has substantially improved with technical advances in imaging and therapeutic endoscopy.

**Conclusion**

Acute pancreatitis in pregnancy is a rare but severe disease. AP usually occurs during the third trimester or early postpartum period. The most common cause for AP is gallstones (65–100 %). The diagnosis of AP in pregnancy is not specific. The signs and symptoms of acute biliary pancreatitis like colicky abdominal pain, nausea, vomiting, and dyspepsia precede the disease. Diagnosis is usually based on the clinical presentation, laboratory investigations, and imaging methods performed cautiously. In mild AP, treatment is conservative and it usually resolves in 7 days. Ten percent of patients have severe pancreatitis. Severe pancreatitis is to be managed in the intensive care unit and with endoscopic and surgical intervention. Endoscopic sphincterotomy, biliary stenting, CBD stone extraction, and laparoscopic cholecystectomy are the major milestones in the management of severe acute pancreatitis in pregnancy. When properly managed, acute pancreatitis does not have bad prognosis as in the past.

## References

1. Ducarne G, Maire F, Chatel P, Luton D, Hammel P. Acute pancreatitis in pregnancy a review. J Perinatol. 2014;34:87–94.
2. Hernandez A, Petrov MS, Brooks DC, Banks P, Ashley SW, Tarakkolizaden A. Acute pancreatitis in pregnancy: a 10 yr single centre experience. J Gastrointest Surg. 2007;11(12):1623–7.
3. Ramin KD, Ramin SM, Richey SD, Cunnigham FG. Acute pancreatitis in pregnancy. Am J Obstet Gynecol. 1995;173(1):187–91.
4. Juneja S, Gupta S, Virk Singh S, Tandon P, Bindal V. Acute pancreatitis in pregnancy: a treatment paradigm based on our hospital experience. Int J Appl Basic Med Res. 2013;3(2):122–5.
5. Pitchumoni C, Yegneswaran B. Acute pancreatitis in pregnancy. World J Gastroenterol. 2009;15(45):5641–6.
6. Wang GJ, Gao CF, Wei D, Wang C, Ding SQ. Acute pancreatitis: etiology and common pathogenesis. World J Gastroenterol. 2009;15(12):1427–30.
7. Augustin G, Majerovic M. Non obstetrical acute abdomen during pregnancy. Eur J Obstet Gynecol Reprod Biol. 2007;131:4–12.
8. Gardner TB, Vege SS, Pearson RK, Chari ST. Fluid resuscitation in acute pancreatitis. Clin Gastroenterol Hepatol. 2008;6(10):1070–6.
9. Sahu S, Raghuvanshi S, Bahl D, Sachan P. Acute pancreatitis in pregnancy. Inter J Surg. 2006;11(2). Cited on 22/11/2015/ispub.com/IJS/11/2/8706.
10. Wilkinson EJ. Acute pancreatitis in pregnancy a series of 98 cases and a report of 8 new cases. Obstet Gynecol Surv. 1973;28:281–303.
11. Talukdar R, Vege SS. Recent development in acute pancreatitis. Clin Gastroenterol Hepatol. 2009;7(11):53–9.

# 10 Complicated Malaria and Dengue During Pregnancy

Haresh U. Doshi

## Complicated Malaria

Malaria continues to be a major global health problem with over 40 % of the world population at risk for malaria. As reported by the National Vector Borne Disease Control Programme (NVBDCP) director in 2013, around 1.5 million laboratory-confirmed cases are annually reported in India. Complicated malaria also known as *severe malaria* is defined by clinical or laboratory evidence of vital organ dysfunction.

Malaria is caused by a malarial parasite, a protozoal parasite of genus *Plasmodium*. Five species can infect human beings. Severe malaria is most commonly caused by infection with *Plasmodium falciparum* although *P. vivax* and *P. knowlesi* [1] can also cause severe disease. Malaria is transmitted by bite of infected female *Anopheles* mosquito which is a definite host for the parasite while a human being is an intermediate host.

Malaria produces hemolytic anemia by (1) rupture of infected RBCs, (2) increased removal of parasitized cells by the spleen, and (3) infected RBCs that become antigenic and produce autoantibodies which can cause hemolysis. Parasite degrades intracellular proteins especially hemoglobin and also alters the permeability of red cell membrane.

H.U. Doshi, MD, PhD
Department of ObGyn, GCS Medical College, Hospital and Research centre, Ahmedabad, India
e-mail: doshiharesh@hotmail.com

**Table 10.1** Chemotherapy of severe and complicated malaria

| **Initial parenteral treatment** for at least 48 h: choose one of following four options | **Follow-up treatment**, when patient can take oral medication following parenteral treatment |
|---|---|
| **Quinine**: 20 mg quinine salt/kg body weight on admission (IV infusion or divided IM injection) followed by maintenance dose of 10 mg/kg 8 hourly; infusion rate should not exceed 5 mg/kg per h. Loading dose of 20 mg/kg should not be given, if the patient has already received quinine | **Quinine** 10 mg/kg three times a day with: **clindamycin** 10 mg/kg 12 hourly to complete 7 days of treatment |
| **Artesunate**: 2.4 mg/kg IV or IM given on admission (time = 0), then at 12 h and 24 h, and then once a day *or* **Artemether**: 3.2 mg/kg bw IM given on admission and then 1.6 mg/kg per day *or* **Arteether**: 150 mg daily IM for 3 days | Full oral course of area-specific ACT: In northeastern states: age-specific ACTAL for 3 days In other states: treat with ACT-SP for 3 days |

*ACTAL* artemisinin-based combination therapy (artemether + lumefantrine), *ACT-SP* artemisinin-based combination therapy (artesunate + sulfadoxine + pyrimethamine)




A. Gandhi et al. (eds.), *Principles of Critical Care in Obstetrics: Volume II*,
DOI 10.1007/978-81-322-2686-4_10

## Clinical Features

Malaria and pregnancy are mutually aggravating conditions. The physiological changes of pregnancy and the pathological changes due to malaria have a synergistic effect on the course of each other. Malaria is more common in pregnancy as compared to the general population. Immunosuppression and loss of acquired immunity could be the causes [2]. A case of uncomplicated malaria usually presents with fever, rigors, headache, body ache, fatigue, anorexia, and nausea. In pregnancy, malaria tends to be more atypical in presentation. This could be due to the hormonal, immunological, and hematological changes of pregnancy. Pregnant mothers are three times more likely to develop severe disease than nonpregnant women acquiring infection from the same area. Primigravida and nonimmune pregnant women are at increased risk for severe falciparum malaria [3]. The parasitemia tends to be ten times higher, and as a result, all the complications of falciparum malaria are more common in pregnancy compared to the nonpregnant population. Apart from severe anemia and severe recurrent hypoglycemia, other clinical features of severe malaria are impaired consciousness, prostration, convulsions, deep breathing and respiratory distress, acute pulmonary edema, circulatory collapse, acute kidney injury, clinical jaundice, and abnormal bleeding.

Severe malaria increases the maternal and perinatal morbidity as well as mortality. Severe falciparum malaria is associated with substantially high mortality in pregnancy (50 %) than in nonpregnant women (15–20 %) [4]. Perinatal complications of malaria include abortion, preterm labor, IUGR, fetal distress and IUFD, and congenital malaria [5]. The newborn with congenital malaria may not present with typical symptoms of malaria such as fever but have other clinical manifestations like jaundice and hemolytic anemia [6].

## Diagnosis

Microscopic examination of the peripheral blood smears is the gold standard for diagnosis. Thick smears are more sensitive than thin smears for diagnosis which is particularly important in low-density malarial parasitemia of *P. falciparum*. Thin smear is important for knowing the species and degree of parasitemia.

Rapid diagnostic tests (RDTs) provide diagnosis of malaria where reliable microscopy is not reliable or practical. RDTs detect antigen produced by malarial parasite. The most widely used RDTs for detecting *P. falciparum* target the HRP2 antigen. RDTs are less sensitive than blood films [7] and cannot diagnose the species or quantify the number of RBCs infected.

PCR: Parasite nucleic acid detection by PCR is more sensitive and specific than microscopy but available in sophisticated laboratories only. PCR is a very useful tool for confirmation of species and detecting of drug resistance mutations.

Laboratory diagnosis of complicated malaria is as follows:

Hypoglycemia (<40 mg/dl)
Metabolic acidosis (plasma bicarbonate <15 mmol/l)
Severe normocytic anemia (Hb <5 g/dl, PCV <20 %)
Hemoglobinuria
Hyperlactatemia (lactate >5 mmol/l)
Hyperparasitemia (>2 % parasitized red blood cells)
Renal impairment
Pulmonary edema confirmed radiologically

## Management

Severe malaria is a medical emergency and treatment should be given as per severity and associated complications which can be best decided by a treating physician. Patients of severe malaria should be admitted in the ICU. Prompt diagnosis and aggressive antimalarial treatment are crucial to prevent mortality in case of severe malaria. Parenteral artemisinin derivatives or quinine should be used irrespective of chloroquine resistance status of the area and irrespective of the species of malaria seen on the blood smear. Oral antimalarial drugs are not recommended for the initial treatment of severe malaria. Treatment advised by the directorate of

National Vector Borne Disease Control Programme in India recently is as follows (Table 10.1):

WHO recommends that IV artesunate is the preferred first-line drug for all severe malaria cases in adults including pregnant women [8]. As compared to quinine, artesunate is associated with 35 % reduction in mortality [9]. Although there is insufficient evidence to support the use of artemisinin in the first trimester, the drug should not be withheld if the life of the woman is endangered [10]. One of the reasons of high mortality in the past was the delay in institution of proper antimalarial drugs [11]. Artesunate is well tolerated with no attributable local or systemic adverse effects. As quinine stimulates insulin secretion, treatment with quinine in pregnancy is associated with severe and recurrent hypoglycemia [12]. Quinine does not induce abortion or labor. Mild side effects known as cinchonism are common with quinine including tinnitus, hearing loss, dizziness, nausea, uneasiness, restlessness, and blurring of vision.

Supportive care in severe malaria [8]

| Manifestation or complication | Management |
|---|---|
| Coma (cerebral malaria) | Monitor using Glasgow Coma Scale. Maintain airway, place patient on her side, and exclude treatable causes of coma (e.g., hypoglycemia, meningitis) |
| Hyperpyrexia | Administer tepid sponging, fanning, and antipyretic drugs |
| Convulsions | Maintain airway, treat promptly with intravenous diazepam |
| Hypoglycemia | Check blood glucose regularly, correct hypoglycemia, and maintain with (blood glucose <40 mg/dl) glucose-containing infusion |
| Severe anemia | Transfuse with packed red cells |
| Acute pulmonary edema | Treat by propping patient up at an angle of 45°, give oxygen, give a diuretic, stop IV fluids, intubate, and add PEEP/CPAP if required |
| Renal failure | Exclude prerenal causes; check fluid balance and urinary sodium; if in established renal failure, add hemofiltration or hemodialysis |
| Spontaneous bleeding and coagulopathy | Transfuse fresh whole blood and blood products; give vitamin K injection |
| Metabolic acidosis | Prevent by careful fluid balance; exclude or treat hypoglycemia, hypovolemia, and septicemia; if severe add hemofiltration or hemodialysis |
| Shock | Suspect septicemia, take blood culture, give broad-spectrum antibiotics, correct hemodynamic disturbances |

Provide good nursing care. This is vital especially if the patient is unconscious. Avoid NSAIDs which increase the risk of gastrointestinal bleeding. For fluid balance urine output should be aimed at >1 ml/kg/h. Give packed cell volume (PCV) transfusion if there is severe anemia. Exchange transfusion to treat severe parasitemia is not proved by evidence.

Role of early cesarean section in severe malaria is unproven. For patients in labor, second stage should be shortened by instrumental delivery.

For prevention of malaria, personal protective measures like long protective clothing, mosquito coils and body repellants (sprays and lotion), and wire screening on windows should be practiced. Treated bed nets (ITN)/long-lasting insecticidal nets (LLIN) should be encouraged for pregnant women. Meta-analysis of intervention trials suggests that successful prevention of these infections reduces the risk of severe maternal anemia by 38 %, low birth weight by 43 %, and perinatal mortality by 27 % among primigravidae [13].

RTS,S is the most recently developed recombinant vaccine for malaria. Phase III clinical trials have shown modest protection against malaria. It might be available for clinical use soon.

## Dengue

Dengue infection is a mosquito-borne viral infection causing a flu-like febrile illness and sometimes causing a potentially lethal complication called severe dengue. Dengue infection is endemic in tropical and subtropical countries including India. The incidence of dengue has increased 30-fold over the past 50 years. This increase is due to many factors like urbanization, population growth, increased international travel, and global warming. About half of the world's population is now at risk [14]. India's National Vector Borne Disease Control Programme reported in 2013 that the country had experienced an annual average of 20,474 dengue cases and 132 dengue-related deaths since 2007 [15]. As dengue is more common in children and young adults, pregnant patients are at increased risk. Also the infection in pregnant mothers is reported to be more severe as compared to nonpregnant females and with higher mortality rates [16].

Dengue virus is an RNA virus of the family Flaviviridae, genus *Flavivirus*. Originally there were four strains of the virus called serotypes DENV-1, DENV-2, DENV-3, and DENV-4. Recently, the fifth type is discovered in 2013. The *Aedes aegypti* mosquito is the primary vector of dengue. The virus is transmitted to humans through the bites of infected female mosquitoes. *Aedes aegypti* is a daytime feeder biting mainly early in the morning and in the evening before dusk. Infected humans are the main carriers and multipliers of virus serving as a source for uninfected mosquitoes.

Recovery from infection by one serotype provides lifelong immunity against that particular serotype but only partial and temporary immunity to the other serotypes. Subsequent infections by other serotypes increase the risk of developing severe dengue.

Dengue can also be transmitted via infected blood products and through organ donation. Vertical transmission during pregnancy is also reported [17]. Otherwise infection does not occur directly from human to human.

Original WHO classification (1997), still in use, divides dengue into undifferentiated fever, dengue fever, and dengue hemorrhagic fever (DHF). Dengue hemorrhagic fever was subdivided into grades I–IV. Grade I is the presence only of easy bruising or a positive tourniquet test in someone with fever, grade II is the presence of spontaneous bleeding into the skin and elsewhere, grade III is the clinical evidence of shock, and grade IV is shock so severe that BP and pulse cannot be recorded. Grades III and IV are referred to as "dengue shock syndrome" (DSS).

The latest WHO 2009 classification [14] divides dengue fever into two groups: uncomplicated and severe. Severe dengue is defined as that associated with severe bleeding, severe organ dysfunction, or severe plasma leakage, while all other cases are classified as uncomplicated.

## Clinical Features

Symptoms usually begin 4–6 days after infection and last for up to 10 days. Symptoms include sudden, high fever, severe headaches, retro-orbital pain, arthralgia, and myalgia. Nausea and vomiting may also occur. Skin rash appears initially as flushed skin and after 3–4 days as measles like rash. Mild bleeding from mucous membranes of the mouth or nose may occur. In some people the disease proceeds to a critical phase as fever resolves. There is leakage of plasma from the blood vessels which typically last 1–2 days. This may result in fluid accumulation in the chest, i.e., pleural effusion, and in the abdominal cavity, i.e., ascites. Depletion of platelets leads to severe bleeding typically from gastrointestinal tract. This is called dengue hemorrhagic fever (DHF).

Depletion of fluid from circulation and hemorrhage leads to profound hypotension and shock. This is called dengue shock syndrome (DSS) which can cause mortality. Patients with weakened immune system as well as those with a second or subsequent dengue infection are at greater risk for developing dengue hemorrhagic fever. With improved diagnosis and treatment, the proportion of DHF cases in dengue fever is decreasing from 20 to <10 % in the last 5 years.

Apart from preterm labor, if pregnant woman delivers at the height of viremia, there is a risk of severe postpartum hemorrhage [18]. Carles et al. reported significant increase in prematurity and fetal death in dengue fever during pregnancy [19]. This may be related to hyperpyrexia. Vertical transmission of 10.5 % was reported in their study. Vertical transmission rate might be dependent on the severity of maternal dengue. Severe dengue affects the newborn only when dengue develops close to term or delivery time, and the mother has no time to produce protective antibodies. Most neonates develop fever within 4–5 days of life and consequently develop thrombocytopenia requiring platelet transfusions [20]. In a study by Fernandes et al., 5-year follow-up of newborns after vertical dengue infection showed no long-term sequelae [21].

Dengue hemorrhagic fever may be confused with HELLP syndrome in a case of preeclampsia in pregnancy, but in HELLP constitutional symptoms are absent and serological tests are negative [22].

## Diagnosis

High index of suspicion is the key for diagnosis when the pregnant patient with fever is from an endemic area or when there are epidemics. A definite diagnosis of dengue can be done by serological tests. IgM capture ELISA is a rapid, simple, and most widely used method. Both IgM and IgG positive suggest secondary infection. Serum sample should be taken 5–10 days after the onset of the disease. Virus isolation in cell cultures and nucleic acid detection by PCR although more accurate are not widely available due to high cost. Viral antigen detection (NS1) is 90 % sensitive in primary infection but less in subsequent infection.

## Treatment

Dengue fever is usually self-limited. There is no specific antiviral treatment available for dengue fever. Most cases only require conservative treatment [23]. Supportive care with antipyretics, bed rest, adequate fluid replacement, and maintenance of electrolyte balance forms are the mainstay of treatment. Paracetamol is preferred. NSAIDs are avoided due to risk of bleeding. Normal saline is preferred to Ringer's lactate for intravenous hydration.

Patients with dengue hemorrhagic fever and dengue shock syndrome are kept in the ICU with monitoring of hematological status and serum albumin levels at timely intervals. The physiological hemodilution of normal pregnancy can mask the criteria of hemoconcentration in DHF. Prophylactic transfusion of platelets or FFP is not recommended. Platelets are given in patients with severe thrombocytopenia who went in labor or who require surgery [24]. PCV and FFPs are required in a dengue patient who has active bleeding. Therapeutic benefit of gamma globulin is reported in nonpregnant patient of DHF, but it is not evaluated in pregnant women [25]. Corticosteroids have no role in treatment.

In the absence of associated fetomaternal complications, infection by itself does not appear to be an indication for obstetric interference.

Prevention: Prevention of dengue fever is by controlling the vector mosquito and avoiding mosquito bites. Controlling the vector can be done by environmental modification. Using of personal household protection measures mentioned under malaria is recommended.

Research: Currently research is under way for (1) development of vaccine against dengue, (2) for antiviral drugs against dengue virus, and (3) finding new methods of vector control.

**Key Points**

1. High index of suspicion in endemic areas and during epidemics helps in the early diagnosis of both malaria and dengue fever.
2. Severe malaria and severe dengue are medical emergencies and patients should be treated in the ICU.
3. For severe malaria parenteral artemisinin derivatives or quinine should be used without delay.
4. There is no specific antiviral treatment for dengue. Supportive therapy with an aim to maintain normothermia and fluid and electrolyte imbalance is the cornerstone of therapy.
5. Pregnant women should be counseled about preventive strategies to avoid mosquito bites.

## References


1. Kantele A, Jokiranta S. Review of cases with the emerging fifth human malaria parasite, Plasmodium knowlesi. Clin Infect Dis. 2011;52:1356–62.
2. www.malariasite.com/pregnancy. Kakkillaya, BS. Updated 11 Mar 2015.
3. Singh N, Shukla MM, Sharma VP. Epidemiology of malaria in pregnancy in central India. Bull World Health Organ. 1999;77(7):567–72.
4. Royal College of Obstetricians & Gynecologists. The diagnosis and treatment of malaria in pregnancy. Green-top Guideline No.54b. 2010. p. 7
5. Poespoprodjo JR, Fobia W, Kenangalem E, Lampah DA, Warikar N, Seal A, et al. Adverse pregnancy outcomes in an area where multidrug-resistant plasmodium vivax and plasmodium falciparum infections are endemic. Clin Infect Dis. 2008;46:1374.
6. Valecha N, Bhatia S, Mehta S, Biswas S, Dash AP. Congenital malaria with atypical presentation: a case report from low transmission area in India. Malar J. 2007;6:43.
7. Chilton D, Malik AN, Armstrong M, et al. Use of rapid diagnostic tests for the diagnosis of malaria in UK. J Clin Pathol. 2006;59:862–6.
8. World Health Organization. Guidelines for the treatment of Malaria. 2nd ed. Geneva: WHO; 2010.
9. Jones KL, Donegan S, Lalloo DG. Artesunate versus quinine for treating severe malaria. Cochrane Database Syst Rev. 2007;(4):CD005967.
10. Dondrop A, Nosten F, Stepneiwska K, Day N, White N. Artesunate versus quinine for treatment of severe falciparum malaria: a randomized trial. Lancet. 2005;366:717–25.
11. Shukla MM, Singh N, Singh MP, et al. Cerebral malaria in Jabalpur. Indian J Malariol. 1995;32:70–5.
12. LooareesuwanS PRE, White NJ, Kietinun S, Karbwang J, Rackow C, et al. Quinine and severe falciparum malaria in late pregnancy. Lancet. 1985;2:4–8.
13. Desai M, ter Kuile FO, Nosten F, McGready R, Asamoa K, Brabin B, Newman RD. Epidemiology and burden of malaria in pregnancy. Lancet Infect Dis. 2007;7:93–104.
14. World Health Organization. Dengue and severe Dengue. Fact sheet No. 17. Geneva: WHO; 2014.
15. National Vector Borne Disease Control Programme. Dengue/dengue hemorrhagic fever. 2013. http://www.nhp.gov.in/nvdcp.
16. Machado CR, Machado CS, Rohloff RD, et al. Is pregnancy associated with severe dengue? a review of data from the Rio de Janeiro surveillance information system. PLoS Negl Trop Dis. 2013;7(5):e2217.
17. Pouliot SH, Xiong X, Harville E, et al. Maternal dengue and pregnancy outcomes: a systematic review. Obstet Gynecol Surv. 2010;65:107–18.
18. Mitra N, Kannan N, Kavita G, Senthil V. Neonatal dengue. Pediatric oncall. [serial online] 2012 [cited 2012 July 1];9. Art #44. Available From: http://www.pediatriconcall.com/Journal/Article/FullText.aspx?artid=494&type=J&tid=&imgid=&reportid=40&tbltype=.
19. Carles G, Talarmin A, Peneau C, et al. Dengue fever and pregnancy. A study of 38 cases in French Guiana. J Gynecol Obstet Biol Reprod. 2000;29:758–62.
20. Fernandez R, Rodriguez T, Borbonet F, et al. Study of the relationship dengue-pregnancy in a group of Cuban mothers. Rev Cubana Med Trop. 1994; 46:76–8.
21. Singh N, Sharma KA, Dadhwal V, Mittal S, Selvi AS. A successful management of dengue fever in pregnancy. Indian J Med Microbiol. 2008;26(4): 377–80.
22. Malhotra N, Chanana C, Kumar S. Dengue infection in pregnancy. Int J Gynaecol Obstet. 2006; 94(2):131–2.
23. Chitra TV, Panicker S. Maternal and fetal outcome of dengue fever in pregnancy. J Vector Borne Dis. 2011;48(4):210–3.
24. Agrawal P, Garg R, Srivastava S, Verma U, Rani R. Pregnancy outcome in women with Dengue infection in Northern India. Ind J Clin Pract. 2014; 24(11):1053–6.
25. Ostronoff M, Ostronoff F, Florencio R, et al. Serious thrombocytopenia due to dengue hemorrhagic fever treated with high dosages of immunoglobulin. Clin Infect Dis. 2003;36:1623–4.

# 11 Neurological Emergencies During Pregnancy

Anuradha Ridhorkar

## Introduction

Acute neurological symptoms in pregnancy could be:

1. Exacerbation of a pre-existing condition, e.g. epilepsy or multiple sclerosis
2. New-onset disease not related to pregnancy, e.g. brain neoplasm
3. New acute-onset condition unique to pregnancy

If the neurological emergencies are not detected and treated promptly, they may result in high morbidity and mortality.

Pregnancy is itself associated with certain pathophysiological changes that may contribute to neurological problems. The physiological changes, which may affect the neurological status, are as follows:

1. Increased levels of oestrogen, which stimulates the production of clotting factors. This in turn increases the risk of thromboembolism.
2. Increased plasma and total blood volume. This increases the risk of hypertension.
3. Increased progesterone in the third trimester enhances venous distensibility and leakage from the small blood vessels.

A. Ridhorkar, MD, DGO. FICMCH
Consultant Obstetrician and Gynecologist,
Nagpur, Maharashtra, India
e-mail: anu.ridhorkar@gmail.com

## Neurological Imaging [1]

CT and MRI have opened new vistas for diagnosis and treatment of neurological emergencies. To get the maximum information from the investigation, there should be a proper discussion between the clinician and the radiologist.

CT scanning of head: Non-contrast CT gives minimum foetal radiation. It is excellent for diagnosing recent haemorrhages.

MRI: This is safe and useful in diagnosing demyelinating diseases, AV malformations and spinal cord lesions. Proper sequences and protocols should be discussed in advance.

IV contrast should be generally avoided in pregnancy. Iodinated contrasts used for CT are better than gadolinium used in MRI. Thyroid functions should be checked in babies exposed to the iodinated contrast agents during pregnancy.

## Conditions That Cause Acute Neurological Emergencies

1. Neurological complications of eclampsia.
2. Acute headache.
3. Seizures.
4. Reversible cerebral vasoconstrictive syndrome (RCVS).
5. Posterior reversible encephalopathy syndrome (PRES).


A. Gandhi et al. (eds.), *Principles of Critical Care in Obstetrics: Volume II*,
DOI 10.1007/978-81-322-2686-4_11

6. Intracerebral and subarachnoid haemorrhage (ICH and SAH).
7. Acute ischaemic stroke (AIS). This may be arterial thrombosis (embolism), cerebral venous sinus thrombosis (CVT) or pre-eclampsia.
8. Rare conditions: amniotic fluid embolism, air embolism and metastatic choriocarcinoma, Wernicke's encephalopathy, pituitary apoplexy and chorea gravidarum.

## Neurological Complications of Eclampsia

Tonic-clonic seizures are the hallmark. Symptoms that may precede seizures are headache, blurred vision, epigastric pain and altered mental status. Exact mechanism for the seizures is not known. The proposed mechanisms resulting in seizures are due to neuronal oedema caused by either of the two causes:

1. Cerebral arterial vasospasm and ischaemia leading to cytotoxic oedema
2. Endothelial dysfunction causing capillary leak and vasogenic oedema

This vasculopathy can also result in PRES, infarction and haemorrhage. Ninety per cent of cases of eclampsia present antepartum. Patients with postpartum eclampsia have high incidence of CVT, ICH and AIS than antepartum eclampsia. Postpartum eclampsia needs thorough diagnostic testing and MRI in the following situations:

1. Focal neurological deficit
2. Persistent visual disturbances
3. Symptoms refractory to magnesium and antihypertensive treatment

The management of these patients of eclampsia is according to the established principles:

1. Control of convulsions using magnesium sulphate
2. Control of hypertension
3. Limitation of IV fluids
4. Prompt delivery

## Acute Headache in Pregnancy [2]

Primary headaches are more common in pregnancy:

1. Tension headache is characterised by mild to moderate pain with muscle tightness. It is not associated with neurological symptoms or nausea. Treatment includes rest, massage, hot fomentation, anti-inflammatory drugs and mild tranquillisers.
2. Migraine usually improves during pregnancy and it returns postpartum. Headache is usually associated with autonomic nervous dysfunction. It is treated with NSAID, IV hydration, parenteral anti-emetics and triptans (serotonin 5-HT receptor agonist). Ergotamine derivatives are potent vasoconstrictors and therefore avoided in pregnancy.
3. Cluster headache is a unilateral, severe, lancinating pain radiating to face and orbit, agitation and associated with autonomic dysfunction. Treatment includes 100 % oxygen and sumatriptan 6 mg subcutaneously.
4. Postdural puncture headache is seen after spinal anaesthesia. It is because of decreased intracranial pressure due to CSF leak. It is occipital and nuchal in location. This headache resolves by lying flat rest, analgesics and hydration. In some refractory cases, blood patch is the treatment.
5. Thunderclap headache is an abrupt onset of a severe, unusual headache. It needs prompt and thorough evaluation to exclude SAH. Increased blood pressure during bearing down may cause aneurysmal SAH. CT and MRI sequences that include vascular studies and lumbar puncture are required for diagnosis.

## Seizures in Pregnancy

Seizures can be seen in one of the three settings:

1. Patients with known seizure disorder before pregnancy. Epilepsy is the most common disorder in this group. There is increased frequency and increased mortality in epileptic patients during pregnancy. Anticonvulsants

like pheneytoin, phenobarbital and valproate are known for teratogenicity. Prevention of seizures by pre-pregnancy folic acid supplementation, promptly treating nausea and vomiting and avoiding provoking stimuli, is of utmost importance. Mono-drug therapy in minimum doses is preferred to avoid congenital malformations. Newer drugs like lamotrigine and oxcarbazepine are more amenable for monitoring.
2. New non-pregnancy related seizure, e.g. hypoglycaemia and brain tumour.
3. Pregnancy-related eclampsia, ICH, CVT, RCVS, thrombotic thrombocytopenic purpura. In PRES, prodromal symptoms are usually absent while in CVT, seizures occur after headache. MRI sequences are required for correct diagnosis.

## Reversible Cerebral Vasoconstriction Syndrome (RCVS)

It is also called as postpartum angiopathy or Call-Fleming syndrome. It develops during puerperium in absence of hypertension. Clinical presentation is abrupt-onset thunderclap headaches and multifocal reversible cerebral vasoconstriction. It is often associated with vomiting, confusion and blurred vision. It leads to complications like brain haemorrhage, infarcts and non-aneurysmal SAH. In patients without infarction, it resolves over a time of 2–3 months. CT, MR angiography and transcranial Doppler are useful for the diagnosis.

## Posterior Reversible Encephalopathy Syndrome (PRES)

This is also known as reversible posterior leukoencephalopathy syndrome (RPLS). The two most common presentations in a pregnant lady are seizures and blindness. It is not a primary diagnosis, but a clinical and imaging syndrome caused by vascular abnormalities. It is seen in pre-eclampsia, acute hypertension, renal disease, sepsis and in patients on immunosuppressants. Patient presents with headache, seizures, encephalopathy and visual disturbances. Symptoms develop without prodrome and progress rapidly over 12–48 h. The cerebral autoregulation of blood pressure is overwhelmed due to a rapid rise in BP. Vasogenic oedema occurs in the posterior circulation since it has a relatively poor ability to autoregulate BP. CT shows vasogenic oedema. Visual symptoms often resolve completely. Control of blood pressure is the mainstay of treatment.

## Intracranial Haemorrhage (ICH) and Subarachnoid Haemorrhage (SAH)

It leads to hemorrhagic stroke and symptoms are similar to ischaemic stroke. ICH is seen in superimposed eclampsia due to rupture of small vessels damaged by chronic hypertension. It has high morbidity and mortality than SAH because of its location. SAH is due to underlying cerebrovascular malformations. In 80 % of cases, the cause is ruptured saccular or berry aneurysms. Other causes are ruptured AV malformations, coagulopathy, drug abuse, trauma and infection. This has got a mortality rate up to 35 %. Ruptured aneurysm causes sudden severe headache with visual changes, cranial nerve abnormalities and altered consciousness. Patients typically show signs of meningeal irritation, nausea, tachycardia and transient hypertension. Prompt diagnosis with CT and MRI is must. Treatment includes bed rest, analgesia, sedation and blood pressure control. Bearing down is not recommended. Repair of the aneurysm is done by surgical clipping or by endovascular coil.

## Acute Ischaemic Stroke (AIS)

Acute occlusion or embolisation of an intracranial vessel causes cerebral ischaemia. Disorders which lead to AIS are pre-eclampsia, arterial and venous thrombosis, antiphospholipid antibodies, sickle-cell disease and vasculitis. Patient presents with sudden-onset severe headache, hemiplegia or other neurological deficit. Evaluation includes echocardiography, CT and MRI. AIS in pre-eclampsia is associated with other signs of PIH. Cerebral embolism usually involves middle cerebral artery, and it is common in the latter half of pregnancy and puerperium. The diagnosis is more certain if an embolic source is identified. Management of embolic stroke consists of supportive measures and antiplatelet therapy. Cerebral artery thrombosis affects older individuals and is caused by atherosclerosis mainly of internal carotid artery. Thrombolytic therapy with recombinant tissue plasminogen activator should be given in first 3 h, after excluding haemorrhage.

## Cerebral Venous Thrombosis (CVT)

More common in late pregnancy and postpartum period. Lateral and superior sagittal sinus is involved in pre-eclampsia, sepsis or thrombophilia. Risk factors are LSCS, dehydration, anaemia, hyperhomocysteinaemia and dural puncture. It is more common in developing countries due to poor nutrition, infections and dehydration. Patient presents with severe, diffuse, thunderclap headache. Other findings are dizziness, nausea, convulsions and papilloedema. MRI venography is diagnostic. Management includes anticonvulsants for seizures and antimicrobials for sepsis. Efficacy of heparinisation is controversial. Prognosis is better in pregnancy than in non-pregnant patient (Table 11.1).

**Table 11.1** Clinical and imaging features of selected conditions

| | PRES | RCVS | CVT | Eclampsia |
|---|---|---|---|---|
| Mode of onset | Rapid, postpartum | Abrupt, postpartum | Third trimester or later, gradual | Antepartum, intrapartum or postpartum |
| Key findings | Seizures. May be accompanied by stupor, visual loss or hallucinations. Headache dull and throbbing | Thunderclap headache. Seizures are less common. Transient focal deficits | Headache is universal, progressive and diffuse. Seizures in 40 % | Seizures, frequent visual symptoms, abdominal pain, hyperreflexia, hypertension and proteinuria |
| Evolution over time | If BP is controlled, resolves within short period | Changes over time. ICH, second week; ischaemic complications, third week | Evolves over several days, non-arterial territorial infarcts and haemorrhages might develop | Can evolve (from pre-eclampsia) gradually or abruptly |
| CSF findings | Usually normal | Often normal. Fifty per cent of cases have pleocytosis and raised proteins | Pressure raised in 80 %; 30–50 % have raised proteins and cell counts | Usually normal unless complicated by haemorrhage |
| Imaging | CT positive in about 50 % of patients; MRI shows prominent T2-weighted and FLAIR abnormalities nearly always in parieto-occipital lobes, but can involve other brain regions; intracerebral haemorrhage in about 15 % of patients | CT usually normal (if no subarachnoid haemorrhage); 20 % show localised convexal subarachnoid haemorrhage on MRI; CT angiogram and magnetic resonance angiogram usually show typical string-of-beads constriction of cerebral arteries; digital subtraction angiogram is more sensitive; might have associated cervical arterial dissection; initial arteriogram might be negative | CT often negative; MRI might show non-arterial territorial infarcts; haemorrhage common; MRV shows intraluminal clot flow voids; although MRV is preferred, CT venogram is also sensitive | Same as for PRES, some patients have coincident acute ischaemic stroke or intracerebral haemorrhage |

Adapted from Edlow et al. [3]

## Rare Conditions

1. Amniotic fluid embolism – it causes agitation, confusion, seizures, encephalopathy and cardiovascular and respiratory collapse during or immediately after delivery.
2. Metastatic choriocarcinoma – tumour causes mass effect and bleeding and invades cerebral vessels. Its clinical presentation and imaging findings are variable.
3. Air embolism – during delivery, air enters venous circulation and right ventricle leading to decreased cardiac output, seizures and abnormal cognition. Presence of air in the retinal veins and mill wheel cardiac murmur suggest the diagnosis.
4. Wernicke's encephalopathy – seen in severe hyperemesis. Abnormal eye movements are always present. Response to IV thiamine confirms the diagnosis.
5. Thrombotic thrombocytopenic purpura (TTP) – commonly seen in late pregnancy. The classic pentad includes thrombocytopenia, microangiopathic haemolytic anaemia, fever and renal and neurological dysfunction. More than half of patients present with fluctuating headache, seizures and focal or generalised neurodeficit. Proper differentiation between TTP and HELLP is must for specific treatment. Haematological consultation is of great value.
6. Chorea gravidarum – characterised by irregular, brief, unpredictable, jerky movements of multiple body parts. This condition is usually associated with rheumatic fever, antiphospholipid syndrome, Wilson's disease and thyrotoxicosis. It typically begins after the first trimester. Symptoms resolve spontaneously over weeks to months.

**Conclusion**

Early diagnosis and specific treatment play a key role in preventing morbidity and mortality in neurological emergencies of pregnancy. Anticipation, prevention, multidisciplinary care and early referral to a higher centre are crucial.

## References

1. Cunningham F, Cunningham FG, et al. Williams obstetrics. 24th ed. New York: Mc Graw Hill; 2014. p. 1187–203.
2. Autumn K, Evans RW. Neurologic clinics, vol. 30. 3rd ed. New York: Elsevier; 2012.
3. Edlow JA et al. Diagnosis of acute neurological emergencies in pregnant and post-partum women. Lancet Neurol. 2013;12:175–85.

# Part III

# Endocrinal Crisis

# Diabetic Ketoacidosis in Pregnancy

12

Vinita Das

## Introduction

Diabetic ketoacidosis (DKA) is a medical emergency and must be treated appropriately and promptly. DKA remains a frequent and life-threatening complication of type I diabetes, and errors in its management are common and are associated with significant morbidity and mortality.

## Pathophysiology

DKA is a complex disordered metabolic state characterized by hyperglycemia, acidosis, and ketonemia. It usually occurs as a consequence of absolute or relative insulin deficiency accompanied by an increase in counter-regulatory hormones (glucagon, cortisol, growth hormone, epinephrine). This type of hormonal balance enhances hepatic gluconeogenesis and glycogenolysis resulting in severe hyperglycemia. Enhanced lipolysis increases serum free fatty acids that are then metabolized as an alternative energy sources in the process of ketogenesis. This results in accumulation of large quantities of ketone bodies and subsequent metabolic acidosis. Ketones include acetone, 3-beta-hydroxybutyrate (predominant ketone), and acetoacetate.

## Diabetic Ketoacidosis in Pregnancy

DKA is a life-threatening emergency observed in 5–10 % of all pregnancies complicated by pregestational diabetes mellitus. Since DKA is caused by an absolute or relative insulin deficiency, it is most commonly observed in women with type I pregestational diabetes mellitus. Enhanced insulin resistance is an important factor during pregnancy for higher incidence of DKA in pregnancy, as well as higher propensity to develop DKA more rapidly and at less severe levels of hyperglycemia and even with normal glucose levels.

Common risk factors for DKA in pregnancy are new-onset diabetes, infections like UTI, influenza, poor patient compliance, insulin pump failure, treatment with β-mimetic tocolytic medications, and antenatal corticosteroids for fetal lung maturity

## Clinical Presentation of DKA in Pregnancy

Abdominal pain, nausea, vomiting, and abnormal sensorium

Abnormal laboratory finding are:

V. Das
Department of Obstetrics and Gynaecology,
King George's Medical University, Lucknow, India
e-mail: das_lko@yahoo.com


A. Gandhi et al. (eds.), *Principles of Critical Care in Obstetrics: Volume II*,
DOI 10.1007/978-81-322-2686-4_12

Ketonemia 3 mmol/L and over or significant ketonuria (more than 2+ on standard urine sticks)
Blood glucose over 11 mmol/L or known diabetes mellitus
Bicarbonate (HCO3 −−) below 15 mmol/L and/or venous pH less than 7.3

Continuous fetal heart rate monitoring commonly demonstrates recurrent late decelerations. Delivery is rarely indicated as FHR pattern resolves as maternal condition improves.

## General Management

HDU/level 2 facility with trained nursing staff and/or insertion of central line is required during pregnancy for management of DKA. Involvement of Diabetes Specialist Team and bedside monitoring is very important in management of DKA. Until recently focus was on lowering the elevated blood glucose with fluids and insulin. Now with the advent of portable ketone meters, bedside measurement of blood ketones has tremendously improved the management. Access to blood gas and blood electrolyte measurement is now relatively easy and available. Therefore, glucose, ketones, and electrolytes including bicarbonate and venous pH should be assessed at bedside.

DKA therapy can lead to frequent complication of hypoglycemia and hypokalemia, so glucose and K concentration monitoring should be done judiciously. Maternal mortality is rare now with proper management, but fetal mortality is still quite high ranging from 10 to 35 %.

## Assessment of Severity

Presence of one or more of the following may indicate severe DKA, and HDU level 2 facilities are mandatory.

| *HDU/level 2 facility and/or insertion of central line may be required in the following circumstances (request urgent senior review in pregnant female)* | |
|---|---|
| Heart or kidney failure<br>Other serious comorbidities<br>Severe DKA by following criteria:<br>Blood ketones above 6 mmol/L<br>Venous bicarbonate below 5 mmol/L | Venous pH below 7.1<br>Hypokalemia on admission (below 3.5 mmol/L)<br>GCS < 12<br>Systolic BP below 90 mmHg<br>Pulse over 100 or below 60 bpm<br>Anion gap above 16 [anion gap = $(Na^+ + K^+) - (Cl^- + HCO3^-)$] |

## Immediate Management upon Diagnosis 0–60 min

### Aim

- Clinical and biochemical assessment of patient
- Expansion of intravascular volume by IV 0.9 % sodium chloride solution
- Correction of deficit in fluids, electrolytes, and acid base status
- Initiation of insulin therapy to correct hyperglycemia
- Monitoring of the patient – hourly blood glucose, hourly ketone measurement and two hourly potassium measurements, 4 hourly plasma electrolyte
- Diabetes specialist team to be involved at the earliest

### Action 1: Rapid Initial Assessment

ABC – respiratory rate, temperature, blood pressure, pulse, oxygen saturation – assessment is to be done as soon as patient arrives in DKA.

Full clinical examination – if patient is drowsy, put NG tube with airway protection to prevent aspiration. Large-bore IV cannula is introduced to start fluid replacement. If systolic BP is below 90 mmHg, 500–1000 ml of 0.9 % saline is infused rapidly over 15–20 min.

Oxygen is to be given to the patients with severe circulatory impairment or shock.

Antibiotics are to be given to febrile patients after obtaining appropriate cultures of body fluids.

Patient is catheterized if unconscious or unable to void on demand Simultaneously.

- Initial investigations to be sent include:
  - Blood ketones
  - Capillary blood glucose
  - Venous plasma glucose
  - Urea and electrolyte
  - Venous blood gases
  - Full blood count
  - Blood cultures
  - ECG
  - Chest radiograph
  - Urine analysis and culture
- Continue cardiac monitoring.
- Continue pulse oximetry.
- Establish usual medication for diabetes.

## Action 2: Fluid Administration

Most important initial step is appropriate fluid replacement and the main aims are:

- Restoration of circulatory volume
- Clearance of ketones
- Correction of electrolyte imbalance

It is recommended that crystalloid rather than colloid is used for fluid resuscitation. 0.9 % sodium chloride solution is the fluid of choice, and it should be cautiously administered as fluid replacement in pregnancy. In a woman of about 70 kg, there may be up to 7 l deficit of fluid. The aim of the first few liters of fluid is to correct any hypotension, replenish the intravascular deficit, and counteract the effects of the osmotic diuresis with correction of electrolyte disturbance. Below is a table outlining typical fluid replacement regimen:

| Fluid | Volume over time |
|---|---|
| .9 % sodium chloride 1 L with potassium chloride | 1000 ml over 1st h |
| .9 % sodium chloride 1 L with potassium chloride | 1000 ml over next 2 h |
| .9 % sodium chloride 1 L with potassium chloride | 1000 ml over next 2 h |
| .9 % sodium chloride 1 L with potassium chloride | 1000 ml over next 4 h |
| .9 % sodium chloride 1 L with potassium chloride | 1000 ml over next 4 h |
| .9 % sodium chloride 1 L with potassium chloride | 1000 ml over next 6 h |
| Reassessment of cardiovascular status at 12 h is mandatory | |

## Action 3: Potassium Replacement

Hypokalemia and hyperkalemia are life-threatening conditions and are common in DKA. Serum potassium is often high on admission (although total body potassium is low) but falls precipitously upon treatment with insulin. Regular monitoring is mandatory.

| Potassium level in first 24 h (mmol/L) | Potassium replacement in mmol/L of infusion solution |
|---|---|
| Over 5.5 | Nil |
| 3.5–5.5 | 40 |
| Below 3.5 | Additional potassium needs to be given as per expert advice |

## Action 4: Commence a Fixed Rate of Intravenous Insulin Infusion (IVII)

- Patient weight in Kg is to be noted (in pregnant state current weight is considered).
- Insulin infusion is to be started 1–2 h after starting fluid replacement therapy.
- 50 units of human soluble insulin (Actrapid Humulin S) made up to 50 ml with .9 % sodium chloride solution are infused at a fixed rate of .1 unit/kg/h (i.e., 7 ml/h if weight is 70 kg) by an infusion pump.
- In case of delay to set up infusion pump, a stat dose of intramuscular insulin (.1 unit/kg) is given.
- Patient's usual dose of insulin should be continued at usual time.

## Follow-Up and Monitoring 60 min to 6 h

### Aim

- Clear the blood of ketones and suppress ketogenesis by achieving a rate of fall of ketones of at least 0.5 mmol/L/h.
- Bicarbonate should rise by 3 mmol/L/h and blood glucose should fall by 3 mmol/L/h.
- Maintain serum potassium in normal range.
- Avoid hypoglycemia.

### Action 1: Reassess

- Monitor vital signs.
- If anuric or incontinent, catheterization is to be done.
- If vomiting is persisting, NG tube is to be put in.
- If oxygen saturation is falling, blood gas analysis is to be done.

### Action 2: Review Metabolic Parameters

- Measure blood ketones and capillary glucose hourly. If blood glucose is high, hourly venous blood is to be sent for measurement.
- Review patient's response by noting the fall of ketone levels, rise in bicarbonate levels, and fall in glucose level (rate of fall of ketones should be at least 0.5 mmol/L/h, rate of rise of bicarbonate by 3 mmol/L/h, and blood glucose fall by 3 mmol/L/h). If desired goal is not achieved, insulin infusion rate is to be increased by 1 unit/h.
- Continue fixed rate of IVII until ketones are less than 0.3 mmol/L, venous pH over 7.3, and/or venous bicarbonate over 18 mmol/L.
- Monitor and replace potassium as it may fall rapidly.
- If glucose falls below 14 mmol/L, 10 % glucose should be given at 125 ml/h along the side of the 0.9 % sodium chloride solution.
- Simultaneously precipitating factor should also be treated.

## Follow-Up and Monitoring 6–12 h

### Aim

- Continue IV fluid replacement.
- Continue insulin administration.
- Assess for complication of treatment, e.g., fluid overload and cerebral edema.
- Avoid hypoglycemia.
- Ensure that clinical and biochemical parameters are improving.

### Action

- Monitoring of vital signs is to be continued.
- At 6 h check for venous pH, bicarbonate, potassium, blood ketones, and glucose.
- Resolution is defined as ketones $<0.3$ mmol/L venous pH $>7.3$.
- Once patient is biochemically stable, oral feeding is allowed, and subcutaneous insulin regimen is restored in consultation with diabetic team.
- At the time of discharge, patient is counseled and reeducated to reduce the chance of recurrence and to facilitate follow-up.

## Follow-Up and Monitoring 12–24 h

### Aim

- Continue IV fluid if patient is not eating and drinking.
- Reassess for complication overload and cerebral edema.
- Subcutaneous insulin is started before IV insulin is discontinued.
- Ensure that clinical and biochemical parameters are normalized.

- At 12 h check for venous pH, bicarbonate, potassium, blood ketones, and glucose.
- By 24 h ketonemia and acidosis should resolve.

**Resolution of DKA**

*Expectation:* Patient should be eating, drinking, and back on normal insulin. If DKA is not resolved, identify and treat the reasons for failure to respond. This situation is unusual and requires senior and specialist inputs.

*Transfer to subcutaneous insulin.*

Convert to subcutaneous regimen when biochemically stable (capillary ketones < 0.3 mmol/L, pH over 7.3) and the patient is ready and able to eat. Do not discontinue insulin infusion until 30 min after subcutaneous short-acting insulin has been given.

Conversion to subcutaneous insulin should be managed by the Specialist Diabetes Team. If the team is not available, use local guidelines. If the patient is newly diagnosed, it is essential that they are seen by a member of the specialist team prior to discharge.

Arrange follow-up with specialist team.

## Serious Complications of DKA and Its Treatment

1. Hypokalemia and hyperkalemia
   - Hypokalemia and hyperkalemia are potentially life-threatening conditions during management of DKA.
   - Initially there is a risk of acute prerenal failure associated with severe dehydration. So if serum potassium remains above 5.5 mmol/L and initial fluid resuscitation is done, there is no need of potassium supplementation.
   - Potassium will always fall as DKA is treated with insulin, so it is recommended that 0.9 % sodium chloride solution with potassium 40 mmol/L (ready mixed) is given as long as potassium level is below 5.5 mmol/L and patient is passing urine.
   - If serum potassium falls below 3.5 mmol/L, more potassium is to be given.
   - If fluid balance does not permit, more concentrated potassium infusion is given.
2. Hypoglycemia
   - Blood glucose may fall very rapidly as ketoacidosis is corrected. It should not be allowed for the blood glucose to drop to hypoglycemic level.
   - Severe hypoglycemia is associated with cardiac arrhythmias, acute brain injury, and death.
   - Hypoglycemia also results in a rebound ketosis driven by counter-regulatory hormones.
   - Once the blood glucose falls to 14 mmol/L, intravenous glucose of 10 % should be commenced to prevent hypoglycemia.
3. Cerebral edema
   - Cerebral edema is more common in children than in adult.
   - Insulin administration in 1st hr and fluid administered over the first 4 h are associated with increased risk of cerebral edema.
   - Symptoms due to cerebral edema are relatively uncommon during DKA although asymptomatic cerebral edema may be a common feature.
   - It is disputed whether subclinical edema is a feature of DKA or is a result of treatment of DKA.
   - The exact cause of this phenomenon is unknown. Recent studies suggest that cerebral hypoperfusion with subsequent reperfusion may be the mechanism operating for development of cerebral edema.
   - Diagnostic criteria
     - Abnormal motor or verbal response to pain
     - Decorticate or decerebrate posture
     - Cranial nerve palsy (specially III, IV, and VI)

  - Abnormal neurogenic respiratory pattern (grunting, tachypnea, Cheyne-Stokes respiration, apneusis)
- Treatment
  - Restrict IV fluids to 2/3 maintenance and replace deficit over 72 h rather than 24 h.
  - Give mannitol 0.5–1 g/kg IV (2.5 ml/kg of 20 % sol) over 20 min and repeat after 6 h, if there is no initial response in 30 min–2 h.
  - Hypertonic saline (3 %), 5–10 ml/kg over 30 min, may be an alternative to mannitol or a second-line therapy if there is no initial response to mannitol.
  - Elevate the head of the bed.
  - Intubation may be necessary for the patient with impending respiratory failure, but aggressive hyperventilation is not recommended.
  - A cranial CT scan should be obtained to rule out other possible intracerebral causes of neurological deterioration.

## Pulmonary Edema

- Pulmonary edema is rarely seen in DKA.
- If it occurs, it usually occurs within few hours of initiation of DKA.
- Rapid infusion of crystalloids over a short period of time increases the likelihood of this complication.

## Conclusion/Summary

Patient should be counseled about the precipitating cause and early warning symptoms of DKA.

- Identification of precipitating factors like infections or omission of insulin should be done. Patient should be educated so that recurrence can be avoided.
- Patient's own insulin may be expired or denatured. This should be checked prior to reuse. Proper counseling is to be done regarding storage and use of insulin.
- Cerebral edema is a major risk causing mortality and morbidity and hence should be identified and managed promptly.

## Further Reading

1. ACOG Practice Bulletin. Clinical Management Guidelines for Obstetrician-Gynecologists. Number 60, 2005.
2. INTECH ©2013 Abdelghaffar. Diabetic Ketoacidosis: clinical practice guidelines. Chapter 11. http://dx.doi.org/10.5772/53020.
3. National Institute for Health & Clinical Excellence (NHS). Diabetes in Pregnancy; Management of diabetes & its complications from pre-conception to the postnatal period. 2008 .Last modified July 2008
4. National Institute for Health & Clinical Excellence (NHS). Joint British Diabetes Societies Inpatient Care Group. 2010.

# 13 Thyroid Dysfunction and Its Emergencies in Pregnancy

Nalini I. Anand and Amita A. Gandhi

## Thyroid Disorders

Thyroid disorders are common in young women. There is an intimate relationship between maternal and fetal thyroid function, and drugs that affect the maternal thyroid also affect the fetal gland. Maternal thyroid dysfunction and thyroid autoimmunity in pregnancy may be associated with adverse obstetric and fetal outcomes. Treatment of overt maternal hyperthyroidism and overt hypothyroidism clearly improves outcomes. To date there is limited evidence that levothyroxine treatment of pregnant women with subclinical hypothyroidism, isolated hypothyroxinaemia or thyroid autoimmunity is beneficial. Thyroid autoantibodies have been associated with increased early pregnancy wastage, and uncontrolled thyrotoxicosis and untreated hypothyroidism are both associated with adverse pregnancy outcomes [1].

N.I. Anand
Department of Obstetrics and Gynaecology, M. P. Shah Govt. Medical College and Hospital, Jamnagar, Gujarat, India

A.A. Gandhi (✉)
Arihant Women's Hospital, Vice President FOGSI, Ahmedabad, Gujarat, India
e-mail: dr.amita67@gmail.com

## Thyroid Physiology and Pregnancy

Physiologic changes of pregnancy cause the thyroid gland to increase production of thyroid hormones by 40–100 % to meet maternal and fetal needs [2].

A number of alterations in thyroid physiology and function during pregnancy are detailed in Fig. 13.1. Beginning early in the first trimester, levels of the principal carrier protein – thyroxine-binding globulin – increases, reaches its zenith at about 20 weeks and stabilizes at approximately double baseline values for the remainder of pregnancy. Total serum thyroxine (T4) increases sharply beginning between 6 and 9 weeks and reaches a plateau at 18 weeks. Free serum T4 levels rise slightly and peak along with hCG levels, and then they return to normal. The rise in total triiodothyronine (T3) is more pronounced up to 18 weeks, and thereafter, it plateaus. Thyroid-releasing hormone (TRH) levels are not increased during normal pregnancy, but this neurotransmitter does cross the placenta and may serve to stimulate the fetal pituitary to secrete thyrotropin [3] (Fig. 13.2).

Interestingly, the secretion of T4 and T3 is not similar for all pregnant women [4]. Approximately a third of women experience relative hypothyroxinaemia, preferential T3 secretion and higher, albeit normal, serum thyrotropin levels. Thus, there may be considerable variability in thyroidal adjustments during normal pregnancy.


A. Gandhi et al. (eds.), *Principles of Critical Care in Obstetrics: Volume II*,
DOI 10.1007/978-81-322-2686-4_13

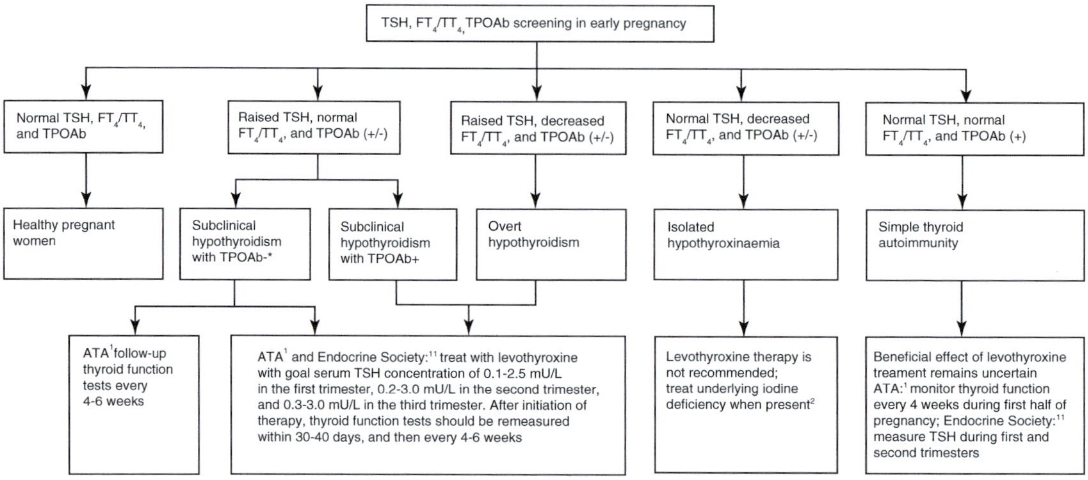


**Fig. 13.1** Correlation of T3, T4 and TSH values with thyroid disorders observed during screening

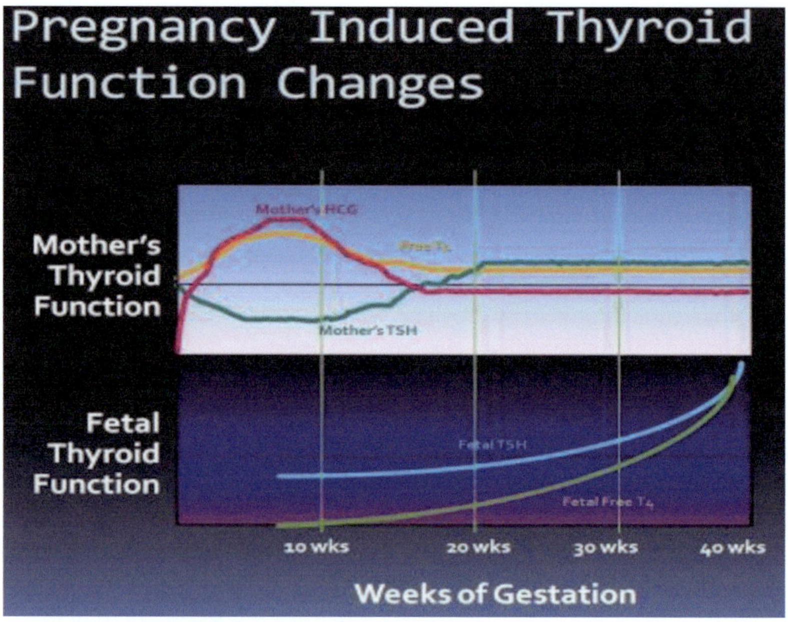


**Fig .13.2** Changes in maternal and foetal thyroid function during pregnancy

Thyrotropin, or thyroid-stimulating hormone (TSH), currently plays central role in screening and diagnosis of many thyroid disorders. Serum thyrotropin levels in early pregnancy decrease because of thyroid stimulation from the weak TSH effects of human chorionic gonadotropin (hCG) [5]. TSH does not cross the placenta. At the same time, hCG serum levels are maximal for the first 12 weeks; free thyroxin levels increase to suppress the pituitary thyrotropin secretion. Accordingly, thyrotropin-releasing hormone (TRH) is undetectable in maternal serum. Fetal serum TRH is detectable beginning at mid-pregnancy, but does not increase.

Throughout pregnancy, maternal thyroxine transferred to the fetus [6]. Maternal thyroxine is important for normal fetal brain development, especially prior to development of fetal thyroid gland function [7]. And even though the fetal thyroid gland begins concentrating iodine and synthesizing thyroid hormone after 12 weeks, maternal thyroxine contribution remains

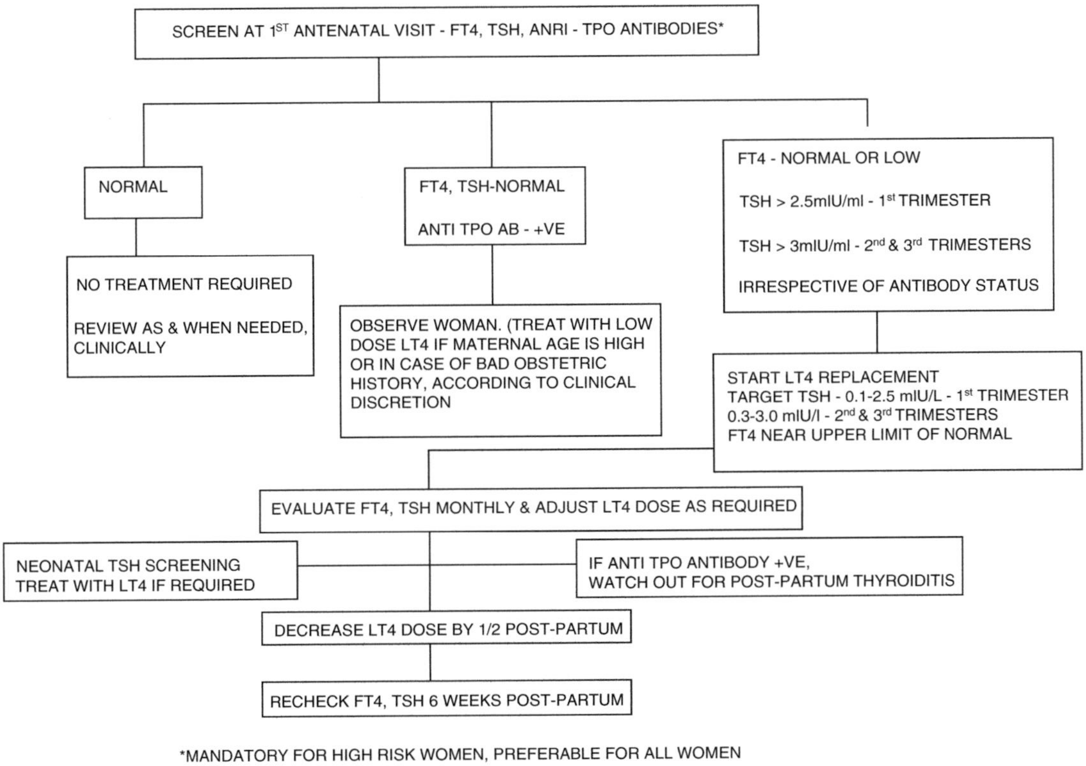


**Fig. 13.3** Flowchart depicting treatment based on screening

important. In fact, maternal thyroxine accounts for 30 % of thyroxine in fetal serum at term [8] (Fig. 13.3).

## TSH: Levels Are Trimester-Dependent

**Ranges [1]**

- 0.2–2.5 mIU/L in the first trimester
- 0.3–3.0 mIU/L in the second trimester
- Up to 3.5 mIU/L in the third trimester

Free T4 varies as albumin and T4-binding globulin change.

Numerous hormonal changes and metabolic demands occur during pregnancy, resulting in profound and complex effects on thyroid function.

Table 13.1 summarizes the main physiologic changes that occur during a normal pregnancy and that relate to thyroid function or thyroid function testing. These changes are discussed below.

**Table 13.1** Factors affecting thyroid physiology during normal pregnancy

| Physiologic change | Thyroid-related consequences |
|---|---|
| Increased renal iodine clearance | Increased 24-h RAIU |
| Decreased plasma iodine and placental iodine transport to the fetus | In iodine-deficient women, decreased T4, increased TSH and goitre formation |
| Increased $O_2$ consumption by fetoplacental unit, gravid uterus and mother | Increased BMR |
| First-trimester increase in hCG | Increased free T4 and T3 and decreased basal TSH (partial blunting of the pituitary-thyroid axis) |
| Increased serum TBG | Increased total T4 and T3 |
| Increased plasma volume | Increased T4 and T3 pool size |
| Inner-ring deiodination of T4 and T3 by placenta | Accelerated rates of T4 and T3 degradation and production |

## Hyperthyroidism

Hyperthyroidism occurs in about 0.2–0.4 % of all pregnancies. Most cases are due to Graves' disease although less common causes (e.g. toxic nodules and thyroiditis) may be seen [9]. Clinical assessment alone may occasionally be inadequate in differentiating hyperthyroidism from the hyperdynamic state of pregnancy. Distinctive clinical features of Graves' disease include the presence of ophthalmopathy, diffuse goitre and pretibial myxoedema. Also, hyperthyroidism must be distinguished from gestational transient thyrotoxicosis, a self-limiting hyperthyroid state due to the thyroid stimulatory effects of beta-hCG . This distinction is important since the latter condition is typically mild and will not usually require specific antithyroid treatment. Hyperthyroidism due to Graves' disease may worsen in the first trimester of pregnancy, remit in later pregnancy and subsequently relapse in the postpartum (Fig. 13.4).

Laboratory confirmation is by a markedly depressed TSH level along with an elevated serum-free T4 (fT4) level. Rarely, hyperthyroidism is caused by abnormally high serum triiodothyronine (T3) levels – the so-called T3 thyrotoxicosis (Fig. 13.5).

## Risks of Hyperthyroidism on Fetal and Maternal Well-Being

Uncontrolled hyperthyroidism in pregnancy is associated with an increased risk of severe

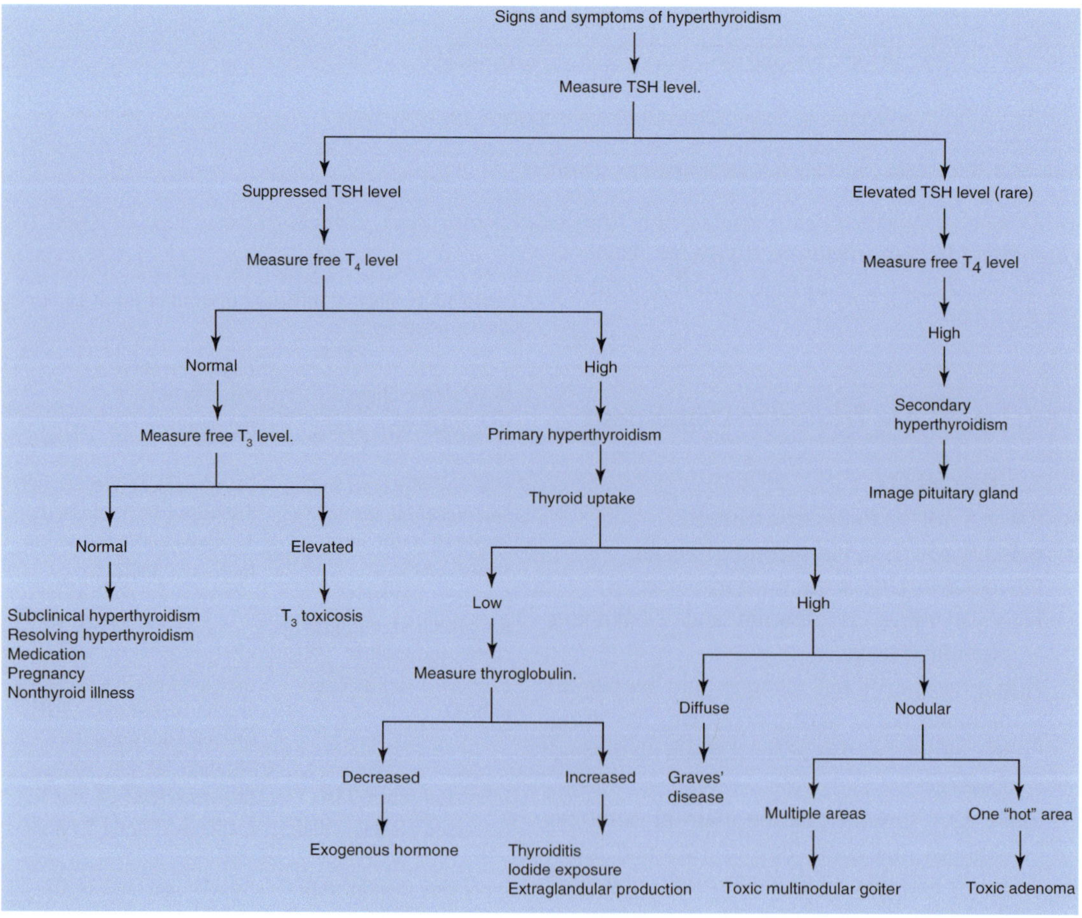


**Fig. 13.4** Signs and symptoms of hyperthyroidism

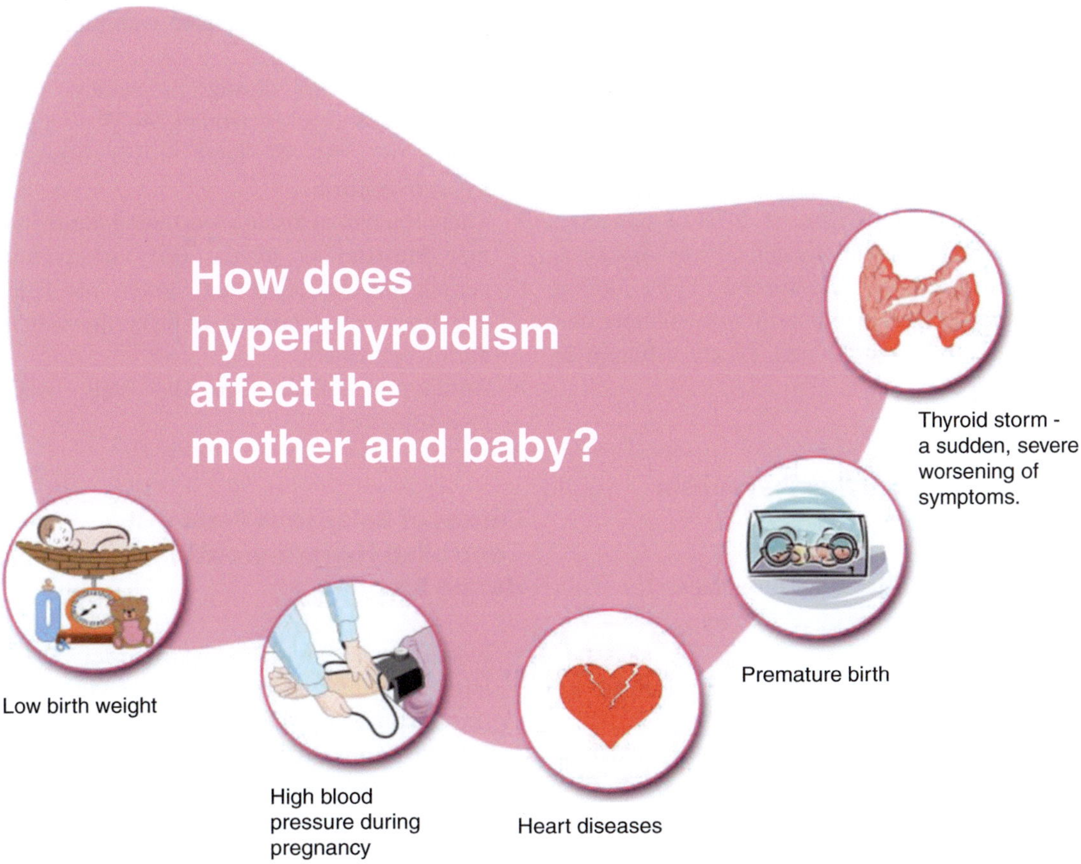


**Fig. 13.5** Effect of hyperthyroidism in mother and baby

pre-eclampsia and up to a fourfold increased risk of low-birth-weight deliveries. Some of these unfavourable outcomes are more marked in women who are diagnosed for the first time in pregnancy.

Uncontrolled and inadequately treated maternal hyperthyroidism may also result in fetal and neonatal hyperthyroidism [10] due to the transplacental transfer of stimulatory TSH-receptor antibodies (TRAbs) [11]. Clinical neonatal hyperthyroidism occurs in about 1 % of infants born to mothers with Graves' disease. Rarely neonatal hypothyroidism may also be observed in the infants of mothers with Graves' hyperthyroidism. This may result from transplacental transfer of circulating maternal anti-thyroid drugs and pituitary-thyroid axis suppression from transfer of maternal thyroxine.

Poorly controlled hyperthyroidism during pregnancy is associated with the following:

- Maternal:
  - Pregnancy-induced hypertension [12]
  - Pre-eclampsia
  - Cardiac failure
  - Premature labour [12]
  - Thyroid storm
  - Abruptio placenta
- Fetal/neonatal:
  - High miscarriage rate is associated with high thyroid hormone and thyrotropin hormone levels (i.e. not due to autoimmunity)
  - Intrauterine growth restriction [12]
  - Low birth-weight baby [12]
  - Stillbirth
  - Thyroid dysfunction

## Investigations

Serum TSH can exclude primary thyrotoxicosis. Confirm diagnosis with free T4 levels. If TSH is suppressed but free T4 levels are normal, then, if not previously supplied, free T3 level is necessary (T3 toxicosis occurs in 5 % of patients). Previously successfully treated Graves' disease is not associated with abnormal TFTs during pregnancy [13]. It is important to remember that the ranges of TSH, T3 and T4 are different in pregnancy [14]:

## Pre-pregnancy Hyperthyroidism Counselling [15]

This should be offered to all women. The main points about which to raise awareness are:

- General pregnancy and pre-conception advice to all women – e.g. folic acid.
- Pre-conception patients may be offered definitive therapy – e.g. ablation with radiotherapy (ideally, the patient should not conceive until 3–6 months later, once the levothyroxine dose has been optimized).
- Monitor thyroid-stimulating hormone (TSH) and thyrotropin receptor-stimulating antibodies (TRAb) – they gradually disappear following surgery, whilst with radiotherapy they rise and then usually fall after 12 months.
- Thus, surgery is usually the therapy of choice in women planning to become pregnant.
- Following definitive therapy, levothyroxine dosage may need to be increased early in pregnancy (increased T4 requirement).
- If definitive therapy is not to be considered, then the importance of adhering to medication must be stressed, as there is risk of multiple complications, both maternal and fetal.
- Reports from America concerning liver toxicity are being investigated [16].Propylthiouracil is, however, less likely to cross the placenta than carbimazole and has been considered the preferred antithyroid drug. These issues should be discussed with the patient. The safest option may be to use propylthiouracil in early pregnancy, changing to carbimazole in the latter months.
- Close follow-up during pregnancy, with TRAb status checked around 24–28 weeks to assess the risk of fetal and/or neonatal hyperthyroidism.
- There is a risk of disease worsening during the first trimester or in the early postpartum period; however, note that women may actually have better control of hyperthyroidism during pregnancy.
- Antithyroid medication is safe when breast-feeding.

## Causes of Relapse of Previously Controlled Hyperthyroidism during Pregnancy

- Increase in TRAb in the first trimester.
- High levels of human chorionic gonadotropin (hCG) stimulating the thyroid gland.
- Impaired drug absorption through vomiting.
- Labour, infection and caesarean section may also worsen thyroid control.

## Management [17, 18]

Hyperthyroidism during pregnancy can present as hyperemesis gravidarum or as thyroid storm – always check the TFTs. These women need urgent admission to hospital [19].

*Note*: Hyperemesis gravidarum is associated with abnormal TFTs which improve once it settles. Control is particularly important as the pregnancy progresses, especially in the third trimester. This is the result of suppression of the fetal pituitary-thyroid axis from maternal transfer of thyroxine when hyperthyroidism is poorly controlled.

## Pregnant Mothers with a New Diagnosis of Hyperthyroidism.

- All pregnant women should be referred urgently for assessment of a new diagnosis.

## Treatment of All Cases of Hyperthyroidism during Pregnancy (New Diagnoses or Worsening of Previously Controlled Hyperthyroidism)

- Antithyroid drugs are the first line for all.
- Radioiodine is contraindicated.
- Surgery is only where absolutely necessary and requires the patient to be rendered euthyroid with drugs to begin with.
- All cases should be discussed with a specialist.
- This needs to be urgently referred if adrenergic symptoms are present which may require treatment.
- Adrenergic symptoms can be treated with short courses of beta-blockers – e.g. propranolol. Use beyond a few weeks may adversely affect the fetus and is not advised.
- Antithyroid drugs:
  - Propylthiouracil may cross the placenta less readily than carbimazole (which has, on rare occasions, been associated with teratogenic affects) and it is the first choice in pregnancy and breast-feeding. However, liver toxicity has been recently reported (see section "Pre-pregnancy hyperthyroidism counselling" above). Current opinion favours using propylthiouracil in early pregnancy and carbimazole in later months [17].
  - Rarely, carbimazole has been associated with teratogenic affects.
  - However, in some countries, carbimazole may be the only choice available and the risks of not treating maternal hyperthyroidism will far outweigh those of potential teratogenicity.
  - The aim is to keep the thyroid hormones in the upper third of the reference range. Once this is achieved, then the dose of propylthiouracil is decreased to prevent effects on neonatal thyroid function (may produce neonatal hypothyroidism). A similar strategy is used in Graves' disease presenting during pregnancy.
  - Block and replace regimen is not recommended and medications need to continue into labour – albeit at a lower dose.
  - Remember that antithyroid drugs may cause neonatal hypothyroidism – thus, a minimal dose required should be used and thyroid hormones should be kept within the upper third of the normal range.
    - All monitoring of pregnant women should take place in secondary care but a full TFT profile should be sent from primary care. Monitoring usually involves the following: Measure TFTs every 4–6 weeks.
    - Serial fetal ultrasonography (looking for intrauterine growth restriction, hydrops fetalis, advanced bone age, goitre, tachycardia and heart failure).
    - Check TRAb.

## Thyrotoxicosis

The overwhelming cause of thyrotoxicosis in pregnancy is Graves' disease, an organ-specific autoimmune process usually associated with thyroid-stimulating antibodies. Such antibody activity declines during pregnancy, and it may become undetectable in the third trimester [20].

### Treatment of Thyrotoxicosis during Pregnancy

Thyrotoxicosis during pregnancy can nearly always be controlled by thionamide drugs. Some clinicians prefer propylthiouracil (PTU) because it partially inhibits the conversion of T4–T3 and crosses the placenta less readily than methimazole. Although not definitely proven, methimazole use in early pregnancy has been associated with a rare methimazole embryopathy characterized by oesophageal or choanal atresia as well as aplasia cutis, which is a congenital skin defect [21, 22]. Although these malformations are uncommon in women treated with methimazole, and despite the lack of epidemiological studies that PTU is safer, PTU is still preferred thionamide in the United States [23].

Transient leukopenia can be documented in up to 10 % of women taking antithyroid drugs but does not require cessation of therapy. In 0.3–0.4 %, agranulocytosis develops suddenly and mandates discontinuance of the drug. It is not dose related, and because of its acute onset, serial leukocyte count during therapy is not helpful. Thus, if fever or sore throat develops, women are instructed to discontinue medication immediately and report for a complete blood count [23]. Hepatotoxicity is another potentially serious side effect that occurs in 0.1–0.2 %. Approximately 20 % of patients treated with PTU develop antineutrophil cytoplasmic antibody (ANCA), but only a small percentage of these go on to develop serious vasculitis [24]. Finally, although thionamides have a potential to cause serious fetal complications, these are uncommon. In some cases, thionamides may even be therapeutic, because thyrotropin receptor antibodies cross the placenta and can stimulate the fetal thyroid gland to cause thyrotoxicosis and goitre.

The initial propylthiouracil dose is empirical. For nonpregnant patients, the American Thyroid Association recommends an initial daily dose of 100–600 mg for PTU or 10–40 mg for methimazole [25]. With a PTU dose that averaged 600 mg daily, only half of women had remission, and in these, the dose was decreased to less than 300 mg daily within 8 weeks. In a third, however, it was necessary to increase the dose. Serum free T4 is considered a better indicator of thyroid status than TSH during first 2–3 months of treatment for hyperthyroidism [26].

Subtotal thyroidectomy can be performed after thyrotoxicosis is medically controlled. This seldom is done during pregnancy but may be appropriate for the very few women who cannot adhere to medical treatment or in whom drug therapy proves toxic [27]. Ablation with therapeutic radioactive iodine is contraindicated during pregnancy. Therapeutic doses for maternal thyroid disease may also cause fetal thyroid gland destruction. Thus, when given unintentionally, most clinicians recommend abortion. Any exposed infant must be carefully evaluated for hypothyroidism [28]. The incidence of fetal hypothyroidism depends on gestational age and radioactive dose [29]. There is no evidence that therapeutic radioiodine given before pregnancy causes fetal anomalies if enough time has passed to allow radiation effects to dissipate and the woman is euthyroid [30, 31]. The International Commission on Radiological Protection has recommended that women avoid pregnancy for 6 months after radioablative therapy [23].

## Thyroid Storm

Only about 1–2 % of women with hyperthyroidism who receive thionamide experience thyroid storm – but it is a devastating complication [32].

Thyroid storm is a rare, life-threatening endocrinologic emergency that can lead to cardiac arrest and death. A total of 20–30 % of all cases are fatal [33]. Maternal mortality for this condition is currently approximately 3 %. Pregnant women with hyperthyroidism are at increased risk for spontaneous pregnancy loss, congestive heart failure, thyroid storm, preterm birth, preeclampsia, fetal growth restriction and associated with increased perinatal morbidity and mortality [34]. Patients can have a wide range of signs and symptoms. The tachycardia is often out of proportion to the hyperthermia. Blood pressure is commonly normal, although a widened pulse pressure is common. Patients with thyroid storm usually appear confused and disoriented. Thyroid storm can be precipitated by surgery, infection, trauma or labour and delivery [35, 36]. Patients with thyroid storm require assessment and management in an intensive care unit where they can be monitored for cardiac status, fluid and electrolyte balance and control of hyperthermia [37]. The underlying cause of thyroid storm must be identified and treated.

## Clinical Features

- Hyperthermia
- Nausea
- Abdominal pain
- Vomiting
- Severe agitation
- Diaphoresis
- Dehydration

- Tachycardia
- Congestive heart failure
- Arrhythmia
- Confusion
- Cardiovascular collapse
- Malignant exophthalmos

## **Management** (Table 13.2)

Patients with thyroid storm should be treated in an ICU setting for close monitoring of vital signs and for access to invasive monitoring and inotropic support, if necessary. Initial stabilization and management of systemic decompensation are as follows:

- If needed, immediately provide supplemental oxygen, ventilatory support and intravenous fluids. Dextrose solutions are the preferred intravenous fluids to cope with continuously high metabolic demand.
- Correct electrolyte abnormalities.
- Treat cardiac arrhythmia, if necessary.
- Aggressively control hyperthermia by applying ice packs and cooling blankets and by administering acetaminophen (15 mg/kg orally or rectally every 4 h).
- Promptly administer antiadrenergic drugs (e.g. propranolol) to minimize sympathomimetic symptoms.
- Correct the hyperthyroid state. Administer antithyroid medications to block further synthesis of thyroid hormones (THs).
- High-dose propylthiouracil (PTU) is preferred because of its early onset of action and capacity to inhibit peripheral conversion of T4–T3. The US Food and Drug Administration (FDA) had added a boxed warning, the strongest warning issued by the FDA, to the prescribing information for PTU.
  - The boxed warning emphasizes the risk for severe liver injury and acute liver failure, some of which have been fatal. The boxed warning also states that PTU should be reserved for use in those who cannot tolerate other treatments such as methimazole, radioactive iodine or surgery.
  - The decision to include a boxed warning was based on the FDA's review of postmarketing safety reports and meetings held with the American Thyroid Association, the National Institute of Child Health and Human Development and the paediatric endocrine clinical community.
  - The FDA has identified 32 cases (22 adult and 10 paediatric) of serious liver injury associated with PTU. Among adults, 12 deaths and 5 liver transplants occurred; among the paediatric patients, 1 death and 6 liver transplants occurred. PTU is indicated for hyperthyroidism due to Graves' disease. These reports suggest an increased risk for liver toxicity with PTU compared with methimazole. Serious liver injury has been identified with methimazole in five cases (three resulting in death).

**Table 13.2** Three-step treatment of thyroid storm

| | Goal | Treatment | Effect |
|---|---|---|---|
| Step 1 | Block peripheral effect of thyroid hormone | Provide continuous intravenous infusion of β-blocking agent | Slows heart rate, increases diastolic filling and decreases tremor |
| Step 2 | Stop the production of thyroid hormone | Provide antithyroid medication (propylthiouracil or methimazole) and dexamethasone | Antithyroids decrease synthesis of thyroid hormone in the thyroid. Propylthiouracil slows conversion of T4 to T3 in periphery. Dexamethasone decreases conversion of T4 to T3 in periphery |
| Step 3 | Inhibit hormone release | Give iodide 1–2 h after antithyroid medication | Decreases release of thyroid hormone from thyroid |

  - PTU is considered as a second-line drug therapy, except in patients who are allergic or intolerant to methimazole, or for women who are in the first trimester of pregnancy. Rare cases of embryopathy, including aplasia cutis, have been reported with methimazole during pregnancy. The FDA recommends the following criteria be considered for prescribing PTU [38]:
    - Reserve PTU use during first trimester of pregnancy or in patients who are allergic to or intolerant of methimazole.
    - Closely monitor PTU therapy for signs and symptoms of liver injury, especially during the first 6 months after initiation of therapy.
    - For suspected liver injury, promptly discontinue PTU therapy and evaluate for evidence of liver injury and provide supportive care.
    - PTU should not be used in paediatric patients unless the patient is allergic to or intolerant of methimazole, and no other treatment options are available.
    - Counsel patients to promptly contact their health-care provider for the following signs or symptoms: fatigue, weakness, vague abdominal pain, loss of appetite, itching, easy bruising or yellowing of the eyes or skin.
- Administer iodine compounds (Lugol's iodine or potassium iodide) orally or via a nasogastric tube to block the release of THs (at least 1 h after starting antithyroid drug therapy). If available, intravenous radiocontrast dyes such as ipodate and iopanoate can be effective in this regard. These agents are particularly effective at preventing peripheral conversion of T4–T3.
- Administer glucocorticoids to decrease peripheral conversion of T4–T3. This may also be useful in preventing relative adrenal insufficiency due to hyperthyroidism.
- Treat the underlying condition, if any, that precipitated thyroid storm and exclude comorbidities such as diabetic ketoacidosis and adrenal insufficiency. Infection should be treated with antibiotics.
- Rarely, as a life-saving measure, plasmapheresis has been used to treat thyroid storm in adults [33].

Iodine preparations should be discontinued once the acute phase resolves and the patient becomes afebrile with normalization of cardiac and neurological status. Glucocorticoids should be weaned and stopped and the dose of thioamides adjusted to maintain thyroid function in the normal range. Beta-blockers may be discontinued once thyroid function normalizes.

If the patient is given PTU during treatment of thyroid storm, this should be switched to methimazole at the time of discharge unless methimazole is contraindicated. If there is a contraindication for the use of methimazole, alternative methods to treat hyperthyroidism should be considered after discharge, such as radioactive iodine or surgery.

## Aims of Therapy

Therapy is aimed (1) ameliorating hyperadrenergic effects of thyroid hormone (TH) on peripheral tissues with use of beta-blockers (e.g. propranolol, labetalol); (2) decreasing further synthesis of THs with antithyroid medications (e.g. propylthiouracil [PTU], methimazole); (3) decreasing hormonal release from the thyroid, using iodides; and (4) preventing further TH secretion and peripheral conversion of T4 to T3, using glucocorticoids or iodinated radiocontrast dyes when available.

## Prevention

The gold standard of treatment of thyroid storm is primary prevention. Prevention of thyroid storm requires careful control and management of the hyperthyroidism. Standard treatment options for Graves' disease include therapy with radioactive iodine, ATDs and thyroid surgery [25]. However, pregnancy limits these treatment options. Because of possible destruction of the thyroid gland in the fetus, radioactive iodine cannot be given, and surgery is avoided because of the increased risk for miscarriage or preterm delivery.

As a result, the standard treatment during pregnancy is the use of ATDs to inhibit the biosynthesis of thyroid hormones. Because of the immunosuppressive effect of pregnancy, ATDs can be given in lower doses in pregnant patients than in nonpregnant patients. Every attempt should be made to treat with the lowest possible effective dose of ATDs because these drugs can cross the placenta, enter the fetal circulation and affect the thyroid gland of the fetus.

Even though propylthiouracil is the drug of choice during pregnancy, it is not given without careful observation, because it results in drug reactions in up to 5 % of treated patients. These reactions include fever, rash, urticaria, arthralgias and leukopenia. A rare adverse effect, agranulocytosis, an acute condition distinguished by a deficit or absolute lack of granulocytes, usually is manifested by fever and sore throat. If fever and sore throat occur, a complete blood cell count should be done, and if agranulocytosis is diagnosed, treatment with thiopropyluracil should be stopped [39].

The starting dose is typically 300–450 mg/day divided into 3 doses. If methimazole is used, the starting dose is 20 mg twice a day. Results of laboratory tests should be monitored carefully, and once a patient becomes euthyroid, the dose can be tapered gradually. Many patients need only 50 mg/day, and some patients may not need any medication by the third trimester; however, the dosage may vary from 50 to 200 mg of propylthiouracil every 8 h or methimazole 10–60 mg/day, depending on the patient's signs and symptoms and laboratory values [40, 41]. Biochemically, the aim is to keep the serum level of total T4 between 154 and 193 nmol/L (12–15 μg/dL) and the serum level of free $T_4$ within the reference range for the laboratory test used. (These values will vary from one laboratory to another [41].)

Fetal and neonatal hypothyroidism, as well as the occurrence of goitres, may occur from passage of thionamides across the placenta [40]. During the first trimester, transfer of ATDs transplacentally can affect thyroid development in the fetus. Fetal exposure to ATDs can produce hypothyroidism and fetal growth restriction [42].

Methimazole therapy may be associated with aplasia cutis (a localized lesion in the parietal area of the scalp, characterized by congenital absence of the skin, punched-out "ulcer" lesions that usually heal spontaneously) in the offspring of treated women and is another reason that propylthiouracil has become the drug of choice during pregnancy [43]. The therapeutic goal is to control the mother's hyperthyroidism by using the smallest possible amount of medication, to avoid suppressing the thyroid gland in the fetus [44].

## Hyperemesis Gravidarum and Gestational Thyrotoxicosis (Fig. 13.6)

Hyperemesis gravidarum is associated with abnormal TFTs which improve once it settles. Control is particularly important as the pregnancy progresses, especially in the third trimester. This is the result of suppression of the fetal pituitary-thyroid axis from maternal transfer of thyroxine when hyperthyroidism is poorly controlled.

## Subclinical Hyperthyroidism and Pregnancy Outcomes [45]

Subclinical hyperthyroidism has long-term sequelae that include osteoporosis, cardiovascular morbidity and progression to overt thyrotoxicosis or thyroid failure.

Subclinical hyperthyroidism is characterized by circulating thyrotropin (thyroid-stimulating hormone; TSH) levels below the reference range and normal serum thyroid hormone levels [46]. The diagnosis is primarily biochemical and depends on the definition of "normal" TSH levels. In 2002, a panel of experts established the reference range for serum THS levels between 0.45 and 4.5 μU/mL.

Whilst interpreting serum TSH levels, physiologic variations as well as presence of occult

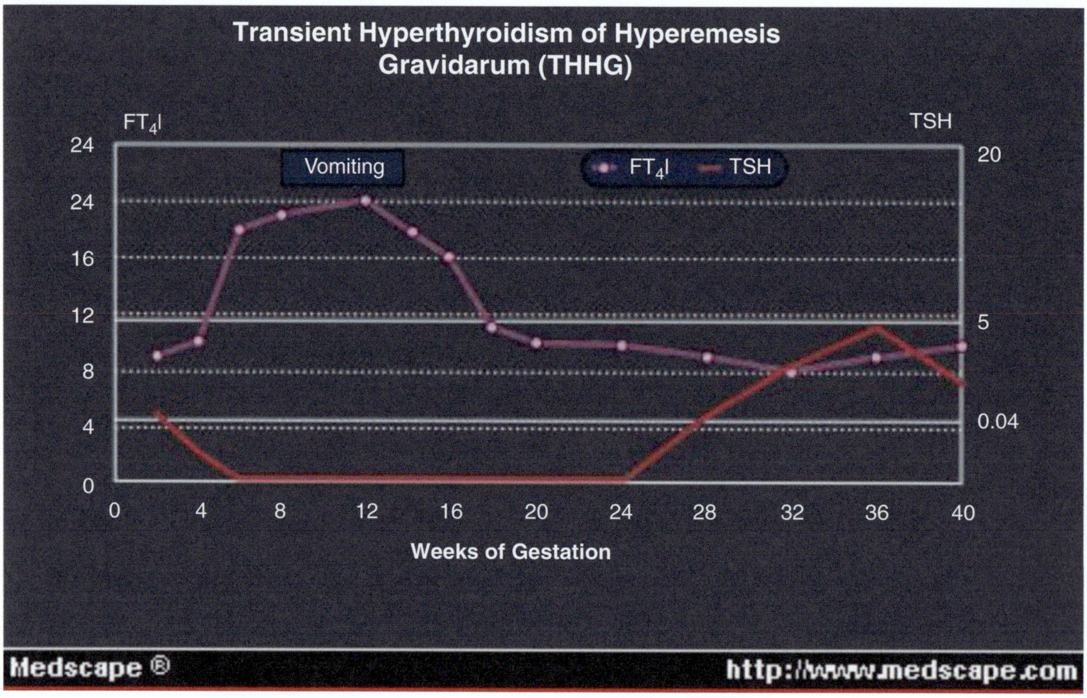


**Fig. 13.6** Relationship of hyperemesis to T.S.H.

thyroid disease should be considered. Several anthropometric variables, including age, gender, race and body mass index (BMI), have a noticeable influence over circulating TSH levels [47–49]. In addition, other factors such as concurrent medication, coexisting pregnancy or concomitant diseases should be considered in order to correctly interpret TSH, thyroxin (T4) and triiodothyronine (T3) status [47].

Additionally, clinicians should consider three important facts whilst interpreting the results of thyroid function tests [50]: (1) TSH secretion follows a circadian rhythm with higher values early in the morning and lowest value in the afternoon, (2) TSH secretion is pulse-regulated and (3) TSH half-life is about 15 min.

A classification system for subclinical hyperthyroidism has been proposed recently, which differentiates between low serum TSH levels (0.1–0.4 μU/mL; Grade I or mild) and suppressed TSH concentration (<0.1 μU/mL; Grade II or severe) [51]. Grade I subclinical hyperthyroidism is three to four times more common than Grade II subclinical hyperthyroidism. The risk of progression from Grade I to overt disease is very low. Conversely, about 2–5 % of the cases of Grade II hyperthyroidism progress to clinical disease per year [51].

In some cases, subclinical hyperthyroidism may present with a normal serum level of free T4 (FT4) whilst the serum T3 level remains above the reference range. This unusual laboratory finding has been called "T3 toxicosis" and may represent the earliest stages of disease, which is normally caused by an autonomously functioning thyroid nodule [46]. All these categories are relevant in clinical practice.

Clinical manifestations of both overt and mild (or subclinical) thyrotoxicosis are similar, but differ in magnitude. Potential complications of untreated subclinical hyperthyroidism are numerous and include weight loss, osteoporosis, atrial fibrillation, embolic events and altered cognition. The most profound consequences of subclinical overactive thyroid dysfunction are observed on the cardiovascular system [52] and the skeleton [53].

2. Severity: In general, patients with Grade I subclinical hyperthyroidism may not be offered

treatment. On the other hand, treatment should be strongly considered in high-risk individuals with persistent endogenous Grade II (TSH level <0.1 μU/mL) subclinical hyperthyroidism [51].

There was an increased risk of TSH above 3 muU/mL in women who consumed 200 mcg or more of iodine supplements daily compared with those who consumed less than 100 mcg/day (adjusted odds ratio = 2.5 [95 % confidence interval = 1.2–5.4]). We observed no association between urinary iodine and TSH levels. Pregnant women from the area with the highest median urinary iodine (168 mcg/L) and highest supplement coverage (93 %) showed the lowest values of serum-free thyroxine (geometric mean = 10.09 pmol/L [9.98–10.19]).

Iodine supplement intake in the first half of pregnancy may lead to maternal thyroid dysfunction in iodine-sufficient or mildly iodine-deficient populations.

**Table 13.3** Clinical signs and symptoms of hypothyroidism

| | |
|---|---|
| Constitutional/general | Fatigue, weight gain, cold intolerance, hoarseness, periorbital oedema |
| Cardiovascular | Bradycardia, diastolic hypertension. Peripheral oedema, hyperlipidaemia, pericardial effusions |
| Pulmonary | Dyspnoea, pleural effusions |
| Gastrointestinal | Constipation |
| Genitourinary | Decreased glomerular filtration rate, elevated creatinine, infertility, menorrhagia |
| Neurological | Poor memory. Difficulty concentrating. Ataxia, muscle weakness. Muscle cramping. Nerve entrapment syndromes (carpal tunnel syndrome), delayed tendon reflex relaxation, paraesthesias, impaired hearing, psychosis |
| Dermatological | Dry coarse skin, diffuse alopecia, yellow skin |

Information from Refs. [1–3]

## Hypothyroidism

The most common cause of hypothyroidism in pregnancy is Hashimoto thyroiditis, characterized by glandular destruction by autoantibodies, particularly antithyroid peroxidase antibodies. Clinical identification of hypothyroidism is especially difficult during pregnancy because many of the signs or symptoms are also common to pregnancy itself. Thyroid testing should be performed on symptomatic women or those with a history of thyroid disease [54]. Severe hypothyroidism with pregnancy is uncommon, probably because it is often associated with infertility and increased miscarriage rates [55] (Table 13.3).

Hypothyroidism is common in pregnancy with an estimated prevalence of 2–3 % and 0.3–0.5 % for subclinical and overt hypothyroidism, respectively [56]. Endemic iodine deficiency accounts for most hypothyroidism in pregnant women worldwide whilst chronic autoimmune thyroiditis is the most common cause of hypothyroidism in iodine-sufficient parts of the world [57]. The presentation of hypothyroidism in pregnancy is not always classical and may sometimes be difficult to distinguish from the symptoms of normal pregnancy. A high index of suspicion is therefore required especially in women at risk of thyroid disease, e.g. women with a personal or family history of thyroid disease, goitre or coexisting primary autoimmune disorder like type 1 diabetes.

### Risks of Hypothyroidism on Fetal and Maternal Well-Being (Fig. 13.7)

Hypothyroidism is diagnosed by noting a high TSH associated with a subnormal T4 concentration. Subclinical hypothyroidism (SCH) is present when the TSH is high but the T4 level is in the normal range but usually low normal. SCH is the most common form of hypothyroidism in pregnancy and is usually due to progressive thyroid destruction due to autoimmune thyroid disease. Several studies, mostly retrospective, have shown an association between overt hypothyroidism and adverse fetal and obstetric outcomes [58]. Maternal complications such as miscarriages, anaemia in pregnancy, pre-eclampsia, abruptio placenta and postpartum haemorrhage can occur in pregnant women with overt hypothyroidism. Also, the offspring of these mothers can have complications such as premature birth, low birth weight and increased neonatal respiratory distress [59]. Similar complications have been reported in mothers with subclinical hypothyroidism. A threefold risk of abruptio placenta and a twofold risk of preterm delivery were reported in mothers with subclinical hypothyroidism [60]. Another study showed a higher prevalence of subclinical hypothyroidism in women with preterm delivery (before 32 weeks) compared to matched controls delivering at term [61]. An association with adverse obstetrics outcome has also been demonstrated in pregnant women with thyroid autoimmunity independent of thyroid function. Treatment of hypothyroidism reduces the risks of these adverse obstetric and fetal outcomes; a retrospective study of 150 pregnancies showed that treatment of hypothyroidism led to reduced rates of abortion and premature delivery. Also, a prospective intervention trial study showed that treatment of euthyroid antibody-positive pregnant women led to fewer rates of miscarriage than nontreated controls [62].

It has long been known that cretinism (i.e. gross reduction in IQ) occurs in areas of severe iodine deficiency due to the fact that the mother is unable to make T4 for transport to the fetus particularly in the first trimester. This neurointellectual impairment (on a more modest scale) has now been shown in an iodine-sufficient area (USA) where a study showed that the IQ scores of 7–9-year-old children, born to mothers with undiagnosed and untreated hypothyroidism in pregnancy, were seven points lower than those of children of matched control women with normal thyroid function in pregnancy [63]. Another study showed that persistent hypothyroxinaemia

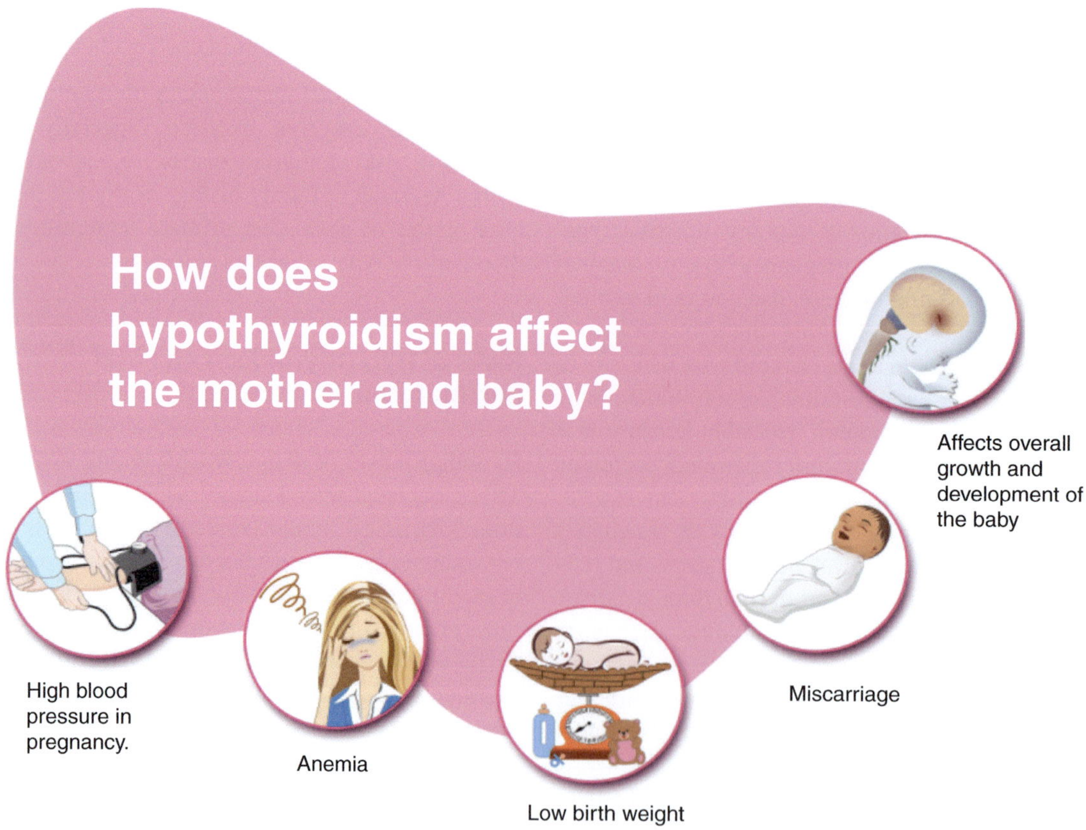


**Fig. 13.7** Effect of hypothyroidism on mother and baby

at 12 weeks gestation was associated with an 8–10-point deficit in mental and motor function scores in infant offspring compared to children of mothers with normal thyroid function [64]. Even maternal thyroid peroxidase SS antibodies were shown to be associated with impaired intellectual development in the offspring of mothers with normal thyroid function [65]. However, no association was found between isolated maternal hypothyroxinaemia and adverse perinatal outcomes in two large US studies [66, 67], although the behavioural outcomes in the children were not tested in these studies.

## Management of Hypothyroidism in Pregnancy

Levothyroxine is the treatment of choice for hypothyroidism in pregnancy. Thyroid function should be normalised prior to conception in women with preexisting thyroid disease. Once pregnancy is confirmed, the thyroxine dose should be increased by about 30–50 % and subsequent titrations should be guided by thyroid function tests (FT4 and TSH) that should be monitored 4–6 weekly until euthyroidism is achieved. It is recommended that TSH levels are maintained below 2.5 mU/l in the first trimester of pregnancy and below 3 mU/l in later pregnancy [68]. The recommended maintenance dose of thyroxine in pregnancy is about 2.0–2.4 μg/kg daily. Thyroxine requirements may increase in late gestation and return to pre-pregnancy levels in the majority of women on delivery. Pregnant patients with subclinical hypothyroidism (normal FT4 and elevated TSH) should be treated as well, since supplementation with levothyroxine in such cases results in significantly higher delivery rate, with a pooled relative chance of 2.76 [69].

## Subclinical Hypothyroidism

Traditionally, overt hypothyroidism cases during pregnancy have been treated due to its adverse effect on fetus as well as on mother. Evidences are now available for the need of treatment of subclinical hypothyroidism (SCH) during pregnancy. SCH is the most common form of hypothyroidism in pregnancy and is usually due to progressive thyroid destruction due to autoimmune thyroid disease. The prevalence and incidence of SCH are found to be more in South Asia than other parts of the world.

Thyroid gland has an important role in brain development of fetus during pregnancy. Subclinical hypothyroidism (SCH) is the most common form of hypothyroidism in pregnancy. SCH is present, when the thyroid-stimulating hormone (TSH) is high or normal but the thyroxine (T4) level is in the normal or low normal range. It is more predominant in South Asia. So, every pregnant women should be ruled out for SCH in first trimester.

Thyroid disease in pregnancy especially SCH during pregnancy results in impaired neurodevelopment in offspring [63, 70]. Further, other reports have associated SCH with preterm delivery, pre-eclampsia and postpartum thyroiditis [60, 71].

The prevalence of SCH could be anticipated to be between 2 and 5 % of women screened, depending on the TSH and free T4 (FT4)-level thresholds applied, and this represents most women who would be identified with thyroid deficiency through routine screening [60]. In North India, there is a high prevalence of hypothyroidism (14.3 %), majority being subclinical in pregnant women during first trimester, necessitating routine screening [72]. Probable causes of SCH are many and chronic autoimmune thyroiditis (e.g. Hashimoto's disease, thyroiditis) with a prevalence of 3–8 % in the general population is said to be the most common cause [73]. High oestrogen states (in pregnancy, it causes decrease in FT4 level) [74] and chronic stress – both physical and mental [75] along with other diseases like diabetes (especially type 1) – are conditions affecting the pituitary or hypothalamus, are some other causes [76]. Women with family history of hypothyroidism or an autoimmune disease are also at increase risk of developing SCH. Serum TSH is the more accurate indication of thyroid status in pregnancy and the gestation age for screening is 12–16 weeks of gestation. Indications for screening of high-risk group include history of thyroid dysfunction or prior thyroid surgery, age >30 years, symptoms of thyroid dysfunction or the presence of goitre, thyroid peroxidase antibody (TPOAb) positivity, type 1 diabetes or other autoimmune disorders, history of miscarriage or preterm delivery (RPL), history of head or neck radiation, family history of thyroid dysfunction, morbid obesity (body mass index [BMI] ≥40 kg/m$^2$), use of amiodarone or lithium or recent administration of iodinated radiologic contrast, history of infertility and residing in an area of known moderate-to-severe iodine sufficiency.

There may be no signs and symptoms or mild general signs and symptoms of hypothyroidism, like depression, weight gain [77], dry or flaky skin, body weakness or feeling cold easily, slow pulse, low body temperature and increased need for sleep. Some women may experience difficulty in concentrating, irritability and anxiety with slow movement, thinking and learning [78] as well as slow circulation and heart rate.

Next step is antithyroid antibodies [79] (maternal thyroid peroxidase) should be done in all cases where serum TSH is out of range. Other least important tests include red cell selenium, urinary T3 (recent studies show that symptoms of hypothyroidism correlate best with 24-hour urinary FT3) [80], urinary iodine concentration, thyroid ultrasound, serum cholesterol (which may be elevated in hypothyroidism), serum prolactin (as a widely available test of pituitary function), testing for anaemia and basal body temperature. These tests are important because the risk complications arising from hypothyroidism either overt or subclinical are very high. These includes a threefold increase in risk of abruptio placenta and a twofold risk of preterm delivery, reported in mothers with SCH [60]. Neuromuscular symptoms and dysfunction are common in patients with SCH and can be reversed by levothyroxine treatment [81]. The overall incidences of hypertension in pregnancy were 6.2 %, 8.5 and 10.9 % in the subclinical hyperthyroid, euthyroid and subclinical hypothyroid groups, respectively [82]; there was a significant association between SCH and severe pre-eclampsia. Therefore, they recommend screening in every case of severe pre-eclampsia. The risk of developing gestational diabetes increases with thyrotropin level. This supports a relationship between SCH and diabetes diagnosed during pregnancy. It may progress to overt hypothyroidism in approximately 2–5 % of cases annually [73]. Pre-eclampsia, eclampsia and pregnancy-induced hypertension have a significantly higher incidence in SCH (15 %; $n=7$ of 45) compared with the incidence in the general population (7.6 %) [83]. Neuromuscular symptoms and dysfunction [82] – postpartum thyroid dysfunction – significantly developed in the presence of antithyroid antibody with a prevalence ranging from 1.1 to 16.7 % with a mean of 7.5 % [84]. Postpartum depression can also occur but no significant difference was found [65]. SCH was found in 19.6 % of women having history of vascular complicated pregnancy. It occurred more often when pregnancy ended before 32 weeks of gestation ($p=0.008$) [85]. Coming to the risk to fetus, 7-point reduction in intelligence quotient was observed in children aged 7–9 years, whose mothers had SCH at pregnancy compared with the children of euthyroid mothers. Even when hypothyroid pregnant women were insufficiently treated with levothyroxine (LT4), the intelligence quotient (IQ) scores of their offspring were not different from those of controls. Pregnant women with SCH have higher incidence of neonatal morbidity and mortality [55].

Twofold risk increase observed in neonate intensive care nursery admission (RR 1.8; 95 % CI 1.1–2.9 %) and incidence of respiratory distress syndrome (defined as ventilator assistance >24 h) [60]. Thyroid hormones are regulators of the mitochondrial activity so hypothesis can be made that all the complications in SCH may be due to mitochondrial dysfunction. It can be prevented providing a minimum of 250 mcg iodine daily to all pregnant and lactating women. Pre-conception ingestion of 150 mg iodine daily along with preconception screening for hypothyroidism can prevent the major complications [86]. The goal of treatment is to normalize maternal serum TSH values within the trimester-specific pregnancy reference range. If trimester-specific reference ranges for TSH are not available in the laboratory, the following reference ranges are recommended by USPSTF [79]: first trimester (0.1–2.5 mIU/L), second trimester (0.2–3.0 mIU/L) and third trimester (0.3–3.0 mIU/L).

Oral levothyroxine is the drug of choice as it is category A drug and has a long half-life (7 days) and is partially converted to T3 in the body, resulting in a constant physiologic level of both T3 and T4 with a single daily dose. It should be started at a low dose of 12.5–25 mg and the maintenance dose should be 2–2.4 mg/kg/day.

The prevalence of SCH in South Asia especially in India is more than in other parts of the world and mostly due to autoimmune thyroiditis and nutrition deficiency. The gravity of the complications like abortion, preterm birth, weight gain, postpartum thyroiditis and converting to overt hypothyroidism in the future outweighs the cost of screening. The child may suffer from low IQ and decreased memory and concentrating power. In this view, we propose screening all pregnant women in the first trimester by doing serum TSH and FT4 followed by antithyroid antibody for diagnosis. It should be made mandatory, so that not a single mother will be deprived of it. Finally, we conclude that treatment should be given to the antibody-positive cases because complications are usually associated with it.

## **Iodine and Pregnancy** [87] (Fig. 13.8)

An adequate iodine intake during pregnancy is essential for the synthesis of maternal thyroid hormones and normal brain development in the

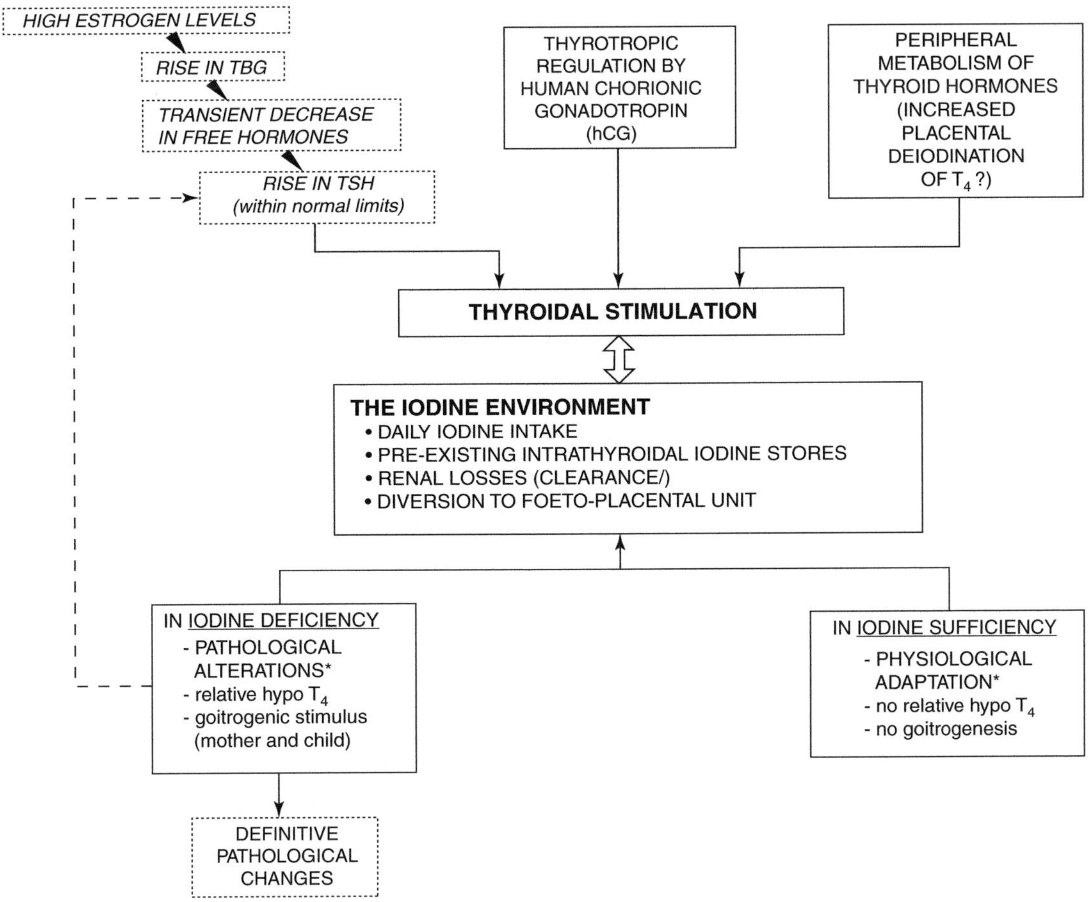


**Fig. 13.8** Effect of iodine on thyroid function

fetus. There was an increased risk of TSH above 3 muU/mL in women who consumed 200 mcg or more of iodine supplements daily compared with those who consumed less than 100 mcg/day (adjusted odds ratio = 2.5 [95 % confidence interval = 1.2–5.4]). We observed no association between urinary iodine and TSH levels. Pregnant women from the area with the highest median urinary iodine (168 mcg/L) and highest supplement coverage (93 %) showed the lowest values of serum-free thyroxine (geometric mean = 10.09 pmol/L [9.98–10.19]).

Iodine supplement intake in the first half of pregnancy may lead to maternal thyroid dysfunction in iodine-sufficient or mildly iodine-deficient populations.

## Myxoedema Coma (Table 13.4)

Myxoedema coma/crisis occurs most commonly in older women with long-standing, undiagnosed or undertreated hypothyroidism who experience an additional significant stress, such as infection, a systemic disease, certain medications and exposure to a cold environment.

When hypothyroidism is long-standing, physiologic adaptations occur. Reduced metabolic rate and decreased oxygen consumption result in peripheral vasoconstriction, which maintains core temperature. The number of beta-adrenergic receptors is reduced, usually with preservation of alpha-adrenergic receptors and circulating catecholamines, causing beta/alpha-adrenergic imbalance, diastolic hypertension and reduced total blood volume.

Myxoedema coma/crisis is a form of decompensated hypothyroidism in which adaptations are no longer sufficient [88]. Essentially, all organ systems are affected.

**Table 13.4** Historical questions in the evaluation of myxoedema coma

| |
|---|
| History of thyroid disease? |
| Symptoms of hypothyroidism: weight gain, hair loss, fatigue, weight gain, dry skin, voice change, depression, constipation, menstrual irregularity? |
| Medication changes often with menometrorrhagia? |
| Physiologic/psychological stressors: infection, trauma, cold exposure, major life changes? |

### Metabolic

Thyroid hormones are critical for cell metabolism and organ function. With an inadequate supply, organ tissues do not grow or mature, energy production declines and the action of other hormones is affected.

Although weight gain is common, severe obesity is rarely secondary to hypothyroidism alone. However, long-standing, untreated hypothyroidism may result in years of inactivity, eventually with a large increase in weight.

Because of decreased drug metabolism, overdoses of medications (e.g. morphine, hypnotics, anaesthetic agents, sedatives) can occur and can even precipitate myxoedema crisis.

### Neurologic

Although the condition is called myxoedema coma, the absence of coma does not exclude the diagnosis of this disorder. The presenting mental status may be lethargy or stupor. The exact mechanisms causing changes in mental status are not known. Brain function is influenced by reductions in cerebral blood flow and oxygen delivery, a lack of thyroxine (T4) and triiodothyronine (T3) and reductions in oxygen and glucose consumption; all of these factors are probably involved. Hyponatraemia brought on by renal dysfunction may be an additional cause of altered mental function.

### Renal

Kidney function may be severely compromised, partly because of low cardiac output and vasoconstriction that causes a low glomerular filtration rate. Reduced levels of $NA^+/K^+$ ATPase decrease sodium reabsorption and impair free-water excretion, resulting in hyponatraemia, which is usually present in myxoedema coma.

## Gastrointestinal

Severe or even mild hypothyroidism decreases intestinal motility. Patients with myxoedema coma can present with gastric atony, megacolon or paralytic ileus. Malabsorption has also been reported. Ascites, whilst uncommon, may occur due to increased capillary permeability, congestive heart failure or other mechanisms.

## Medical Care

Myxoedema crisis/coma is a life-threatening condition; therefore, patients with this disorder must be stabilized in an intensive care unit. The first 24–48 h is critical. If the diagnosis is considered likely, immediate and aggressive administration of multiple interventions is necessary to lower an otherwise high-rate mortality. Initial priorities include the following:

- Mechanical ventilation if respiratory acidosis/hypercapnia/hypoxia is significant
- Immediate intravenous thyroid hormone replacement whilst awaiting confirmatory test results (T4 and TSH), even if the diagnosis of myxoedema coma is only probable.
- Because GI absorption is compromised, intravenous therapy is mandatory. Whether to use T4 alone, combined T4 and T3 or T3 alone remains a subject of controversy. Deiodinase conversion of T4 to the active hormone T3 is reduced in these patients, and T3 administration may be advisable. However, T3, because of its more immediate action and short half-life, may be more likely to cause arrhythmias, particularly if myocardial function is compromised. The usual conversion to an intravenous dose of T4 is approximately one half to two thirds of the oral dose.
- An intravenous loading dose of 500–800 mcg of levothyroxine is followed by a daily intravenous dose of 50–100 mcg; the daily dose is administered until the patient is able to take medication by mouth. Use caution in elderly persons and in patients with coronary artery disease or myocardial infarction, because full-dose T4 therapy may worsen myocardial ischemia by increasing myocardial oxygen consumption [89]. Some authorities advocate the use of additional intravenous T3 at 10–20 mcg every 8–12 h, especially in young patients with low cardiovascular risk.
- Because of the rarity of the condition, randomized trials comparing different treatment modalities are not available. Observational studies are not in agreement regarding whether low- [90, 91] or high-dose T4 or T3 replacement reduces mortality [92].
- In light of the possibility of adrenal insufficiency, stress steroid replacement *after* a cortisol level is obtained [93].
- After a baseline cortisol level is ascertained, initiate hydrocortisone at 5–10 mg/h. Continue therapy unless the random cortisol level on admission indicates adrenal function without abnormalities, in which case, hydrocortisone may be stopped without tapering.
- Passive rewarming using ordinary blankets and a warm room (rapid and external rewarming are contraindicated).
- Treatment of associated infection.
- Correction of severe hyponatraemia (sodium level <120 mEq/L) with saline, free-water restriction.
- Broad-spectrum antibiotics with modification of the antibiotic regimen based on culture results.
- Correction of hypoglycaemia with intravenous dextrose.
- Treatment of severe hypotension with cautious administration of 5–10 % glucose in half-normal or normal saline (or hypertonic saline if severely hyponatraemic, i.e. <120 mEq/L).
- Dose adjustment of any medication to compensate for decreased renal perfusion, drug metabolism, etc.
- Infection.
  - The precipitating event in myxoedema coma/crisis is often overt or occult bacterial infection.
  - Fever and elevated white blood cell (WBC) count are usually absent, although a left shift and/or bands may be observed.

- Pan-culture and initiate empiric broad-spectrum antibiotic treatment, which can be narrowed if the source of infection is identified.
- If culture results remain negative, antibiotics may be discontinued.

- Myocardial ischaemia [94].
  - Myocardial infarction may be the precipitating event in older patients, or it may subsequently occur.
  - Serial CK determinations with fractionation assist in the diagnosis and treatment of an acute coronary event. CK levels are often elevated in myxoedema coma/crisis but are usually of muscle origin.
  - If ischemia or infarction is diagnosed, or if the patient has significant risk factors for coronary artery disease, institute thyroid replacement at low doses.
- Volume status.
  - Intravenous glucose and normal saline should be carefully administered, because patients are usually volume overloaded and prone to congestive heart failure from the reduced cardiac function of hypothyroidism. If severely hyponatraemic (sodium level <120 mEq/L), consider administration of small amounts of hypertonic saline followed by intravenous furosemide to improve volume status.
  - Generally, hypotension is resistant to the usual drugs until thyroid hormone and glucocorticoids (if insufficient) are administered. If hypotension does not improve with prudent fluid replacement, whole blood can be transfused. Finally, cautious administration of dopamine can be used.

## Further Outpatient Care

Follow-up care is necessary to ensure compliance with thyroid hormone replacement.

- If primary hypothyroidism was diagnosed, assess the TSH level every 6 weeks and adjust the T4 dose. Once a normal TSH level is obtained, it may be monitored yearly. If compliance is an issue, check the patient every 3–6 months.
- In hypothyroidism secondary to pituitary dysfunction, monitor free T4 levels. The TSH level is not an accurate measure of thyroid function.
- Obtain assurance that the precipitants of the initial presentation will not recur.
- Patients with risk factors for coronary artery disease should be carefully monitored to ensure that an acute ischaemic event is neither a precipitant of myxoedema coma/crisis nor a consequence of treatment.

## Postpartum Thyroditis

Postpartum thyroiditis is a phenomenon observed following pregnancy [95] and may involve hyperthyroidism, hypothyroidism or the two sequentially. It affects about 5 % of all women within a year after giving birth. The first phase is typically hyperthyroidism. Then, the thyroid either returns to normal or a woman develops hypothyroidism. Of those women who experience hypothyroidism associated with postpartum thyroiditis, one in five will develop permanent hypothyroidism requiring lifelong treatment.

Postpartum thyroiditis is believed to result from the modifications to the immune system necessary in pregnancy and histologically is a subacute lymphocytic thyroiditis. The process is normally self-limiting, but when conventional antibodies are found, there is a high chance of this proceeding to permanent hypothyroidism. Postpartum thyroiditis is a member of the group of thyroiditis conditions known as resolving thyroiditis.

## Signs and Symptoms

The initial phase of hyperthyroid symptoms occurs transiently about 2–6 months postpartum [84]. Typical symptoms include fatigue, irritability, nervousness, palpitations and heat intolerance.

Hormonal disturbances during this phase tend to occur with lower intensity compared with the hypothyroid phase [84]. As a result, the hyperthyroid phase may pass undetected. The second phase of hypothyroid symptoms is also transient and can occur anytime within the 3- to 12-month period postpartum [84]. Women in this phase experience low energy, poor memory, impaired concentration, carelessness, dry skin, cold intolerance and general aches and pains. After 1 year postpartum, euthyroid function resumes. Any case with hypothyroid symptoms extending beyond 1 year postpartum is not considered postpartum thyroiditis [84].

Women who test positive for thyroid antibodies may be at increased risk of developing symptoms associated with postpartum depression than women without thyroid antibodies [96].

## Prevalence

Worldwide reporting of postpartum thyroiditis cases is highly varied. This variation may be due to methodological discrepancies in assessing women for this condition [97]. Factors such as length of follow-up after delivery, diagnostic criteria, frequency of postpartum blood sampling and thyroid hormone assay methodology [98] likely contribute to this variation. On average, 5–7 % of pregnant women from most iodine-replete populations develop this condition [97].

Women with type I diabetes mellitus have a threefold increase in the prevalence of postpartum thyroiditis than nondiabetic women in the same region [84].

## Etiology

During pregnancy, immunologic suppression occurs which induces tolerance to the presence of the fetus [97]. Without this suppression, the fetus would be rejected causing miscarriage [97]. As a result, following delivery, the immune system rebounds causing levels of thyroids antibodies to rise in susceptible women [98].

Specifically, the immunohistological features of susceptible women are indicated by [97]:

- Antibodies to thyroglobulin (TgAb)
- Antibodies to thyroid peroxidase (TPOAb)
- Increase in TPOAb subclasses IgG1–IgG3
- Lymphocyte infiltration and follicle formation within thyroid gland (Hashimoto's thyroiditis)
- T-cell changes (increased CD4:CD8 ratio)
- TSH-receptor antibodies (TSH-R Abs)

## Diagnosis

This condition is commonly undiagnosed by physicians due to either unfamiliarity with the disease, the subtlety of symptoms or the attribution of the symptoms to the stresses of having a newborn [99]. Usual screening begins with assessing the thyroid-stimulating hormone (TSH) level. A suppressed TSH could represent the hyperthyroid phase but warrants further testing to investigate for possible Graves' disease [99]. A normal TSH with persistent symptoms could represent the shift between phases and requires repeat testing 4–6 weeks later; an elevated TSH at this time could indicate the hypothyroid phase [99].

## Treatment

For most women, the hyperthyroid phase presents with very mild symptoms or is asymptomatic; intervention is usually not required. If symptomatic cases require treatment, a short course of beta-blockers would be effective [84].

Assessing treatment for the hypothyroid is more complex. Women with symptoms or a very high TSH level or both are usually prescribed a course of levothyroxine [84]. Asymptomatic women with slightly elevated TSH levels who are planning subsequent pregnancies should consider a course of treatment until completion of the family to avoid possible developmental complications in future children [84]. Otherwise, treatment could be discontinued after 1 year postpartum.

## Conclusion

Pregnancy has profound effects on the regulation of thyroid function in healthy women and patients with thyroid disorders. These effects need to be recognized, precisely assessed, clearly interpreted and correctly managed. For healthy pregnant women who reside in areas with a restricted iodine intake, relative hypothyroxinaemia and goitrogenesis occur frequently, indicating that pregnancy constitutes a challenge for the thyroidal economy.

Overt thyroid dysfunction occurs in 2–3 % of pregnancies, but subclinical thyroid dysfunction (both hyper- and hypothyroidism) is probably more prevalent and frequently remains undiagnosed, unless specific screening programs are initiated to disclose thyroid function abnormalities in early gestation. Maternal alterations of thyroid function due to iodine deficiency, hypothyroidism and hyperthyroidism have important implications for fetal/neonatal outcome. In recent years, particular attention has been focused on potential developmental risks for the fetuses of women with subclinical hypothyroidism during early gestation. These include obstetric problems and the possibility of impaired neurodevelopment.

Pregnancy increases the metabolic rate, blood flow, heart rate and cardiac output and various subjective sensations such as fatigue and heat intolerance that may suggest the possibility of coexistent thyrotoxicosis. Other metabolic changes which also impact the hypothalamic pituitary-thyroid system are the potential direct stimulation of the maternal thyroid by hCG, as well as the accelerated metabolism of thyroxine, presumably due to increased placental deiodination enzymes.

In patients with hypothyroidism, it is important to recognize that therapeutic requirements for exogenous thyroxine are increased by 50 % on average during pregnancy. This should be taken into account in the management of such patients.

Main causes of thyrotoxicosis in pregnancy include Graves' disease (uncommon, but potentially pregnancy-threatening) and gestational non-autoimmune transient hyperthyroidism (more common, but remaining mild usually). The natural history of Graves' disease is altered during pregnancy, with a tendency for exacerbation in 1st trimester, amelioration during 2nd and 3rd trimesters and typically a rebound during the postpartum period. These changes are the consequences of partial immune suppression during gestation with a rebound during the postpartum period. This must be kept in mind when treating thyrotoxic patients, since all ATD cross the placenta and may affect fetal thyroid function. PTU is now recommended only for 1st trimester and MMI for the rest of pregnancy.

Fetal and neonatal hyperthyroidism is due to the transplacental transfer of maternal stimulating TSH-receptor antibodies (TRAb). The diagnosis of fetal (and neonatal) hyperthyroidism is usually made on the basis of fetal tachycardia, accelerated bone age and intrauterine growth retardation. It may occur in infants born to women with active Graves' disease, but also to women who have had prior definitive cure of their disease by surgery or radioactive iodine, but maintain high titres of TRAb. The proper management of pregnant patients with Graves' disease remains a difficult challenge in clinical endocrinology.

Thyroid nodules discovered during pregnancy should be aspirated for cytological diagnosis. If a malignancy is diagnosed, surgery should be performed during pregnancy or shortly thereafter. Pregnancy by itself does may not adversely affect the natural history of differentiated thyroid carcinoma.

During the postpartum period, particular attention should be given to women with thyroid autoimmunity, since hypothyroidism and hyperthyroidism are frequently exacerbated in the months following the delivery.

Antenatal screening for thyroid dysfunction is being actively discussed by the thyroid community. At present evidence-based studies are very limited and do not support this strategy. However many clinics worldwide are currently screening for thyroid dysfunction. Dialogue between endocrinologist and obstetrician is important in this regard. The results of further randomized trials are awaited.

## References


1. Mannisto T, Vaarasmaki M, Pouta A, et al. Perinatal outcome of children born to mothers with thyroid dysfunction or antibodies: a prospective population based cohort study. J Clin Endocrinal Metabol. 2009;94:772.
2. Smallridge RC, Glinoer D, Hollowell JG, Brent G. Thyroid function inside and outside of pregnancy: what do we know and what don't we know? Thyroid. 2005;15:54. Fig 1 http://www.houstonendocrine.com/.
3. Thorpe-Beeston JG, Nicolaides KH, Snijders RJM, et al. Fetal thyroid stimulating hormone response to maternal administration of thyrotropin releasing hormone. Am J Obstet Gynecol. 1991;164:1244.
4. Glinoer D, de Nayer P, Bourdoux P, et al. Regulation of maternal thyroid during pregnancy. J Clin Endocrinol Metab. 1990;71:276.
5. Grossman M, Weintraub BD, Szkudlinski MW. Novel insights into the molecular mechanisms of human thyrotropin action: structural, physiological and therapeutic implications for the glycoprotein family. Endocr Rev. 1997;18:476.
6. Calvo RM, Jauniaux E, Gulbis B, et al. Fetal tissues are exposed to biologically relevant free thyroxin concentrations during early phases of development. J Clin Endocrinol Metab. 2000;160:526.
7. Bernal J. Thyroid hormone receptors in brain development and function. Nat Clin Pract Endocrinol Metab. 2007;3(3):249.
8. Thorpe-Beeston JG, Nicolaides KH, Snijders RJM, et al. Thyroid function in small for gestational age foetuses. Obstet Gynecol. 1991;77:701. Table -1 www.thyroidmanager.org/chapter/thyroid-regulation-and-dysfunction-in-the-pregnant-patient/.
9. Marx H, Amin P, Lazarus JH. Hyperthyroidism and pregnancy. BMJ (Clin Res Ed). 2008;336(7645):663–7. doi:10.1136/bmj.39462.709005.AE.PMC 2270981.
10. Zimmerman D. Fetal and neonatal hyperthyroidism. Thyroid. 1999;9:727–33.
11. Polak M, Le Gac I, Vuillard E, et al. Fetal and neonatal thyroid function in relation to maternal Graves' disease. Best Pract Res Clin Endocrinol Metab. 2004;18:289–302.
12. Luewan S, Chakkabut P, Tongsong T. Outcomes of pregnancy complicated with hyperthyroidism: a cohort study. Arch Gynecol Obstet. 2010;20.
13. Luton D, Le Gac I, Noel M, et al. Thyroid function during pregnancy in women with past Graves' disease. BJOG. 2005;112(11):1565–7.
14. Gartner R. Thyroid diseases in pregnancy. Curr Opin Obstet Gynecol. 2009;21(6):501–7.
15. Patil Sisodia K, Mestman JH. Graves hyperthyroidism and pregnancy: a clinical update. Endocr Pract. 2010;16(1):118–29.
16. Glinoer D, Cooper DS. The propylthiouracil dilemma. Curr Opin Endocrinol Diabetes Obes. 2012;19(5):402–7. doi:10.1097/MED.0b013e3283565b49.
17. Marx H, Amin P, Lazarus JH. Hyperthyroidism and pregnancy. BMJ. 2008;336(7645):663–7.
18. Azizi F, Amouzegar A. Management of hyperthyroidism during pregnancy and lactation. Eur J Endocrinol. 2011;164(6):871–6. Epub 2011 Mar 9.
19. Maguire D, et al. Hyperemesis gravidarum and gestational hyperthyroidism. Endocr Abstr. 2007;13:342.
20. Kung AWC, Jones BM. A change from stimulatory to blocking antibody activity in Graves' disease during pregnancy. J Clin Endocrinol Metab. 1998;83:514.
21. Diav-Citrin O, Ornoy A. Teratogen update: antithyroid drugs-methimazole, carbimazole, and propylthiouracil. Teratology. 2002;65:38.
22. Di Gianantonio E, Schaefer C, Mastroiacovo PP, et al. Adverse effects of prenatal methimazole exposure. Teratology. 2001;64(5):262.
23. Brent GA. Graves' disease. N Engl J Med. 2008;358:2594.
24. Helfgott SM. Weekly clinicopathological exercises: case 21–2002. N Engl J Med. 2002;347:122.
25. Singer PA, Cooper DS, Levy EG, et al. Treatment guidelines for patients with hyperthyroidism and hypothyroidism. Standards of Care Committee, American Thyroid Association. JAMA. 1995;273:808–12.
26. National Academy of Clinical Biochemistry, NACB. Laboratory support for the diagnosis and monitoring of thyroid disease. Washington: National Academy of Clinical Biochemistry; 2002. p. 125.
27. Davison S, Lennard TWJ, Davison J, et al. Management of a pregnant patient with Graves' disease complicated by thionamide induced neutropenia in the first trimester. Clin Endocrinol. 2001;54:559.
28. Berg GEB, Nystrom EH, Jacobson L, et al. Radioiodine treatment of hyperthyroidism in a pregnant woman. J Nucl Med. 1998;39:357.
29. Berlin L. Malpractice issues in radiology: Iodine-131 and the pregnant patient. AJR Am J Roentgenol. 2001;176:869.
30. Ayala C, Navarro E, Rodriguez JR, et al. Conception after iodine-131 therapy for differentiated thyroid cancer. Thyroid. 1998;8:1009.
31. Casara D, Rubello D, Saladini G, et al. Pregnancy after high therapeutic doses of iodine-131 in differentiated thyroid cancer: potential risks and recommendations. Eur J Nucl Med. 1993;20:192.
32. Weetman AP. Graves' disease. N Engl J Med. 2000;343:1236–48 (Level III).
33. Tietgens ST, Leinung MC. Thyroid storm. Med Clin North Am. 1995;79:169–84.
34. Wing DA, Leung AS, et al. Low birth weight and preeclampsia in pregnancies complicated by hyperthyroidism. Obstet Gynecol. 1994;84:946–9.
35. Sherwen LN, Scoloveno MA, Weingarten CT. Maternity nursing: care of the childbearing family. 3rd ed. Stamford: Appleton & Lange; 1999.
36. Gabbe SG, Niebyl JR, Simpson JL. Obstetrics: normal and problem pregnancies. 3rd ed. New York: Churchill Livingstone; 1996.

37. Cunningham FG, Leveno KJ, Gilstrap LC, Hauth JC, Wenstrom KD. Williams obstetrics. 21st ed. New York: McGraw-Hill; 2000.
38. Fisher D. Fetal thyroid function: diagnosis and management of fetal thyroid disorders. Clin Obstet Gynecol. 1997;40:16–21.
39. American College of Obstetrics and Gynecology. ACOG practice bulletin: thyroid disease in pregnancy. No. 37, August 2002. American College of Obstetrics and Gynecology. Int J Gynaecol Obstet. 2002;79:171–80.
40. Mestman JH. Hyperthyroidism in pregnancy. Endocrinol Metab Clin North Am. 1998;27:127–49.
41. Levin RM. Thyroid disease in pregnancy [on-line course]. January 15, 2001. Available at:http://www.bumc.bu.edu/www/busm/cme/modules/thyroid_10–99/bcs.htm. Accessed 2 July 2002.
42. Mestman JH. Diagnosis and management of maternal and fetal thyroid disorders. Curr Opin Obstet Gynecol. 1999;11:167–75.
43. Mazzaferri EL. Evaluation and management of common thyroid disorders in women. Am J Obstet Gynecol. 1997;176:507–14.
44. Ecker JL, Musci TJ. Treatment of thyroid disease in pregnancy. Obstet Gynecol Clin North Am. 1997;24:575–89.
45. http://www.ncbi.nlm.nih.gov/pubmed/16449121.
46. Bahn Chair RS, Burch HB, Cooper DS, Garber JR, Greenlee MC, Klein I, et al. Hyperthyroidism and other causes of thyrotoxicosis: management guidelines of the American Thyroid Association and American Association of Clinical Endocrinologists. Thyroid. 2011;21(6):593–646. doi:10.1089/thy.2010.0417.
47. Fatourechi V. Upper limit of normal serum thyroid-stimulating hormone: a moving and now an aging target? J Clin Endocrinol Metab. 2007;92(12): 4560–2. doi:10.1210/jc.2007-2285.
48. Surks MI, Hollowell JG. Age-specific distribution of serum thyrotropin and antithyroid antibodies in the US population: implications for the prevalence of subclinical hypothyroidism. J Clin Endocrinol Metab. 2007;92(12):4575–82. doi:10.1210/jc.2007-1499.
49. Galofré JC, Frühbeck G, Salvador J. Obesity and thyroid function: pathophysiological and therapeutic implications. Hot Thyroidal. 6/10, Online ISSN: 2075–2202, p 7.
50. Brabant G, Prank K, Ranft U, Schuermeyer Th, Wagner TOF, Hauser H, Kummer B, Feistner H, Hesch RD, and von zur Mühlen A. Physiologic regulation of circadian and pulsatile thyrotropin secretion in normal men and women. J Clin Endocrinol Metab. 2013:70(2). doi:10.1210\jcem-70-2-403.
51. Mitchell AL, Pearce SH. How should we treat patients with low serum thyrotropin concentrations? Clin Endocrinol (Oxf). 2010;72(3):292–6. doi:10.1111/j.1365-2265.2009.03694.x.
52. Klein I, Danzi S. Thyroid disease and the heart. Circulation. 2007;116(15):1725–35. doi:10.1161/CIRCULATIONAHA.106.678326.
53. Wartofsky L. Management of subclinical hyperthyroidism. J Clin Endocrinol Metab. 2011;96(1): 59–61. doi:10.1210/jc.2010-2409.
54. American College of Obstetricians and Gynecologists. Thyroid disease in pregnancy. Practice Bulletin No. 37. London: COLLEGE Publication; 2002.
55. Abalovich M, Gutierrez S, Alcaraz G, Maccallini G, Garcia A, Levalle O. Overt and subclinical hypothyroidism complicating pregnancy. Thyroid. 2002;12:63.
56. Klein RZ, Haddow JE, Faix JD, Brown RS, Hermos RJ, Pulkkinen A, Mitchell ML. Prevalence of thyroid deficiency in pregnant women. Clin Endocrinol (Oxf). 1991;35(1):41–6. doi:10.1111/j.1365-2265.1991.tb03494.x.
57. Mandel SJ. Hypothyroidism and chronic autoimmune thyroiditis in the pregnant state: maternal aspects. Best Pract Res Clin Endocrinol Metab. 2004;18(2):213–24. doi:10.1016/j.beem.2004.03.006.
58. Glinoer D, Soto MF, Bourdoux P, Lejeune B, Delange F, Lemone M, Kinthaert J, Robijn C, Grun JP, de Nayer P. Pregnancy in patients with mild thyroid abnormalities: maternal and neonatal repercussions. J Clin Endocrinol Metab. 1991;73(2):421–7. doi:10.1210/jcem-73-2-421.PMID 1906897.
59. Davis LE, Leveno KJ, Cunningham FG. Hypothyroidism complicating pregnancy. Obstet Gynecol. 1988;72(1):108–12.
60. Casey BM, Dashe JS, Wells CE, McIntire DD, Byrd W, Leveno KJ, Cunningham FG. Subclinical hypothyroidism and pregnancy outcomes. Obstet Gynecol. 2005;105(2):239–45. doi:10.1097/01.AOG.0000152345.99421.22.PMID 15684146.
61. Stagnaro-Green A, Chen X, Bogden JD, Davies TF, Scholl TO. The thyroid and pregnancy: a novel risk factor for very preterm delivery. Thyroid: Off J Am Thyroid Assoc. 2005;15(4):351–7. doi:10.1089/thy.2005.15.351.PMID 15876159.
62. Negro R, Formoso G, Mangieri T, Pezzarossa A, Dazzi DH, Hassan H. Levothyroxine treatment in euthyroid pregnant women with autoimmune thyroid disease: effects on obstetrical complications. J Clin Endocrinol Metab. 2006;91(7):2587–91. doi:10.1210/jc.2005-1603.
63. Haddow JE, Palomaki GE, Allan WC, Williams JR, Knight GJ, Gagnon J, O'Heir CE, Mitchell ML, Hermos RJ, Waisbren SE, Faix JD, Klein RZ. Maternal thyroid deficiency during pregnancy and subsequent neuropsychological development of the child. N Engl J Med. 1999;341(8):549–55. doi:10.1056/NEJM199908193410801.
64. Pop VJ, Brouwers EP, Vader HL, Vulsma T, van Baar AL, de Vijlder JJ. Maternal hypothyroxinaemia during early pregnancy and subsequent child development: a 3-year follow-up study. Clin Endocrinol (Oxf). 2003;59(3):282–8. doi:10.1046/j.1365-2265.2003.01822.x.
65. Pop VJ, de Vries E, van Baar AL, Waelkens JJ, de Rooy HA, Horsten M, Donkers MM, Komproe IH,

van Son MM, Vader HL. Maternal thyroid peroxidase antibodies during pregnancy: a marker of impaired child development? J Clin Endocrinol Metab. 1995;80(12):3561–6. doi:10.1210/jcem.80.12.8530599.
66. Casey BM, Dashe JS, Spong CY, McIntire DD, Leveno KJ, Cunningham GF. Perinatal significance of isolated maternal hypothyroxinemia identified in the first half of pregnancy. Obstet Gynecol. 2007;109(5):1129–35. doi:10.1097/01.AOG.0000262054.03531.24.
67. Cleary-Goldman J, Malone FD, Lambert-Messerlian G, Sullivan L, Canick J, Porter TF, Luthy D, Gross S, Bianchi DW, D'Alton ME. Maternal thyroid hypofunction and pregnancy outcome. Obstet Gynecol. 2008;112(1):85–92. doi:10.1097/AOG.0b013e3181788dd7.
68. Abalovich M, Amino N, Barbour LA, Cobin RH, De Groot LJ, Glinoer D, Mandel SJ, Stagnaro-Green A. Management of thyroid dysfunction during pregnancy and postpartum: an Endocrine Society Clinical Practice Guideline. J Clin Endocrinol Metab. 2007;92(8 Suppl):S1–47. doi:10.1210/jc.2007-0141. PMID 17948378.
69. Velkeniers B, Van Meerhaeghe A, Poppe K, Unuane D, Tournaye H, Haentjens P. Levothyroxine treatment and pregnancy outcome in women with subclinical hypothyroidism undergoing assisted reproduction technologies: systematic review and meta-analysis of RCTs. Hum Reprod Update. 2013;19(3):251–8. doi:10.1093/humupd/dms052.
70. Pop VJ, Kuijpens JL, van Baar AL, Verkerk G, van Son MM, de Vijlder JJ, et al. Low maternal free thyroxine concentrations during early pregnancy are associated with impaired psychomotor development in infancy. Clin Endocrinol (Oxf). 1999;50(2):149–55.
71. Stagnaro-Green A, Chen X, Bogden JD, Davies TF, Scholl TO. The thyroid and pregnancy: a novel risk factor for very preterm delivery. Thyroid. 2005;15(4):351–7.
72. Dhanwal DK, Prasad S, Agarwal AK, Dixit V, Banerjee AK. High prevalence of subclinical hypothyroidism during first trimester of pregnancy in North India. Indian J Endocrinol Metab. 2013;17(2):281–4.
73. Fatourechi V. Subclinical hypothyroidism: an update for primary care physicians. Mayo Clin Proc. 2009;84(1):65–71.
74. Steingold KA, Matt DW, DeZiegler D, Sealey JE, Fratkin M, Reznikov S. Comparison of transdermal to oral estradiol administration on hormonal and hepatic parameters in women with premature ovarian failure. J Clin Endocrinol Metab. 1991;73(2):275–80.
75. Sapolsky RM, Krey LC, McEwen BS. The neuroendocrinology of stress and aging: the glucocorticoid cascade hypothesis. Endocr Rev. 1986;7(3):284–301.
76. Ongphiphadhanakul B, Fang SL, Tang KT, Patwardhan NA, Braverman LE. Tumor necrosis factor-alpha decreases thyrotropin-induced 5′-deiodinase activity in FRTL-5 thyroid cells. Eur J Endocrinol. 1994;130(5):502–7.
77. Yeum CH, Kim SW, Kim NH, Choi KC, Lee J. Increased expression of aquaporin water channels in hypothyroid rat kidney. Pharmacol Res. 2002;46(1):85–8.
78. Samuels MH. Cognitive function in untreated hypothyroidism and hyperthyroidism. Curr Opin Endocrinol Diabetes Obes. 2008;15(5):429–33.
79. Gharib H, Cobin RH, Dickey RA. Subclinical hypothyroidism during pregnancy: position statement from the American Association of Clinical Endocrinologists. Endocr Pract. 1999;5(6):367–8.
80. Baisier WV, Hertoghe J, Eeckhaut W. Thyroid insufficiency. Is TSH measurement the only diagnostic tool? J Nutr Environ Med. 2000;10(2):105–13.
81. Christ-Crain M, Meier C, Huber PR, Staub JJ, Muller B. Effect of l-thyroxine replacement therapy on surrogate markers of skeletal and cardiac function in subclinical hypothyroidism. Endocrinologist. 2004;14(3):161–6.
82. Wilson KL, Casey BM, McIntire DD, Halvorson LM, Cunningham FG. Subclinical thyroid disease and the incidence of hypertension in pregnancy. Obstet Gynecol. 2012;119(2 Pt 1):315–20.
83. Wier FA, Farley CL. Clinical controversies in screening women for thyroid disorders during pregnancy. J Midwifery Womens Health. 2006;51(3):152–8.
84. Stagnaro-Green A. Postpartum thyroiditis. Best Pract Res Clin Endocrinol Metab. 2004;18(2):303–16. doi:10.1016/j.beem.2004.03.008.
85. van der Zanden M, Hop-de Groot RJ, Sweep FC, Ross HA, den Heijer M, Spaanderman ME. Subclinical hypothyroidism after vascular complicated pregnancy. Hypertens Pregnancy. 2013;32(1):1–10.
86. Stagnaro-Green A, Abalovich M, Alexander E, Azizi F, Mestman J, Negro R, et al.; American Thyroid Association Taskforce on Thyroid Disease During Pregnancy and Postpartum. Guidelines of the American Thyroid Association for the diagnosis and management of thyroid disease during pregnancy and postpartum. Thyroid. 2011;21(10):1081–125.
87. http://www.ncbi.nlm.nih.gov/pubmed/19940773.
88. Nicoloff JT, LoPresti JS. Myxedema coma. A form of decompensated hypothyroidism. Endocrinol Metab Clin North Am. 1993;22(2):279–90.
89. Rehman SU, Cope DW, Senseney AD, et al. Thyroid disorders in elderly patients. South Med J. 2005;98(5):543–9.
90. Yamamoto T, Fukuyama J, Fujiyoshi A. Factors associated with mortality of myxedema coma: report of eight cases and literature survey. Thyroid. 1999;9(12):1167–74.
91. Hylander B, Rosenqvist U. Treatment of myxoedema coma – factors associated with fatal outcome. Acta Endocrinol (Copenh). 1985;108(1):65–71.

92. Rodríguez I, Fluiters E, Pérez-Méndez LF, et al. Factors associated with mortality of patients with myxoedema coma: prospective study in 11 cases treated in a single institution. J Endocrinol. 2004; 180(2):347–50.
93. Jordan RM. Myxedema coma. Pathophysiology, therapy, and factors affecting prognosis. Med Clin North Am. 1995;79(1):185–94.
94. Taguchi T, Iwasaki Y, Asaba K, et al. Myxedema coma and cardiac ischemia in relation to thyroid hormone replacement therapy in a 38-year-old Japanese woman. Clin Ther. 2007;29(12): 2710–4.
95. Muller AF, Drexhage HA, Berghout A. Postpartum thyroiditis and autoimmune thyroiditis in women of childbearing age: recent insights and consequences for antenatal and postnatal care. Endocr Rev. 2001;22(5):605–30. doi:10.1210/er.22.5.605.
96. Bokhari R, Bhatara VS, Bandettini F, McMillan JM. Postpartum psychosis and postpartum thyroiditis. Psychoneuroendocrinology. 1998;23(6):643–50. doi:10.1016/S0306-4530(98)00034-1.
97. Premawardhana LDKE, Parkes AB, Lazarus JH. Thyroiditis, postpartum. In: Martini L, editor. Encyclopedia of endocrine diseases. New York: Elsevier; 2004. p. 509–14. doi:10.1016/B0-12-475570-4/01299-3.
98. http://www.thyroidmanager.org/Chapter6/Ch-6-2.htm.
99. Stagnaro-Green A. Recognizing, understanding, and treating postpartum thyroiditis. Endocrinol Metab Clin N Am. 2000;29(2):417–30. doi:10.1016/S0889-8529(05)70140-7.

# 14 Other Endocrine Emergencies in Pregnancy

Anita Singh and Shipra Singh

## Introduction

Endocrine emergencies in pregnancy are rare and are more likely to occur in the absence of good obstetric care. Because of their rare occurrence, these entities are often not suspected and diagnosed timely, thus leading to serious consequences in the form of increased fetal and maternal morbidity and mortality. Thyroid- and diabetes-related events in pregnancy are more common because of their higher prevalence in the normal population. Pituitary, adrenal, and parathyroid hormonal complications in pregnancy are relatively rare. A high index of suspicion is needed for early diagnosis, and medical treatment is directed primarily at maintaining maternal hemodynamic stability. A close liaison between an endocrinologist, maternal-fetal specialist, and intensivist is critical in optimizing both maternal and fetal outcomes. A brief description of prevalence, etiology, clinical features, diagnosis, and management of parathyroid, pituitary, and adrenal diseases presenting as emergencies in pregnancy has been dealt with in the following chapter.

A. Singh (✉)
Ex. Professor Department of Obstetrics and Gynaecology, Patna Medical College, Patna, India

Chief Consultant, Jyoti Punj Hospital, Boring Road, Patna, India
e-mail: anitasinghob@gmail.com

S. Singh
Consultant, Jyoti Punj Hospital, Boring Road, Patna, India

## Hyperparathyroidism

Primary hyperparathyroidism occurs rarely during pregnancy; its true incidence remains unknown because it may remain unnoticed and go undiagnosed in uncomplicated pregnancies. Hyperparathyroidism in a pregnant patient can cause considerable morbidity in the mother and the fetus. Complications have been reported in 67 % of mothers and 80 % of fetus and neonates [1].

The diagnosis of hyperparathyroidism is difficult during pregnancy because of normal pregnancy-induced changes that decrease total serum calcium and suppress parathormone. An increased serum ionized calcium level and detectable parathormone indicate primary hyperparathyroidism in most cases.

**Etiology:** a series of 100 cases of hyperparathyroidism diagnosed during pregnancy or post delivery revealed adenomas in 89 %, hyperplasia in 9 %, and carcinoma in 2 % [2].


A. Gandhi et al. (eds.), *Principles of Critical Care in Obstetrics: Volume II*,
DOI 10.1007/978-81-322-2686-4_14

## Manifestations and Complications in Pregnant Women

Symptoms include nausea, vomiting abdominal pain, renal colic, generalized muscular weakness, and mental disturbances. Other symptoms include hyperemesis gravidarum, weight loss, and generalized seizures. Many of these symptoms can be attributed to pregnancy itself. Objective findings include nephrolithiasis and nephrocalcinosis, urinary tract infections, bone disease on radiograph, and pancreatitis. Pancreatitis usually occurs in second and third trimesters and may be associated with hypercalcemic crisis [3]. Acute parathyroid crisis has been reported during pregnancy and postpartum which may prove fatal [4, 5]. Susceptibility to fractures increases drastically. Bilateral femoral neck fractures and rib fractures have been reported [6, 7].

## Complications in Fetus

The most frequently reported serious complications include stillbirths, miscarriages, and neonatal tetany. However the incidence of these complications has declined over the decades due to early recognition of maternal disease and proper management. Neonatal tetany mainly presents in cases of unrecognized maternal hyperthyroidism.

## Management

Parathyroidectomy performed during pregnancy prevents fetal and neonatal morbidities. Surgery is best performed during second trimester, after completion of organogenesis in fetus and to avoid poor outcome of surgery in the third trimester [8, 9]. Mild asymptomatic disease diagnosed in the third trimester may be managed expectantly until after delivery.

Medical treatment includes adequate hydration and correction of electrolyte abnormalities [1]. Calcitonin, a pregnancy category B drug of US FDA, does not cross the placenta and has been used safely in pregnancy [1]. Oral phosphate a pregnancy category C medication has been used in pregnancy; its most common side effects are diarrhea and hypokalemia. It should be avoided in patients with renal failure or high serum phosphate because of the risk of soft tissue calcification [1]. Parathyroidectomy is recommended postpartum in cases that were followed medically during pregnancy. Lactation is not contraindicated in women with untreated hyperparathyroidism, but worsening of hypercalcemia and accelerated skeletal losses may be anticipated.

Neonatal hypoparathyroidism, secondary to maternal hyperparathyroidism, is usually transient. Treatment includes supplementation with calcium and calcitriol. These neonates should be fed with milk formulas high in calcium and low in phosphate to minimize the risk of hypocalcemia.

The prevalence and severity of complications from hyperparathyroidism in mother and neonates have and will continue to decrease overtime as a result of increased awareness, surveillance, timely intervention, improved surgical skills, and anesthetic technology [10].

# Pituitary Disorders during Pregnancy

Pituitary adenomas are common in women of reproductive age group, constituting 5.7 % of intracranial (malignant and nommalignant) neoplasms [11]. These adenomas may cause problems either due to oversecretion of hormones by the tumor or hypopituitarism. Hormonal dysfunction caused by pituitary adenomas may affect fertility and pregnancy outcome if pregnancy does ensue. In addition, the pregnancy itself alters hormone secretion and pituitary function, complicating the evaluation of patients with pituitary neoplasms.

During pregnancy, the normal pituitary gland enlarges considerably as a result of estrogen-mediated hyperplasia and hypertrophy of prolactin-producing lactotrophs [12, 13]. Concomitantly, prolactin levels increase gradually throughout gestation [14].

MRI scans of the pituitary during pregnancy show an increase in size secondary to lactotroph hyperplasia, with the peak size occurring in the first 3 days postpartum [15, 16]. This stimulatory effect of pregnancy on the pituitary has important implications for a patient with prolactinoma who desires pregnancy.

## Prolactinoma

In women with prolactinomas, the hormonal milieu of pregnancy may result in significant tumor enlargement during gestation. In an analysis of 376 women, only 1.3 % with microadenomas had symptoms of tumor enlargement. Symptomatic tumor enlargement was reported in 23.2 % with macroadenomas, while 2.8 % of previously surgically treated cases reported symptomatic tumor enlargement [17–19]. When tumor enlargement occurs, patients may present with acute severe headache and visual disturbances.

### Management

When there is evidence of tumor enlargement during pregnancy, bromocriptine and cabergoline therapy is usually successful in reducing the tumor size. If there is no response to medical therapy, transsphenoidal surgery or delivery should be considered [20, 21].

## Acromegaly

Reports of pregnancy in patients with acromegaly are uncommon. Hyperprolactinemia is seen in 30–40 % of cases of acromegaly [22]. Correction of hyperprolactinemia by bromocriptine might lead to pregnancy in these cases [23].

Diagnosis becomes difficult in pregnancy due to production of growth hormone by placenta. However, the pulsatile secretion of pituitary GH and its response to TRH helps to differentiate between the two [24].

### Effect of Pregnancy on Tumor Size in Acromegaly

Tumor enlargement and its manifestations are similar to that seen in cases of prolactinoma. Patients with acromegaly should be monitored for signs of tumor enlargement. There is some evidence that pregnancy may cause an exacerbation of acromegaly in a few cases [23], but the risk is not significant enough to advise against pregnancy.

### Effect of Acromegaly on Pregnancy

Carbohydrate intolerance occurs in up to 50 % of patients with acromegaly while 10–20 % of cases have overt diabetes [22]. Increased salt retention and subsequent hypertension are seen in 25–30 % of patients. Cardiac involvement is present in about a third of cases in the form of cardiomyopathy and coronary artery disease [22].

### Management

The considerations regarding the use of bromocriptine and cabergoline in women with prolactinomas also apply to women with acromegaly. These drugs should be discontinued during pregnancy in most cases. Octreotide and other somatostatin analogues should be largely discontinued if pregnancy is considered. Complications during pregnancy should be recognized early and managed accordingly.

## Cushing's Syndrome

Cushing's syndrome is uncommon in pregnancy and only a little more than 100 cases have been reported so far [25].

**Etiology:** <50 % – pituitary adenoma
<50 % – adrenal adenoma
>10 % – adrenal carcinoma
Rest – ectopic ACTH syndrome [26, 27]

In many cases, hypercortisolism first becomes apparent during pregnancy and improves after parturition. Rarely, recurrent Cushing's syndrome may only manifest during pregnancy but remits completely after delivery.

### Diagnosis of Cushing's Syndrome during Pregnancy

Diagnosing Cushing's syndrome may be difficult during pregnancy. Both conditions may be associated with weight gain in central distribution, fatigue, edema, emotional upset, glucose intolerance, and hypertension. The striae associated with weight gain are usually white in normal pregnancy and red or purple in Cushing's syndrome. Elevated levels of both total and free cortisol, ACTH levels, and urinary free cortisol excretion are present in normal pregnancy. The persistent circadian variation of elevated levels of total and free cortisol seen in pregnancy is characteristically absent in Cushing's syndrome. MRI of the pituitary (without contrast enhancement) or ultrasound scan of the adrenals may aid in diagnosis.

### Effect of Cushing's Syndrome on Pregnancy

Hypertension develops in most cases. Diabetes and myopathy are frequent. Postoperative wound infection and dehiscence are common after caesarean section [27, 28].

Cushing's syndrome is associated with fetal wastage, as high as 25 % from spontaneous abortions, still births, and early neonatal deaths because of extreme prematurity [25, 29]. Premature labor occurs in more than 50 % of cases regardless of cause [25, 29].

### Management of Cushing's Syndrome during Pregnancy

Treatment during pregnancy has been advocated to improve neonatal survival. Medical therapy for Cushing's syndrome during pregnancy is not very effective. A few case reports have documented the efficacy of metyrapone [25]. Transsphenoidal resection of pituitary ACTH secreting adenoma has been performed successfully in several patients during the second trimester [25]. The risks of not operating a case of Cushing's syndrome seem to be considerably higher than the risks of proceeding with surgery [30].

## Sheehan's Syndrome

Sheehan's syndrome consists of pituitary necrosis secondary to ischemia occurring within hours of delivery [31, 32]. It is usually secondary to hypovolemia and shock from an obstetric hemorrhage. Pituitary enlargement during pregnancy apparently predisposes to the risk of ischemia with intense spasm of the arteries to the anterior pituitary and stalk. Modern obstetric techniques have resulted in Sheehan's syndrome being rarely found in current practice [33].

Acute necrosis may present as an obstetric emergency in the form of hypotension and tachycardia persisting even after adequate replacement of blood products. The woman fails to lactate and may have hypoglycemia [31, 32].

Investigations include estimation of levels of ACTH, cortisol, prolactin, and free thyroxine. Thyroxine levels may be normal initially because the hormone has a half-life of 7 days. Prolactin levels are usually found to be low.

Treatment should be instituted promptly without waiting for laboratory reports. Saline infusion should be started and stress dose of corticosteroids administered.

Diabetes insipidus may also occur secondary to vascular occlusion with atrophy and scarring of neurohypophysis [34].

## Adrenal Disorders

The adrenal gland is a mixture of steroid hormone producing adrenal cortex (cortisol and aldosterone) and the adrenal medulla, responsible for secretion of catecholamines. The hypothalamic-pituitary axis is responsible for cortisol production while the renin-angiotensin system is vital for aldosterone secretion.

The hypothalamic-pituitary-adrenal axis and renin-angiotensin system are upregulated during normal pregnancy. There is hypercortisolism as a result of interaction of the maternal HPA axis and feto-placental unit. The RAS maintains normal sodium balance and volume homeostasis.

Adrenal disorders that occur during pregnancy cause significant maternal and fetal morbidity. The following adrenal disorders may present as an acute emergency during pregnancy, labor, and puerperium:

Cushing's syndrome
Primary adrenal insufficiency
Hyperaldosteronism
Pheochromocytoma

## Cushing's Syndrome

It has been dealt with earlier in the chapter.

## Adrenal Insufficiency in Pregnancy

Adrenal insufficiency may be attributed to primary adrenal disease or caused by a wide variety of pituitary hypothalamic disorders. Diseases causing primary adrenal insufficiency usually destroy the total adrenal cortex, thereby causing a deficiency of glucocorticoids, mineralocorticoids, and adrenal androgens. Occasionally the adrenal medulla also gets involved. Primary adrenal insufficiency therefore usually has an acute onset and characteristically prominent signs and symptoms than in cases of secondary insufficiency. Secondary adrenal insufficiency selectively causes glucocorticoid deficiency while mineralocorticoid function is better maintained. Secondary adrenal insufficiency thus rarely causes an acute-onset adrenal insufficiency crisis.

### Etiology of Adrenal Insufficiency

| Primary adrenal insufficiency | Secondary adrenal insufficiency |
|---|---|
| Autoimmune disease | Pituitary surgery, pituitary/brain trauma |
| Adrenal infections and inflammation | Acute interruption of prolonged glucocorticoid therapy |
| After adrenalectomy | |
| Adrenal hemorrhagic necrosis caused by meningococcal sepsis or coagulation disorders | |

### Presentation of Acute Adrenal Insufficiency (Adrenal Crisis)

Adrenal crisis is attributable to mineralocorticoid deficiency. The clinical presentation is dominated by hypotension or hypotensive shock, caused by sodium and plasma volume depletion. The associated prostaglandin excess (prostacyclin) and decreased responsiveness to norepinephrine and angiotensin II may aggravate the circulatory collapse. This clinical presentation is often preceded by acute abdominal pain or symptoms attributable to the etiology of acute adrenal insufficiency (e.g., sepsis, pituitary or adrenal hemorrhage or necrosis, surgery, or trauma).

### Atypical Presentations

A new case of adrenal insufficiency may present as excessive fatigue, malaise, weight loss, vomiting, orthostasis, abdominal pain, hyperpigmentation, or biochemical disturbances. Hypoglycemia, salt craving, malaise, seizures, and even coma may be the presenting symptoms. Severe hyponatremia or metabolic acidosis is associated with poor outcomes and fetal death, if not recognized and managed promptly.

### Maternal and Fetal Morbidity and Mortality

Adrenal insufficiency recognized in the antenatal period and managed properly does not cause severe maternal morbidity. Unrecognized adrenal insufficiency in pregnancy manifests in puerperium at the time when there is disruption of transplacental transfer of cortisol from fetus to mother [26]. Gestational adrenal insufficiency has been associated with high rates of intrauterine growth restriction [35, 36] and fetal mortality.

### Diagnosis of Acute Adrenal Insufficiency

One should be highly suspicious of adrenal crisis in case of unexplained hypotension, especially in high-risk patients (e.g., AIDS patients, patients with autoimmune disease, patients on prior glucocorticoid therapy). If acute adrenal insufficiency is suspected, simple diagnostic screening procedures should be used based on what is rapidly available. Immediate therapeutic intervention is required even before the diagnosis is formally confirmed. The following laboratory investigations should be done:

A. Serum analysis of:
   - Sodium, potassium, and bicarbonate
   - Plasma cortisol
   - Plasma corticotrophin, renin, and aldosterone

B. Corticotrophin stimulation test: 250 mcg of corticotrophin is administered IV followed by measurement of cortisol 30 min later. Adrenal crisis is highly unlikely if:
   - Basal total cortisol is greater than 20 mcg/dl.
   - Post corticotrophin cortisol is greater than 20 mcg/dl.

### Treatment of Adrenal Insufficiency

The immediate treatment of acute adrenal crisis rests upon correction of fluid and electrolyte imbalance and hydrocortisone replacement. Treatment should be started promptly after sending the lab samples. Initial therapeutic intervention includes the following:

- Infusion of sodium chloride 0.9 % and dextrose 5 %
- Hydrocortisone 100 mg IV or IM repeated every 8 h until the results of diagnostic screening tests are available.
- If diagnostic screening indicates:
  - Basal or post corticotrophin cortisol greater than 20 mcg/dl: further hydrocortisone therapy is stopped unless the patient is still critically ill.
  - Cortisol less than 20 mcg/dl: hydrocortisone therapy is continued by IV or IM route (150–300 mg/day for 2–3 days) until full recovery.
- Final diagnosis and evaluation of etiology are done after resolution of acute crisis.

### Management during Labor and Postpartum Period

Normal vaginal delivery can be expected for women with adrenal insufficiency. Indication for a caesarean section is similar to that in a normal pregnancy. During labor, the patient's normal dose of hydrocortisone is doubled. Alternatively, a single dose of hydrocortisone, 50 mg IV, may be administered during the second stage of labor. Before caesarean section, stress dose of hydrocortisone, 100 mg, is administered by IV or IM route at the onset of surgery and continued at intervals of 6–8 h following delivery. The dose is tapered over 48 h to regular replacement dose. Breast-feeding is not contraindicated for patients on treatment.

## Hyperaldosteronism

Primary hyperaldosteronism is rare in pregnancy with approximately 31 cases reported worldwide [37, 38]. The majority of reported cases may be due to an adrenal adenoma or hyperplasia.

Hyperaldosteronism in pregnancy is associated with hypertension and hypokalemia in a high proportion of cases. Symptoms include headache, fatigue, weakness, dizziness, and muscle cramps [39]. Pregnancy is characterized by moderate to severe hypertension, proteinuria, placental abruption, intra uterine fetal deaths, or preterm births which is mostly iatrogenic.

### Diagnosis

The diagnosis of hyperaldosteronism in pregnancy is challenging. The physiological rise of aldosterone in normal pregnancy overlaps the values seen in hyperaldosteronism. However, suppressed renin levels in this setting are confirmatory of hyperaldosteronism. Findings that aid in reaching a diagnosis include the following: elevated aldosterone levels and suppressed renin levels (imaging with MRI or ultrasonography).

### Management

Unilateral adrenalectomy in midtrimester is advocated for unilateral macroadenoma. Successful surgery results in normalization of elevated blood pressure as well as serum potassium in majority of cases. Medical therapy is advocated in cases of adrenal hyperplasia or adrenal adenoma identified late in pregnancy. Conventional antihypertensive therapy, otherwise considered safe in pregnancy, like methyldopa and calcium channel blockers, is not very effective. Drugs with specific aldosterone receptor blockade activity, e.g., spironolactone and amiloride, are largely contraindicated in pregnancy.

## Pheochromocytoma

Pheochromocytoma is a paraganglioma, a rare catecholamine-producing tumor derived from chromaffin cells that can be fatal if left untreated. They occur mainly in adrenals and less commonly in extra adrenal sites. Twenty-four percent of pheochromocytomas have hereditary basis.

The prevalence of pheochromocytoma at term is approximately 1 in 54,000 [40, 41].

Characteristically, patients present with sustained or paroxysmal episodes of hypertension, headache, palpitations, and pallor. The triad of headache, palpitations, and sweating is often seen. Emergency situations occur owing to high levels of catecholamines secreted by the tumor. Antenatal diagnosis results in improved outcomes but pheochromocytoma can be missed because of unexpectedly normal blood pressure during gestation [40, 42].

Pheochromocytoma can be present as an acute emergency in varied ways:

1. Multisystem failure: a temperature greater than 40° centigrade, encephalopathy, hypertension or hypotension, pulmonary edema, acute renal failure, and DIC. The clinical features may be mistaken for septicemia.
2. Cardiovascular emergencies: hypertensive crisis, shock, hypotension, acute heart failure, myocardial infarction, arrhythmias, cardiomyopathy, myocarditis, dissection of aortic aneurysm, and acute peripheral edema.
3. Pulmonary emergencies: infrequently, pulmonary edema is the presenting feature of pheochromocytoma which may be cardiogenic or noncardiogenic in origin.
4. Gastrointestinal emergencies: severe abdominal pain and vomiting may indicate hemorrhage of the tumor or spasm of mesenteric arteries causing bowel ischemia.
5. Nephrogenic emergencies: rarely pheochromocytoma may present as acute renal failure.
6. Neurological emergencies: cerebral hemorrhage, subarachnoid hemorrhage, and seizures have been reported during attacks of paroxysmal hypertension.

If pheochromocytoma is unsuspected in pregnancy, it can lead to very high rates of morbidity and mortality. Pregnancy-related life-threatening situations can occur owing to tumor stimulation by pressure from enlarging uterus, by fetal movements, by abdominal palpation, or during labor in a patient with unsuspected pheochromocytoma. In one series, diagnosis made in antenatal period reduced maternal and fetal mortality to 1 and 15 %, respectively [43].

### Diagnosis

Diagnosis of pheochromocytoma in pregnancy can be difficult because the clinical features resemble preeclampsia. But in contrast to preeclampsia, hypertension in pheochromocytoma can occur throughout pregnancy. Edema and proteinuria are often absent. Furthermore, pheochromocytoma-associated hypertension is paroxysmal and may be accompanied by postural hypotension [41]. New sensitive and specific biochemical tests and imaging aid in reaching the diagnosis.

Fractionated urinary metanephrines and plasma metanephrines estimation are sensitive tests for diagnosis of pheochromocytoma in nonpregnant patients, but their values in pregnancy have yet to be fully evaluated in pregnancy [44].

MRI (without gadolinium) has better sensitivity than an ultrasound scan. Pheochromocytoma is typically bright on T2-weighted MRI with a sensitivity of 93–100 % [45].

### Treatment

If diagnosis is made early in pregnancy, adrenalectomy is the preferred definitive treatment of pheochromocytoma following adequate alpha and beta blockade for at least 2 weeks before surgery. The optimal timing of adrenalectomy is late in first trimester or early second trimester. In the third trimester, a combined caesarean section followed by adrenalectomy may be considered.

Primary medical therapy is indicated in patients if diagnosed after 24 weeks of gestation. Alpha blockade with phenoxybenzamine, 10–20 mg BD, is administered initially and titrated gradually till hypertension is controlled. After several days of alpha blockade, beta blockers are added to minimize tachycardia. Metyrosine, a specific inhibitor of catecholamine synthesis, is an FDA category C agent. Short-term emergency use of metyrosine is advocated in cases late in third trimester with refractory hypertension or arrhythmia [46]. Phentolamine

(1–5 mg) is the agent of choice for the treatment of hypertensive crisis [47].

### Obstetric Management

Labor and vaginal delivery should be avoided because this may cause tumor stimulation and further catecholamine secretion with severe hypertensive crisis in spite of adrenergic blockade. Hypertensive crisis typically presents as severely elevated blood pressure, arrhythmia, or pulmonary edema. Hypertensive crisis most frequently occurs at the time of delivery. Caesarean section is the method of choice for delivering the fetus as it avoids the risk of hypertensive crisis and adrenalectomy may be done in the same sitting.

#### Conclusion

Pituitary and adrenal disorders may rarely present as acute emergency in pregnancy. An interdisciplinary approach is required for appropriate management of patients. Diagnosis and treatment before pregnancy lead to better outcomes. Endocrine insufficiency requires continuation of supplementary dose in pregnancy. Patients on steroids need increased dose to cover the stress of labor and delivery. Surgery if necessary is best performed in the second trimester. Most cases in third trimester are managed medically and surgery deferred until the pregnancy is complete. Appropriate and timely diagnosis and management of cases have a definite impact on reducing maternal and perinatal morbidity and mortality.

## References


1. Schnatz PF, Curry SL. Primary hyperparathyroidism in pregnancy: evidence-based management. Obstet Gynecol Surv. 2002;57:365–76.
2. Kelly TR. Primary hyperparathyroidism during pregnancy. Surgery. 1991;110:1028–34.
3. Croom RD, Thomas CG. Primary hyperparathyroidism during pregnancy. Surgery. 1984;96:1109–18.
4. Clarke D, Seeds JW, Cefalo RC. Hyperparathyroid crisis and pregnancy. Am J Obstet Gynecol. 1981;140:840–2.
5. Matthias GS, Helliwell TR, Williams A. Postpartum hyperparathyroid crisis: cases report. Br J Obstet Gynaecol. 1987;94:807–10.
6. Negishi H, Kobayashi M, Nishida R, et al. Primary hyperparathyroidism and simultaneous bilateral fracture of the femoral neck during pregnancy. J Trauma. 2002;52:367–9.
7. Hess HM, Dickson J, Fox HE. Hyperfunctioning parathyroid carcinoma presenting as acute pancreatitis in pregnancy. J Reprod Med. 1980;25:83–7.
8. Kristoffersson A, Dahlgren S, Lithner F, Jarhult J. Primary hyperparathyroidism in pregnancy. Surgery. 1985;97:326–30.
9. Shangold MM, Dor N, Welt SI, et al. Hyperparathyroidism and pregnancy: a review. Obstet Gynecol Surv. 1982;37:217–28.
10. Wagner G, Transhol L, Melchior JC. Hyperparathyroidism and pregnancy. Acta Endocrinol. 1964;47:549–64.
11. Central Brain Tumor Registry of the United States (CBTRUS). Statistical report: primary brain tumors in the US 1997–2001. Available at: http://www.cbtrus.org/. Accessed 8 Apr 2005.
12. Goluboff LG, Ezrin C. Effect of pregnancy on the somatotroph and the prolactin cell of the human adenohypophysis. J Clin Endocrinol Metab. 1969;29:1533–8.
13. Scheithauer BW, Sano T, Kovacs KT, et al. The pituitary gland in pregnancy: a clinicopathologic and immunohistochemical study of 69 cases. Mayo Clin Proc. 1990;65:461–74.
14. Rigg LA, Lein A, Yen SSC. Pattern of increase in circulating prolactin levels during human gestation. Am J Obstet Gynecol. 1977;129:454–6.
15. Elster AD, Sanders TG, Vines FS, Chen MYN. Size and shape of the pituitary gland during pregnancy and postpartum: measurement with MR imaging. Radiology. 1991;181:531–5.
16. Dinc H, Essen F, Demircy A, et al. Pituitary dimensions and volume measurements in pregnancy and postpartum: MR assessment. Acta Radiol. 1998;39:64–9.
17. Kupersmith MJ, Rosenberg C, Kleinberg D. Visual loss in pregnant women with pituitary adenomas. Ann Intern Med. 1994;121:473–7.
18. Rossi AM, Vilska S, Heinonen PK. Outcome of pregnancies in women with treated or untreated hyperprolactinemia. Eur J Obstet Gynecol Reprod Biol. 1995;63:143–6.
19. Musolino NRC, Bronstein MD. Prolactinomas and pregnancy. In: Bronstein MD, editor. Pituitary tumors

and pregnancy. Norwell: Kluwer Academic Publishers; 2001. p. 91–108.
20. Molitch ME. Pregnancy and the hyperprolactinemic women. N Engl J Med. 1985;312:1364–70.
21. Liu C, Tyrrell JB. Successful treatment of a large macroprolactinoma with cabergoline during pregnancy. Pituitary. 2001;4:179–85.
22. Molitch ME. Clinical manifestations of acromegaly. Endocrinol Metab Clin North Am. 1992;21:597–614.
23. Herman-Bonert V, Seliverstow M, Melmed S. Pregnancy in acromegaly: successful therapeutic outcome. J Clin Endocrinol Metab. 1998;83:727–31.
24. Beckers A, Stevenaert A, Foidart J-M, et al. Placental and pituitary growth hormone secretion during pregnancy in acromegalic women. J Clin Endocrinol Metab. 1990;71:725–31.
25. Lindsay JR, Jonklass J, Oldfield EH, Nieman LK. Cushing's syndrome during pregnancy: personal experience and review of the literature. J Clin Endocrinol Metab. 2005;90:3077–83.
26. Aron DC, Schnall AM, Sheeler LR. Cushing's syndrome and pregnancy. Am J Obstet Gynecol. 1990;162(1):244–52.
27. Guilhaume B, Sanson ML, Villaud L, et al. Cushing's syndrome and pregnancy: aetiologies and prognosis in 22 patients. Eur J Med. 1992;1:83–9.
28. Bevan JS, Gough MH, Gillmer MD, Burke CW. Cushing's syndrome in pregnancy; the timing of definitive treatment. Clin Endocrinol Oxf. 1987;27: 225–33.
29. Madhun ZT, Aron DC. Cushing's disease in pregnancy. In: Bronstein MD, editor. Pituitary tumors and pregnancy. Norwell: Kluwer Academic Publishers; 2001. p. 149–72.
30. Brodsky JB, Cohen EN, Brown Jr BW, et al. Surgery during pregnancy and fetal outcome. Am J Obstet Gynecol. 1980;138:1165–7.
31. Sheehan HL, Davis JC. Pituitary necrosis. Br Med Bull. 1968;24:59–70.
32. Kelestimur F. Sheehan's syndrome. Pituitary. 2003;6:181–8.
33. Feinberg E, Molitch M, Peaceman A. Frequency of Sheehan's syndrome. Fertil Steril. 2005;84:975–9.
34. Sheehan HL. The neurohypophysis in post-partum hypopituitarism. J Pathol Bacteriol. 1963;85: 145–69.
35. Osler M, Pedersen J. Pregnancy in a patient with Addison's disease and diabetes mellitus. Acta Endocrinol. 1962;4:79–87.
36. O'Shaughnessy RW, Hackett KJ. Maternal Addison's disease and fetal growth retardation: a case report. J Reprod Med. 1984;29(10):752–6.
37. Okawa T, Asano K, Hashimoto T, et al. Diagnosis and management of primary aldosteronism in pregnancy: case report and review of the literature. Am J Perinatol. 2002;19(1):31–6.
38. Crane MG, Andes JP, Harris JJ, et al. Primary aldosteronism in pregnancy. Obstet Gynecol. 1964;23:200–8.
39. Fujiyama S, Mori Y, Matsubara H, et al. Primary aldosteronism with aldosterone-producing adrenal adenoma in a pregnant woman. Intern Med. 1999;38(1): 36–9.
40. Botchan A, Hauser R, Kutfermine M, et al. Pheochromocytoma in pregnancy: case report and review of the literature. Obstet Gynecol Surv. 1995;50(4):321–7.
41. Lyman DJ. Paroxysmal hypertension, pheochromocytoma, and pregnancy. J Am Board Fam Pract. 2002;15(2):153–8.
42. Cermakova A, Knibb AA, Hoskins C, et al. Post partum phaeochromocytoma. Int J Obstet Anesth. 2003;12(4):300–4.
43. Harper MA, Murnaghan GA, Kennedy L, et al. Phaeochromocytoma in pregnancy: five cases and a review of the literature. Br J Obstet Gynaecol. 1989;96(5):594–606.
44. Lenders JW, Pacak K, Eisnhofer G. New advances in the biochemical diagnosis of pheochromocytoma: moving beyond catecholamines. Ann N Y Acad Sci. 2002;970:29–40.
45. Ilias I, Pacak K. Current approaches and recommended algorithm for the diagnostic localization of pheochromocytoma. J Clin Endocrinol Metab. 2004;89(2):479–91.
46. Devoe LD, O'Dell BE, Castillo RA, et al. Metastatic pheochromocytoma in pregnancy and fetal biophysical assessment after maternal administration of alpha-adrenergic, beta adrenergic, and dopamine antagonists. Obstet Gynecol. 1986;68(Supll 3):S15–8.
47. Strachan AN, Claydon P, Caunt JA. Phaeochromocytoma diagnosed during labour. Br J Anaesth. 2000;85(4): 635–7.

# Part IV

# Special Conditions Requiring Critical Care

# Severe Anemia in Critically Ill Obstetric Patients

# 15

Kavita N. Singh and Jitendra Bhargava

## Introduction

Severe anemia poses enough challenges to cure for a clinician, and in the setting of pregnancy, it assumes more significance as both maternal and fetal aspects need equal considerations. It is estimated that 0.07–0.08 % of all pregnant women can find themselves into conditions that necessitate admission in the ICU [1].

Pregnancy associated with any serious illness including severe anemia can lead to acute organ failures, and both situations in the critically ill patients require special medical attention from experts in a specialized setup to improve maternal and fetal survival.

## Definition of Anemia and Severity

The World Health Organization (WHO) defines anemia in pregnancy as a hemoglobin concentration of <11 g/dL [2]. However there is variation in definition of normal hemoglobin levels in pregnancy. Classification derived from an iron-supplemented population lists the following levels as anemic: hemoglobin (g/dL) and hematocrit (percentage) levels below 11 g/dL and 33 %, respectively, in the first trimester; 10.5 g/dL and 32 %, respectively, in the second trimester; and 11 g/dL and 33 %, respectively, in the third trimester [3] (Table 15.1).

WHO defines anemia in postpartum period as hemoglobin concentration of <10 g/dL [2]. The Indian Council of Medical Research categorizes severity of anemia on the basis of hemoglobin levels as shown in Table 15.2 [4].

## Prevalence of Anemia in Pregnancy

Anemia affects 1.62 billion people globally, corresponding to 24.8 % of the world population. According to WHO survey, the global prevalence of anemia (1993–2005) among pregnant women is at 42 %, that is, 56 million [5]. WHO has estimated that the prevalence of anemia in pregnant women is 14 % in developed countries and 51 % in developing countries and 65–75 % in India. Anemia prevalence in rural and urban India was found to be 32.4 and 27.3 % in the third National Family Health Survey in 2005 and 2006 [6]. The relative prevalence of mild, moderate, and severe anemia is 13 %, 57 %, and 12 % respectively in India [4].

K.N. Singh, MS, PhD (✉)
Department of Obstetrics and Gynaecology, NSCB Medical College, Jabalpur, MP, India
e-mail: drkavitasingh@rediffmail.com

J. Bhargava, MD, DTCD
Department of Pulmonary and Sleep Medicine, NSCB Medical College, Jabalpur, MP, India
e-mail: jitendrabhargav@gmail.com


A. Gandhi et al. (eds.), *Principles of Critical Care in Obstetrics: Volume II*,
DOI 10.1007/978-81-322-2686-4_15

**Table 15.1** Anemia classification based on hemoglobin and hematocrit

| Trimester | Hemoglobin g/dL | Hematocrit % |
|---|---|---|
| First | <11 | <33 |
| Second | <10.5 | <32 |
| Third | <11 | <33 |

**Table 15.2** Anemia – categories of severity [ICMR]

| Category | Anemia severity | Hemoglobin concentration in gram/dL |
|---|---|---|
| 1 | Mild | 10–10.9 |
| 2 | Moderate | 7–10 |
| 3 | Severe | <7 |
| 4 | Very severe | <4 |

## Causes of Anemia in Pregnancy

Anemia is most commonly categorized by the underlying causative mechanisms:

1. Decreased red blood cell production mainly due to dietary deficiency or malabsorption
   - Iron deficiency
   - $B_{12}$ deficiency
   - Folate deficiency
   - Bone marrow disorder or suppression
   - Thyroid disorders
   - Low erythropoietin levels
2. Increased red blood cell destruction or blood loss: acquired or inherited hemolytic anemia
   Inherited:
   - Sickle cell anemia
   - Thalassemia major
   - Hereditary spherocytosis

   Acquired:
   - Autoimmune hemolytic anemia
   - Anemia associated with thrombocytopenic purpura
   - Anemia associated with hemolytic uremic syndrome
   - Hemolytic anemia associated with malaria
   - Hemorrhagic anemia

Iron deficiency is the most common cause, and even in the developed world an estimated 30–40 % of preschool children and pregnant women have iron depletion (WHO, 2001). In a study from India, of the 120 pregnant women, 65 % had iron deficiency, 18.3 % had dimorphic anemia, and 11.6 % had hemolytic anemia [7].

## Risk Factors for Development of Anemia

Iron deficiency is the major cause of anemia followed by folate and $B_{12}$ deficiencies. In India, the prevalence of anemia is high because of (1) low dietary intake and poor iron (less than 20 mg/day) and folic acid intake (less than 70 mg/day), (2) poor bioavailability of iron (3–4 % only) in phytate- and fiber-rich Indian diet, and (3) chronic blood loss due to infection such as malaria and hookworm infestations [8]. In addition, teenage pregnancy, short birth intervals, and too many childbirths contribute to development of anemia in reproductive age group females.

## Maternal Consequences of Anemia

Women with chronic mild anemia may go through pregnancy and labor without any adverse consequences, but those who had moderate anemia have reduced working capacity. Premature births are more common in women with moderate anemia and have higher morbidity and mortality due to antepartum and postpartum hemorrhage, pregnancy-induced hypertension, and sepsis [ICMR 1989]. Severe anemia may be decompensated and associated with circulatory failure. Cardiac decompensation usually occurs when Hb falls below 5.0 g/dl. The cardiac output is raised even at rest, and there is palpitations and breathlessness even at rest. Because of very low hemoglobin level, there is tissue hypoxia and lactic acid accumulation, leading to circulatory failure. If untreated, it may lead to pulmonary edema and death of the patient. A blood loss of even 200 ml in the third stage of labor produces shock and death. India data indicate that maternal morbidity rates are higher in women with Hb below 8.0 g/dl. Maternal mortality rates show a steep increase when maternal hemoglobin levels fall below 5.0 g/dl [8].

## Fetal Consequences of Anemia

Irrespective of maternal iron stores, the fetus still obtains iron from maternal transferrin, which is trapped in the placenta and which, in turn, removes and actively transports iron to the fetus. Gradually, however, such fetuses tend to have decreased iron stores due to depletion of maternal stores. Adverse perinatal outcome in form of preterm and small-for-gestational-age babies and increased perinatal mortality rates have been observed in the neonates of anemic mothers. Iron supplementation to the mother during pregnancy improves perinatal outcome. Mean weight, Apgar score, and hemoglobin level 3 months after birth were significantly greater in babies of the supplemented group than the placebo group [9]. Most of the studies suggest that a fall in maternal hemoglobin below 11.0 g/dl is associated with a significant rise in perinatal mortality rate. There is usually a two- to threefold increase in perinatal mortality rate when maternal hemoglobin levels fall below 8.0 g/dl and eight- to tenfold increase when maternal hemoglobin levels fall below 5.0 g/dl. A significant fall in birth weight due to increase in prematurity rate and intrauterine growth retardation has been reported when maternal hemoglobin levels were below 8.0 g/dl [10].

## Clinical Features

### Symptoms

Patients are largely asymptomatic in mild and moderate anemia.

- Weakness.
- Exhaustion and lassitude.
- Palpitation.
- Dyspnea.
- Giddiness.
- Edema and rarely.
- Anasarca and even congestive cardiac failure can occur in severe cases.

### Signs

There may be no signs especially in mild anemia. Common signs that may be present are:

- Pallor.
- Glossitis.
- Stomatitis.
- Edema due to hypoproteinemia.
- Soft systolic murmur can be heard in mitral area due to hyperdynamic circulation.

## Assessment of Fetal Well-Being

Maternal anemia could have a direct bearing on child's growth and can lead to growth restrictions, premature rupture of membrane, increased chances of preterm labor, and premature births, so these aspects should be duly looked into.

## Lab Diagnosis of Anemia

Lab diagnosis of anemia requires assessment of serum iron levels, total iron-binding capacity, serum ferritin levels, and iron and iron-binding capacity ratio and is indicative of causative factor (Table 15.3) [11].

## Evaluation of Patients with Anemia

1. Evaluation is done by assessment of hematocrit levels less than 33 % in the first and third trimesters and less than 32 % in the second trimester.
2. Apart from medical history, physical examination; investigations like the complete blood count, red blood cell indices, serum iron levels, and ferritin levels; and peripheral smear exam are needed to rule out hemolytic or parasitic disease as the cause of anemia. Hemoglobin electrophoresis is useful in some ethnic populations [12].
3. To diagnose severe anemia in ICU settings, one must look for active hemorrhage, persistent

**Table 15.3** Lab diagnosis of anemia

| Type | Serum iron level | Total iron-binding capacity (TIBC) | Ferritin level | Iron/iron-binding capacity |
|---|---|---|---|---|
| Iron deficiency | Decreased | Increased | Decreased | <18 % |
| Thalassemia | Normal | Normal | Normal | Normal |
| Anemia of chronic disease | Decreased | Decreased | Increased | >18 % |

inflammatory condition like sepsis, phlebotomy and increased use of blood products, decreased or inadequate erythropoietin level, and in some case a combination of these, and assessment of severe anemia should include detailed workup of all the above conditions. In addition, coagulopathy, nutritional deficiency due to critical illness, and drug-induced platelet dysfunction due to use of aspirin or clopidogrel or a combination of both must be kept in mind. Mental status changes due to low oxygenation as a result of reduced hemoglobin, radiological assessment for search of active bleeding, and pulmonary artery catheterization to assess hemodynamic status and tissue oxygenation. While testing hemoglobin level daily trends, hydration status must be kept in mind as volume-overloaded patients may show low hemoglobin levels and dehydrated patients may falsely show high levels.

## Severe Anemia in Comorbid Critical Conditions

Anemia is a common problem in critically ill and mostly it is due to anemia of chronic inflammation, phlebotomy, and reduced erythropoietin levels. A hemoglobin level of 100 g/L (10 g/dL) is needed to be maintained in critically ill patients. Patients who are not actively hemorrhaging should be treated with conservative transfusion strategy as a rule. Anemia in patients with cardiovascular diseases can worsen quickly and lead to decompensation and myocardial infarction. A hematocrit level below 28 % and hemoglobin level below 8–10 g/dL are associated with increased mortality. Acute renal failure is usually precipitated by hypoperfusion and/or nephrotoxic agents; acute tubular necrosis is the main pathologic event. Patients with antepartum active hemorrhage should be considered for transfusion. Aplastic anemia may occur during pregnancy and can disappear with delivery or abortion.

*Management*: Strategy should be based on the following principles:

1. Detection of anemia in critically ill obstetric patients and assessment through lab markers
2. Assessment of various treatment plans and risk-benefit analysis
3. Preparation of patient-specific plan
4. Maintenance of tissue oxygenation
5. Appropriate use of blood or blood components
6. Use of hemostatic drugs
7. Use of antifibrinolytic drugs for stopping active bleeding
8. Use of recombinant factor VII
9. Maximum enhancement of hemoglobin level
10. Minimization of blood loss
11. Reversal of drug-induced coagulopathy
12. Prevention of anemia

## Role of Iron Therapy in Final Outcome of Delivery

Prevalence of maternal anemia at the time of delivery in patients who are on the weaker side or malnourished is reduced by iron therapy, but it is not clear whether well-nourished non-anemic pregnant women get any benefit from iron therapy and their perinatal outcome improves [13]. Side effects of iron therapy usually are gastrointestinal symptoms and do not cause any significant morbidity; however patients with hemochromatosis and with certain other genetic disorders should be put on treatment with great caution.

## Role of Transfusion in Antepartum or at the Time of Delivery

Indications for transfusions are few and include severe blood loss leading to hypovolemia or surgical intervention is needed for a secured delivery in patients with anemia. Only 24 % of women who are predicted to require transfusion actually need by the time delivery is completed [14]. Trauma associated with surgery, placenta previa, coagulation problems, and uterine atony are the conditions where transfusion should be considered. Fetal conditions like abnormal heart rate, low amniotic fluid volume, and fetal cerebral vasodilatation in the setting of severe maternal anemia should be treated with maternal transfusion.

*Role for erythropoietin:* Oral iron preparations serve adequately in most clinical settings. Patients who cannot tolerate oral iron and patients with malabsorption syndrome and severe iron deficiency anemia should receive parenteral iron. Erythropoietin together with parenteral iron has shown to improve hemoglobin and hematocrit levels and increase reticulocyte counts in 2 weeks or lesser time, but erythropoietin alone has not shown any significant benefit [15]. Hemorrhage remains the leading cause of mortality during pregnancy. A significant proportion of these women need blood transfusion. Patients expected to have blood loss more than 1000 ml should be admitted where blood transfusion and ICU facility are readily available [16–19]. Due care about infections related to transfusion, immunological events like red cell alloimmunization, and errors about incorrect blood transfusion must be taken, and decision about choice of blood component must be made with adequate caution. Minimizing blood loss is of paramount importance [20].

*Autologous transfusion:* Hematocrit level greater than 32 % at 32 weeks of gestation is considered to be an indication for autologous transfusion in high-risk case like placenta previa but does not have the universal consensus and also is not found to be cost-effective as it remains difficult to predict the future need for transfusion [21].

## Choice of Therapy

1. Oral iron should be given for hematinic deficiencies.
2. When oral iron is not indicated, absorbed, or tolerated, parenteral iron is indicated. Iron dextran in single dose and iron sucrose can be given in multiple doses.
3. Hemoglobinopathies and bone marrow failures should be treated with blood transfusion.
4. Recombinant human erythropoietin (rHuEPO) can also be used during pregnancy and in the postpartum period [18, 19].
5. Active management of third stage of labor is integral to minimize blood loss [20].
6. Patients with concurrent illness and patients on anticoagulation need optimization of their regimens.

## Prevention

1. Screening for iron deficiency anemia in all pregnant women.
2. Universal iron supplementation to all pregnant women except with genetic condition like hemochromatosis is helpful in maintaining maternal iron stores and can also be helpful in building neonatal iron stores. It is also useful in preventing maternal anemia at delivery and low birth weight, premature delivery, and perinatal mortality.
3. Cooking and dietary advice: Cooking should be encouraged in iron pots/vessels. Jaggery, green leafy vegetables should be included in meals. Parboiled rice and tea should be avoided.
4. Treatment for malaria should be instituted when required and deworming medicines should be given if infestation is a possibility.
5. 100 mg of supplemental iron daily should be given from second trimester onwards.

## Conclusion

- Screening of all pregnant women for anemia should be a routine part of assessment.
- Women found to have iron deficiency anemia should be treated with supplemental iron and prenatal vitamins.
- Patients with non-iron-deficiency anemia and those with iron deficiency anemia who fail to respond to therapy should be subjected to deeper evaluation.
- Approximately 75 % patients in the ICU suffer from severe anemia.
- The cause of severe anemia is multifactorial in the ICU setting and includes active blood loss, inflammation, nutritional deficiencies, drug-induced coagulopathy, etc.
- Tissue oxygenation, arrest of persistent inflammation, and stopping of active bleeding is key to management of severe anemia in the ICU.

**Acknowledgment** Dr Rahul Rai, MD, DM, Associate Professor of Medicine, NSCB Medical College, Jabalpur, MP, INDIA.

## References

1. Irene YV, Vaneet K, et al. Critical care in obstetrics-scenario in a developing country. J Obstet Gynecol India. 2008;58(3):217–20.
2. WHO. Iron deficiency anemia: assessment, prevention and control. WHO/NHD/01.3, Geneva. 2001.
3. 47(RR-3):1–36. http://www.cdc.gov/mmwr/preview/mmwrhtml/00051880.htm. 3 Apr 1998. 47(RR-3);1–36.
4. Indian Council of Medical Research. Evaluation of the National Nutritional Anemia Prophylaxis Programme. Task Force Study. New Delhi: ICMR; 1989.
5. World Health Organization. Worldwide prevalence of anaemia 1993-2005: WHO global database on anaemia. Edited by Bruno de Benoist, Erin McLean, Ines Egli and Mary Cogswell. 2008.
6. Perumal V. Reproductive risk factors assessment for anaemia among pregnant women in India using a multinomial logistic regression model. Trop Med Int Health. 2014;19(7):841–51. doi:10.1111/tmi.12312. Epub 2014 Apr 7.
7. Sinha M, Panigrahi I, Shukla J, Khanna A, Saxena R. Spectrum of anemia in pregnant Indian women and importance of antenatal screening. Indian J Pathol Microbiol. 2006;49(3):373–5.
8. Kalaivani K. Prevalence & consequences of anaemia in pregnancy. Indian J Med Res. 2009;130(5):627–33.
9. Prema K, Neela Kumari S, Ramalakshmi BA. Anaemia and adverse obstetric outcome. Nutr Rep Int. 1981;23:637–43.
10. Adebisi OY, Strayhorn G. Anemia in pregnancy and race in the United States: blacks at risk. Fam Med. 2005;37:655–62 (Level III).
11. Angastiniotis M, Modell B. Global epidemiology of hemoglobin disorders. Ann N Y Acad Sci. 1998;850: 251–69 (Level II-3).
12. Pena-Rosas JP, Viteri FE. Effects of routine oral iron supplementation with or without folic acid for women during pregnancy. Cochrane Database Syst Rev. 2006;(3);CD004736. doi:10.1002/14651858.CD004736.pub2. (Level III).
13. Sherman SJ, Greenspoon JS, Nelson JM, Paul RH. Obstetric hemorrhage and blood utilization. J Reprod Med. 1993;38:929–34 (Level II-2).
14. Wagstrom E, Akesson A, Van Rooijen M, Larson B, Bremme K. Erythropoietin and intravenous iron therapy in postpartum anaemia. Acta Obstet Gynecol Scand. 2007;86:957–62 (Level I).
15. Perez EM, Hendricks MK, Beard JL, Murray-Kolb LE, Berg A, Tomlinson M, et al. Mother-infant interactions and infant development are altered by maternal iron deficiency anemia. J Nutr. 2005;135:850–5 (Level I).
16. Snow CF. Laboratory diagnosis of vitamin B12 and folate deficiency: a guide for the primary care physician. Arch Intern Med. 1999;159:1289–98 (Level III).
17. Bothwell TH, Charlton RW. Iron deficiency in women. Washington DC: The Nutrition Foundation; 1981 (Level III).
18. Baynes RD. Iron deficiency. In: Brock JH, Halliday JW, Pippard MJ, Powell LW, editors. Iron metabolism in health and disease. Philadelphia: W.B. Saunders; 1994. p. 189–225 (Level III).
19. Agency for Healthcare Research and Quality. Screening for iron deficiency anemia in childhood and pregnancy: update of the 1996 U.S. Preventive Task Force review. AHRQ Publication No. 06-0590-EF-1. Rockville (MD): AHRQ; 2006. (Level III).
20. Johnson-Spear MA, Yip R. Hemoglobin difference between black and white women with comparable iron status: justification for race-specific anemia criteria. Am J Clin Nutr. 1994;60:117–21 (Level III).
21. Etchason J, Petz L, Keeler E, Calhoun L, Kleinman S, Snider C, et al. The cost effectiveness of preoperative autologous blood donations. N Engl J Med. 1995;332: 719–24 (Level III).

# Management of Sickle Cell Crisis in Pregnancy

16

Sadhana Gupta and Hema J. Shobhane

## Introduction

Sickle cell disease is a group of inherited single-gene autosomal recessive disorders caused by the 'sickle' gene, which affects haemoglobin structure. SCD has its origins in sub-Saharan Africa and the Middle East; hence, it is most prevalent in individuals of African descent as well as in the Caribbean, Middle East, parts of India and the Mediterranean and South and Central America. Owing to population migration, SCD is now of increasing importance worldwide [1].

All over the world, about 300,000 children with these disorders are born each year. Acute sickle cell pain episodes are the most common cause of hospitalisation. Pregnancy in women with sickle cell disease is associated with an increased incidence of maternal and fetal morbidity and mortality.

The term SCD includes sickle cell anaemia (HbSS) and the heterozygous conditions of haemoglobin S and other clinically abnormal haemoglobins. These include combination with haemoglobin C (giving HbSC), combination with beta thalassaemia (giving HbSB thalassaemia) and combination with haemoglobin D, E or O-Arab. All of these genotypes will give a similar clinical phenotype of varying severity [2]. Haemoglobin S combined with normal haemoglobin (A), known as sickle trait (AS), is asymptomatic, except for a possible increased risk of urinary tract infections and microscopic haematuria.

S. Gupta, MS (Gyn), FICOG, FICMU, FICMCH (✉)
Senior Consultant Obstetrician and Gynecologist, Jeevan Jyoti Hospital and Medical Research Centre, Jeevan Jyoti Test Tube Baby Centre, Bobina Road, Gorakhpur, UP, India
e-mail: drguptasadhana@gmail.com

H.J. Shobhane, MD (Obs & Gyn), FICOG, FICMCH
Associate Professor, Maharani Laxmi Bai Medical College, Jhansi, UP, India
e-mail: dr.hemashobhane3@gmail.com

## Pathophysiology

The sickle cell syndrome is caused by a mutation in the beta globin gene that changes the sixth amino acid from glutamic acid to valine. HbSS when deoxygenated form a gelatinous network of fibrous polymers that stiffen the RBC membrane, increase viscosity and cause dehydration due to potassium leakage and calcium influx. Sickled RBC has life span of about 2–3 weeks that is much lower than the normal RBC, that is 120 days. Sickled cells lose the pliability needed to traverse small capillaries. They possess altered sticky membranes that are abnormally adherent to the endothelium of small venules. These abnormalities provoke unpredictable episodes of microvascular vaso-occlusion and premature RBC destruction (haemolytic anaemia). Haemolysis occurs because the spleen destroys the abnormal RBC. The rigid adherent cells clog small capillaries and venules, causing tissue ischaemia, acute pain, and gradual end-organ damage. Prominent


A. Gandhi et al. (eds.), *Principles of Critical Care in Obstetrics: Volume II*,
DOI 10.1007/978-81-322-2686-4_16

manifestations include episodes of ischaemic pain that is painful crisis, acute chest syndrome and infarction or ischaemia in CNS and acute anaemia but can give infarction or ischaemia of any part in body like the spleen, bones, liver, kidneys, etc.

**Pathophysiology of sickle cell crisis in pregnancy**

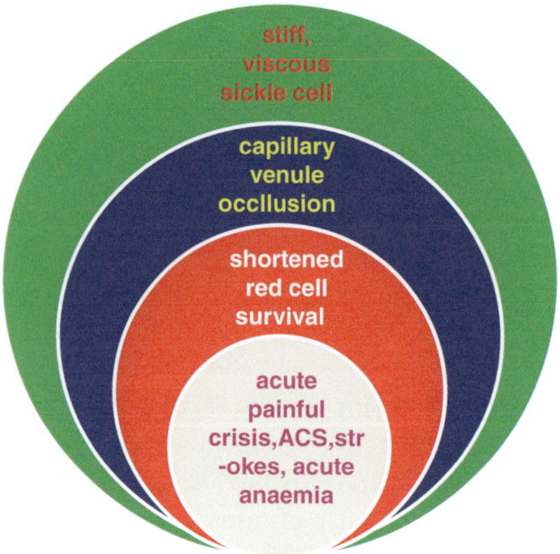


## Clinical Features

Any woman with pregnancy, who is with refractory anaemia and who originally belongs to the Eastern India, especially with good social class, presenting with signs and symptoms of anaemia, in such cases haemoglobinopathies should be excluded.

Any pregnant woman with HbSS can present with shortness of breath, dizziness, headaches, coldness in the hands and feet and palor than normal skin or mucous membranes; jaundice with sudden pain throughout the body is a common symptom of sickle cell anaemia, and this pain is called a sickle cell crisis. Sickle cell crises often affect the bones, lungs, abdomen and joints. These crises occur when sickled red blood cells block blood flow to the limbs and organs. This can cause pain and organ damage. The pain from sickle cell anaemia can be acute or chronic, but acute pain is more common. Acute pain is sudden and can range from mild to very severe. The pain usually lasts from hours to as long as a week or more. Next common presentation of sickle cell crisis is acute chest syndrome characterised by chest pain, tachypnoea, fever, cough and arterial oxygen desaturation. Other presentations of sickle cell crisis, abnormal neurological presentation as a case of stroke or a case of acute anaemia.

## Prevention and Management

### Primary Prevention

Prevention of the sickle cell anaemia or sickle cell syndrome in offsprings by avoiding marriage of sickle cell trait to another sickle cell trait or any other haemoglobinopathies, such as beta thalassaemia. The inheritance when both parents have sickle cell trait, there is a 1:4 chances with each pregnancy that the offspring will have sickle cell anaemia.

**Possible Genotype of offspring of parents with sickle cell trait**

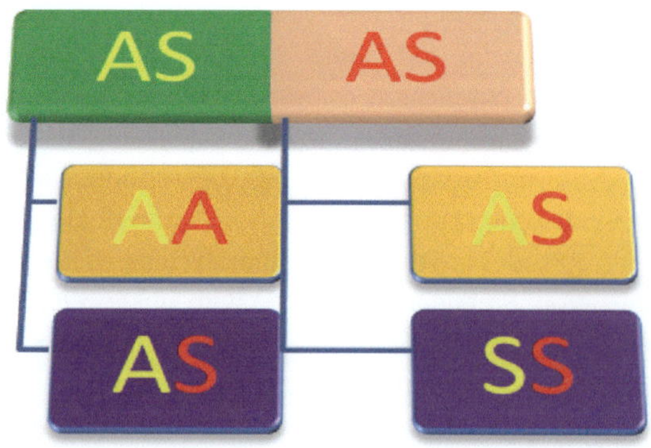


### Secondary Prevention

#### Preconception Care

SCD is associated with both maternal and fetal complications and is associated with an increased incidence of perinatal mortality, premature labour, fetal growth restriction and acute painful crises during pregnancy [3]. Some studies also describe an increase in spontaneous miscarriage, antenatal hospitalisation, pre-eclampsia, PIH, maternal mortality, delivery by caesarean section, infection, thromboembolic events and antepartum haemorrhage and infection in postpartum period [4].

**Information That Is Particularly Relevant for Women Planning to Conceive Includes** The role of dehydration, cold, hypoxia, overexertion and stress in the frequency of sickle cell crises, how nausea and vomiting in pregnancy can result in dehydration and the precipitation of crises, risk of worsening anaemia, the increased risk of crises and acute chest syndrome (ACS) and the risk of increased infection (especially urinary tract infection) during pregnancy

**The Assessment for Chronic Disease Complications Should Include** Screening for blood pressure and urinalysis should be performed to identify women with hypertension and/or proteinuria.

- Renal and liver function tests should be performed to identify sickle nephropathy and/or deranged hepatic function.
- Screening for pulmonary hypertension with echocardiography. The incidence of pulmonary hypertension is increased in patients with SCD and is associated with increased mortality. A tricuspid regurgitant jet velocity of more than 2.5 m/s is associated with a high risk of pulmonary hypertension.
- Retinal screening. Proliferative retinopathy is common in patients with SCD, especially patients with HbSC, and can lead to loss of vision [5].
- Screening for iron overload by serum ferritin level. In women who have been multiple transfused in the past or who have a high ferritin level, T2* cardiac magnetic resonance imaging may be helpful to assess body iron loading. Aggressive iron chelation before conception is advisable in women who are significantly iron loaded.
- Screening for red cell antibodies. Red cell antibodies may indicate an increased risk of haemolytic disease of the newborn.
- Women should be encouraged to have the haemoglobinopathy status of their partner.

**Antibiotic Prophylaxis and Immunisation** Penicillin prophylaxis or the equivalent should be prescribed. Vaccination status should be determined and updated before pregnancy. Patients with SCD are hyposplenic and are at risk of infection, in particular from encapsulated bacteria such as *Neisseria meningitides*, *Streptococcus pneumonia* and *Haemophilus influenzae*. Daily penicillin prophylaxis is given to all patients with SCD, in line with the guidelines for all hyposplenic patients. People who are allergic to penicillin should be recommended erythromycin. In addition, women should be given *H. influenza* type b and the conjugated meningococcal C vaccine as a single dose if they have not received it as part of primary vaccination. The pneumococcal vaccine (Pneumovax®, Sanofi Pasteur MSD Limited, Maidenhead, UK) should be given every 5 years. Hepatitis B vaccination is recommended, and the woman's immune status should be determined preconceptually. Women with SCD should be advised to receive the influenza and 'swine flu' vaccine annually [6].

**Supplementation of Folic Acid** Folic acid should be given once daily both preconceptually and throughout pregnancy.

Folic acid, 5 mg, is recommended in all pregnant women to reduce the risk of neural tube defect and to compensate for the increased demand for folate during pregnancy.

**Prevention of Hydroxycarbamide (Hydroxyurea)** Hydroxyurea should be stopped at least 3 months before conception. In spite of hydroxycarbamide decreases the incidence of acute painful crises and ACS, it should be stopped due to its teratogenic effects in animal.

## Antenatal Care

Antenatal care should be provided by a multidisciplinary team including an obstetrician and midwife with experience of high-risk antenatal care and a haematologist.

Women with SCD should undergo medical review by the haematologist and be screened for end-organ damage (if this has not been undertaken preconceptually).

Women with SCD should aim:

- Document baseline oxygen saturation, blood pressure and urinalysis at each visit and midstream urine for culture performed monthly.

- Avoid precipitating factors of sickle cell crises such as exposure to extreme temperatures, dehydration and overexertion. Persistent vomiting can lead to dehydration and sickle cell crisis, and women should be advised to seek medical advice early.
- The influenza vaccine should be recommended if it has not been administered in the previous year. Many women become pregnant without preconceptual care. Therefore, all of the actions in preconception care, including vaccinations, review of iron overload and red cell autoantibodies, should take place as early as possible during antenatal care.
- Iron supplementation should be given only if there is laboratory evidence of iron deficiency.
- Women with SCD should be considered for low-dose aspirin 75 mg once daily from 12 weeks of gestation in an effort to reduce the risk of developing pre-eclampsia.
- Women with SCD should be advised to receive prophylactic low-molecular-weight heparin during antenatal hospital admissions. The use of graduated compression stockings of appropriate strength is recommended in pregnancy for women considered to be at risk of venous thromboembolism,
- Non-steroidal anti-inflammatory drugs (NSAIDs) should be prescribed only between 12 and 28 weeks of gestation owing to concerns regarding adverse effects on fetal development.
- Women should be offered the routine first-trimester scan (11–14 weeks of gestation) and a detailed anomaly scan at 20 weeks of gestation. In addition, women should be offered serial fetal biometry scans (growth scans) every 4 weeks from 24 weeks of gestation.
- Routine prophylactic transfusion is not recommended during pregnancy for women with SCD.
- If acute exchange transfusion is required for the treatment of a sickle complication, it may be appropriate to continue the transfusion regimen for the remainder of the pregnancy. Blood should be matched for an extended phenotype including full rhesus typing (C, D and E) as well as Kell typing. Blood used for transfusion in pregnancy should be cytomegalovirus negative.
- Subsequent visits at 16, 20, 24, 26, 28, 30, 32, 34, 36, 38 and 40 weeks of gestation for prevention or early diagnosis and management of complications and crisis.
- Offer information and advice about: timing, mode and management of the birth, analgesia and anaesthesia, induction of labour or caesarean section between 38 and 40 weeks of gestation.

## Management of Sickle Cell Crisis during Pregnancy and Peripartum Period

### Acute Painful Crisis

Women with SCD who become unwell should have sickle cell crisis excluded as a matter of urgency. Painful crisis is the most frequent complication of SCD during pregnancy, with between 27 and 50 % of women having a painful crisis during pregnancy, and it is the most frequent cause of hospital admission. Avoidance of precipitants such as a cold environment, excessive exercise, dehydration and stress is important. Primary care physicians should have a low threshold for referring women to secondary care; all women with pain which does not settle with simple analgesia, who are febrile, have atypical pain or chest pain or symptoms of shortness of breath should be referred to hospital.

On presentation, the woman in sickle crisis should be assessed rapidly for medical complications requiring intervention such as ACS, sepsis or dehydration. History should ascertain if this is typical sickle pain or not and if there are precipitating factors. Examination should focus on the site of pain, any atypical features of the pain and any precipitating factors, in particular whether there are any signs of infection. Pregnant women presenting with acute painful crisis should be rapidly assessed by the multidisciplinary team, and appropriate and prompt management should be started.

**Investigation** Initial investigations should include full blood count, reticulocyte count and renal function. Other investigations will depend on the clinical scenario but may include blood cultures, chest X-ray, urine culture and liver function tests.

**Management** *Oxygen therapy*: The requirement for fluids and oxygen should be assessed and fluids and oxygen administered if required. Oxygen saturations should be monitored, and facial oxygen should be prescribed if oxygen saturation falls below the woman's baseline or below 95 % [7]. There should be early recourse to intensive care if satisfactory oxygen saturation cannot be maintained by facial or nasal prong oxygen administration.

*Fluid therapy*: The requirement for fluids and oxygen should be assessed and fluids and oxygen administered if required. Fluid intake of at least 60 ml/kg/24 h should be ensured; this can be taken either orally or intravenously if the woman is not able to take adequate oral fluids. There is a risk of fluid overload in women with pre-eclampsia; senior experienced staff should be involved in managing the fluid balance of these women.

*Pain and palliative care*: Analgesia should be administered. Initial analgesia should be given within 30 min of arriving at hospital, and effective analgesia should be achieved within 1 h. The World Health Organisation analgesic ladder should be used, starting with paracetamol for mild pain; NSAIDs can be used for mild to moderate pain between 12 and 28 weeks of gestation. Weak opioids such as co-dydramol, co-codamol or dihydrocodeine can be used for moderate pain, and stronger opiates such as morphine can be used for severe pain. Morphine or diamorphine can be given by oral, subcutaneous, intramuscular or intravenous route depending on the woman's preference and local expertise. Parenteral opiates can be given by intermittent bolus or patient-controlled administration systems. Pethidine should be avoided because of the risk of toxicity and pethidine-associated seizures in patients with SCD. Women presenting with pain should initially be monitored at 20-min intervals for pain severity, respiratory rate and sedation. Assessments of pain score, sedation score and oxygen saturation should be performed at least 2-hourly using a modified obstetric early warning chart [8]. While women are receiving parenteral opiates, they should be nursed in an area where they can undergo hourly observations for rapid clinical assessment. If pain is severe and oral analgesia is not effective, give strong opioids (e.g. morphine). Give adjuvant non-opioid analgesia: paracetamol or NSAID (if 12–28 weeks of gestation). Prescribe laxatives, antipruritic and antiemetic if required. Monitor pain, sedation, vital signs, respiratory rate and oxygen saturation every 20–30 min until pain is controlled and signs are stable and then monitor every 2 h (hourly if receiving parenteral opiates).

Give a rescue dose of analgesia if required. If respiratory rate is less than 10/min, omit maintenance analgesia; consider naloxone. Consider reducing analgesia after 2–3 days and replacing injections with equivalent dose of oral analgesia.

Other adjuvants may be required to treat the adverse effects of opiates, such as antihistamines to treat itching or laxatives to prevent opiate-induced constipation, and antiemetics may be required. As the painful crisis resolves, most women are able to reduce their opiate requirement rapidly, but this should be guided by the woman's previous experience. Opiates are not associated with teratogenicity or congenital malformation but may be associated with transient suppression of fetal movement and a reduced baseline variability of the fetal heart rate. Where a mother has received prolonged administration of opiates in late pregnancy, the neonate should be observed for signs of opioid withdrawal.

*Thromboprophylaxis*: Thromboprophylaxis should be provided to women with SCD who are admitted to hospital with painful crises.

*Antibiotic*: The woman should be assessed for infection. Therapeutic antibiotics should be prescribed if the woman is febrile or there is a high clinical suspicion of infection. White blood cell counts are often raised in SCD and do not necessarily indicate infection.

*Discharge*: Discharge the woman when pain is controlled and improving without analgesia or on acceptable doses of oral analgesia. If the women need strong opiate therapy, they will need to be admitted to a hospital: to a medical ward in early pregnancy or to a level 2 antenatal bed in later pregnancy, under the joint care of obstetricians and haematologists.

*Care after discharge*

Arrange any necessary home care and outpatient follow-up appointment.

*Blood transfusion*

## Acute Chest Syndrome

Each hospital should have a *protocol in place for the management of ACS in pregnancy, including the use of transfusion therapy.* After acute pain, ACS is the most common complication, reported in 7–20 % of pregnancies [9]. ACS is characterised by respiratory symptoms such as tachypnoea, chest pain, cough and shortness of breath in the presence of a new infiltrate on the chest X-ray. The signs and symptoms of ACS are the same as those of pneumonia, so both should be treated simultaneously. Acute severe infection with the H1N1 virus in pregnancy can cause a similar clinical picture, and investigation and treatment for this should be instituted. Early recognition of ACS is key.

*Management*: Treatment is with intravenous antibiotics, oxygen and blood transfusion, as in non-pregnant women.

*Blood transfusion*: Top-up blood transfusion may be required if the haemoglobin is falling, and certainly if the haemoglobin is less than 6.5 g/dl, but in severe hypoxia, and if the haemoglobin level is maintained, exchange transfusion will be required. If ACS is suspected, the woman should be reviewed urgently by the haematology team to advise on transfusion. If the woman has hypoxia, she should be reviewed by the critical care team, and ventilatory support may be required.

*Thromboprophylaxis*: There is an increased risk of pulmonary embolism among women with SCD. In women presenting with acute hypoxia, there should be a low threshold for considering pulmonary embolism. In this situation, therapeutic low-molecular-weight heparin should be commenced until the woman has been reviewed by senior staff and definitive investigations have been undertaken.

## Acute Stroke

Acute stroke, both infarctive and haemorrhagic, is associated with SCD [10], and this diagnosis should be considered in any woman with SCD who presents with acute neurological impairment.

*Blood transfusion*: Acute stroke is a medical emergency, and a rapid-exchange blood transfusion can decrease long-term neurological damage. If a stroke is suspected, the woman should have urgent brain imaging, and the haematologist should be called for consideration of urgent exchange transfusion.

*Thomboprophylaxis*: Thrombolysis is not indicated in acute stroke secondary to SCD [6].

## Acute Anaemia

Acute anaemia in women with SCD may be attributable to erythrovirus infection. Infection with erythrovirus in SCD causes a red cell maturation arrest and an aplastic crisis characterised by a reticulocytopenia. Therefore, a reticulocyte count should be requested in any woman presenting with an acute anaemia and, if low, may indicate infection with erythrovirus.

**Management** *Blood transfusion*: Treatment is with blood transfusion and the woman must be isolated. With erythrovirus infection there is the added risk of vertical transmission to the fetus, which can result in hydrops fetalis; hence, a review by a fetal medicine specialist is indicated [11]. Women with SCD can develop anaemia owing to bleeding or any other causes of anaemia incidental to the SCD. Rare causes of anaemia in SCD include malaria and, occasionally, splenic sequestration in women with a mild phenotype.

*Top-up transfusion*: is indicated for women with acute anaemia [6]. Acute anaemia may be attributable to transient red cell aplasia, acute splenic sequestration or the increased haemolysis and volume expansion encountered in SCD. There is no absolute level at which transfusion should be undertaken, and the decision must be made in conjunction with clinical findings, but haemoglobin under 6 g/dl or a fall of over 2 g/dl from baseline is often used as a guide to transfusion requirement.

*Exchange transfusion*: for ACS was demonstrated to be effective in one prospective randomised trial and is accepted as best practice [12].

*Alloimmunisation*: The formation of antibodies to red cell antigens is common in SCD, occurring in 18–36 % of patients. Alloimmunisation is clinically important as it can lead to delayed haemolytic transfusion reactions or haemolytic disease of the newborn [13] and can render patients untransfusable. The most common antibodies are to the C, E and Kell antigens. The risk of alloimmunisation is significantly reduced by giving red cells matched for the C, E and Kell antigens [12], and this should be standard practice for all patients with SCD whether they are pregnant or not.

## Intrapartum Care

The risks of abruption, pre-eclampsia, peripartum cardiomyopathy and acute sickle cell crisis are increased and unpredictable. The relevant multidisciplinary team (senior midwife in charge, senior obstetrician, anaesthetist and haematologist) should be informed as soon as labour is confirmed. Women with SCD should be advised to give birth in hospitals that are able to manage both the complications of SCD and high-risk pregnancies.

*Elective birth*: Pregnant women with SCD who have a normally growing fetus should be offered elective birth through induction of labour or by elective caesarean section if indicated, after 38+0 weeks of gestation. The labour should be carefully supervised; caesarean section should be considered if labour is not progressing well and delivery is not imminent [4]. SCD should not in itself be considered a contraindication to attempting vaginal delivery or vaginal birth after caesarean section. It is the opinion of the developers that, like most 'high-risk' conditions, delivery of the baby at 38–40 weeks of gestation will prevent late pregnancy complications and associated adverse perinatal events.

*Warmth*: Women should be kept warm and avoid cold stimulus.

*Fluid therapy*: Women should be given adequate fluid during labour. There is an increased frequency of sickle cell crisis and ACS in the intrapartum period. There is an increased risk of painful crisis with protracted labour (more than 12 h), but this is often secondary to dehydration. In this situation, if the woman is well hydrated and labour is progressing, During labour, if oral hydration is not tolerated or is inadequate, intravenous fluids should be administered using a fluid balance chart to prevent fluid overload. Venous access can be difficult, especially if they have had multiple previous admissions, and as such anaesthetic review/intravenous access should be obtained early.

*Oxygen therapy*: The demand for oxygen is increased during the intrapartum period, and the use of pulse oximetry to detect hypoxia in the mother is appropriate during labour. Arterial blood gas analysis should be performed and oxygen therapy instituted if oxygen saturation is 94 % or less.

*Electronic fetal monitoring*: Continuous intrapartum electronic fetal heart rate monitoring is recommended owing to the increased risk of fetal distress which may necessitate operative delivery. Continuous electronic fetal heart rate monitoring is recommended because of the increased rate of stillbirth, placental abruption and compromised placental reserve [14]. Women with SCD should be offered anaesthetic assessment in the third trimester of pregnancy.

*Blood transfusion*: Blood should be crossmatched for delivery if there are atypical antibodies present (since this may delay the availability of blood); otherwise a 'group and save' will suffice.

*Position*: In women who have hip replacements (because of avascular necrosis), it is important to discuss suitable positions for delivery.

*Antibiotics*: Routine antibiotic prophylaxis in labour is currently not supported by evidence, but hourly observations of vital signs should be performed. A raised temperature (over 37.5 °C) requires investigation. The clinician should have a low threshold to commence broad-spectrum antibiotics.

*Analgesia and anaesthesia*: Avoid the use of pethidine, but other opiates can be used. Regional analgesia is recommended for caesarean section. Pregnant women with SCD are at risk of end-organ damage as well as experiencing a higher rate of caesarean section. General anaesthesia carries additional risks beyond the normal obstetric case and should be avoided where possible. Regional anaesthesia during labour may reduce the necessity of general anaesthesia for delivery. It is also likely to reduce the need for high doses of opioids if the woman has sickle-related pain in the lower body. An anaesthetic assessment in the third trimester is warranted. Pethidine should be avoided because of the risk of seizures when administered to a woman with SCD [7]; other opiates can be used. Indications for epidural analgesia in labour are the same as routine case. Sickle cell crisis in labour should be treated as per the guidance for antepartum crisis above.

## Postpartum Care

The same level of care and vigilance should be maintained as has been described for antenatal care, since acute crisis and other complications of SCD remain a risk in the puerperium.

In pregnant women where the baby is at high risk of SCD (i.e. the partner is a carrier or affected), early testing for SCD should be offered. Capillary samples should be sent to laboratories where there is experience in the routine analysis of SCD in newborn samples. This will usually be at a regional centre.

*Oxygen therapy and fluid balance*: Maintain maternal oxygen saturation above 94 % and adequate hydration based on fluid balance until discharge. The risk of sickle cell crisis remains increased: in one study it occurred in 25 % of women and was more common following general anaesthesia. Hydration and oxygenation should be maintained.

*Thromboprophylaxis*: Low-molecular-weight heparin should be administered while in hospital and 7 days post-discharge following vaginal delivery or for a period of 6 weeks following caesarean section. Antithrombotic stockings are recommended in the puerperium; early mobilisation should be encouraged.

*Pain ad palliative care*: Crises should be managed as for non-pregnant women. NSAIDs are routinely administered in the postpartum period and can be used during breastfeeding.

*Breast feeding*: Breastfeeding should be encouraged, as in women without SCD.

*Postpartum contraception*: Progestogen-containing contraceptives such as the progesterone-only pill, injectable contraceptives and the levonorgestrel intrauterine system are safe and effective in SCD. Oestrogen-containing contraceptives should be used as second-line agents.

Barrier methods are as safe and effective in women with SCD as in the general population. Women taking intramuscular depot medroxyprogesterone acetate (DMPA) were less likely to have a painful episode. Progestogens to be effective and safe in SCD [15].

## References

1. Stuart MJ, Nagel RL. Sickle cell disease. Lancet. 2004;364:1343–60.
2. Weatherall D, Akinyanju O, Fucharoen S, Olivieri N, Musgrove P, et al. Inherited disorders of haemoglobin. In: Jamison DT, Breman JG, Measham AR, Alleye G, Claeson M, Evans DB, editors. Disease control priorities in developing countries. 2nd ed. Washington, DC/New York: The World Bank/Oxford University Press; 2006. p. 663–80.
3. Powars DR, Sandhu M, Niland-Weiss J, Johnson C, Bruce S, Manning PR. Pregnancy in sickle cell disease. Obstet Gynecol. 1986;67:217–28.
4. Villers MS, Jamison MG, De Castro LM, James AH. Morbidity associated with sickle cell disease in pregnancy. Am J Obstet Gynecol. 2008;199:125.e1–5.
5. Clarkson JG. The ocular manifestations of sickle-cell disease: a prevalence and natural history study. Trans Am Ophthalmol Soc. 1992;90:481–504.

6. Sickle Cell Society. Standards for the clinical care of adults with sickle cell disease in the UK. London: Sickle Cell Society; 2008.
7. Rees DC, Olujohungbe AD, Parker NE, Stephens AD, Telfer P, Wright J, British Committee for Standards in Haematology General Haematology Task Force by the Sickle Cell Working Party. Guidelines for the management of acute painful crisis in sickle cell disease. Br J Haematol. 2003;120:744–52.
8. National Confidential Enquiry into Patient Outcome and Death. A sickle crisis? A report of the national confidential enquiry into patient outcome and death. London: NCEPOD; 2008.
9. Howard RJ, Tuck SM, Pearson TC. Pregnancy in sickle cell disease in the UK: results of a multicentre survey of the effect of prophylactic blood transfusion on maternal and fetal outcome. Br J Obstet Gynaecol. 1995;102:947–51.
10. Ohene-Frempong K, Weiner SJ, Sleeper LA, Miller ST, Embury S, Moohr JW, et al. Cerebrovascular accidents in sickle cell disease: rates and risk factors. Blood. 1998;91:288–94.
11. Smith-Whitley K, Zhao H, Hodinka RL, Kwiatkowski J, Cecil R, Cecil T, et al. Epidemiology of human parvovirus B19 in children with sickle cell disease. Blood. 2004;103:422–7.
12. Styles LA, Abboud M, Larkin S, Lo M, Kuypers FA. Transfusion prevents acute chest syndrome predicted by elevated secretory phospholipase A2. Br J Haematol. 2007;136:343–4.
13. Tuck SM, Studd JW, White JM. Sickle cell disease in pregnancy complicated by anti-U antibody. Case report. Br J Obstet Gynaecol. 1982;89:91–2.
14. Anyaegbunam A, Morel MI, Merkatz IR. Antepartum fetal surveillance tests during sickle cell crisis. Am J Obstet Gynecol. 1991;165:1081–3.
15. Legardy JK, Curtis KM. Progestogen-only contraceptive use among women with sickle cell anemia: a systematic review. Contraception. 2006;73:195–204.

# 17 HIV in Critical Pregnancy

Atul Munshi and Sujal Munshi

## Introduction

In India, approximately 49,000 women living with HIV become pregnant and deliver each year which is about 6–10 % of the total world figure [1].

Most of the pregnant women are unaware of their HIV status at the time of diagnosis of pregnancy and some of them even are not aware of their status until labour. Maternal HIV-1 infection has been associated with an increased risk of PTB, but mechanisms underlying this association are undefined [2].

HIV-infected women were more likely than HIV-uninfected women to have pregnancy-induced hypertension, anaemia, breech presentations, stillborn babies and foetal deaths [Indian Study] [3].

Pregnancy does not appear to influence the progression of HIV disease [4, 5].

A. Munshi, MD, DGO, FICOG (✉)
Department of OB-GYN, GCS Medical College, Ahmedabad, Gujarat, India

Munshi Hospital Ahmedabad, Ahmedabad, Gujarat, India
e-mail: munshiap@gmail.com

S. Munshi, MD, DNB, MICOG, DIAGE (Kiel)
Munshi Hospital and Pulse Hospital, Ahmedabad, Gujarat, India

Department of OB-GYN, Visiting Endoscopist, P.S. Medical College, Karamsad, Gujarat, India
e-mail: sujalmunshi@gmail.com

Furthermore, pregnancy does not seem to affect survival of women infected with HIV [6].

Testing pregnant women for HIV at the time of labour and delivery is the last opportunity for prevention of mother-to-child HIV transmission (PMTCT) measures, particularly in settings where women do not receive adequate antenatal care. However, HIV testing and counselling of pregnant women in labour is a challenge, especially in resource-constrained settings. In India, many rural women present for delivery without any prior antenatal care. Those who do get antenatal care are not always tested for HIV, because of deficiencies in the provision of HIV testing and counselling services [7].

HIV impacts on direct (obstetrical) causes of maternal mortality by an associated increase in pregnancy complications such as *anaemia, postpartum haemorrhage and puerperal sepsis.*

HIV is also a major indirect cause of maternal mortality by an increased susceptibility to *opportunistic infections like tuberculosis and malaria* [8].

## Impact on Mother and Foetus

Antiretroviral therapy (ART) during pregnancy should focus on the reduction of perinatal transmission and the treatment of maternal human immunodeficiency virus (HIV) disease.

ART can reduce perinatal transmission by several mechanisms, including lowering maternal


A. Gandhi et al. (eds.), *Principles of Critical Care in Obstetrics: Volume II*,
DOI 10.1007/978-81-322-2686-4_17

antepartum viral load and preexposure and post-exposure prophylaxis of the infant. Therefore, for prevention of perinatal transmission of HIV, combined antepartum, intrapartum and infant antiretroviral prophylaxis is recommended.

Combination drug regimens are considered the standard of care for treatment of HIV infection and for prevention of perinatal HIV transmission [9].

Assuming that due diligence has been observed in the diagnosis and treatment of anaemia and the patient has been on ART, we are left with the modalities of treating the critical stage when an active mode is to be employed.

While prevention measures are preferred to emergency management, in a resource-poor setting, it is not always possible.

*That is when critical care management assumes importance in the reduction of maternal morbidity and mortality.*

*We will focus on some of these conditions like postpartum haemorrhage, sepsis and malaria in the context of HIV-positive pregnant women in a resource-poor setting.*

## HIV/AIDS Precautions: CDC Recommendations

### Isolation of Patient during Treatment and Incineration of Disposables Recommended

All used syringes or other sharp instruments should be routinely placed in "sharps" containers for proper disposal to prevent accidental injuries and risk of HIV transmission.

For most HIV exposures that warrant PEP, a basic 4-week, two-drug (there are several options) regimen is recommended, starting as soon as possible after exposure. For HIV exposures that pose an increased risk of transmission (based on the infection status of the source and the type of exposure), a three-drug regimen may be recommended. Special circumstances, such as a delayed exposure report, unknown source person, pregnancy in the exposed person, resistance of the source virus to antiretroviral agents and toxicity of PEP regimens, are also discussed in the guidelines. Occupational exposures should be considered urgent medical concerns, and PEP should be started within 72 h—the sooner the better; every hour counts.

## WHO Recommendations for the Treatment of PPH (Specially for HIV-Positive Patients)

1. *Intravenous oxytocin alone is the recommended uterotonic drug for the treatment of PPH.*
2. If intravenous oxytocin is unavailable, or if the bleeding does not respond to oxytocin, the use of intravenous ergometrine, oxytocin-ergometrine fixed dose or a prostaglandin drug (including sublingual misoprostol, 800 μg) is recommended.
3. The use of isotonic crystalloids is recommended in preference to the use of colloids for the initial intravenous fluid resuscitation of women with PPH.
4. The use of tranexamic acid is recommended for the treatment of PPH if oxytocin and other uterotonics fail to stop bleeding or if it is thought that the bleeding may be partly due to trauma.
5. Uterine massage is recommended for the treatment of atonic PPH.
6. If women do not respond to treatment using uterotonics, or if uterotonics are unavailable, the use of intrauterine balloon tamponade is recommended for the treatment of PPH due to uterine atony.
7. If other measures have failed and if the necessary resources are available, the use of uterine artery embolization is recommended as a treatment for PPH due to uterine atony.
8. If bleeding does not stop in spite of treatment using uterotonics and other available conservative interventions (e.g. uterine massage, balloon tamponade), the use of surgical interventions is recommended.
9. The use of bimanual uterine compression is recommended as a temporizing measure until appropriate care is available for the

treatment of PPH due to uterine atony after vaginal delivery.
10. The use of external aortic compression for the treatment of PPH due to uterine atony after vaginal birth is recommended as a temporizing measure until appropriate care is available.
11. The use of non-pneumatic anti-shock garments is recommended as a temporizing measure until appropriate care is available.
12. The use of uterine packing is not recommended for the treatment of PPH due to uterine atony after vaginal birth.
13. If the placenta is not expelled spontaneously, the use of IV/IM oxytocin (10 IU) in combination with controlled cord traction is recommended.
14. The use of ergometrine for the management of retained placenta is not recommended as this may cause tetanic uterine contractions which may delay the expulsion of the placenta.
15. The use of prostaglandin E2 alpha (dinoprostone or sulprostone) for the management of retained placenta is not recommended.
16. A single dose of antibiotics (ampicillin or first-generation cephalosporin) is recommended if manual removal of the placenta is required.

## Malaria and Pregnancy

Although the prevalence of malaria in pregnancy in Asia and Latin America is presumed to be high, there is an absence of longitudinal data on:

- Effect of single plasmodium infection or asymptomatic infections on the burden of malaria in pregnancy
- Effect of malaria in pregnancy on newborn baby and infant health, as well as true cumulative effect of malaria in pregnancy
- Prevalence of malaria in pregnancy in the first trimester and its correlation with adverse outcomes
- Direct and indirect effect of malaria on severe maternal morbidity and mortality, hypertensive disorders of pregnancy and postpartum complications [10]

HIV increases the degree to which malaria is associated with maternal severe anaemia and low birth weight beyond the effect of HIV itself on anaemia and birth weight (interaction) [11].

- Mefloquine is the agent of choice for chloroquine-resistant areas, and evidence suggests it is not associated with an increased risk to the foetus.
- Although the atovaquone-proguanil drug combination is not currently recommended for use during pregnancy, limited data suggest that it is not harmful to the foetus.
- Doxycycline and primaquine are not recommended during pregnancy [12].

## GOI Guidelines

*In the first trimester of pregnancy, parenteral quinine is the drug of choice.*

*However, if quinine is not available, artemisinin derivatives may be given.*

*In the second and third trimesters, parenteral artemisinin derivatives are preferred.*

## Puerperal Sepsis

The most common site of infection in puerperal sepsis is the placental site. Other sites of infection are abdominal and perineal wounds following surgery and lacerations of the genital tract, e.g. cervix, vagina and perineum.

HIV-positive patients are at higher risk of sepsis due to immunocompromised status.

## Symptoms and Signs

- Fever – temperature 38 °C or more
- Chills and general malaise
- Lower abdominal pain
- Ender uterus
- Subinvolution
- Purulent, foul-smelling lochia

There may also be light vaginal bleeding/shock.

## Tests/Investigations to Confirm Diagnosis

- Midstream specimen of urine wound swab, e.g. perineal or abdominal, or high vaginal swab
- Blood culture, in the presence of chills or evidence of severe infection

WHO recommends.

Prevention:

For puerperal sepsis prevention, three main strategies have been described:

- Hand hygiene
- Intravaginal application of antiseptics
- Use of prophylactic antibiotics

*Management*:

- Sepsis in pregnancy is often insidious in onset but can progress very rapidly. Regular monitoring of pulse, blood pressure and respiratory rate may assist with early identification.
- If sepsis is suspected in a patient in the community, urgent referral to hospital is indicated.
- *In hospital, high-dose intravenous broad-spectrum antibiotics should be started immediately after obtaining appropriate cultures; septicaemia can develop rapidly and has a high mortality rate. Treatment should not be delayed unduly by collection of clinical samples and can be adjusted after results of investigations become available.*
- *If GAS is isolated, IV penicillin is the treatment of choice.*
- Aggressive fluid resuscitation and close monitoring of fluid balance may be required; early involvement of critical care staff may be necessary.

### Conclusion

Critical pregnancy in presence of HIV infection poses greater challenge and requires special care. Timely diagnosis of risk factor and proper management will do wonders for the mother and the newborn.

## References


1. Madhivanan P1, Krupp K, Kulkarni V, Kulkarni S, Vaidya N, Shaheen R, Philpott S, Fisher C. HIV testing among pregnant women living with HIV in India: are private healthcare providers routinely violating women's human rights? BMC Int Health Hum Rights. 2014;14:71.
2. Slyker JA, et al. Correlates and outcomes of preterm birth, low birth weight, and small for gestational age in HIV-exposed uninfected infants. BMC Pregnancy Childbirth. 2014;14:7.
3. Lionel J, et al. HIV and obstetric complications and fetal outcomes in Vellore, India. Trop Doct. 2008; 38(3):144–6.
4. Heather watts. Management of human immunodeficiency virus infection in pregnancy. N Engl J Med. 2002;346(24):1879–91.
5. Minkoff H, et al. The relationship of pregnancy to human immunodeficiency virus disease progression. Am J Obstet Gynecol. 2003;189(2):5529.
6. French R, Brocklehurst P. The effect of pregnancy on survival in women infected with HIV: a systematic review of the literature and meta-analysis. Br J Obstet Gynaecol. 1998;105(8):82735.
7. Pai NP, et al. Impact of round-the-clock, rapid oral fluid HIV testing of women in labor in rural India. PLoS Med. 2008;5(5):e92.
8. McIntyre J. Mothers infected with HIV. Br Med Bull. 2003;67:127–35.
9. Chaudhry, et al. http://emedicine.medscape.com/article/2042311overview
10. Desai M, et al. Epidemiology and burden of malaria in pregnancy. Lancet Infect Dis. 2007;7:93–104.
11. ter Kuile FO, et al. The burden of co-infection with human immunodeficiency virus type 1 and malaria in pregnant women in sub-saharan Africa. Am J Trop Med Hyg. 2004;71 (suppl):41–54.
12. Marie-Hélène Irvine et al. vol 57: noveMBER noveMBRE 2011|Canadian Family Physician.

# Antiphospholipid Syndrome

# 18

Mala Arora

The antiphospholipid syndrome (APS) is an autoimmune condition characterized by recurrent arterial or venous thrombosis and recurrent pregnancy loss. The autoantibodies are targeted to negatively charged phospholipids, in the cell membrane. The prevalence of APS in general obstetric population is 2 %. However in women with autoimmune disorders like systemic lupus erythematosus (SLE), it is as high as 30 %. Among obstetric patients with early-onset severe pre-eclampsia, the prevalence can be as high as 30 %.

This syndrome was first described in 1983 by Harris [1] and Hughes [2] who observed that patients with SLE had high levels of anticardiolipin antibodies of at least one immunoglobulin class, IgG, IgM or IgA. There were strong correlations between raised anticardiolipin levels and the lupus anticoagulant (LA), venous and arterial thrombosis and thrombocytopenia. In their original study, of the 15 patients with the highest anticardiolipin titres, six had a history of venous thrombosis, five had cerebral thrombosis, five had thrombocytopenia and two each had pulmonary hypertension and recurrent miscarriages. They originally named it anticardiolipin (aCL) syndrome or Hughes' syndrome. It is ironic that APS was discovered largely by the aCL test, but the clinical value of this test is now considered marginal, as a host of other antibodies are also associated with this condition.

This syndrome was initially described in patients with SLE, but it was later recognized that most patients with primary APS do not fulfil the diagnostic criteria of SLE and that those with primary APS do not progress to SLE. Hence we recognized that APS syndrome may be classified as:

- Primary APS or PAPS
- Secondary APS or SAPS which is associated with SLE

The two have similar clinical presentations (Table 18.1).

## Laboratory Testing (Table 18.2)

### Antibody Testing

It is recommended that in APS syndrome both the lupus anticoagulant and the antiphospholipid antibody and/or the anticardiolipin antibody should be tested as they are heterogeneous in nature [3].

Antibody testing in APS syndrome is not simple, as patients may exhibit antibodies to cardiolipin (CL), phospholipids (PL) or to one of the cofactors, beta 2 glycoprotein I ($\beta_2$GPI) [4], which is a natural anticoagulant protein.

M. Arora, FRCOG, FICOG, FICMCH, DA (UK)
Director Noble IVF Centre, Sector 14,
Senior Consultant, Fortis La Femme GK2,
Faridabad, New Delhi, India
e-mail: malanarinder@yahoo.com



A. Gandhi et al. (eds.), *Principles of Critical Care in Obstetrics: Volume II*,
DOI 10.1007/978-81-322-2686-4_18

**Table 18.1** Classification of APS

| | |
|---|---|
| Primary APS | No associated autoimmune disorder |
| Secondary APS | Associated with SLE, ITP |
| Familial APS | Runs in families with a complex inheritance pattern |
| Catastrophic APS | Multiple-vessel thrombosis – life-threatening |

**Table 18.2** Antibody testing in APS

| Antibody type | Subtype |
|---|---|
| Anticardiolipin ACL | IgG and IgM |
| Antiphospholipid APL | Antiphosphatidylserine |
| IgG and IgM | Antiphosphatidylcholine |
| | Antiphosphatidylethanolamine |
| Cofactors | Anti-beta 2 glycoprotein I |
| | Antiprothrombin |
| | Anti-annexin V |
| | Anti-protein C |
| Lupus anticoagulant | PTT, APTT, DRVVT |

Hence, there are a host of antibodies that can be tested, which add to the cost of testing. Antibodies tested by ELISA may be IgG, IgM or IgA classes alone or in combination. In APS, positive IgG antibodies are diagnostic. IgM antibodies found alone may be transient and may be stimulated by viral infections or drugs described below. They are generally innocuous or non-thrombogenic. Hence it is necessary to repeat antibody titres after 6–12 weeks. The antibody titres are reported as low, medium or high positive.

The antiphospholipid antibodies (aPL) are a group of heterogeneous antibodies of which the most commonly tested are phosphatidylcholine (PC), phosphatidylserine (PS) and phosphatidylethanolamine (PE). In addition phosphatidylglycerol and phosphatidylinositol are also recognized but less commonly used in the clinical setting.

It was realized in 1990 that a positive ELISA test for aCL depends on a protein cofactor, $\beta_2$GPI, to exert their action and aPL antibodies need this plasma cofactor. They do not bind directly to the anionic phospholipid but to the protein/phospholipids and prothrombin [5].

Hence antibodies to beta 2 glycoprotein I are also diagnostic for APS syndrome. Many additional cofactors have been identified since then, like antiprothrombin, anti-annexin V and anti-protein C and S [5].

Recently antiphosphatidylserine-dependent antiprothrombin antibody (aPS/aPT) has also been detected in these patients [6]. This is a new marker antibody reported in 2006.

The definition of aPL antibody now appears to be *an antibody that targets not just phospholipids but also PL-binding proteins*. The antibody may react preferentially with the PL-bound form or may bind to the free antigen in plasma as an immune complex (IC) to potentiate binding to a given PL.

## Lupus Anticoagulant

Apart from antibody testing by ELISA, these patients test positive for lupus anticoagulant (LA). It tests for derangement of coagulation profile. Contrary to what its name implies, the LA is powerfully thrombotic in vivo. Its name has been derived from the observation that it prolongs all phospholipid-dependent coagulation tests, including the prothrombin time, partial thromboplastin time and Russell viper venom time.

ACL and LA although related antibodies are distinct, and many individuals with aCL do not have LA and vice versa [7]. Although majority of patients are positive for aCL and LA, about 10–16 % are positive for LA and negative for aCL, and 25 % are positive for aCL and negative for LA [8, 9]. Thus it is important to test for both antibodies while investigating for APS.

## Mechanism of Pregnancy Loss

APS is associated with very early pregnancy loss, first-trimester miscarriages, second-trimester intrauterine deaths and third-trimester complications like pre-eclampsia, intrauterine growth restriction, oligohydramnios, placental abruption and intrauterine fetal death. It is also associated with neonatal morbidity related to prematurity and growth retardation, like necrotizing enterocolitis, intraventricular haemorrhage and even neonatal deaths.

Pregnancy is a hypercoagulable state. In 1856, the Prussian pathologist Rudolf Virchow first proposed his hypothesis, to explain the pathogenesis of thrombosis [10], which holds true even today. He suggested that three factors were necessary to produce thrombosis:

(i) Hypercoagulability
(ii) Stasis
(iii) Endothelial damage

In pregnancy there is an increase in certain clotting factors leading to hypercoagulability and there is stasis in the pelvic and lower limb veins. There is however no endothelial damage. In APS syndrome endothelial damage is widespread due to antigen-antibody binding and complement activation which adds fuel to the fire and increases the thrombogenic potential manifold. Available data indicate that the thrombogenic function of aPL antibodies involves their general effect on platelets, endothelial cells, anticoagulant mechanisms and fibrinolytic pathways, as well as their local effect on trophoblasts and villi cells, leading to reduction of annexin V (placental anticoagulant protein-I) production and inhibition of its anticoagulant function [11, 12].

Thrombogenic effects of APS in pregnancy include:

- Recognition of cofactor beta 2 glycoprotein I on the endothelial cells and trophoblastic surface that allows deposition of aPL antibodies at these sites promoting thrombosis.
- Activation of endothelial cells like monocytes and platelets at the antibody-binding site.
- Vasculopathy of the spiral arteries of the uterus that are the feeder vessels to the placenta. This leads to placental infarction and thrombosis, which is a triggering factor for pre-eclampsia and intrauterine growth restriction.

In addition APS slows the mechanisms that aid in dissolving intravascular clots like:

- Inhibition of natural anticoagulants like protein C and tissue factor pathway inhibitor
- Inhibition of fibrinolytic system

All of the above mechanisms increase thrombogenic complications in pregnancy and can also result in arterial and venous thrombosis in pregnancy.

Besides thrombogenesis, APS also exerts harmful non-thrombogenic effects which are as follows:

1. Antiphospholipid antibodies exert a direct effect on trophoblast function resulting in direct cellular injury and inhibition of syncytia formation, which results in decreased trophoblastic invasion. This will result in trophoblastic dysfunction and account for very early pregnancy losses as well as poor implantation leading to subfertility.
2. Antiphospholipid antibodies affect human chorionic gonadotrophin secretion by trophoblast cells by abolishing GnRH-induced hCG stimulation of human trophoblastic cells. They also decrease the placental hormone production, secondary to trophoblastic dysfunction [13]. This will account for early and mid-trimester losses.
3. Recent studies have defined an important inflammatory role of antiphospholipid antibodies with activation of the complement system. RPL may be the result of this inflammatory condition and that *complement inhibitors* may be the preferred therapy. The efficacy of heparin in APS may rely on its complement inhibitory action as well as its anticoagulant potential. Thus, it is possible that the unifying feature of the many aPL antibodies which have been linked to RPL is the propensity of a given aPL to fix and activate the complement, particularly in an inflammatory setting. Furthermore, the complement in conjunction with specific antibody can elicit a wide array of clinical features, including thrombosis, and therefore may be a common denominator in aPL disorders [14].

It is now well recognized that aPL antibodies exert both thrombogenic and non-thrombogenic detrimental effects on pregnancy in the early mid- and late trimesters and may be implicated in recurrent implantation failures in patients undergoing assisted reproductive techniques (ART).

## Indications for Testing

The obstetric clinical criteria for testing had been defined at an international antiphospholipid symposium, held in 1999. These include [15]:

1. One or more unexplained deaths of a morphologically normal fetus more than 10 weeks of gestation documented by ultrasound or direct examination
2. One or more preterm births at or before 34 weeks of gestation due to severe pre-eclampsia or placental insufficiency
3. Three or more consecutive abortions before 10 weeks gestation with no maternal hormonal, anatomic abnormalities, normal maternal and paternal chromosomes and other causes of recurrent losses being ruled out
4. History of vascular thrombosis:
   Unexplained venous thrombosis
   Unexplained arterial thrombosis
   Small-vessel thrombosis

These criteria have been revised in 2006 at a workshop in Sydney, Australia. The revised criteria are mentioned in Table 18.3 [16].

There is currently a debate over screening the high-risk obstetric population for APS [17]. It

**Table 18.3** Revised classification of APS syndrome

| |
|---|
| Revised classification criteria for the antiphospholipid syndrome: |
| Antiphospholipid antibody syndrome (APS) is present if at least one of the clinical criteria and one of the laboratory criteria that follow are met. |
| *Clinical criteria* |
| 1. Vascular thrombosis |
| One or more clinical episodes of arterial, venous or small-vessel thrombosis, in any tissue or organ. Thrombosis must be confirmed by objective validated criteria (i.e. unequivocal findings of appropriate imaging studies or histopathology). For histopathologic confirmation, thrombosis should be present without significant evidence of inflammation in the vessel wall. |
| 2. Pregnancy morbidity |
| (a) One or more unexplained deaths of a morphologically normal fetus at or beyond the 10th week of gestation, with normal fetal morphology documented by ultrasound or by direct examination of the fetus |
| (b) One or more premature births of a morphologically normal neonate before the 34th week of gestation because of (i) eclampsia or severe pre-eclampsia defined according to standard definitions or (ii) recognized features of placental insufficiency |
| (c) Three or more unexplained consecutive spontaneous abortions before the 10th week of gestation, with maternal anatomic or hormonal abnormalities and paternal and maternal chromosomal causes excluded |
| In studies of populations of patients who have more than one type of pregnancy morbidity, investigators are strongly encouraged to stratify groups of subjects according to a, b or c above. |
| *Laboratory criteria* |
| 1. Lupus anticoagulant (LA) present in plasma, on two or more occasions at least 12 weeks apart, detected according to the guidelines of the International Society on Thrombosis and Haemostasis (Scientific Subcommittee on LAs/phospholipid-dependent antibodies) |
| 2. Anticardiolipin (aCL) antibody of IgG and/or IgM isotype in serum or plasma, present in medium or high titre (i.e. >40 GPL or MPL or > the 99th percentile), on two or more occasions, at least 12 weeks apart, measured by a standardized ELISA |
| 3. Anti-$\beta_2$ glycoprotein I antibody of IgG and/or IgM isotype in serum or plasma (in titre > the 99th percentile), present on two or more occasions, at least 12 weeks apart, measured by a standardized ELISA, according to recommended procedures |
| Classification of APS should be avoided if less than 12 weeks or more than 5 years separate the positive aPL test and the clinical event. |

has been proposed that in patients with history of thrombotic episodes prior to pregnancy or patients with previous thromboembolic episodes during pregnancy or gestational problems likely to be thrombotic in nature, the significant association with predisposing thrombophilic conditions could justify screening for APS syndrome, homocysteine levels and perhaps factor V Leiden mutation, activated protein C resistance (APCR) and antithrombin III deficiency. However routine screening of the general obstetric population is not recommended as it is not cost-effective.

## Diagnosis

At least one clinical and one laboratory criteria are required to classify a patient with APS [18]. These must be positive on two occasions 6–12 weeks apart. This is because transient positive results for aPL IgM may occur in the presence of viral infections such as chickenpox, adenovirus, mumps, HIV and also syphilis [19]. Certain drugs such as procainamide, chlorpromazine, sodium valproate, phenytoin, hydralazine and propranolol may induce aPL antibodies which are transient and non-thrombogenic. Because of the heterogeneity of antibodies tested and the fluctuating antibody levels, the diagnosis of APS syndrome is difficult to establish, although once diagnosed the treatment is non-controversial.

## **Classification of APS** (Table 18.1)

*Primary APS (PAPS)* Patients with LA or medium-to-high levels of IgG or IgM aCL antibodies and fetal death, recurrent pre-embryonic or embryonic pregnancy loss, thrombosis, or neonatal death after delivery for severe pre-eclampsia or fetal distress.

*Secondary APS (SAPS)* Patients with systemic lupus erythematosus (SLE) who have antiphospholipid antibodies (aPL) and or lupus antibodies are classified as secondary APS. There are no major differences in the clinical presentation in primary and secondary APS except that secondary APS has a greater than 40 % risk of thrombosis than those without SLE and conveys a worse prognosis.

*Familial APS Syndrome* Goel [20] studied families with more than one affected member, examined possible modes of inheritance and determined linkage to potential candidate genes. In seven families, 30 of 101 family members met the diagnostic criteria for the syndrome. Segregation studies rejected both environmental and autosomal recessive models, and the data fitted best, either a dominant or a codominant model. Linkage analysis showed independent segregation of antiphospholipid syndrome and several candidate genes.

*Catastrophic APS (CAPS)* Recently described in 280 patients, catastrophic APS is an uncommon but potentially life-threatening condition that needs high clinical awareness. The first clinical manifestation at the time of the catastrophic episode was a pulmonary complication in 24 % of the cases, a neurologic feature in 18 % and a renal feature in 18 %. During the catastrophic episode, multiple-vessel thrombosis may lead to multi-organ failure. Intraabdominal involvement was identified in the majority of patients, mainly consisting of renal (71 %), hepatic (33 %), gastrointestinal (25 %), splenic (19 %), adrenal (13 %) and pancreatic (8 %) manifestations. One hundred twenty-three (44 %) patients died at the time of the catastrophic APS event, but higher recovery rate was achieved by the combination of anticoagulants plus corticosteroids along with plasma exchange (PE) and/or intravenous immunoglobulins (IVIG) (69 % versus 54 %) [21].

## Management

### Preconception Counselling

Therapy needs to be started early in pregnancy hence preconception counselling is necessary. In patients with implantation failures and very early pregnancy loss, low-dose aspirin may be started in the preconception period along with folic acid.

The need for close surveillance of the pregnancy, with a multidisciplinary approach, should be explained. Delivery should be planned at a centre with advanced neonatal intensive care facilities.

Medical and obstetric risks should also be explained. Pre-eclampsia, fetal growth restriction, preterm labour and fetal losses are the obstetric complications seen. In a study of APS treated with heparin, 40 % had growth restriction and 25 % delivered at less than 32 weeks [22]. Other studies have also shown that the complication rates in treated patients with moderate to high levels of aPL are high [23].

## Low-Dose Aspirin

Low-dose aspirin 60–80 mg/day has significant antiplatelet action thereby preventing platelet adhesion which is the first step in clot formation. Hence low-dose aspirin is recommended in the prevention of pre-eclampsia and intrauterine growth restriction [24, 25] in high-risk gravidas. There are many non-randomized studies suggesting that low-dose aspirin is effective and it can prevent pregnancy loss in experimental APS mice. Randomized controlled trials of aspirin as a single agent in APS do not support any benefit over placebo; however, such studies have been undertaken in low-risk women. Most centres now advocate treatment with low-dose aspirin for all women with APS, prior to conception in the belief that trophoblastic dysfunction occurs early in gestation and aspirin may prevent failure of placentation. It is then continued throughout pregnancy along with low molecular weight heparin (LMWH).

Caution needs to be exercised in its use in the third trimester as it is associated with closure of fetal ductus arteriosus in utero and possible pulmonary hypertension of the newborn, jaundice and kernicterus. It also crosses the placenta. There have been recent case reports of fetal intracranial bleeding with the use of low-dose aspirin [26].

Patients with APS and stroke are probably best treated with aspirin, while those with other forms of arterial thromboembolism (TE) are likely best treated with moderate-intensity warfarin plus aspirin.

## Heparin

Heparin has been used effectively during pregnancy to avert complications of APS syndrome. It is a potent anticoagulant, but as early as 1929 it was shown to have "anti-complementary effects" [27]. It is now postulated that this may play an important role in preventing obstetric complications in APS syndrome. It is important to realize that heparin does not alter binding of aPL-IgG to decidual tissue, but it can only prevent complement-activated damage. Given the importance of complement-split products as mediators of aPL antibody-induced fetal injury, it was considered that heparin prevents pregnancy loss by inhibiting complement activation on trophoblast and that anticoagulation, in and of itself, is not sufficient to prevent pregnancy complications in APS. In the mice model, treatment with unfractionated or low molecular weight heparins (LMWH) protected pregnancies from aPL antibody-induced damage, whereas treatment with hirudin or fondaparinux (anticoagulants without anti-complement effects) was not protective. Mice that received unfractionated heparin (UFH) 20U, LMWH, fondaparinux or hirudin were all anticoagulated, as demonstrated by increased partial thromboplastin time (PTT) or decreased factor Xa activity. However mice receiving hirudin and fondaparinux although well anticoagulated did not show a decline in pregnancy loss. Conversely, mice treated with a low dose of heparin, 10 U, were also protected against APL-induced pregnancy complications in spite of not showing detectable anticoagulant effect [14] (Table 18.4).

The increased circulating blood volume in pregnancy necessitates a higher dose of heparin 10,000 units twice daily subcutaneously preferably self-administered. During labour this may be reduced to 5,000–7,500 units twice daily. For elective abdominal deliveries, heparin is stopped 48 h prior to the procedure.

The main danger of heparin therapy in pregnancy is osteoporosis, firstly because its use in pregnancy is prolonged and secondly pregnancy and lactation cause reversible bone demineralization. There have been several reports of verte-

**Table 18.4** Heparins prevent pregnancy loss and inhibit complement activation [14]

| | Anticoagulation | Prevention of pregnancy loss | Complement inhibition |
|---|---|---|---|
| UFH (10 U) | – | + | + |
| UFH (20 U) | + | + | + |
| LMWH | + | + | + |
| Fondaparinux | + | – | – |
| Hirudin | + | – | – |

Salmon [14], The American Clinical and Climatological Association
*LMWH* low molecular weight heparin, *UFH* unfractionated heparin

bral collapse associated with heparin use in pregnancy. It must be emphasized that to prevent this dreaded complication there should be adequate calcium and vitamin D3 intake as well as moderate exercise. Bed rest should be strictly avoided as it accelerates bone loss. Fortunately bone density improves once heparin therapy is discontinued.

Another rare but dreaded complication is thrombocytopenia and a complete blood count should be done one week after starting heparin therapy. If platelet counts drop, heparin should be discontinued with immediate effect, and low molecular weight heparin (LMWH) should be substituted.

## Low Molecular Weight Heparin

Low molecular weight heparins (LMWHs) have fewer complications than conventional heparin and are being more frequently used in pregnancy safely [28, 29]. LMWH inhibits factor Xa and therefore has an antithrombotic effect, while heparin has, in addition, an anticoagulant effect through its action on antithrombin III and factor IIa. Thus bleeding complications with LMWH are few with little alteration of PT and aPTT. Other advantages include increased bioavailability and a longer half-life necessitating a once-daily administration and a lower risk of thrombocytopenia and osteoporosis. The major factor precluding routine long-term use in pregnancy is the cost. Both heparin and LMWH do not cross the placenta and fetal complications have not been reported. A number of low molecular weight heparins are available which have a molecular weight of 4000–6000 daltons. The various fractions have different pharmacological profiles and the properties, and the dose of one LMWH cannot be extrapolated to another. Enoxaparin in the dose of 40 mg/day subcutaneously and dalteparin 5,000 units per day are recommended during pregnancy. It has been used successfully in pregnancy with a live birth rate of 85–95 % [30]. Some women may develop a local allergic reaction to LMWH.

Enoxaparin (Clexane) 40 m mg per day subcutaneously or dalteparin (Fragmin) 5,000 units per day is injected from the confirmation of pregnancy till delivery. During labour LMWH should be discontinued at least 8 h prior to instituting regional analgesia like epidurals. It can be recommenced after delivery. Its action can be reversed by an intravenous injection of protamine sulphate for emergency surgery. One milligram of protamine sulphate neutralizes 80–100 units of heparin when given 15 min after the heparin injection. If longer time has elapsed, less protamine sulphate is required as heparin is rapidly excreted.

Management options in varied clinical scenarios of APS are discussed in Table 18.5 [31].

## Fetal Monitoring (Table 18.6)

Close fetal monitoring is essential in each trimester.

In the *first trimester* serial monitoring with serum beta HCG and transvaginal ultrasound scan will ensure the progress of pregnancy.

During the *second trimester*, Doppler waveform analysis of the uterine artery at 20–24 weeks gestation to look for diastolic notching will help predict the high-risk pregnancy.

In high-risk pregnancy the *third trimester* is closely monitored with serial growth scans and Doppler interrogation of the fetal vessels especially the middle cerebral artery (MCA) in patients with oligohydramnios and IUGR. This will allow timely delivery and improve fetal outcome.

**Table 18.5** Management options for APS

| Feature | Management |
|---|---|
| APS with prior fetal death or recurrent pregnancy loss, fetal death, neonatal death, pre-eclampsia, IUGR, abruption | Low-dose aspirin preconception with unfractionated heparin 20,000 units/day or LMWH 5,000 units /day when pregnancy is confirmed<br>Calcium and vitamin D3 supplementation |
| APS with prior thrombosis or stroke | On warfarin, transfer to LMWH+ aspirin prior to 6 weeks of pregnancy<br>Heparin/LMWH to achieve full anticoagulation with low-dose aspirin<br>Calcium and vitamin D3 |
| APS without prior pregnancy loss or thrombosis | Optimal management uncertain<br>Low-dose aspirin daily and/or prophylactic heparin daily |
| aPL antibodies without APS<br>LA positive or aCL positive medium to high titres | Optimal management uncertain<br>No treatment or low-dose aspirin or<br>LMWH + low-dose aspirin |

**Table 18.6** Fetal monitoring in APS

| | |
|---|---|
| First trimester | Serial beta HCG<br>Transvaginal scan |
| Second trimester | Uterine artery Doppler at 20–24 weeks<br>Microalbuminuria<br>Blood pressure(BP) monitoring |
| Third trimester | BP monitoring + albuminuria<br>Serial ultrasound scan for growth<br>Fetal Doppler of umbilical/MCA |

Regular monitoring of blood pressure and urine analysis for proteinuria are done at each antenatal visit. Testing for microalbuminuria will help in the detection of early-onset pre-eclampsia.

## Postpartum Prophylaxis

- Women on long-term warfarin treatment may recommence this on the second or third postpartum day, and the low molecular weight heparin is discontinued when the INR is >2.
- Women with previous thrombosis should receive postpartum heparin or warfarin for 6 weeks.
- Women with no previous thrombosis should receive postpartum prophylactic heparin for 5 days.

Neither heparin nor warfarin is excreted in breast milk; hence, breastfeeding is not contraindicated with the use of these drugs.

## Other Drugs Used in APS Syndrome

### Warfarin

Warfarin crosses the placenta and causes embryopathy hence is contraindicated in the first trimester of pregnancy. The teratogenic risks include chondrodysplasia punctata, nasal hypoplasia, growth restriction and short proximal limbs. The period of risk is between 6 and 12 weeks; hence, conception on warfarin is not dangerous provided that warfarin is replaced by LMWH within 2 weeks of a missed period. The risk of miscarriage and stillbirth is also increased. When used in the third trimester, there is a significant risk of maternal retroplacental and fetal intracranial bleeding.

If the bleeding is severe, the action of warfarin can be reversed by injection of vitamin K 5 mg by slow intravenous injection supplemented with fresh frozen plasma 15 ml/kg to replenish the clotting factors. The use of warfarin in pregnancy is only justified in the presence of prosthetic heart valves and perhaps prior arterial thrombosis.

In patients with pregestational arterial or venous thrombosis, warfarin is the drug of choice and may have to be continued in the second and early third trimester of pregnancy as well as postpartum period. However it should be substituted with LMWH and low-dose aspirin in the first trimester of pregnancy, and the switch should be done prior to 6 weeks of pregnancy.

Among patients with aPL antibodies, the absolute risk of developing new thrombosis is low (<1 % per year) in otherwise healthy patients without prior thrombotic events. It may be moderately increased (up to 10 % per year) in women with recurrent pregnancy loss without prior thrombosis and is highest (>10 % in the first year) in patients with a history of venous thrombosis who have discontinued anticoagulant drugs within 6 months of getting pregnant. Compared with placebo or untreated control, anticoagulation with moderate-intensity warfarin (adjusted to a target international normalized ratio [INR] of 2.0–3.0) reduces the risk of recurrent venous thrombosis by 80–90 % irrespective of the presence of aPL antibodies and may be effective for preventing recurrent arterial thrombosis. No evidence exists that high-intensity warfarin (target INR, >3.0) is more effective than moderate-intensity warfarin [30]. For patients with a single positive aPL antibody test result and prior stroke, aspirin and moderate-intensity warfarin appear equally effective for preventing recurrent stroke. Treatment issues that have not been addressed in clinical trials, or for which the evidence is conflicting, include:

- Role of antithrombotic prophylaxis in patients with antiphospholipid antibodies without prior thrombosis
- Optimal treatment of non-cerebrovascular arterial thrombosis
- Recurrent thrombosis despite warfarin therapy [30]

Based on the available data, the American College of Chest Physicians recommends for patients with APS and a venous thromboembolic event warfarin therapy with a target INR of 2.5 (Grade 1A) for 12 months (Grade 1C+) and suggests that indefinite anticoagulant therapy should be considered (Grade 1C) especially for recurrent events [32].

## Corticosteroids

Oral prednisolone (40–60 mg/day) along with low-dose aspirin (75 mg/day) was used in the mid-1990s to treat APS-associated recurrent pregnancy loss [33], but was soon abandoned in favour of anticoagulant regimes because of complications such as hypertension, diabetes, osteoporosis, steroid psychosis, preterm rupture of membranes and preterm labour. Subsequently controlled clinical trials showed that prednisolone is ineffective and possibly detrimental in the treatment of recurrent pregnancy loss [34]. Hence it is no longer used in pregnancy. However, pregnant patients with SLE and APS may require corticosteroids for control of SLE under the guidance of a physician. Short-course parenteral steroids are used to induce fetal lung maturity if delivery is imminent prior to 34 weeks in APS syndrome. Steroids are also used in life-threatening situations such as in the management of catastrophic APS [21].

## Intravenous Immunoglobulins

Several reports exist on successful pregnancy outcome when high-dose IVIG was used in conjunction with heparin or LDA or alone. In patients treated with IVIG, unfractionated heparin and LDA, fewer pregnancy complications like IUGR and pre-eclampsia were noted [35, 36]. However a recent prospective, randomized, controlled study of women with definite APS on heparin and LDA found no additional benefit of IVIG [37]. Thus IVIG may be indicated when pregnancy failure has occurred despite judicious heparin use. A dose of 0.3 g/kg immunoglobulin given every 4 weeks till 32 weeks is a commonly employed regime.

## Plasmapheresis or Plasma Exchange

In patients with catastrophic APS, one may need to resort to plasma exchange to lower the antibody levels.

## Fluvastatin

Fluvastatin has been shown to revert pro-inflammatory/prothrombotic effects of antiphospholipid antibodies (aPL) in vitro and in mice. Here, we examined whether fluvastatin affects the levels of pro-inflammatory/prothrombotic markers in antiphospholipid syndrome (APS) patients. Vascular endothelial growth factor (VEGF), soluble tissue factor (sTF), tumour necrosis factor-alpha (TNF-alpha), soluble intercellular adhesion molecule-1 (sICAM-1), sE-selectin (sE-sel), C-reactive protein (CRP) and soluble vascular cell adhesion molecule (sVCAM-1) were measured in the sera of 93 APS patients and 60 controls and in the sera of nine patients with APS before and after 30 days of treatment with fluvastatin. Elevated levels of VEGF, sTF and TNF-alpha were found in APS patients. Fluvastatin significantly reduced those markers in the majority of treated subjects. The data from this study show that statins may be beneficial in aPL-positive patients and warrant larger clinical trials to confirm the efficacy of the drug for the treatment of clinical manifestations of APS [38].

In obstetrics APS is regarded as the most important prothrombotic cause of recurrent pregnancy loss, with pregnancy success improving from below 20 % in the past to a current live birth rate of over 80 % with the introduction of anticoagulant therapy.

In summary APS syndrome is a treatable cause of pregnancy loss and implantation failure.

- Suspicious cases should be screened by antibody testing and/or testing for lupus anticoagulant.
- Therapy with low-dose aspirin is started at the pre-pregnancy counselling clinic, and heparin/low molecular weight heparin is added when the diagnosis of pregnancy is confirmed on ultrasound scan.
- Therapy is continued till at least 34 weeks of pregnancy.
- Pregnancy is closely monitored for pre-eclampsia, IUGR and abruption.
- Postpartum anticoagulation is important to prevent DVT.
- Corticosteroids are only used in APS that is concomitant with SLE.
- In patients with recurrent arterial/venous thrombosis, long-term warfarin therapy may be required.

## References

1. Harris EN, Charavi AE, Boey ML, Patel BM, Mackworth-Young CG, Loizou S, Hughes GRV. Anticardiolipin antibodies: detection by radioimmunoassay and association with thrombosis in systemic lupus erythematosus. Lancet. 1983;2:1211–4.
2. Hughes GRV, Harris EN, Gharavi AE. The anticardiolipin syndrome. J Rheumatol. 1985;13:486–9.
3. Shoenfeld Y, Meroni PL. The beta-2 glycoprotein I and antiphospholipid antibodies. Clin Exp Rheumatol. 1992;10:205–9.
4. Bevers EM, Galli M, Barbui T, Comfurius P, Zwaal RF. Lupus anticoagulants IgG's (LA) are not directed to phospholipids only but to a complex of lipid-bound human prothrombin. Thromb Haemost. 1991;66:629–32.
5. Horstman LL, Jy W, Bidot CJ, Ahn YS, Kelley RE, Zivadinov R, Maghzi AH, Etemadifar M, Mousavi SA, Minagar A. Antiphospholipid antibodies: paradigm in transition. J Neuroinflammation. 2009;6:3.
6. Ieko M, Nakabayashi T, Tarumi T, Yoshida M, Naito S, Atsumi T, Koike T. Phosphatidylserine dependent anti prothrombin antibody as a new marker for the diagnosis of antiphospholipid syndrome. Rinsho Byori. 2006;54(3):256–62 (article in Japanese).
7. McNeil HP, Chesterman CN, Krilis SA. Anticardiolipin antibodies and lupus anticoagulants comprise separate antibody subgroups with different phospholipids binding characteristics. Br J Haematol. 1989;73:506–13.
8. Kandiah DA, Krilis SA. Laboratory detection of antiphospholipid antibodies. Lupus. 1996;5:160–2.
9. Pierangeli SS, Gharavi AE. Testing for antiphospholipid antibodies: problems and solutions. Clin Obstet Gynecol. 2001;44:48–57.
10. Lowe GD. Virchow's triad revisited: abnormal flow. Pathophysiol Haemost Thromb. 2004;33:455–7.
11. Gharavi AE, Pierangeli SS, Levy RA, Harris EN. Mechanisms of pregnancy loss in antiphospholipid syndrome. Clin Obstet Gynecol. 2001;44(1):11–9.
12. Geis W, Branch DW. Obstetric implications of antiphospholipid antibodies: pregnancy loss and other complications. Clin Obstet Gynecol. 2001;44:2–10.
13. Caruso A, De Carolis S, Di Simon N. Antiphospholipid antibodies in obstetrics: new complexities and sites of action. Hum Reprod Update. 1999;5(3):267–76.
14. Salmon JE. Antiphospholipid antibodies revisited: a disorder initiated by inflammation [Theodore E Woodward Award]. Trans Am Clin Climatol Assoc. 2007;118:99–114.
15. Wilson WA. Classification criteria for antiphospholipid syndrome. Rheum Dis Clin North Am. 2001;27(3):499–505, v.
16. Miyakis S, Lockshin MD, Atsumi T, Branch DW, Brey RL, Cervera R, Derksen RH, DE Groot PG, Koike T, Meroni PL, Reber G, Shoenfeld Y, Tincani A, Vlachoyiannopoulos PG, Krilis SA. International

consensus statement on an update of the classification criteria for definite antiphospholipid syndrome (APS). J Thromb Haemost. 2006;4(2):295–306.
17. Salvagno GL, Lippi G, Franchini M, Targher G, Montagnana M, Franchi M, Guidi GC. The cost-benefit ratio of screening pregnant women for thrombophilia. Blood Transfus. 2007;5(4):189–203.
18. Levine JS, Branch DW, Rauch J. The antiphospholipid syndrome. N Engl J Med. 2002;346:752–63.
19. Vaarala O, Palosuo T, Kleemola M, Aho K. Anticardiolipin response in acute infections. Clin Immunol Immunopathol. 1986;41:8–15.
20. Goel N, Ortel TL, Bali D, Anderson JP, Gourley IS, Smith H, Morris CA, DeSimone M, Branch DW, Ford P, Berdeaux D, Roubey RAS, Kostyu DD, Kingsmore SF, Thiel T, Amos C, Seldin M. Familial antiphospholipid antibody syndrome: criteria for disease and evidence for autosomal dominant inheritance. Arthritis Rheum. 1999;42:318–27.
21. Cervera R, Bucciarelli S, Plasín MA, Gómez-Puerta JA, Plaza J, Pons-Estel G, Shoenfeld Y, Ingelmo M, Espinos G, Catastrophic Antiphospholipid Syndrome (CAPS) Registry Project Group (European Forum On Antiphospholipid Antibodies). Catastrophic antiphospholipid syndrome (CAPS): descriptive analysis of a series of 280 patients from the "CAPS Registry". J Autoimmun. 2009;32(3–4):240–5. Epub 2009 Mar 26.
22. Tuthill JI, Khamashta MA. Management of antiphospholipid syndrome. J Autoimmun. 2009;33(2):92–8. Epub 2009 Jun 25.
23. Erkan D, Lockshin MD. Antiphospholipid syndrome. Curr Opin Rheumatol. 2006;18(3):242–8.
24. CLASP: a randomised trial of low-dose aspirin for the prevention and treatment of pre-eclampsia among 9364 pregnant women. CLASP (Collaborative Low-dose Aspirin Study in Pregnancy) Collaborative Group. Lancet. 1994;343(8898):619–29.
25. Knight M, Duley L, Henderson-Smart DJ, King JF. WITHDRAWN: antiplatelet agents for preventing and treating pre-eclampsia. Cochrane Database Syst Rev. 2007;18;(2):CD000492.
26. Sasidharan CK, Kutty PM, Ajithkumar, Sajith N. Fetal intracranial hemorrhage due to antenatal low dose aspirin intake. Indian J Pediatr. 2001;68(11):1071–2.
27. Ecker E, Gross P. Anticomplementary power of heparin. J Infect Dis. 1929;44:250.
28. Bar J, Cohen-Sacher B, Hod M, et al. Low molecular weight heparin for thrombophilia in pregnant women. Int J Gynaecol Obstet. 2000;69:209–13.
29. Brenner B, Hoffman R, Blumenfeld Z, et al. Gestational outcome in thrombophilic women with recurrent pregnancy loss treated by enoxaparin. Thromb Haemost. 2000;83:693–7.
30. Lim W, Crowther MA, Eikelboom JW. Management of antiphospholipid antibody syndrome: a systematic review. JAMA. 2006;295(9):1050–7.
31. Nelson-Piercy C. Handbook of obstetric medicine, 4th ed, Informa health care. 2011, p 150.
32. Schünemann HJ, Cook D, Grimshaw J, Liberati A, Heffner J, Tapson V, Guyatt G. Antithrombotic and thrombolytic therapy: from evidence to application: the Seventh ACCP Conference on Antithrombotic and Thrombolytic Therapy. Chest. 2004;126:401S–512.
33. Cowchock FS, Reece AE, Balaban D, Branch DW, Plouffe L. Repeated fetal losses associated with antiphospholipid antibodies: a collaborative randomized trial comparing prednisone with low-dose aspirin. Am J Obstet Gynecol. 1992;166:1318–23.
34. Khamastha MA. Management of thrombosis and pregnancy loss in antiphospholipid syndrome. Lupus. 1998;7 Suppl 2:S162–5.
35. Clark AL, Branch DW, Silver RM, et al. Pregnancy complicated by the antiphospholipid syndrome: outcomes with intravenous immunoglobulin therapy. Obstet Gynecol. 1999;93:437–41.
36. Spinnato JA, Clark AL, Pierangeli SS, et al. Intravenous immunoglobulin therapy for antiphospholipid syndrome in pregnancy. Am J Obstet Gynecol. 1995;172:690–4.
37. Branch DW, Peaceman AM, Druzin M, et al. A multicenter, placebo-controlled pilot study of intravenous immune globulin treatment of antiphospholipid syndrome during pregnancy. The pregnancy loss study group. Am J Obstet Gynecol. 2000;182:122–7.
38. Jajoria P, Murthy V, Papalardo E, Romay-Penabad Z, Gleason C, Pierangeli SS. Statins for the treatment of antiphospholipid syndrome? Ann N Y Acad Sci. 2009;1173:736–45.

# 19 Systemic Lupus Erythematosus and Pregnancy

Hiralal Konar and Picklu Chaudhuri

## Overview

Systemic lupus erythematosus (SLE) is a multi-system connective tissue disease characterized by multi-organ involvement; characteristic inflammatory lesions of the skin, joints, serous membranes, kidneys and CNS; and its association with high titres of autoantibodies to an array of autoantigens. Its clinical course is often one of the disease flares followed by variable periods of remission. Approximately 90 % of the affected population are young women in their second or third decades of life. Therefore, SLE is the commonest connective tissue disorder encountered during pregnancy, and it has been widely studied by researchers across the globe. Evidence shows the foetal and maternal outcomes are adversely affected by the disease.

A multidisciplinary team comprising of obstetrician with experience in high-risk care, rheumatologist, nephrologists and haematologist is essential for monitoring and managing women with SLE during pregnancy and puerperium [1].

H. Konar, MD, DNB, FACS, FRCOG (✉)
Department of Obstetrics & Gynaecology, Calcutta National Medical College & Hospital, CD-55, Sector-1, Salt Lake City, Kolkata 700 064, India
e-mail: h.kondr@gmail.com

P. Chaudhuri, DGO, MS
Department of Obstetrics & Gynaecology, N.R.S. Medical College, Kolkata, West Bengal, India

## Epidemiology

The prevalence of the disease shows wide variation in relation to geographical and racial background.

A point prevalence of 3/100,000 population was observed by researchers in India [2]. This was much lower than data available from the western countries (12.5/100,000 in England [2a], 39/100,000 in Finland [2b], 124/100,000 in the USA [2c]).

Evidence suggests that SLE is more common in African American and Hispanic groups than in Caucasians. The incidence of lupus is much higher in women than in men. During the childbearing years, the female-to-male ratio is about 12:1.

## Pathophysiology

### Effect of Pregnancy on SLE

There is no consensus of opinion whether pregnancy results in exacerbations or "flare-ups" of SLE. Earlier studies conducted before 1980 showed very high (up to 6 times higher) incidences of flare during pregnancy especially during puerperium in comparison to non-pregnant controls [3, 4]. A number of recent case control studies however found a modest rise of such flares (15–60 %) during pregnancy [5, 6]. Some investigators believe that the rate of flares during


A. Gandhi et al. (eds.), *Principles of Critical Care in Obstetrics: Volume II*, DOI 10.1007/978-81-322-2686-4_19

pregnancy may be similar to the frequency of exacerbation while not pregnant, while other researchers maintain that pregnancy is a time of vulnerability to increased disease activity [7, 8].

Risk of SLE flares was found to be proportional to disease activity at the onset of pregnancy. Women who had sustained remission prior to pregnancy had lesser chance of having flares. In contrast women who discontinued maintenance therapy before pregnancy suffered more exacerbations during pregnancy.

Renal disease flare-up is the most common presentation of SLE aggravation in pregnancy. Combining all published data on women with lupus nephropathy, it was evident that one third of them had exacerbations, 21 % of them had deterioration of renal function during pregnancy, and 7 % had permanent deterioration of the same [9]. Chorea is a rare complication of SLE which was found to aggravate during pregnancy.

## Effect of SLE on Pregnancy

Pregnancy and its outcome are affected by SLE in the following manner.

### Gestational Hypertension and Pre-eclampsia

Twenty to 30% of women with SLE develop gestational hypertension or pre-eclampsia during pregnancy [10]. Women with lupus nephropathy develop this complication more frequently. SLE associated with chronic hypertension, antiphospholipid syndrome and long-term steroid use are also vulnerable to develop pre-eclampsia.

### Secondary Antiphospholipid Syndrome and Thrombosis

Women with SLE who have antiphospholipid antibodies (anticardiolipin antibody and lupus anticoagulant) carry additional risk of thrombosis during pregnancy and especially during puerperium.

### Pregnancy Loss

Women with SLE have higher rates of miscarriages and intrauterine foetal death than the general healthy obstetric population. In a meta-analysis of various prospective studies on foetal outcome of women with SLE, it was found that 8–23 % (median 14 %) had miscarriages, 2–12 % (median 5 %) had foetal deaths, and 15–34 % (median 24 %) had overall pregnancy losses. Women with nephropathy and antiphospholipid syndrome were found to have higher rates of pregnancy loss [9].

The cause of miscarriages and foetal death is uncertain. Inflammation and altered compliment regulation, poor placentation and placental infarction are some of the possible causes.

### Preterm Birth

Although the preterm birth rate in women with SLE and in healthy controls were compared in a few studies, available evidence shows a higher incidence of preterm birth in women with SLE, more so in women with active disease [11]. It may be attributed to higher incidence of pre-eclampsia and foetal growth restriction needing premature termination.

### Foetal Growth Restriction

Co-morbidities as hypertension and renal disease and also steroid therapy lead to high incidence of foetal growth restriction in women with SLE.

### Neonatal Lupus Syndrome

Neonatal lupus is the occurrence of SLE symptoms in an infant born from a mother with SLE, most commonly presenting with a rash resembling discoid lupus erythematosus, and sometimes with systemic abnormalities such as heart block or hepatosplenomegaly or haematological complications as haemolytic anaemia, leucopenia and thrombocytopenia. Cause of neonatal lupus may be due to transplacental passage of antibodies from mother.

Neonatal lupus is highly associated with maternal anti-Ro/SSA (usually also with anti-La/SSB) antibodies, although the rash may occur with anti-ribonucleoprotein (RNP) antibodies.

## Diagnosis

Revised American Rheumatism Association (1997) [12] criteria have been widely used for diagnosis of SLE. According to it, the women should have at least four of the following features, either simultaneously or serially.

1. Facial butterfly rash
2. Discoid lupus
3. Photosensitivity rash as a result of sunlight exposure
4. Oral or nasopharyngeal ulceration
5. Nonerosive arthritis involving two or more peripheral joints
6. Pleurisy or pericarditis
7. Proteinuria >0.5 g/day or cellular cast
8. Psychosis or convulsion
9. One haematologic problem
10. Hemolytic anaemia
11. Leucopenia, WBC <4000/μL on two or more occasions
12. Lymphopenia <1500/μL on two or more occasions
13. Thrombocytopenia <100,000/μL (in absence of drug)
14. Immunologic problem
15. Abnormal ANA titre
16. Abnormal anti-DNA titre
17. Anti-SM nuclear antigen

Abnormal serum level of IgG or IgM anticardiolipin antibody or positive test for lupus anticoagulant

## Diagnostic Dilemma during Pregnancy

SLE and its exacerbations pose diagnostic difficulty during pregnancy as they mimic some pregnancy-associated conditions.

Malar rash needs to be differentiated from chloasma.

Differentiation from pre-eclampsia is often challenging as both conditions are characterized by proteinuria [13]. Severe pre-eclampsia with HELLP syndrome with thrombocytopenia also mimics SLE flare. Presence of leucopenia, hematuria, cellular cast in urine and abnormal ANA and anti-ds DNA in serum clinches the diagnosis in favour of SLE nephritis/flare. On the other hand, elevated serum levels of liver enzymes and uric acid and decreased urinary excretion of calcium are more prominent in pre-eclampsia than lupus nephritis. Flares of systemic lupus erythematosus (SLE) are likely to be associated with hypocomplementemia; in comparison, complement levels are usually (but not always) increased in patients with pre-eclampsia [14].

## Management

### Pre-pregnancy

Women and her partner need to be counselled regarding postponement of pregnancy till good control of SLE for at least 6 months. Risk of exacerbation, pre-eclampsia and foetal and neonatal problems is to be explained. Baseline pre-pregnancy evaluation in terms of haemoglobin, platelet count, urine for protein, serum creatinine and 24 h urine for creatinine clearance should be done to assess haematologic and renal conditions. Antiphospholipid antibody titre, anti-Ro/SSA and anti-La/SSB titres are also measured for predicting prognosis.

Azathioprine, cyclophosphamide and methotrexate are to be discontinued before contemplating pregnancy. Maintenance therapy with optimum doses of hydroxychloroquine or steroids need not be discontinued.

### Prenatal

Multidisciplinary approach is essential for successful outcome. Women need to be evaluated and managed by obstetrician with expertise in high-risk pregnancy. Frequent monitoring, repeated investigations to diagnose disease activity and adverse effects and prompt intervention of complications are the essential steps in management.

## Monitoring and Investigation

Women need frequent antenatal checks, two weekly in first and second trimesters and weekly in the third.

*The schedule for monitoring includes:*

First visit:

At the first visit after (or at which) pregnancy is confirmed, the following investigations are recommended:

- Physical examination, including blood pressure
- Renal function (glomerular filtration rate, urinalysis, urine protein/urine creatinine ratio)
- Complete blood count (haemoglobin and platelet count)
- Anti-Ro/SSA and anti-La/SSB antibodies
- Lupus anticoagulant (LA) and anticardiolipin antibody (aCL) assays
- Anti-double-stranded DNA antibodies
- Complement (CH50, or C3 and C4)
- Uric acid level

A platelet count (or CBC) is recommended on a monthly basis. Urine protein should be done in all visits after 20 week to detect pre-eclampsia. Renal function needs to be repeated on the basis of clinical findings (more frequently in women with nephritis/pre-eclampsia). Women with lupus and the APS require more frequent monitoring than those with SLE alone.

## Foetal Monitoring

Dating scan and anomaly scans are to be done routinely. Growth scans for foetal biometry and amniotic fluid volume need to be done 3–4 weekly from 18 to 20 weeks onward.

Foetal surveillance is recommended to start at 30–32 weeks with Doppler studies and biophysical profile scoring. Indications to start early surveillance at 26–28 weeks are worsening disease/flare, APS, renal disease, pre-eclampsia, clinical/biometric foetal growth restriction and previous poor outcome of pregnancy.

Foetal echocardiography weekly between 16 and 26 weeks is recommended in women with added risk for foetal heart block (women who have antibodies to Ro/SSA and/or La/SSB).

## Drug Therapy

None of the medications used in the treatment of systemic lupus erythematosus (SLE) are absolutely safe during pregnancy. Hence, whether to use medications should be decided after careful assessment of the risks and benefits in consultation with the patient. Any medication during first trimester should be avoided.

Antimalarials (hydroxychloroquine) and glucocorticoids may be administered for maintaining remissions. Data from observational studies of the infants of patients with SLE and other rheumatic disorders who received antimalarials during pregnancy suggest that these agents are safe [15–17].

Glucocorticoids are relatively safe to use during pregnancy. Prednisone, prednisolone and methylprednisolone cross the placenta at very low concentration, whereas dexamethasone and betamethasone reach the foetus at higher concentration. Human and animal studies have suggested an increased risk of cleft palate in offspring exposed to glucocorticoids in utero.

Azathioprine and cyclophosphamide are better avoided except in women unresponsive to steroids. Foetal loss is a likely outcome of cyclophosphamide administration during pregnancy, as a result of cyclophosphamide toxicity, severe disease or a combination these factors. In one retrospective review of four such pregnancies, there were no live births [18].

Methotrexate is contraindicated during pregnancy. Use of NSAIDs in the third trimester may cause premature closure of the ductus arteriosus and is usually avoided.

Low-dose aspirin should be started in women with previous history of early-onset pre-eclampsia, foetal growth restriction and women with positive lupus anticoagulant and/or high levels of anticardiolipin antibodies even in the absence of classical history of APS. Some suggest the use of low-dose heparin and aspirin for such patients, even in the absence of previous pregnancy complications.

## Prenatal Therapy of Complete Congenital Heart Block (CCHB)

Dexamethasone, beta-mimetics and IVIG have been tried in CCHB diagnosed prenatally by echocardiography. However, no definite beneficial effect was evidenced.

## Labour and Delivery

Mode and time of delivery need to be individualized on the basis of associated complicating factors as pre-eclampsia or foetal growth restriction. However, all women irrespective of complicating factors should be delivered at term, and continuous foetal monitoring should be done. Women who were on chronic steroid during pregnancy should receive intravenous glucocorticosteroids.

## Puerperium and Breastfeeding

Some women experience exacerbations of SLE in the post-partum period. Thus, assessment of disease activity is warranted post-partum by the usual tests as:

Urinalysis, urine protein/urine creatinine ratio, renal function (if the urinalysis is abnormal), complete blood count, anti-double-stranded DNA (anti-dsDNA) and complement (CH50, or C3 and C4). Maintenance therapy can be started as used during pregnancy.

Women are advised to breastfeed if they are not taking azathioprine, methotrexate, cyclophosphamide or mycophenolate. Hydroxychloroquine and NSAIDs are also secreted in breast milk and, therefore, should be used with caution. Prednisone (<15–20 mg/day) can be used safely during breastfeeding because small amounts (5 % of the glucocorticoid dose) are secreted in breast milk. At doses of prednisone higher than 20 mg once or twice daily, breast milk should be pumped and discarded 4 h after the dose to minimize drug exposure to the infant.

## Treatment of SLE Flare

Prednisolone is the drug of choice for SLE flare. The dose of prednisolone depends on the severity of the exacerbation. Mild to moderate exacerbation without renal or CNS involvement can be treated with an oral dose of 30–40 mg/day. Severe flares involving the kidney or CNS need aggressive treatment with intravenous methylprednisolone, 30–50 mg/kg/day (500–1000 mg/day) for 3–6 days. Thereafter, the dose of prednisolone should be tapered to the maintenance dose.

Cyclophosphamide and azathioprine are the second-line drugs for SLE flare. Plasmapheresis and IVIG may be used in life-threatening conditions.

## Prognosis

As the survival rate in patients with SLE has improved dramatically over the past 50 years due to early diagnosis, increased potency of pharmaceutical agents and improved treatments (e.g. dialysis, kidney transplantation), more women are contemplating pregnancy. Successful pregnancy with live birth was recorded in 75 % women in a meta-analysis [8]. However, hypertension, preterm delivery, caesarean delivery, post-partum haemorrhage and maternal venous thromboembolism were more common in women with SLE than in women without SLE. In addition, foetal growth restriction/retardation and neonatal deaths were most often seen in association with SLE.

The long-term effect of pregnancy in patients with systemic lupus erythematosus (SLE) is unknown. Current evidences suggest no clinically significant adverse or positive effect of pregnancy on the course of SLE.

**Key Points**

- The prognosis for both mother and child is best when systemic lupus erythematosus (SLE) has been quiescent for at least 6 months prior to the pregnancy. Renal disease should be in remission for at least 6 months prior to conception.
- The incidence of SLE exacerbation with pregnancy, which may occur at any time during the pregnancy or the post-partum period, has progressively decreased in the past few decades, especially in those in remission at the beginning of pregnancy.
- Complications as hypertension/pre-eclampsia, miscarriages, preterm labour and foetal growth restriction are commonly associated with SLE during pregnancy.
- Multidisciplinary management in tertiary care centre is essential for successful outcome.
- Frequent antenatal check-ups and repeated investigation are required to detect disease flare and deteriorating renal function. Foetal growth and well-being need to be monitored closely.
- Less harmful drugs in optimum dosage should be administered for maintenance of remission.
- Close monitoring is essential during puerperium. Breastfeeding is possible if women receive compatible drugs.

## References


1. Mintz G, Niz J, Gutierrez G, et al. Prospective study of pregnancy in systemic lupus erythematosus. Results of a multidisciplinary approach. J Rheumatol. 1986;13:732.
2. Malaviya AN, Singh RR, Singh YN, Kapoor SK, Kumar A. Prevalence of systemic lupus erythematosus in India. Lupus. 1993;2:115–8.

2a. Hochberg MC. Prevalence of systemic lupus erythematosus in England and Wales (1981–82). Ann Rheum Dis. 1987;46:664–6.

2b. Jonsson H, Nived O, Surfelt G. Outcome in systemic lupus erythematosus: a prospective study of patients from a defined population. Medicine (Baltimore). 1989;68:141–50.

2c. Uramoto KM, Michet Jr CJ, Thumboo J, et al. Trends in the incidence and mortality 1950–1992. Arthritis Rheum. 1992;42:46–50.

3. Fraga A, Mintz G, Orozco J, Orozco JH. Sterility and fertility rates, foetal wastage and maternal morbidity in Systemic lupus erythematosus. J Rheumatol. 1974;1:1293–8.
4. Garsenstein M, Pollak VE, Karik RM. Systemic lupus erythematosus and pregnancy. N Engl J Med. 1962;267:165–9.
5. Lockshin MD. Pregnancy does not cause systemic lupus erythematosus to worsen. Arthritis Rheum. 1989;32:665.
6. Urowitz MB, Gladman DD, Farewell VT, et al. Lupus and pregnancy studies. Arthritis Rheum. 1993;36:1392.
7. Petri M, Howard D, Repke J. Frequency of lupus flare in pregnancy. The Hopkins Lupus Pregnancy Center Experience. Arthritis Rheum. 1991;34:1538.
8. Lockshin MD, Reinitz E, Druzin ML, et al. Lupus pregnancy. Case–control prospective study demonstrating absence of lupus exacerbation during or after pregnancy. Am J Med. 1984;77:893.
9. Denney JM, Porter TF, Branch DW. Autoimmune disease, Chapter 43, High risk pregnancy, management options, 4th ed. Elsevier Saunders. Egerman RS, Ramsey RD.
10. Kao LW, et al. Hypertensive disease in pregnancies complicated by systemic lupus erythematosus. Am J Obstet Gynecol. 2005;193:1676.
11. Johnson MJ, Petri M, Witter FR, Repke JT. Evaluation of preterm delivery in a systemic lupus erythematosus pregnancy clinic. Obstet Gynecol. 1995;86:396.
12. Hochberg MC. Updating The American College of Rheumatology revised criteria for the classification of Systemic lupus erythematosus. Arthritis Rheum. 1997;40:1725.
13. Repke JT. Hypertensive disorders of pregnancy. Differentiating preeclampsia from active systemic lupus erythematosus. J Reprod Med. 1998; 43:350.
14. Buyon JP, Cronstein BN, Morris M, et al. Serum complement values (C3 and C4) to differentiate between systemic lupus activity and pre-eclampsia. Am J Med. 1986;81:194.
15. Al-Herz A, Schulzer M, Esdaile JM. Survey of antimalarial use in lupus pregnancy and lactation. J Rheumatol. 2002;29:700.
16. Costedoat-Chalumeau N, Amoura Z, Duhaut P, et al. Safety of hydroxychloroquine in pregnant patients with connective tissue diseases: a study of one hundred thirty-three cases compared with a control group. Arthritis Rheum. 2003;48:3207.
17. Clowse ME, Magder L, Witter F, Petri M. Hydroxychloroquine in lupus pregnancy. Arthritis Rheum. 2006;54:3640.
18. Clowse ME, Magder L, Petri M. Cyclophosphamide for lupus during pregnancy. Lupus. 2005;14:593.

# DVT and Pregnancy

# 20

Vijayalakshmi G. Pillai

## Introduction

Deep venous thrombosis (DVT) represents a serious manifestation of venous thromboembolism (VTE), the other manifestations being pulmonary thromboembolism or pulmonary embolism (PE) and cerebral venous thrombosis (CVT). Often, the clinical suspicion of this disease is overlooked in pregnancy and the puerperium and hence leads to diagnostic delays. Venous thrombosis leads to considerable, but potentially preventable, morbidity and mortality among pregnant women. Serious sequelae of survived patients of severe DVT and PE are postthrombotic syndrome, venous insufficiency, and pulmonary hypertension.

## Epidemiology of Pregnancy-Associated Thrombosis

In pregnant women, the risk of venous and arterial thromboembolic events is increased. Approximately 80 % of these thromboembolic events are venous [58]. Studies have agreed that during pregnancy, the risk of DVT is increased 4–5 times [91] compared to nonpregnant women of same age. This risk is present in all trimesters of pregnancy more or less equally. One such data quotes the overall incidence of VTE as 167.7/100,000 births with an average case fatality rate of 0.41 % [1]. Data on the true incidence of DVT in different trimesters of pregnancy are limited. Compared to nonpregnant state, puerperium holds a further 20–60-fold higher risk, which is maximum at the first week of postpartum [51]. Pulmonary embolism (PE) remains the leading direct cause of maternal deaths due to VTE.

Although the true incidence of DVT is unknown, it is accepted that it occurs in 1–2 per 1000–20,000 pregnancies and accounts for maternal deaths of 1.2–4.7 per 100,000 pregnancies in developed countries [6, 56, 105]. The best recorded Indian data into the causes of maternal deaths is documented in the "Second Report of Confidential Review of Maternal Deaths, Kerala" [125], which quotes the incidence of fatal VTE at 2.6 % of all maternal deaths in the years 2006–2009. Data from other regions, as in a prospective large cohort study from Western India [121], has put the incidence of VTE at par with that of the developed counties. An accurate data of the incidence of pregnancy-related DVT, fatal or treated, is difficult to get as we do not have a national registry.

Seventy-five percent to 80 % of pregnancy-associated VTE is deep vein thrombosis (DVT), and 20–25 % is pulmonary embolism (PE). Half of these venous thromboembolic events occur

V.G. Pillai, DGO, MRCOG
Department of Obstetrics and Gynecology,
Vijayalakshmi Medical Centre,
NH-Bypass, Vennala P.O., Kochi, Kerala, India
e-mail: drvijayalakshmi@hotmail.com


A. Gandhi et al. (eds.), *Principles of Critical Care in Obstetrics: Volume II*,
DOI 10.1007/978-81-322-2686-4_20

during pregnancy and half postpartum [105]. Two percent (2 %) of pregnancy-associated DVT occurs in the upper extremity [59]. Cerebral venous thrombosis (CVT) is a rare entity in pregnancy and the postpartum period, with an incidence of 1:10,000–1:25,000 [8, 76].

DVT occurring in pregnancy is more likely to be seen in the left lower extremity and is more proximal than in calf, and it tends to be massive. Pelvic vein thrombosis is another site, which accounts for 10–12 % of DVT during the postpartum period. But they form less than 1 % of all cases of reported DVT [46] confirmed by venous ultrasound. Involvement of the left leg was reported in around 85 % for which the affected side was known, and 70 % cases were restricted to the proximal veins without involvement of the calf veins. Among the cases of proximal deep vein thrombosis, 65 % were restricted to the iliac and/or femoral vein [22, 44, 94]. In spite of the increased risk of venous thromboembolism (VTE) during pregnancy and the postpartum period, most women are considered low risk and they do not require anticoagulation.

## Pathophysiology of Thrombosis

Rudolf Virchow, more than 150 years ago, had described three factors that are primarily important in the development of venous thrombosis: (1) venous stasis, (2) activation of blood coagulation, and (3) endothelial damage of veins. These factors have come to be known as the Virchow triad.

"In pregnancy, venous stasis can occur as a result of anything that slows or obstructs the flow of venous blood," like increased venous capacitance or reduced smooth muscle tone which is hormonally induced, decreased venous return, and mechanical obstruction by the gravid uterus [57, 115]. The left-sided predominance is presumed to be due to a relative stenosis of the left common iliac vein, where it lies between the lumbar vertebral body and the right common iliac artery (May-Thurner syndrome, Fig. 20.1). The true mechanism is unknown.

Pregnant women are many a times advised bed rest and hence decreased mobility [46, 62]. They also have a tendency to be dehydrated due to excessive vomiting, sweating, etc. This leads to an increase viscosity of blood and the formation of microthrombi inside veins, which are not washed away by the sluggish venous return in pregnancy. The thrombus thus formed may grow and propagate.

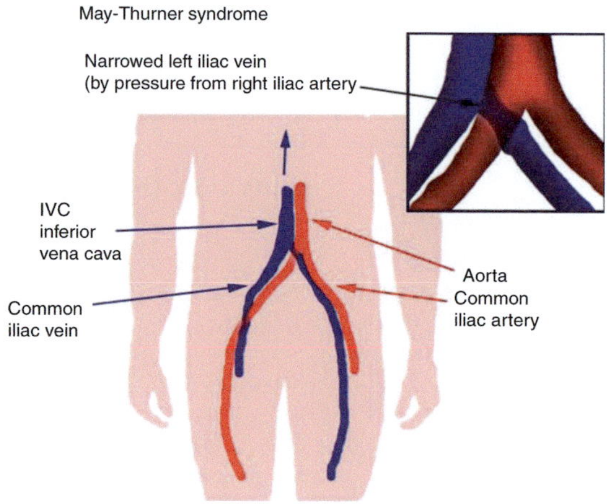


**Fig. 20.1** Diagrammatic/Schematic representation of May-Thurner syndrome (Courtesy (http://emedicine.medscape.com/article/2056380) [34])

Pregnancy is a hypercoagulable state [15]. This is due to the physiological changes in pregnancy. These changes are in both coagulation and fibrinolytic systems. There is an increase in endogenous thrombin generation, combined with a decrease in circulating plasma antithrombin and fibrinolysins. Normal pregnancy-associated changes in coagulation are increased concentrations of factors VII, VIII, and X and von Willebrand factor and marked increases in fibrinogen. Factors II, V, and IX are relatively unchanged [15]. The only blood coagulation factor that is decreased in pregnancy is factor XI. There is acquired resistance to activated protein C (an endogenous anticoagulant). Free protein S, which is its active and unbound form, is decreased during pregnancy. Plasminogen activator inhibitor type 1 (PAI-1) levels are increased almost five times in pregnancy. Toward the third trimester, levels of PAI-2 produced by the placenta increase drastically [82]. Prothrombin fragments (PF1+2), which are the markers of thrombin generation and thrombin–antithrombin (TAT) complexes, are also increased in pregnancy. These changes start to increase at conception and may take up to 8 weeks postpartum to return to baseline [20].

**Risk Factors Associated with an Increased Risk for Thromboembolism**

- Age >35
- Infection
- Malignancy
- Obesity
- Personal/family history of thrombosis
- Smoking
- Surgery
- Varicose veins
- Blood loss >1 L
- Cesarean birth
- Forceps (midcavity or rotational)
- Hyperemesis/dehydration
- Multiparity >3
- Multiple pregnancy
- Preeclampsia
- Pregnancy/puerperium
- Prolonged labor >24 h
- Cardiac disease
- Nephrotic syndrome
- Ovarian hyperstimulation syndrome
- Paraplegia/pelvic trauma/long-distance travel
- Prolonged immobilization
- Sickle cell disease
- Thrombophilia

This hypercoagulable state is indeed a protection against hemorrhage during abortion and delivery. Hemorrhage still accounts for the majority of maternal deaths in India. Endothelial (intimal) damage in the blood vessel may be intrinsic or secondary to external trauma. It may be from accidental injury or surgical insult.

## Natural Inhibitors of Coagulation during Pregnancy

Antithrombin (AT) is a serine proteinase inhibitor which acts by interaction with its cofactor heparin [89, 109]. Thrombin is inactivated by AT either directly or by inactivating factors IX, X and XI by forming a covalent complex. These factors are inhibited very slowly. This process can be accelerated by the binding of heparin and heparin-like compounds to AT. Protein C gets activated by thrombin. The process is enhanced by the interaction of thrombin with thrombomodulin [26]. Activated protein C inactivates factors Va and VIIIa on the platelet and endothelial cell surface and hence serves to block thrombin generation. Protein C requires protein S, which is another vitamin K-dependent molecule as a cofactor. The imbalance between reduced inhibitors of coagulation and/or increased activation of coagulation factors can lead to thrombosis in pregnancy [20, 26, 114].

## Fibrinolysis

Enzymes like plasmin are involved in the removal of thrombus from the circulation. The main role of plasmin is to degrade fibrin. Plasmin is present in its inactive form as plasminogen. The activation of plasminogen is by serine enzymes known as tissue-type plasminogen activator (t-PA) and urokinase (u-PA) [14]. This activity is regulated by specific inhibitors, plasminogen activator inhibitor (PAI)-1 and PAI-2. Plasminogen deficiencies can also lead to thrombophilia in patients.

## Specific Types of Inherited Thrombophilias

The list of inherited thrombophilias well studied [4, 12, 17, 27, 31–33, 37, 41, 43, 45, 48, 60, 63–65, 67, 68, 73, 75, 78, 81, 83, 87, 88, 92, 95, 102, 103, 119, 120, 129] includes established genetic factors such as factor V Leiden mutation, prothrombin gene mutation; protein C, protein S, and antithrombin deficiencies; activated protein C resistance; prothrombin gene mutation; rare genetic factors like dysfibrinogenemia and hyperhomocysteinemia; elevated factors VIII, IX, and XI; elevated lipoprotein a; platelet glycoprotein gene polymorphisms; plasminogen deficiency; tissue plasminogen activator (tPA); plasminogen activator inhibitor (PAI); thrombomodulin gene defect; heparin cofactor II; and histidine-rich glycoprotein deficiency.

The lifetime probability of developing thrombosis in individuals with inherited thrombophilias compared to those with no defect shows that the highest incidence occurred with carriers of protein S deficiency, next with antithrombin deficiency, followed by protein C deficiency, and the least for factor V Leiden mutation. We have advanced a lot in our knowledge of congenital defects that predispose to thrombosis. This has made us understand the disease process of inherited thrombophilias as well as helped us recommend appropriate screening, detection, diagnosis, and treatment of selected patients effectively, to prevent morbid VTE in pregnancy [10].

## Acquired Thrombophilias

Among the acquired thrombophilic disorders, anticardiolipin antibody, annexin V antibodies, lupus anticoagulant, and anti-beta-2 glycoprotein1 ($\beta_2$GPI) antibodies were more frequently seen in the Indian study on DVT in antenatal period [121]. The main acquired form of thrombophilia leading to increased risk of DVT in pregnancy is the antiphospholipid antibody syndrome (APLA). The patients with this disease present with venous and/or arterial thrombosis together with laboratory evidence for antibodies in blood that recognize anionic phospholipid–protein complexes [54]. The hypothesis of etiology of thrombosis in antiphospholipid syndrome is described elsewhere in this book.

In patients with APLA syndrome, vascular occlusions [23] are seen. Renal, celiac, and intracerebral artery stenoses [97, 98, 127] have been reported. In APLA syndrome, vascular changes reported include thrombosis, vascular intimal and smooth muscle hyperplasia, activation of platelets, and APLA antibodies-stimulating platelet aggregation [35]. Tissue factor activity by leukocytes is promoted by these antibodies. Protein C pathway is interfered by oxidation, thereby enhancing the anticoagulant activity of activated protein C [38]. Many patients with APLA syndrome are seen to have concurrent protein S deficiency as well [30]. The prevalence of APLA syndrome is estimated to be 5 % of the general population [21]. They are seen in >50 % of pregnancy-associated thrombosis.

Acquired and familial thrombophilic disorders are known to be involved in the pathophysiology of DVT. The knowledge of this disorder and understanding their mechanism of action [58, 59] are helpful in the selection of cases for anticoagulant therapy, thereby preventing VTE in pregnancy.

## Management of Deep Vein Thrombosis/Venous Thromboembolism

### Diagnosis of DVT

Diagnosis of deep vein thrombosis (DVT) requires both clinical assessment and objective testing. The clinical features are mostly nonspecific. Investigations can either be falsely positive or negative.

Table 20.1 gives management principles of DVT/PE in general.

The initial step in the diagnostic process is to stratify patients into risk assessment categories using a validated clinical model:

- High risk
- Intermediate risk
- Low risk

Refer Table 20.2 for risk categorization of VTE in pregnancy.

Screening for thrombophilias should be done if the results are likely to alter management of DVT. Screening is unnecessary when clinical suspicion of DVT is very high.

**Table 20.1** Guideline for management of VTE

| |
|---|
| Assess risk of VTE for all pregnant women at booking or at the earliest opportunity |
| Consider whether antenatal thromboprophylaxis is required |
| Consider postnatal thromboprophylaxis liberally |
| Reassess risk throughout the pregnancy and puerperium |
| Make an individualized plan with the patient |
| Ensure all women mobilize early postpartum and the puerperium |
| Avoid dehydration all through pregnancy; encourage GCS usage liberally |

**Table 20.2** Risk Assessment of VTE in Pregnancy

| |
|---|
| *High risk*: |
| Prior VTE is the most important risk factor, especially when unprovoked/estrogen related |
| Previous recurrent VTE >1 |
| The inherited and acquired thrombophilias. Family history of thrombophilia is identified in less than 50 % of patients with unprovoked VTE [10] |
| *Intermediate risk*: |
| Single previous VTE with no family history of thrombophilia |
| Thrombophilia + no previous VTE |
| Other medical conditions like SLE, cancer, inflammatory conditions, nephrotic syndrome, sickle cell disease, intravenous drug users, surgical conditions in pregnancy like appendectomy, etc. [25, 108] |
| *Low risk*: |
| Elective Cesarean delivery, which has twice the risk as vaginal delivery [108] |
| Obesity, BMI >30 |
| Age >35 years |
| Smoking |
| Current systemic infection |
| Parity >3 |
| Long-distance travel |
| Dehydration, prolonged immobilization in pregnancy |
| Multiple pregnancies |
| Premature delivery |
| ART |
| Preeclampsia |

*For all risk categories*:

Consider clinical surveillance, encourage mobilization, and avoid dehydration.

*If with intermediate or high risk, consider the following*:

Graduated compression stockings (GCS), intermittent pneumatic compression (IPC) if hospitalized, and low-molecular-weight heparin (LMWH) prophylaxis. Avoid dehydration at all stages of pregnancy.

Long-haul flights require particular counseling and probably DVT prophylaxis.

Management of VTE in pregnancy is by a tertiary team, where a referral system has to be developed. The tertiary management team comprises of multidisciplinary personals. This team includes obstetricians, senior physicians, hematologists, interventional radiologists, intensivists, and thoracic surgeons. Figure 20.2 is a flowchart of management of VTE. This is particularly relevant to Indian scenario.

## Signs and Symptoms of DVT and PE

Signs and symptoms of DVT and PE are generally nonspecific and hence overlooked. Refer to Table 20.3 for general signs and symptoms of VTE in pregnancy.

## Principles of Treatment of DVT in Pregnancy

Pregnant women are more prone to have DVT. The clots form mostly in the lower limb veins and can break up to form emboli. These emboli can move to the lungs causing pulmonary embolism. This has serious consequences including maternal death. Anticoagulants are used to treat clots and are given to pregnant women with increased risk to clotting. These medications reduce the risk of further thrombosis and thereby reduce the risk of pulmonary embolism. An important complication of treatment with anticoagulants is hemorrhage. When a woman is anticoagulated, this risk of hemorrhage is present all through the pregnancy, i.e., in antepartum, intrapartum, and postpartum period.

During pregnancy heparin is the most common anticoagulant used, either the conventional unfractionated heparin (UFH) which is cheaper or the low-molecular-weight heparin (LMWH). Neither of these cross the placenta, and both have been shown to be safe during pregnancy. Oral anticoagulants like warfarin are generally considered unsafe in pregnancy as it may affect the fetus.

## History and Physical Examination of DVT

Diagnosis of first episode of DVT is often difficult as most of the signs and symptoms are atypical and are seen commonly in pregnancy with

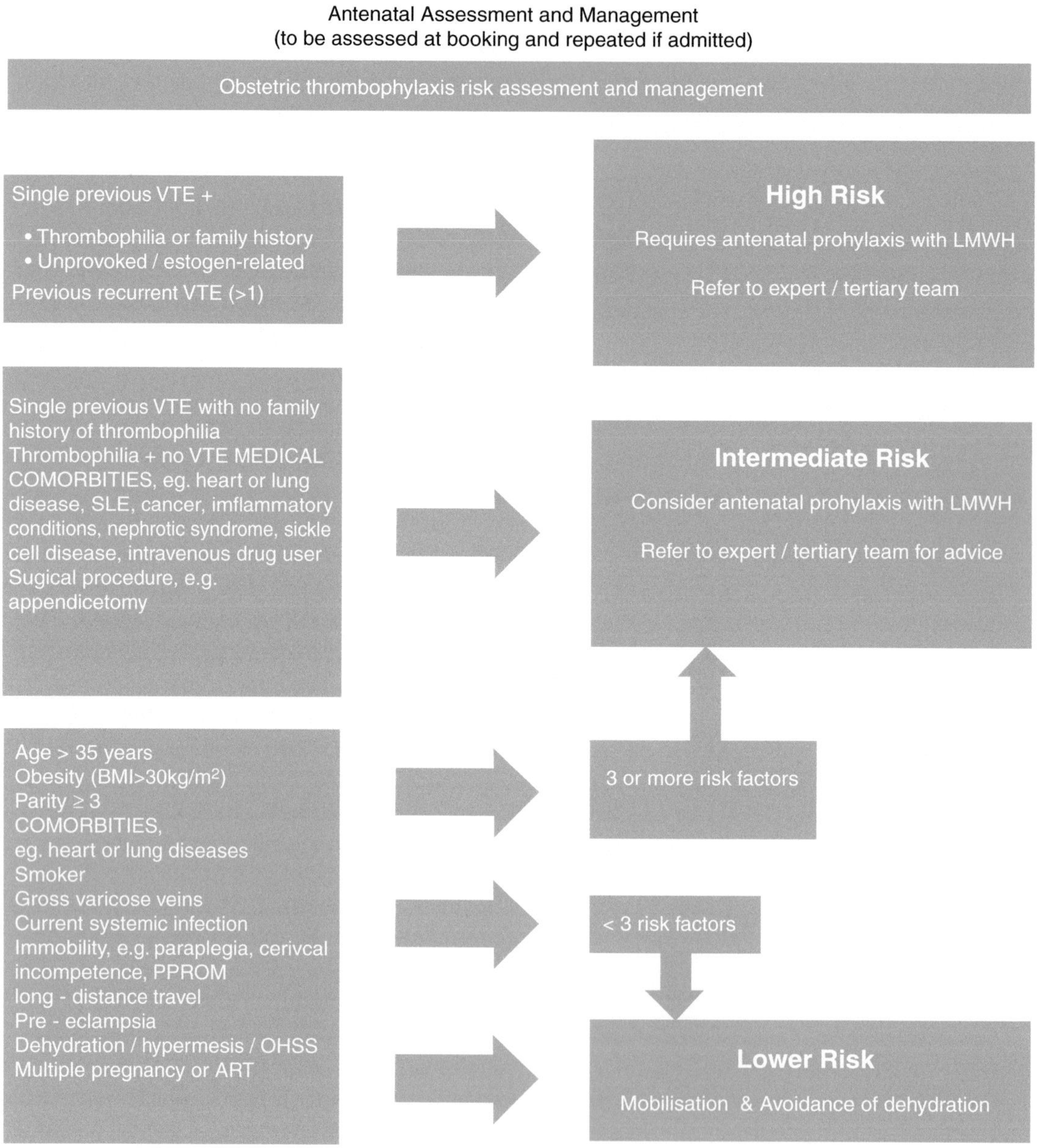


**Fig. 20.2** Flowchart for the management of VTE in pregnancy (Adapted from "Thrombosis and Embolism during Pregnancy and the Puerperium, Reducing the Risk", RCOG Green-top Guideline No. 37a. Nov. 2009) [113]

non-thrombotic conditions as well. Symptoms like mild tachypnea, dyspnea, tachycardia, lower extremity edema, and cramps are common in most pregnant women. Hence, diagnosis of VTE by physical examination is frequently inaccurate or overlooked.

The two most common symptoms of DVT are unilateral *pain and swelling* of the lower extremity. Among the 80 % of pregnant women who experience these symptoms, only a few have true DVT. So also among 70 % of women with dyspnea, only a few have PE.

Examination findings of the following are important for the diagnosis of DVT:

- Mid-calf circumference difference of ≥2 cm
- Symptoms in the left lower extremity
- First trimester presentation

**Table 20.3** Signs and symptoms of DVT and PE

| |
|---|
| *Symptoms of DVT*: |
| Pain and swelling of the lower extremity |
| Back pain and swelling of lower extremity in iliac vein thrombosis |
| *Symptoms of PE*: |
| Dyspnea – 82 % |
| Abrupt onset of chest pain – 49 % |
| Cough – 20 % |
| *The common presenting signs of PE*: |
| Tachypnea |
| Crackles |
| Tachycardia |
| *Patients with massive PE*: |
| Syncope |
| Hypotension |
| Pulseless cardiac electrical activity |
| Death |

Since the risks of VTE are increased in pregnancy and postpartum and the morbidity and mortality are great, a low threshold for initiation of evaluation with the above findings is recommended for the prevention of serious catastrophe. Until excluded, these women should begin anticoagulation therapy.

## History and Signs and Symptoms of Pulmonary Thromboembolism

Risk assessment is essential, as deaths due to PE are mainly from overlook or not having clinical suspicion [11, 47] of the condition. This should start prepregnancy.

Clinical signs and symptoms of PE as with DVT are nonspecific. The classic symptoms of PE are dyspnea (82 %), abrupt-onset chest pain (49 %), and cough (20 %) and sometimes hemoptysis. The most common presenting signs are tachypnea, crackles, and tachycardia.

Pulmonary embolism is more often fatal, has a higher recurrence rate, and presents with less specific symptoms in comparison to DVT. Most of these signs and symptoms are common in "normal" pregnancies. PE is an enigma in pregnancy, in that all these signs and symptoms are rarely seen together. PE is usually a consequence of DVT. About 40 % of patients with proximal DVT are found to have an associated pulmonary embolism by lung scan; about 70 % of patients presenting with pulmonary embolism are found to have DVT in the legs [84].

Diagnosis is a real challenge to the clinician [126]. The clinician has to make an accurate judgment of this life-threatening condition. Therefore, if there is a suspicion of PE, anticoagulation therapy and appropriate immediate diagnostic testing should be performed until the diagnosis is made or ruled out as early as possible [69]. Patients with massive PE may present with syncope, hypotension, pulseless cardiac electrical activity, or death.

## Electrocardiogram in PE

An electrocardiogram pattern suggestive of pulmonary embolism is a right ventricular strain and the S1Q3T3 [116]. These findings are mostly nonspecific and infrequent. Seventy percent of patients with PE have nonspecific ECG abnormalities.

## Laboratory Evaluation for DVT/PE

D-dimer value of <500 ng/mL has been shown to have 99 % negative predictive value in patients with low and intermediate probability for VTE in the nonpregnant patients. D-dimer levels are increased in pregnancy if there is a concomitant problem such as preeclampsia [124]. At term and in the postnatal period, in most healthy pregnant women, D-dimer levels are raised [42]. The specificity of this test in pregnancy is hence low. In spite of that, it remains a test with good negative predictive value even in pregnancy [124]. DVT may be safely excluded if the D-dimer is negative [18] and the compression duplex ultrasonography (CUS) is normal. The sensitivity of compression duplex ultrasonography test is 100 % when put together with a low D-dimer test value.

Other laboratory testing, e.g., cardiac enzyme, arterial blood gas analysis, etc. [112], are useful to rule out possible differential diagnosis to PE. Before anticoagulation therapy is initiated, a full blood count, coagulation profile, urea, creatinine, electrolytes and liver function tests [113] should be performed. Performing thrombophilia screening for an acute episode of PE prior to treatment is not recommended.

## Imaging in PE

A chest X-ray is the first image to be taken in suspected PE. CXR helps for differential diagnosis of other pulmonary conditions like pneumonia, pneumothorax, or lobar collapse. The most common chest radiography findings associated with pulmonary embolism are enlarged pulmonary arteries, peripheral wedge of airspace opacity which implies lung infarction (atelectasis or parenchymal density), pleural effusion, regional oligemia, and elevation of a hemidiaphragm. In several cases, CXR maybe normal. They are again nonspecific [39]. If CXR is normal, a bilateral CUS of lower limbs should be performed. If both tests are negative, but clinical suspicion is high, a ventilation–perfusion (V/Q) lung scan has to be performed. This can also detect other pathologies like a dissecting aorta. A computed tomography pulmonary angiography (CTPA) is the diagnostic test of choice when the technology is available and appropriate for the patient [85]. Even when the tests come negative, anticoagulation treatment should be continued if the clinical suspicion is high [5]. Magnetic resonance direct thrombus imaging (MRDTI) may be performed if the diagnosis still remains uncertain [107].

It is necessary to understand that the diagnostic strategy for pulmonary embolism (PE) during pregnancy is not based on strong evidence. Neither is it accepted unanimously. Most of the clinical scores are not validated. The diagnostic value of D-dimer is low and is rarely negative in pregnant women.

## Imaging for DVT

The initial test of choice in the evaluation of DVT is compression duplex ultrasound (CUS) of the lower extremity veins [8, 74, 79, 86, 90, 100]. Sensitivity and specificity for proximal lower extremity DVT is more than 95 % for CUS. CUS is to be performed with the patient in the left lateral decubitus position. Doppler analysis of flow variation during respiration needs to be assessed as well, so as to maximize the study's ability to diagnose pelvic DVT [5]. Veins have to be easily compressible and collapse completely. The normal venous blood flow should be spontaneous and phasic; cease with the Valsalva maneuver, and show augmentation with distal compression. Absence of this usually indicates the presence of a substantial clot (Fig. 20.3).

If CUS results are negative and if we have no suspicion of iliac (pelvic) vein thrombosis (usual symptoms are back pain and swelling of lower extremity), she may be left for routine observation. CUS can be done with reasonable accuracy for pelvic vein thrombosis in the first and second trimesters of pregnancy and with difficulty in the third trimester.

If the study is equivocal or abnormal, or if pelvic vein thrombosis is suspected, further evaluation is recommended. Magnetic resonance venography is the image of choice [70, 90, 107]. Conventional contrast venography may also be performed if MRI is not available [86]. The risk of radiation exposure to the fetus has to be discussed with the patient in such instances [85]. The choice of imaging testing is based on availability and in consultation with the radiologist (Table 20.4).

## Treatment of DVT in Pregnancy and the Puerperium

If clinical suspicion of DVT or PE is high, empirical treatment with LMWH should be given until the diagnosis is excluded by objective testing. LMWH is considered equally effective as unfractionated heparin in the initial treatment of VTE. Advantages of LMWH over UFH include the following: it does not cross placenta just as UFH, it lowers the risk of hemorrhagic complications, it lowers mortality compared to UFH, and there is no risk of heparin-induced thrombocytopenia [9, 36, 40, 66, 72, 93, 99]. Different LMWH preparations have

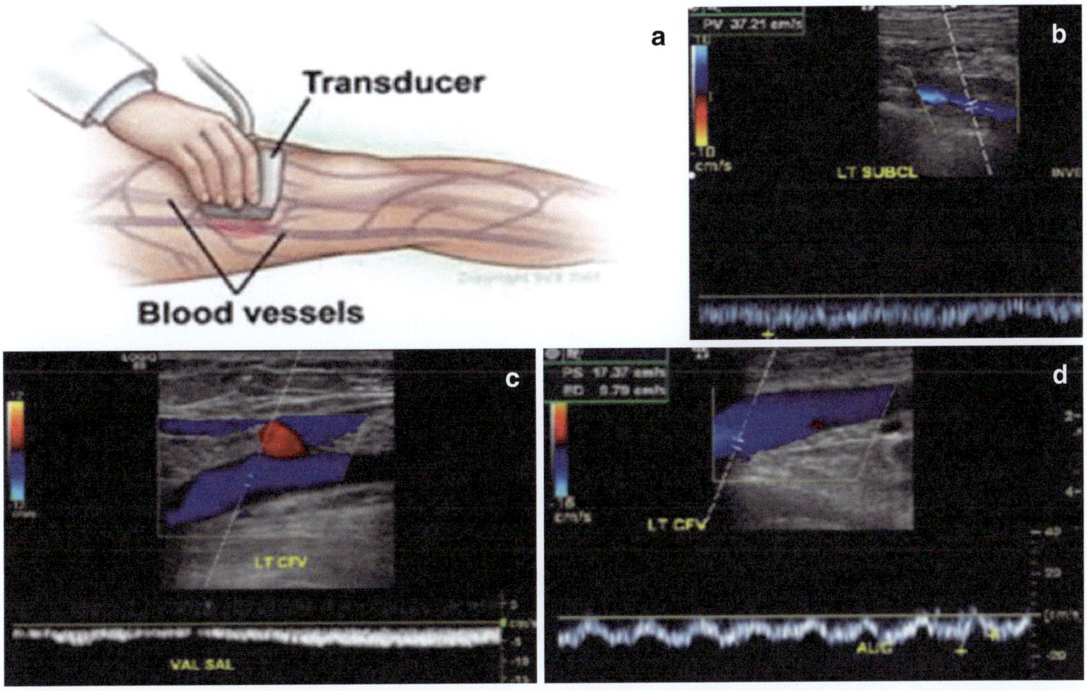


**Fig. 20.3** Compression duplex ultrasound (CUS). (**a**) Patient in the left lateral decubitus position, flow variation during respiration needs to be assessed. http://www.vascularweb.org/vascularhealth. (**b**) Veins have to be easily compressible and collapse completely. Blood flow should be spontaneous and phasic, cease with Valsalva maneuver, and show augmentation with distal compression. (**c**) Duplex ultrasound showing abnormal Valsalva response. (**d**) Duplex ultrasound showing absence of augmentation with distal compression. (**b–d**) http://www.surgery.wisc.edu/referring-physicians

**Table 20.4** Diagnosis of lower extremity deep vein thrombosis

| Diagnosis of lower extremity deep vein thrombosis |
|---|
| Compression ultrasound (US) is highly sensitive and specific for the detection of deep vein thrombosis (DVT) in the upper leg |
| Lower extremity US can give indirect evidence of pelvic DVT. However, MR venography is recommended for direct diagnosis of suspected pelvic DVT |
| US is not sufficiently sensitive to rule out thrombosis below the knee, and, if clinical suspicion remains high, US examination should be repeated after a week because of the danger of thrombus propagation into the thigh veins |
| CT pulmonary angiography combined with CT venography of the lower extremity is recommended for patients with symptoms of pulmonary embolism to detect emboli in the lung and to screen for DVT |

been compared for their efficacy in the treatment of VTE in pregnancy, and the data are now available [55, 71, 96, 106]. There seems to be no particular advantage of one preparation over the other. The risk of recurrent VTE after treatment with LMWH in pregnancy is comparable to that in nonpregnant state when VTE was treated with similar LMWH (1.15 % vs. 5–8 %) [52]. It is also comparable to patients treated with unfractionated heparin or coumarin, especially when followed up over 3–6 months of initial episode [128]. LMWH does not increase peripartum bleeding and hence particularly useful where hemorrhage accounts for major peripartum morbidity and even mortality. No case of heparin-induced thrombocytopenia has been recorded with LMWH [16, 128]. Heparin-induced osteoporosis [49] is hardly seen with LMWH.

To summarize, comparing LMWH to unfractionated heparin (UFH), LMWH decreased the risk of mortality, recurrent VTE, and hemorrhage. Disadvantages of LMWH include cost and longer half-life (Fig. 20.4).

## The Therapeutic Dose of LMWH in Pregnancy

Subcutaneous low-molecular-weight heparin (LMWH) is the preferred treatment [118] for most patients with acute VTE [10]. LMWH should be given daily in two subcutaneous divided doses [80]. The most commonly used LMWH is enoxaparin. Enoxaparin 1 mg/kg twice daily or dalteparin 100 units/kg twice daily is the recommended dose. Tinzaparin 175 units/kg is also considered equivalent in the treatment of VTE in pregnancy [49]. This is called weight-adjusted, fixed-dosage regime. Routine platelet count monitoring is not required in women who receive only LMWH. Occasionally, the dosing of LMWH may have to be monitored and adjusted by anti-Xa assay because of the effects of increased plasma volume and glomerular filtration rate in pregnancy [19]. Monitoring anti-Xa is expensive. But it is beneficial in extremes of body weight [61], (below 50 kg or above 90 kg) or for patients with renal disorders or if there is a recurrent VTE episodes. Deciding the dose of LMWH with anti-Xa measurement is called adjusted-dose regime. If anti-Xa level is measured, it should be 3–6 h after the third or fourth dose of enoxaparin or third or fourth dose after dose adjustments. The target is to achieve an optimal peak anti-Xa level of 0.5–1.2 IU/ml. The LMWH dose may have to be increased or decreased 10–25 % to achieve the optimal anti-Xa level [10, 80].

For patients greater than 150 kg, UFH maybe preferred, or otherwise, a closer monitoring of anti-Xa levels should be performed to ensure therapeutic effect. Unfractionated heparin (UFH) may also be preferred if the patient is likely to have immediate surgery or delivery because of its shorter half-life and its reversibility with protamine. However, due to cost, some patients may have limited access to LMWH especially in a country like India. UFH should not be denied to such patients. Monitoring of heparin therapy is usually by measurement of the activated partial thromboplastin time (aPTT) [10]. A therapeutic range of aPTT ratio (international normalized ratio or INR) of 1.5–2.5 is recommended [50]. UFH is administered by IV bolus, followed by IV infusion, with titration of the dose to a standard aPTT. The heparin infusion is typically increased or decreased by 10–30 % to titrate to goal aPTT [10].

After reaching a therapeutic and stable aPTT, the heparin can be converted to either subcutaneous UFH or LMWH. The disadvantage of subcutaneous UFH is that it is less predictable for anticoagulation as dosing variability exists to maintain therapeutic response. The platelet count needs to be monitored every 2–3 days from day 4 to day 14 or until heparin is stopped, whichever occurs first [10, 34, 112].

Prophylaxis dose with UFH [10, 34, 112]:

- 5000 units SC q8–12 h
- 7500 units SC q12 h

Treatment dose of UFH for DVT and PE [10, 34, 112] 80 units/kg IV bolus and then continuous infusion of 18 units/kg/h:

- 5000–10,000 units IV bolus and then continuous infusion of 1300 units/h
- 17,500 units SC
- Then 250 units/kg q12 h SC

(Refer to Table 20.5 for summary.)

Heparinization can be a problem, especially in late pregnancy as heparin resistance may happen because of increased fibrinogen and factor VIII [24]. If such a problem is seen, get hematologist's support.

If a PE is suspected, an urgent CXR, an electrocardiogram, or CTPA (computed tomography pulmonary angiogram) as early as possible [34, 85, 112], preferably within 1 h of presentation, should be done.

## Management of Life-Threatening PE in Pregnancy

Expedited treatment of patients should be initiated if brought in collapse and in whom PE is strongly considered. A multidisciplinary resuscitation team has to be set up in all referral hospitals managing high-risk obstetrics [112]. This

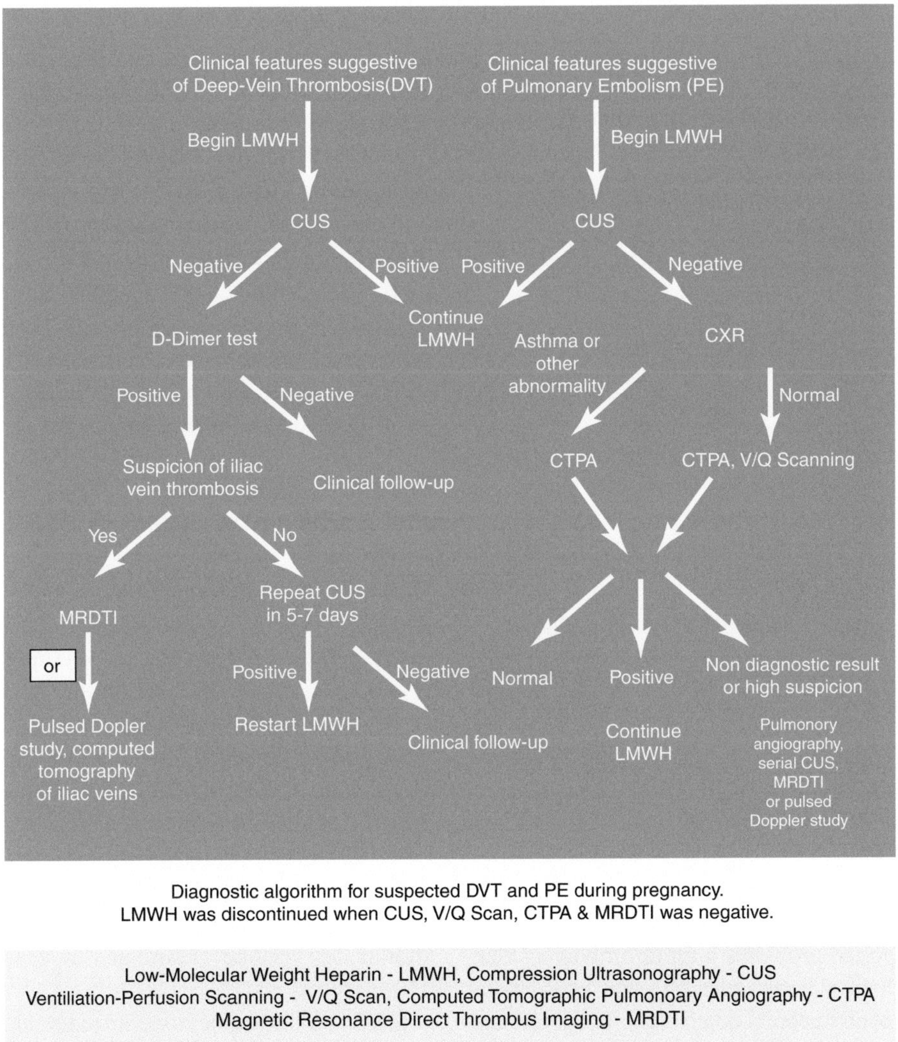


**Fig. 20.4** Flow chart for the management of DVT/PE. *LMWH* low-molecular-weight heparin, *CUS* compression ultrasonography, *V/Q Scan* ventilation–perfusion scanning, CTPA computed tomographic pulmonary angiography, *MRDTI* magnetic resonance direct thrombus imaging (Courtesy, Medscape CME and Education, Thromboembolism in Pregnancy, April 2014) [34]

team should include, other than the obstetricians, senior physician, hematologist, interventional radiologist, intensivist and thoracic surgeon. They should have collective responsibility in the management. They should start immediate workup. The treatment should be on an individual basis. The treatment modalities may include thrombolytic therapy or thoracotomy and surgical embolectomy [29, 110, 111].

Immediate treatment is to start intravenous unfractionated heparin [10]. The loading dose of UFH is 5000–10,000 U or 80 units/kg intravenous. After a loading dose of UFH, an infusion of 18 U/kg is started. Monitor and keep the activated partial thromboplastin time (aPTT) in the therapeutic range of 1.5–2 (refer to Table 20.5 for summary).

If massive PE is confirmed, immediate thrombolysis [122] should be considered. Thrombolysis with streptokinase, urokinase, and recombinant tissue plasminogen activator has been documented in pregnancy [80]. They are found to be more effective than heparin in massive PE to reduce the

**Table 20.5** The various regimens of UFH and LMWH [10]

| |
|---|
| Prophylactic UFH: UFH 5000 U subcutaneously q12h |
| Intermediate-dose UFH: UFH subcutaneously q12h in doses adjusted to target an anti-Xa level of 0.1–0.3 U/ml |
| Adjusted-dose UFH:UFH subcutaneously q12h in doses adjusted to target a mid-interval aPTT into the therapeutic range of 1.5–2 |
| Treatment dose of UFH for DVT and PE [34, 94, 112] 80 units/kg IV bolus, then continuous infusion of 18 units/kg/h OR 5000 units IV bolus, then continuous infusion of 1300 units/h OR 17,500 units SC. Then 250 units/kg q12h. SC |
| Prophylactic LMWH: *e.g.*, dalteparin 5000 U subcutaneously q24h, tinzaparin 4500 U subcutaneously q24h, or enoxaparin 40 mg subcutaneously q24h (although at extremes of body weight modification of dose may be required) |
| Intermediate-dose LMWH: *e.g.*, dalteparin 5000 U subcutaneously q12h or enoxaparin 40 mg subcutaneously q12h |
| Therapeutic adjusted-dose LMWH: weight-adjusted, full treatment doses of LMWH, given once or twice daily (e.g., dalteparin 200 U/kg or tinzaparin 175 U/kg qd or dalteparin 100 U/kg q125h or enoxaparin 1 mg/kg q12h) |
| Postpartum anticoagulants: vitamin K antagonists for 4–6 weeks with a target INR of 2.0–3.0, with initial UFH or LMWH overlap until the INR is ≥2.0, or prophylactic LMWH for 4–6 weeks |

clot burden and to improve hemodynamics [3, 122]. Reported problems with thrombolysis treatment include maternal bleeding and fetal deaths. But to date no maternal deaths have been reported.

If thrombolytic therapy has been given, an infusion of unfractionated heparin can be given but the initial loading dose is avoided. If the woman is not fit for thrombolysis or is moribund, a cardiothoracic surgeon must be involved with a view to urgent thoracotomy or embolectomy [28].

Over and above this, a rigid clinical vigilance and appropriate objective testing of women with symptoms suspicious of DVT, for new episode, or for extension of the disease or for pulmonary embolism (PE) is pertinent.

## Additional Therapies

Graduated elastic compression stockings [13, 112] and leg elevation should be done immediately if a woman is suspected to have DVT. Intermittent pneumatic compression can be used, if available and if in hospital. This helps to reduce edema. Mobilization and wearing graduated elastic compression stockings should be encouraged throughout pregnancy and puerperium. There is no need for bed rest for patients with DVT on anticoagulation therapy. Avoid dehydration all through pregnancy.

A retrievable temporary inferior vena caval filter can be placed [2, 28] in the perinatal period if a woman presents with PE or a woman has iliac vein DVT or if anticoagulant therapy has to be interrupted due to bleeding concerns.

## Maintenance Treatment of VTE

Once a woman is diagnosed to have DVT in pregnancy, for the rest of pregnancy LMWH twice daily therapeutic dose should be continued [49]. If anti Xa is tested, once the optimal anti Xa level of 0.5–1.2 IU/mL is reached and stable, repeat testing of the levels in 1–3 months is sufficient [9, 104]. After the initiation of anticoagulant therapy, patient can be followed up as an outpatient. Clinical monitoring for progression or refractory VTE, bleeding, heparin allergies, and heparin-induced thrombocytopenia (HIT) if UFH is used should be verified. Estimated risk of HIT is 1/1000 [123].

HIT is a thrombocytopenic state which is iatrogenic. Paradoxically it is more likely to cause both arterial and venous thromboembolism. Be alert when platelet count drops 50 % or more of baseline or falls below $100\times10^9$/L or if a new venous or arterial thrombosis occurs after initiation of heparin. If anaphylactoid reactions occur after intravenous UFH infusion, or if skin necrosis occurs even in the absence of thrombocytopenia, heparin should be discontinued and alternate therapy should be discussed.

Alternate therapy in HIT or for those who have heparin allergy and require continuing anticoagulant therapy with UFH is management with the heparinoids: danaparoid sodium (a heparinoid glycosaminoglycuronan antithrombotic agent) or fondaparinux (a synthetic heparin pentasaccharide, with selective inhibition of factor Xa). Anecdotal successful case reports of usage of these drugs in VTE in pregnancy have been reported. This requires expert hematologists' consideration.

Oral anticoagulants like warfarin [101] are not recommended in pregnancy as it crosses the placenta and can cause fetal hemorrhage or neonatal hemorrhage. Warfarin embryopathy characterized by chondromalacia punctata, midface hypoplasia, stippled chondral calcification, scoliosis, short proximal limbs, congenital heart defects, short fingers, agenesis of the corpus callosum, etc., has been described when it is given in the first trimester. Warfarin is rarely used in pregnancy. But more studies are coming up for its comparative safety in the second trimester. This would help countries with poor resources like India. Its selective use in midtrimester has to be studied well in India. One exception where warfarin is still used in pregnancy is when it is used in women with prosthetic heart valves, usually after the first trimester.

## Peripartum Anticoagulation

Managing patients in labor while on complete dose of therapeutic anticoagulants is described now. Most of these patients do not have increased delivery-related bleeding or PPH. Several options of management are available for maintaining anticoagulation prior to delivery. Patients can be converted from LMWH to subcutaneous UFH at 36–37 weeks. If delivery is expected earlier, this can be timed as per case. If delivery can be planned, especially planned Cesarean section, subcutaneous LMWH or UFH can be withheld 24–36 h prior to delivery. If anticoagulation has to be prolonged for some unexpected reasons, subcutaneous LMWH or UFH can be discontinued and the patient can be anticoagulated with intravenous UFH because of its shorter half-life. Intravenous UFH can be discontinued 4–6 h prior to delivery [10, 34, 112].

Consultation with anesthesiologists quite early to assess risks will help the patient. Before neuraxial anesthesia, intravenous UFH should be stopped and aPTT checked to ensure clearance. Regional anesthesia or analgesia is not recommended until at least 24 h after the last therapeutic dose of LMWH [5, 113]. Neuraxial anesthesia is not recommended in women who are fully anticoagulated. Women with high risk of hemorrhage should be on intravenous UFH until the risk is resolved (APH, coagulopathy, progressive hematoma, suspected intra-abdominal bleeding, and PPH). Surgical drains inserted under the rectus sheath and intra-abdominal should be considered as good surgical practice in patients on heparin.

Post-delivery, prophylactic or therapeutic heparin has to be resumed. In women who had neuraxial anesthesia, once hemostasis is ensured, treatment can be resumed [5, 53, 112]. A minimum of 4 h after neuraxial catheter removal, anticoagulant treatment can be resumed. Therapeutic UFH or LMWH can be started 4–6 h after vaginal delivery or 6–12 h after Cesarean delivery [112]. Pregnant patients with acute VTE are usually treated with therapeutic anticoagulation for a minimum of at least 6 weeks postpartum [10]. This can be continued use of heparin or LMWH, or more cost-effective would be to bridge her to warfarin. Both are not contraindicated in breast feeding. Abrupt discontinuation of heparin in the transition to warfarin may cause increased risk of VTE. During conversion to warfarin, the patient should remain on therapeutic anticoagulation with heparin for at least 4–5 days while the warfarin is titrated to a goal INR of 2.0–3.0 [101]. Daily INR monitoring is needed until the therapeutic dose is reached. In all cases, dehydration should be avoided and early ambulation wearing GCS should be encouraged.

## Postnatal Clinic Visit

At the postnatal visit, a clinical assessment should be made of possible postthrombotic venous damage. The rare instances of venous insufficiency and pulmonary hypertension as sequelae of PE should not be overlooked. Hereditary and acquired thrombophilia tests should be reviewed and may have to be repeated. The need for thromboprophylaxis in future pregnancies and also at other occasions with increased risk of VTE has to be counseled. Patients who are considered as high risk category for VTE are the ones who have hereditary or acquired thrombophilia, morbid obesity, recurrent VTE episodes, who delivered by Cesarean section and who are above 40 years of age. The risk associated with hormonal contraceptives should be explained.

## Prevention of Postthrombotic Syndrome

Postthrombotic syndrome [77, 117] is a group of symptoms comprising of chronic leg swelling, discoloration, pain on walking or standing, a feeling of heaviness, telangiectasis, dependent cyanosis, varicose veins, eczema, and in some cases lipodermatosclerosis and chronic ulceration. It improves with rest and in recumbent posture. It is more common where there is recurrent DVT with obesity. It occurs in 60 % of patients [77] who develop a proximal DVT when followed over 4–5 years. Graduated elastic compression stockings (GCS) are considered the treatment for postthrombotic syndrome.

## Prophylaxis for Venous Thromboembolic Disease in Pregnancy and the Early Postnatal Period

Currently available literature reviews on prevention of VTE in pregnancy, e.g., Cochrane pregnancy and childbirth group [7], have not shown enough good-quality evidence to point out which are the best ways to prevent VTE (including DVT and PE) during or following pregnancy, even with a Cesarean birth. Most studies didn't find enough evidence to be sure of these preventive treatments. This clearly shows our management dilemmas in preventing VTE in pregnancy. Most women are considered low risk for this disease. Almost all the cases of maternal mortality and near-misses data from all across the world suggest that VTEs (DVT, PE, and CVT) occurred in unexpected patients.

The need to understand risk stratification of all patients who could be prone to such an event and the knowledge of management of acute DVT and PE, developing an efficient team for the purpose, are the core essentials in reducing maternal mortality and serious morbidity of this condition.

**Conclusion**

Proposed scope for improvement in diagnosing VTE and preventing maternal deaths from VTE should start by developing a reporting format of every case. Several major medical registries and noninterventional studies have been initiated to assess real-world outcomes in patients with VTE. A few such registries are *IMPROVE (International Medical Prevention Registry on Venous Thromboembolism), RIETE (the Computerized Registry of Patients with Venous Thromboembolism),* and *ENDORSE* (*E*pidemiologic I*n*ternational *D*ay for the Evaluation *o*f Patients at *R*isk of Venous Thromboembolism in the Acute Hospital Care *Se*tting). These registries help to contribute to the development of strategies to improve patient care with venous thromboembolic diseases.

Often we have serious doubts on how to manage a specific patient, e.g., she is pregnant with thrombocytopenia, she has cerebral metastasis, or she has GI ulcer or even hepatic cirrhosis. There is no clinical evidence to show us how to manage these patients when they develop DVT or PE. Individualization of treatment is the crux to its management. The bibliography available is not of much help. Only if we have a database with sufficient number of cases, we may be able to make evidence-based decisions. It is our duty to have a good reporting format for a serious preventable condition as VTE in pregnancy.

## References

1. Abbasi N, Balayla J, Laporta DP, Kezouh A, Abenhaim HA. Trends, risk factors and mortality among women with venous thromboembolism during labour and delivery: a population-based study of 8 million births. Arch Gynecol Obstet. 2014;289(2):275–84.
2. Aburahma AF, Mullins DA. Endovascular caval interruption in pregnant patients with deep vein thrombosis of the lower extremity. J Vasc Surg. 2001;33(2):375–8.

3. Ahearn GS, Hadjiliadis MD, Govert JA, Tapson VF. Massive pulmonary embolism during pregnancy successfully treated with recombinant tissue plasminogen activator. Arch Int Med. 2002;162:1221–7.
4. Ambruso DR, Leonard BD, Bies RD, Jacobson L, Hathaway WE, Reeve EB. Antithrombin III deficiency: decreased synthesis of a biochemically normal molecule. Blood. 1982;60:78–83.
5. American College of Obstetricians and Gynecologists. Practice Bulletin No. 137: Gestational diabetes mellitus. Committee on Practice Bulletins—Obstetrics. Obstet Gynecol. 2013;122(2 Pt 1):406–16.
6. Andersen BS, Steffensen FH, Sorensen HT, et al. The cumulative incidence of venous thromboembolism during pregnancy and puerperium—an 11 year Danish population-based study of 63,300 pregnancies. Acta Obstet Gynecol Scand. 1998;77:170–3.
7. Bain E, Wilson A, Tooher R, Gates S, Davis L-J, Middleton P. Prophylaxis for venous thromboembolic disease in pregnancy and the early postnatal period. Published online 11 Feb 2014. Editorial Group: Cochrane pregnancy and childbirth group.
8. Bansal BC, Gupta RR, Prakash C. Stroke during pregnancy and puerperium in young females below the age of 40 years as a result of cerebral venous/venous sinus thrombosis. Jpn Heart J. 1980;21:171–83.
9. Bates SM, Greer IA, Hirsh J, Ginsberg JS. Use of antithrombotic agents during pregnancy: the Seventh ACCP Conference on Antithrombotic and thrombolytic therapy. Chest. 2004;163:627S–44.
10. Bates SM, Greer IA, Pabinger I, Sofaer S, Hirsh J. Venous thromboembolism, thrombophilia, antithrombotic therapy, and pregnancy: American College of Chest Physicians Evidence-Based Clinical Practice Guidelines (8th Edition). Chest. 2008;133(6 Suppl):844S–86.
11. Battinelli EM, Marshall A, Connors JM. The Role of Thrombophilia in Pregnancy. Thrombosis. vol. 2013. 2013. Article ID 516420, 9 pages, http://dx.doi.org/10.1155/2013/516420. Review Article.
12. Bertina RM, Koeleman BP, Koster T, Rosendaal FR, Dirven RJ, de Ronde H, van der Velden PA, Reitsma PH. Mutation in blood coagulation factor V associated with resistance to activated protein C. Nature. 1994;369(6475):64–7.
13. Brandjes DP, Buller HR, Heijboer H, Huisman MV, de Rijk M, Jagt H, et al. Randomised trial of effect of compression stockings in patients with symptomatic proximal–vein thrombosis. Lancet. 1997;349:759–62.
14. Brandt JT. Plasminogen and tissue-type plasminogen activator deficiency as risk factors for thromboembolic disease. Arch Pathol Lab Med. 2002;126:1376–81.
15. Bremme KA. Haemostatic changes in pregnancy. Best Pract Res Clin Haematol. 2003;16:153–68.
16. Brill-Edwards P, Ginsberg JS, Gent M, Hirsh J, Burrows R, Kearon C, et al. Safety of withholding heparin in pregnant women with a history of venous thromboembolism. N Engl J Med. 2000;343:1439–44.
17. Broekmans AW, Veltkamp JJ, Bertina RM. Congenital protein C deficiency and venous thromboembolism. A study of three Dutch families. N Engl J Med. 1983;309:340–4.
18. Brown MD, Lau J, Nelson RD, Kline JA. Turbidimetric D-dimer test in the diagnosis of pulmonary embolism: a metaanalysis. Clin Chem. 2003;49:1846–53.
19. Casele HL, Laifer SA, Woelkers DA, Venkataramanan R. Changes in the pharmacokinetics of the low-molecular-weight heparin enoxaparin sodium during pregnancy. Am J Obstet Gynecol. 1999;181(5 Pt 1):1113–7.
20. Cerneca F, Ricci G, Simeone R, Malisano M, Alberico S, Guaschino S. Coagulation and fibrinolysis changes in normal pregnancy. Increased levels of procoagulants and reduced levels of inhibitors during pregnancy induce a hypercoagulable state, combined with a reactive fibrinolysis. Eur J Obstet Gynecol Reprod Biol. 1997;73:31–6.
21. Cervera R, Piette J, Font J, et al. Antiphospholipid syndrome: clinical and immunologic manifestations and patterns of disease expression in a cohort of 1,000 patients. Arthritis Rheum. 2002;46(4):1019–27.
22. Chan W-S, Spencer FA, Ginsbergm JS. Anatomic distribution of deep vein thrombosis in pregnancy. Can Med Assoc J. 2010;182(7):657–60.
23. Christodoulou C, Sangle S, D'Cruz DP. Vasculopathy and arterial stenotic lesions in the antiphospholipid syndrome. Rheumatology (Oxford). 2007;46:907–10.
24. Chunilal SD, Young E, Johnston MA, et al. The aPTT response of pregnant plasma to unfractionated heparin. Thromb Haemost. 2000;87:92–7.
25. Clark SL, Belfort MA, Dildy GA, Herbst MA, Meyers JA, Hankins GD. Maternal death in the 21st century: causes, prevention, and relationship to cesarean delivery. Am J Obstet Gynecol. 2008;199(1):36e1–e5.
26. Clark P, Brennand J, Conkie JA, McCall F, Greer IA, Walker ID. Activated protein C sensitivity, protein C, protein S and coagulation in normal pregnancy. Thromb Haemost. 1998;79:1166–70.
27. Clouse LH, Comp PC. The regulation of hemostasis: the protein C system. N Engl J Med. 1986;314:1298.
28. Condliffe R, Elliot CA, Hughes RJ, Hurdman J, Maclean RM, Sabroe I, van Veen JJ, Kiely DG. Management dilemmas in acute pulmonary embolism. Thorax. 2014;69(2):174–80.
29. Conti E, Zezza L, Ralli E, Comito C, Sada L, Passerini J, Caserta D, Rubattu S, Autore C, Moscarini M, Volpe M. Pulmonary embolism in pregnancy. J Thromb Thrombolysis. 2014;37(3):251–70.
30. Crowther MA, Johnston M, Weitz J, Ginsberg JS. Free protein S deficiency may be found in patients with antiphospholipid antibodies who do not have systemic lupus erythematosus. Thromb Haemost. 1996;76:689–91.

31. Dahlbäck B, Carlsson M, Svensson PJ. Familial thrombophilia due to a previously unrecognized mechanism characterized by poor anticoagulant response to activated protein C: prediction of a cofactor to activated protein C. Proc Natl Acad Sci U S A. 1993;90(3):1004–8.
32. Demarmels Biasiutti F, Sulzer I, Stucki B, Wuillemin WA, Furlan M, Lammle B. Is plasminogen deficiency a thrombotic risk factor? A study on 23 thrombophilic patients and their family members. Thromb Haemost. 1998;80:167–70.
33. den Heijer M, Kostor T, Blom HJ, et al. Hyperhomocysteinemia as a risk factor for deep-vein thrombosis. N Engl J Med. 1996;334:759–62.
34. Edward Henry Springel, Thomas Chih Cheng Peng; Thromboembolism in Pregnancy Workup, Medscape CME and education. Reference Apr 30, 2014.
35. Emmi L, Bergamini C, Spinelli A, Liotta F, Marchione T, Caldini A, Fanelli A, De-Cristofaro MT, Dal-Pozzo G. Possible pathogenetic role of activated platelets in the primary antiphospholipid syndrome involving the central nervous system. Ann N Y Acad Sci. 1997;823:188–200.
36. Ensom MHH, Stephenson MD. Low molecular weight heparins in pregnancy. Pharmacotherapy. 1999;19:1013–25.
37. Esmon CT, Esmon NL, Harris KW. Complex formation between thrombin and thrombomodulin inhibits both thrombin-catalyzed fibrin formation and factor V activation. J Biol Chem. 1982;257:7944–7.
38. Esmon NL, Safa O, Smirnov MD, Esmon CT. Antiphospholipid antibodies and the protein C pathway. J Autoimmun. 2000;15:221–5.
39. Forbes KP, Reid JH, Murchison JT. Do preliminary chest X-ray findings define the optimum role of pulmonary scintigraphy in suspected pulmonary embolism? Clin Radiol. 2001;56(5):397–400.
40. Forestier F, Daffos F, Capella-Pavlovsky M. Low molecular weight heparin (PK 10169) does not cross the placenta during the second trimester of pregnancy: study by direct fetal blood sampling under ultrasound. Thromb Res. 1984;34:557–60.
41. Foster DC, Yoshitake S, Davie EW. The nucleotide sequence of the gene for human protein C. Proc Natl Acad Sci. 1985;82:4673–7.
42. Francalanci I, Comeglio P, Alessandrello Liotta A, Cellai AP, Fedi S, Parretti E, Mecacci F, Mello G, Prisco D, Abbate R. D-dimer plasma levels during normal pregnancy measured by specific ELISA. Int J Clin Lab Res. 1997;27(1):65–7.
43. Francis C. Plasminogen activator inhibitor-1 levels and polymorphisms: association with venous thromboembolism. Arch Pathol Lab Med. 2002;126: 1401–4.
44. Ginsberg JS, Brill-Edwards P, Burrows RF, et al. Venous thrombosis during pregnancy: leg and trimester of presentation. Thromb Haemost. 1992;67(5):519–20.
45. Girolami A, Randi ML, Gavasso S, Lombardi AM, Spiezia F. The occasional venous thromboses seen in patients with severe (homozygous) FXII deficiency are probably due to associated risk factors. J Thromb Thrombolysis. 2004;17:139–43.
46. Goldhaber SZ, Tapson VF. A prospective registry of 5,451 patients with ultrasound-confirmed deep vein thrombosis. Am J Cardiol. 2004;93:259–62.
47. Goldhaber SZ, Visani L, De Rosa M. Acute pulmonary embolism: clinical outcomes in the International Cooperative Pulmonary Embolism Registry (ICOPER). Lancet. 1999;353(9162):1386–9.
48. Greer IA. Inherited thrombophilia and venous thromboembolism. Best Pract Res Clin Obstet Gynaecol. 2003;17:413–25.
49. Greer IA, Nelson-Piercy C. Low-molecular-weight heparins for thromboprophylaxis and treatment of venous thrombo-embolism in pregnancy: a systematic review of safety and efficacy. Blood. 2005;106:401–7.
50. Guidelines on diagnosis and management of acute pulmonary embolism. Task Force on Pulmonary Embolism, European Society of Cardiology. Eur Heart J. 2000;21(16):1301–36.
51. Heit JA, Kobbervig CE, James AH, et al. Trends in the incidence of venous thromboembolism during pregnancy or postpartum: a 30-year population-based study. Ann Intern Med. 2005;143: 697–706.
52. Hirsh J, Warkentin TE, Shaughnessy SG, Anand SS, Halperin JL, Raschke R, et al. Heparin and low-molecular weight heparin: mechanism of action, pharmacokinetics, dosing, monitoring, efficacy, and safety. Chest. 2001;119(1 Suppl):64S–94.
53. Horlocker TT, Wedel DJ, Rowlingson JC, Enneking FK. Executive summary: regional anesthesia in the patient receiving antithrombotic or thrombolytic therapy: American Society of Regional Anesthesia and Pain Medicine Evidence-Based Guidelines (Third Edition). Reg Anesth Pain Med. 2010;35(1): 102–5.
54. Jacob H. Rand, molecular pathogenesis of the antiphospholipid syndrome. Circ Res. 2002;90: 29–37.
55. Jacobsen AF, Qvigstad E, Sandset PM. Low molecular weight heparin (dalteparin) for the treatment of venous thrombo-embolism in pregnancy. BJOG. 2003;110:139–44.
56. Jacobsen AF, Skjeldestad FE, Sandset PM. Incidence and risk patterns of venous thromboembolism in pregnancy and puerperium—a register-based case-control study. Am J Obstet Gynecol. 2008;198:233.e1–7.
57. James AH. Venous thromboembolism: mechanisms, treatment, and public awareness. Arterioscler Thromb Vasc Biol. 2009;29:326–31.
58. James AH, Jamison MG, Brancazio LR, Myers ER. Venous thromboembolism during pregnancy and the postpartum period: incidence, risk factors, and mortality. Am J Obstet Gynecol. 2006; 194(5):1311–5.
59. James AH, Tapson VF, Goldhaber SZ. Thrombosis during pregnancy and the postpartum period. Am J Obstet Gynecol. 2005;193:216–9.

60. Khan S. Hereditary thrombophilia. Thromb J. 2006;4:15.
61. Konstantinides S, Torbicki A, Agnelli G, Danchin N, Fitzmaurice D, Galie` N, Simon J, Gibbs R, et al. 2014 ESC Guidelines on the diagnosis and management of acute pulmonary embolism. DOI: http://dx.doi.org/10.1093/eurheartj/ehu283. First published online: Aug 30 2014.
62. Kovacevich GJ, Gaich SA, Lavin JP, et al. The prevalence of thromboembolic events among women with extended bed rest prescribed as part of the treatment for premature labor or preterm premature rupture of membranes. Am J Obstet Gynecol. 2000;182:1089–92.
63. Kunicki TJ. The influence of platelet collagen receptor polymorphisms in hemostasis and thrombotic disease. Arterioscler Thromb Vasc Biol. 2002;22:14–20.
64. Lane DA, Bayston T, Olds RJ, et al. Antithrombin mutation database: 2nd (1997) update. For the Plasma Coagulation Inhibitors Subcommittee of the Scientific and Standardization Committee of the International Society on Thrombosis and Haemostasis. Thromb Haemost. 1997;77:197.
65. Lane DA, Mannucci PM, Bauer KA, et al. Inherited thrombophilia: part 2. Thromb Haemost. 1996;76:824.
66. Lepercq J, Conard J, Borel-Derlon A, Darmon JY, Boudignat O, Francoual C, et al. Venous thromboembolism during pregnancy: a retrospective study of enoxaparin safety in 624 pregnancies. BJOG. 2001;108:1134–40.
67. Lijnen HR, Holylaerts M, Collen D. Heparin binding properties of human histidine-rich glycoprotein. Mechanism and role in the neutralization of heparin in plasma. J Biol Chem. 1983;258:3803.
68. Lijnen HR, Soria J, Soria C, et al. Dysfibrinogenemia (fibrinogen Dusard) associated with impaired fibrin-enhanced plasminogen activation. Thromb Haemost. 1984;51:108.
69. Lindqvist P, Dahlbäck B, Marsál K. Thrombotic risk during pregnancy: a population study. Obstet Gynecol. 1999;94(4):595–9.
70. Macklon NS, Greer IA, Bowman AW. An ultrasound study of gestational and postural changes in the deep venous system of the leg in pregnancy. Br J Obstet Gynaecol. 1997;104(2):191–7.
71. Makatsaria AD, Bitsadze VO, Dolgushina NV. Use of the low-molecular-weight heparin nadroparin during pregnancy. A review. Curr Med Res Opin. 2003;19:4–12.
72. Malcolm JC, Keely EJ, Karovitch AJ, Wells PS. Use of low molecular weight heparin in acute venous thromboembolic events in pregnancy. J Obstet Gynaecol Can. 2002;24:568–71.
73. Marcucci R, Liotta AA, Cellai AP, Rogolino A, Gori AM, Giusti B, Poli D, Fedi S, Abbate R, Prisco D. Increased plasma levels of lipoprotein(a) and the risk of idiopathic and recurrent venous thromboembolism. Am J Med. 2003;115:601–5.
74. Marik PE, Plante LA. Venous thromboembolic disease and pregnancy. N Engl J Med. 2008;359(19):2025–33.
75. Martinelli I, Mannucci PM, De Stefano V, Taioli E, Rossi V, Crosti F, Paciaroni K, Leone G. Different risks of thrombosis in four coagulation defects associated with inherited thrombophilia: a study of 150 families. Blood. 1998;92:2353–8.
76. McCaulley JA, Pates JA. Postpartum cerebral venous thrombosis. Obstet Gynecol. 2011;118(2 Pt 2):423–5.
77. McColl MD, Ellison J, Greer IA, Tait RC, Walker ID. Prevalence of the post thrombotic syndrome in young women with previous venous thromboembolism. Br J Haematol. 2000;108:272–4.
78. McCully KS. Homocysteine and vascular disease. Nat Med. 1996;2:386–9.
79. McLintock C, Brighton T, Chunilal S, Dekker G. Recommendations for the diagnosis and treatment of deep venous thrombosis and pulmonary embolism in pregnancy and the postpartum period. Aust N Z J Obstet Gynaecol. 2012;52(1):14–22.
80. McRae SJ, Ginsberg JS. Treatment of venous thromboembolism; initial treatment of venous thromboembolism. Circulation. 2004;110:I-3-I-9.
81. Meade TW, Ruddock V, Stirling Y, Chakrabarti R, Miller GJ. Fibrinolytic activity, clotting factors, and long-term incidence of ischaemic heart disease in the Northwick Park Heart Study. Lancet. 1993;342:1076–9.
82. Medcalf RL, Stasinopoulos SJ. The undecided serpin. The ins and outs of plasminogen activator inhibitor type 2. Febs J. 2005;272:4858–67.
83. Meijers JCM, Tekelenburg WLH, Bouma BN, Rogier BM, Rosendaal FR. High levels of coagulation factor XI as a risk factor for venous thrombosis. N Engl J Med. 2000;342:696–701.
84. Moser KM, Fedullo PF, LitteJohn JK, Crawford R. Frequent asymptomatic pulmonary embolism in patients with deep venous thrombosis [published correction appears in JAMA. 1994;271(24)1908]. JAMA. 1994;271(3):223–5.
85. Niemann T, Nicolas G, Roser HW, Müller-Brand J, Bongartz G. Imaging for suspected pulmonary embolism in pregnancy—what about the fetal dose? A comprehensive review of the literature. Insights Imaging. 2010;1(5–6):361–72.
86. Nijkeuter M, Ginsberg JS, Huisman MV. Diagnosis of deep vein thrombosis and pulmonary embolism in pregnancy: a systematic review. J Thromb Haemost. 2006;4(3):496–500.
87. O'Donnell J, Tuddenham EG, Manning R, Kemball-Cook G, Johnson D, Laffan M. High prevalence of elevated factor VIII levels in patients referred for thrombophilia screening: role of increased synthesis and relationship to the acute phase reaction. Thromb Haemost. 1997;77:825–8.
88. Ohlin AK, Norlund L, Marlar RA. Thrombomodulin gene variations and thromboembolic disease. Thromb Haemost. 1997;78:396–400.
89. Perry DJ. Antithrombin and its inherited deficiencies. Blood Rev. 1994;8(1):37–55.
90. Polak JF, Wilkinson DL. Ultrasonographic diagnosis of symptomatic deep venous thrombosis in preg-

nancy. Am J Obstet Gynecol. 1991;165(3):625–9.
91. Pomp ER, Lenselink AM, Rosendaal FR, et al. Pregnancy, the postpartum period and prothrombotic defects: risk of venous thrombosis in the MEGA study. J Thromb Haemost. 2008;6(4):632–7.
92. Poort SR, Rosendaal FR, Reitsma PH, Bertina RM. A common genetic variation in the 3′-Untranslated region of the prothrombin gene is associated with elevated plasma prothrombin levels and an increase in venous thrombosis. Blood. 1996;88:3698–703.
93. Quinlan DJ, McQuillan A, Eikelboom JW. Low-molecular-weight heparin compared with intravenous unfractionated heparin for treatment of pulmonary embolism: a meta-analysis of randomized, controlled trials. Ann Intern Med. 2004; 140:175–83.
94. Ray JG, Chan WS. Deep vein thrombosis during pregnancy and the puerperium: a meta-analysis of the period of risk and the leg of presentation. Obstet Gynecol Surv. 1999;54:265–71.
95. Reiner Alexander P, Siscovick David S, Rosendaal FR. Platelet glycoprotein gene polymorphisms and risk of thrombosis: facts and fancies. Rev Clin Exp Hematol. 2001;5:262–87.
96. Rowan JA, McLintock C, Taylor RS, North RA. Prophylactic and therapeutic enoxaparin during pregnancy: indications, outcomes and monitoring. Aust N Z J Obstet Gynaecol. 2003;43:123–8.
97. Sangle SR, D'Cruz DP, Jan W, Karim MY, Khamashta MA, Abbs IC, Hughes GR. Renal artery stenosis in the antiphospholipid (Hughes) syndrome and hypertension. Ann Rheum Dis. 2003;62:999–1002.
98. Sangle SR, Jan W, Lau IS, Bennett AN, Hughes GRV, D'Cruz DP. Coeliac artery stenosis and antiphospholipid (Hughes) syndrome/antiphospholipid antibodies. Clin Exp Rheumatol. 2006;24:349.
99. Sanson BJ, Lensing AW, Prins MH, Ginsberg JS, Barkagan ZS, Lavenne-Pardonge E, et al. Safety of low molecular weight heparin in pregnancy: a systematic review. Thromb Haemost. 1999;81:668–72.
100. Scarsbrook AF, Evans AL, Owen AR, Gleeson FV. Diagnosis of suspected venous thromboembolic disease in pregnancy. Clin Radiol. 2006;61:1–12.
101. Schaefer C, Hannemann D, Meister R, Eléfant E, Paulus W, Vial T. Vitamin K antagonists and pregnancy outcome. A multi-centre prospective study. Thromb Haemost. 2006;95(6):949–57.
102. Schmidel DK, Tatro AV, Phelps LG, Tomczak JA, Long GL. Organization of the human protein S genes. Biochemistry. 1990;29:7845–52.
103. Schulman S, Wiman B. The significance of hypofibrinolysis for the risk of recurrence of venous thromboembolism. Duration of Anticoagulation (DURAC) Trial Study Group. Thromb Haemost. 1996;75:607–11.
104. Sephton V, Farquharson RG, Topping J, Quenby SM, Cowan C, Back DJ, Toh CH. A longitudinal study of maternal dose response to low molecular weight heparin in pregnancy. Obstet Gynecol. 2003;101(6):1307–11.
105. Simpson EL, Lawrenson RA, Nightingale AL, et al. Venous thromboembolism in pregnancy and the puerperium: incidence and additional risk factors from a London perinatal database. BJOG. 2001;108:56–60.
106. Smith MP, Norris LA, Steer PJ, Savidge GF, Bonnar J. Tinzaparin sodium for thrombosis treatment and prevention during pregnancy. Am J Obstet Gynecol. 2004;190:495–501.
107. Spritzer CE, Norconk Jr JJ, Sostman HD, Coleman RE. Detection of deep venous thrombosis by magnetic resonance imaging. Chest. 1993;104(1):54–60.
108. Sultan AA, Tata LJ, West J, Fiaschi L, Fleming KM, Nelson-Piercy C, Grainge MJ. Risk factors for first venous thromboembolism around pregnancy: a population-based cohort study from the United Kingdom. Blood. 2013;121(19):3953–61.
109. Tait RC, Walker ID, Perry DJ, Islam SI, Daly ME, McCall F, Conkie JA, Carrell RW. Prevalence of antithrombin deficiency in the healthy population. Br J Haematol. 1994;87:106–12.
110. Tawfik MM, Taman ME, Motawea AA, Abdel-Hady E. Thrombolysis for the management of massive pulmonary embolism in pregnancy. Int J Obstet Anesth. 2013;22(2):149–52.
111. te Raa GD, Ribbert LS, Snijder RJ, Biesma DH. Treatment options in massive pulmonary embolism during pregnancy; a case-report and review of literature. Thromb Res. 2009;124(1):1–5.
112. The Acute Management of Thrombosis and Embolism During Pregnancy and the Puerperium, RCOG Green-top Guideline No. 37b Reviewed 2010.
113. Thrombosis and Embolism during Pregnancy and the Puerperium, Reducing the Risk, RCOG Green-top Guideline No. 37a, Nov 2009.
114. Uchikova EH, Ledjev II. Changes in haemostasis in normal pregnancy. Eur J Obstet Gynecol Reprod Biol. 2005;119:185–8.
115. Ulander VM, Lehtola A, Kaaja R. Long-term outcome of deep venous thrombosis during pregnancy treated with unfractionated heparin or low molecular weight heparin. Thromb Res. 2003;111:239–42.
116. Ulman E, Brady WJ, Perron AD. Electrocardiographic manifestations of pulmonary embolism. Am J Emerg Med. 2001;19(6):514–9.
117. van Dongen CJJ, Prandoni P, Frulla M, Marchiori A, Prins MH, Hutten BA. Relation between quality of anticoagulant treatment and the development of the postthrombotic syndrome. J Thromb Haemost. 2005;3:939–42.
118. van Dongen CJ, van den Belt AG, Prins MH, Lensing AW. Fixed dose subcutaneous low molecular weight heparins versus adjusted dose unfractionated heparin

for venous thromboembolism. Cochrane Database Syst Rev. 2004;(4):CD001100.
119. van Hylckama VA, et al. High levels of factor IX increase the risk of venous thrombosis. Blood. 2000;95:3678–82.
120. Villa P, Aznar J, Vaya A, Espana F, Ferrando F, Mira Y, Estelles A. Hereditary homozygous heparin cofactor II deficiency and the risk of developing venous thrombosis. Thromb Haemost. 1999;82:1011–4.
121. Vora S, Ghosh K, Shetty S, Salvi V, Satoskar P. Deep venous thrombosis in the antenatal period in a large cohort of pregnancies from western India. Thromb J. 2007;5:9.
122. Wan S, Quinlan DJ, Agnelli G, Eikelboom JW. Thrombolysis compared with heparin for the initial treatment of pulmonary embolism: a meta-analysis of the randomized controlled trials. Circulation. 2004;110:744–9.
123. Warkentin TE, Greinacher A. Heparin-induced thrombo-cytopenia: recognition, treatment, and prevention; the Seventh ACCP Conference on Antithrombotic and Thrombolytic Therapy. Chest. 2004;126(3 Suppl):311S–37.
124. Wells PS, Anderson DR, Rogers M, et al. Evaluation of d-dimer in the diagnosis of suspected deep venous thromboembolism. N Engl J Med. 2003;349:1227–35.
125. Why Mothers Die Kerala – 2006–09 Second Report of Confidential Review of Maternal Deaths, Kerala Maternal Fetal Medicine Committee, Kerala Federation of Obstetrics & Gynaecology Editors: VP Paily, K Ambujam, Betsy Thomas.
126. Wilbur J, Shian B. Diagnosis of deep venous thrombosis and pulmonary embolism. Am Fam Physician. 2012;86(10):913–9.
127. Wong M, Sangle S, Jan W, Hughes GR, D'Cruz DP. Intracerebral arterial stenosis with neurological events associated with antiphospholipid syndrome. Rheumatology (Oxford). 2005;44:948–9.
128. Yusen RD, Gage BF. Outpatient treatment of acute thrombo- embolic disease. Clin Chest Med. 2003;24:46–61.
129. Zoller B, Svensson PJ, He X, Dahlback B. Identification of the same factor V mutation in 47 out of 60 thrombosis-prone families with inherited resistance to activated protein C. J Clin Invest. 1994;94:2521–4.

# Gestational Trophoblastic Disease 21

P.K. Sekharan

## Introduction

Gestational trophoblastic disease (GTD) is a spectrum of abnormal trophoblastic hyperplasia resulting from abnormal conception; there is imbalance in the genetic input from the ovum and sperm. The genetic makeup in complete hydatidiform mole (CHM) and partial hydatidiform mole (PHM) is different. In both types of mole, there is an excess of paternal chromosomes resulting in rapidly multiplying trophoblastic cells of both the cytotrophoblastic and the syncytiotrophoblastic layers, which is capable of producing excess of human chorionic gonadotropin (hCG) with potential to progress to gestational trophoblastic neoplasia (GTN). Gestational trophoblastic neoplasia can also develop from previously normal trophoblasts as in cases of choriocarcinoma and placental site trophoblastic tumor (PSTT) following term delivery and abortion. All types of GTN, irrespective of their genetic origin, share the feature of producing high level of hCG. Gestational trophoblastic neoplasia is one of the most chemosensitive and highly curable cancers, even in the presence of widespread metastatic disease, and in most cases with preservation of fertility. GTD is unique because the maternal lesions arise from the fetal tissue.

P.K. Sekharan, MD
Department of Obstetrics and Gynaecology,
Medical College, Calicut, India
e-mail: drsekharanpk@hotmail.com

## Classification

### Hydatidiform Mole

- Complete Hydatidiform Mole (CHM)
- Androgenetic Complete Mole
- Homozygous – Two identical chromosome compliments derived from duplication of paternal haploid set of chromosome, monospermic fertilization –80 %, always 46XX
- Heterozygous – All chromosomes are paternal, dispermic fertilization, can be 46XX or 46XY
- Biparental complete mole – Both paternal and maternal chromosomes, failure of maternal imprinting
- Partial hydatidiform mole (PHM) – Fertilization of ovum containing 23 haploid set by dispermy 69XXY/69XXX or duplication of sperm with haploid set 23X to result in 69XXX

### Gestational Trophoblastic Neoplasia (GTN)

GTN comprises a group of tumors with the potential for local invasion and metastases:

- Invasive mole
- Gestational choriocarcinoma
- Placental site trophoblastic tumor (PSTT)
- Epithelioid trophoblastic tumor (ETT)


A. Gandhi et al. (eds.), *Principles of Critical Care in Obstetrics: Volume II*,
DOI 10.1007/978-81-322-2686-4_21

## Genetics of Hydatidiform Mole

Hydatidiform moles have excess of paternal chromosomes, and imprinting has a role in the development of gestational trophoblastic diseases. Paternal genes have control over growth and development of trophoblast and placenta while maternal gene has more control over growth and development of embryo and fetus. Thus with excess influence of paternal genes in hydatidiform moles, there is excessive trophoblastic proliferation and invasion.

Studies by Vassilakos et al. [1] in 1977 and by Szulman and Surti [2, 3] in 1978 have shown that CHM and PHM are two separate entities. Complete hydatidiform moles have a normal chromosome number of 46, but they are genetically abnormal as all the chromosomes are paternally derived and hence androgenetic, as the maternal haploid set of 23X is inactivated. Partial hydatidiform moles are diandric triploid (69XXY, 69XXX, or 69XYY) and are formed by dispermic fertilization of a haploid oocyte, resulting in a conceptus with two paternal and one maternal haploid set of chromosomes.

## Paternal Origin of Complete Hydatidiform Mole

A complete hydatidiform mole results by the abnormal fertilization of an "empty egg" (absent or inactivated maternal chromosomes) by a sperm containing haploid set of 23X chromosomes which duplicates to form 46XX (monospermic fertilization), the androgenic CHM (AnCHM, homozygous). Although majority of CHM results from duplication of a haploid sperm, about 20 % of AnCHM result from fertilization of an empty ovum with an inactivated genome by two sperms and can have a 46XY or 46XX karyotype, the heterozygous CHM [1, 2, 4]. Heterozygous moles are at higher risk of developing malignancy. Since absence of the X chromosome is not compatible with early development, 46YY karyotype has never been observed in CHM. The mitochondrial DNA is derived from the mother [5, 6]. CHM by dispermic fertilization (heterozygous) containing Y chromosome shows high malignant potential [7] (Diagram 21.1).

## Paternal Origin of Partial Hydatidiform Mole

Partial hydatidiform moles are triploid and may have a 69XXX, 69XXY, or 69XYY karyotype [3]. PHM results from dispermic fertilization of ovum containing haploid set of 23X chromosome by two sperms containing haploid sets of 23X or 23Y, a diandric triploidy. Fertilization by diploid sperm resulting in partial mole is also suggested (Diagram 21.2).

## Biparental CHM

The rare type of biparental CHM (BiCHM) is seen in patients with recurrent mole and occurs in families with two or more members of the family developing molar pregnancies. There is contribution from both parents, but due to defect in genomic imprinting, molar pregnancy develops and resembles complete hydatidiform mole. Genetic studies of such families have shown evidence of mutations in the leucine-rich regions of NLRP7 at chromosome 19q13.3-13.4 [8–10]. The mode of inheri-

**Diagram 21.1** Fertilization of an empty ovum by sperm containing 23X haploid set of chromosome which duplicates to form 46XX

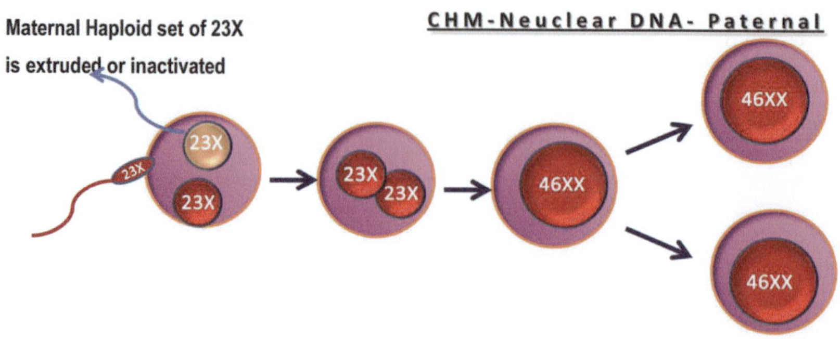

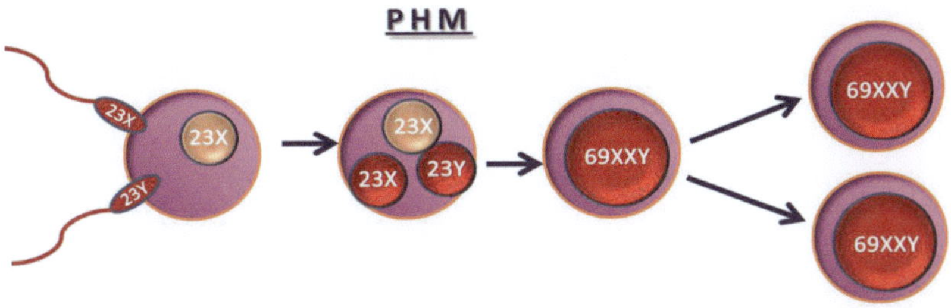


**Diagram 21.2** Fertilization of ovum with haploid set of 23X by two sperms with haploid sets of 23X or 23X and 23Y to result in 69XXX or 69XXY. Diandric triploidy

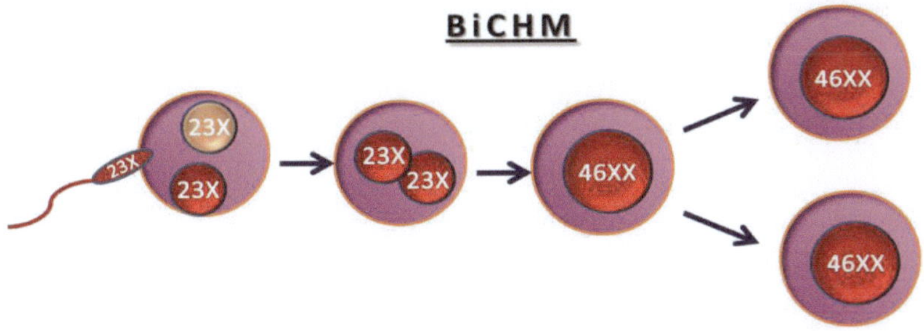


**Diagram 21.3** BiCHM is seen in patients with recurrent mole and occurs in families with two or more members developing molar pregnancies. Defect in genomic imprinting, risk of malignancy. Genetic defect – 19q13.3-13.4, NLRP7

tance in familial biparental recurrent mole is by an autosomal recessive disorder. The probable mechanism of biparental recurrent moles seems to be a defect in the methylation process in the paternal and maternal alleles in the H19 gene; the paternal allele is methylated and maternal allele is unmythelated. The defective methylation process can sometimes be partial or even may overcome which would explain why in certain woman with the disorder had a normal pregnancy, despite a theoretical recurrence risk of 100 % (Diagram 21.3).

## Risk Factors

Pregnancy at extremes of age is an important risk factor for development of hydatidiform mole; the risk is doubled in teenage and at age above 35 years. Women older than 40 years experience a 5- to 10-fold increase in risk compared to younger women [11]. Parity does not affect the risk for developing molar pregnancy. Relative deficiency of carotene and animal fat intake is reported as a risk factor. History of previous molar pregnancy is an important risk factor, a reported risk of ten times compared to the normal population. Cigarette smoking, history of infertility, contraceptive use, and induction of ovulation are reported to increase the risk of having molar pregnancy.

## Pathology of Trophoblastic Lesions

All types of gestational trophoblastic diseases exhibit proliferation of both syncytiotrophoblast and cytotrophoblast which maintain secretion of hCG. Placental site trophoblastic tumor arising from the intermediate trophoblast cells produces low levels of hCG and hPL.

## Complete Hydatidiform Mole

The histological features of complete hydatidiform include:

- Generalized diffuse hyperplasia of both cytotrophoblast and syncytiotrophoblast.
- Generalized edema of chorionic villi with central cistern formation of varying sizes, which resembles the macroscopic description of the hydatidiform mole, the "bunch of grapes."
- Absenc e of an embryo resorption occurs before development of fetal circulation, and no nucleated fetal erythrocytes are observed in the villous.

Fisher and others in 1997 [12] reported the presence of fetal blood cells in seven complete hydatidiform moles by polymerase chain reaction

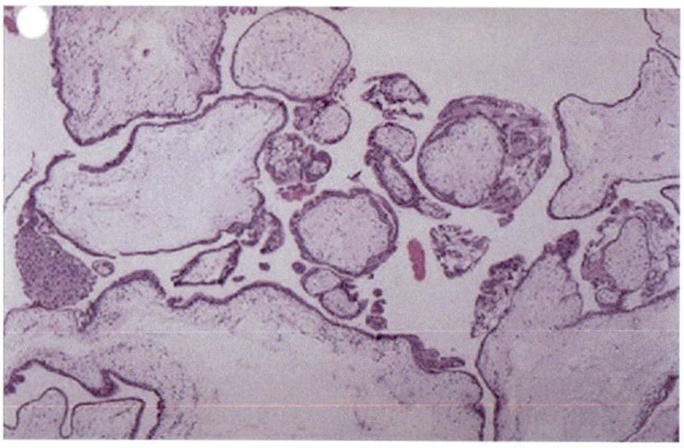

**Fig. 21.1** The chorionic villi of complete mole are diffusely hydropic with central cistern formation with no blood vessels and hyperplasia of trophoblastic layers

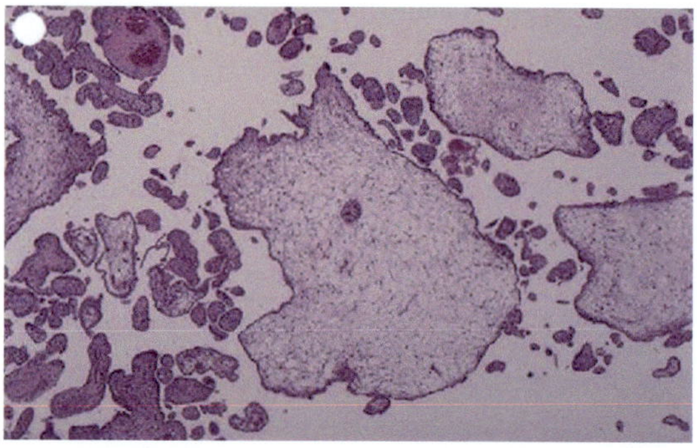

**Fig. 21.2** Focal hydropic degeneration with focal hyperplasia of trophoblast with normal villi in between and fetal parts

amplification of DNA. Their conclusion was that fetal blood cells may be present in the villi of complete hydatidiform moles, and the presence of fetal erythrocytes alone should not be considered indicative of a diagnosis of partial hydatidiform mole.

With the availability of ultrasonography for early pregnancy evaluation, many moles are evacuated before the classical development of mole as a case of failed pregnancy. It is important to submit all products evacuated for histopathological study. The classical findings of the complete mole may not be seen in such early cases. Abnormal trophoblastic hyperplasia is a constant finding in early CHM, and the generalized hydrops may not be evident. Early CHM may exhibit stromal blood vessels and stromal karyorrhexis.

Complete moles show overexpression of several growth factors, including c-myc, epidermal growth factor, and c-erb B-2, compared with normal placenta. Immunostaining using p57KIP2 will be absent in complete mole (Fig. 21.1).

## Partial Hydatidiform Mole

The partial hydatidiform mole (PHM) results by fertilization of an ovum containing haploid set of 23X by two sperms with haploid sets of 23X or 23X and 23Y, a Diandric Triploidy. The characteric features of partial mole are:

- Mild focal variable hydropic villi.
- Mild trophoblastic hyperplasia, predominantly confined to syncytium.
- Fetal vessels are usually present and contain nucleated fetal erythrocytes.
- Embryo/fetus will be present often with congenital anomalies.
- Runs a milder course and the diagnosis is often missed as “missed abortion”.

It was thought that partial mole does not transform into choriocarcinoma. Recently, Newlands et al. have reported three cases of choriocarcinoma following partial mole [13]. Many other reports of malignant sequelae following PHM were reported by other authors also subsequently [14–16].

The distinction between a hydatidiform mole and an abortion with hydropic villi can be difficult. Like hydatidiform mole, a hydropic abortion may show villous edema with hydropic swelling, although a hydropic abortion lacks the marked trophoblastic hyperplasia. With the introduction of p57kip2 immunohistochemistry, a better differentiation between complete and partial mole has become possible. The p57kip2 gene (CDKN1C) is paternally imprinted and expressed from the maternal allele. Since complete moles lack a maternal genome, p57kip2 immunostaining is absent, whereas hydropic abortus and partial moles show positive staining (Figs. 21.1 and 21.2).

## Invasive Mole

Invasive mole is the penetration of molar villi most often from CHM into the myometrium or the uterine vasculature and may spread to the

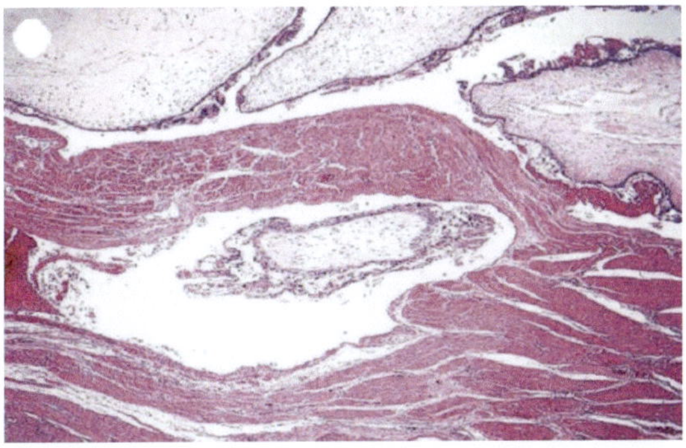

**Fig. 21.3** Invasive mole – trophoblastic element is invading into the myometrium maintaining the villous pattern

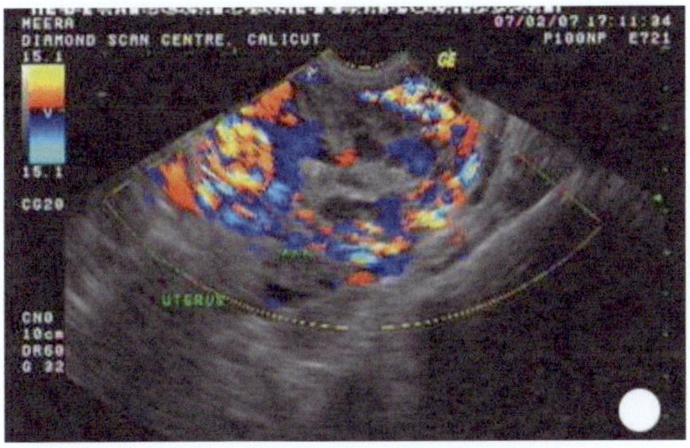


**Fig. 21.4** Color Doppler study showing highly vascularized area in the myometrium in invasive mole

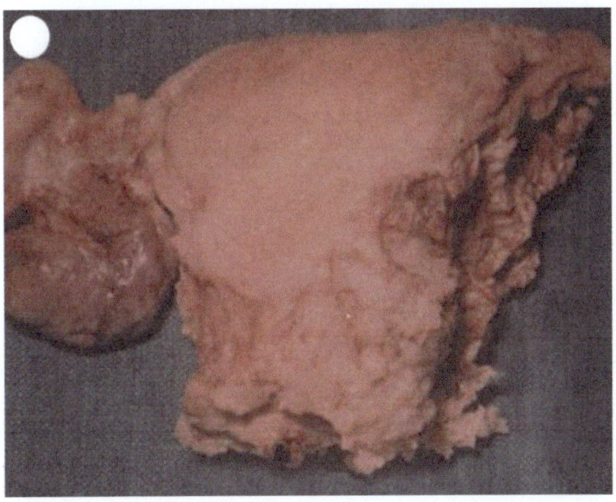

**Fig. 21.5** Subtotal hysterectomy done as a life-saving procedure for perforation of uterus by invasive mole which leads to severe intraperitoneal bleeding

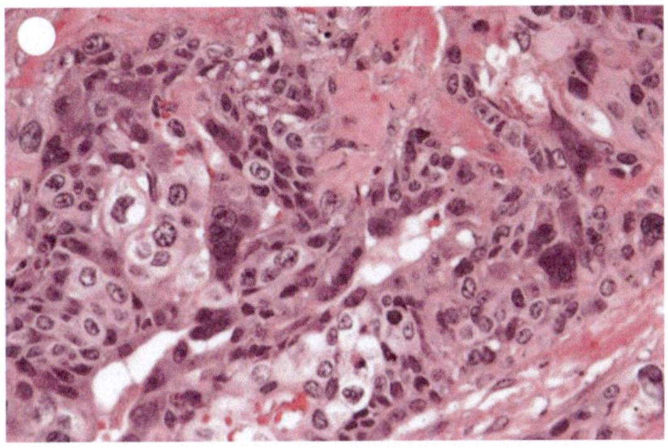

**Fig. 21.6** Choriocarcinoma showing both cytotrophoblastic and syncytiotrophoblastic hyperplasia with atypia

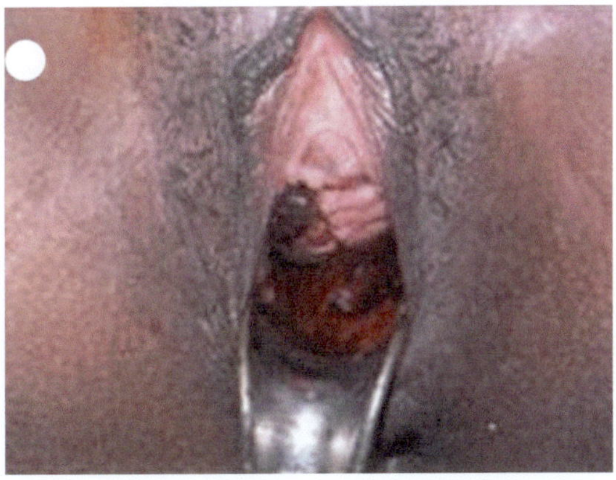

**Fig. 21.7** Suburethral nodule causing vaginal bleeding in GTN

vagina or lungs. It is locally invasive and can penetrate the full thickness of the myometrium leading to severe intraperitoneal hemorrhage. The lesion is characterized microscopically by trophoblastic invasion of the myometrium with identifiable villous structures. Most invasive moles show moderate to marked trophoblastic activity and persistence of villous structure. The histological diagnosis of invasive mole is rarely made, as hysterectomy is seldom done and it is difficult to identify from curetting. On ultrasound examination it shows focal areas of increased echogenicity within the myometrium. The lesion is heterogeneous containing small fluid-filled cavities, and Doppler color flow mapping shows high vascularity. It is associated with uterine subinvolution, persistent heavy vaginal bleeding, and rising hCG level. Chemotherapy may be started on the basis of rising hCG level, and it is not necessary to confirm the histopathological diagnosis of invasive mole or choriocarcinoma (Figs. 21.3, 21.4, 21.5, 21.6, and 21.7).

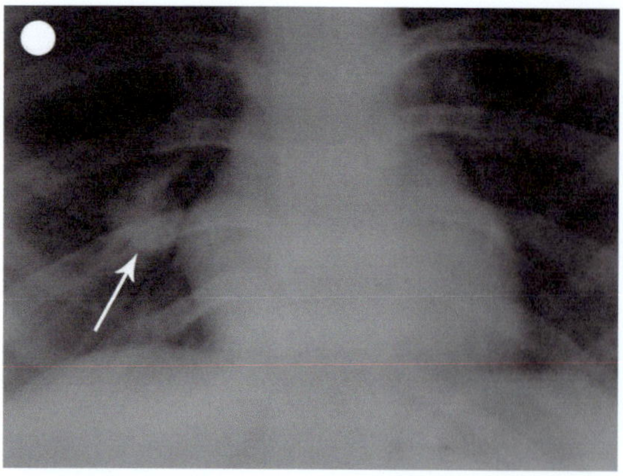

**Fig. 21.8** Chest X-ray showing secondary in the lung

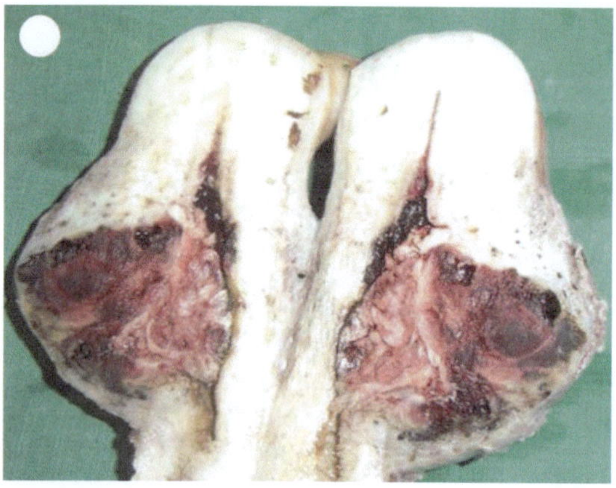

**Fig. 21.9** Choriocarcinoma of the uterus

## Ectopic Hydatidiform Mole

Rarely molar pregnancy may develop in the fallopian tube. The criteria for diagnosis are the same as for hydatidiform mole present in the uterine cavity. Sonographically it will be seen as an ectopic pregnancy.

## Gestational Choriocarcinoma

Choriocarcinoma is a malignant neoplasm consisting of sheets of anaplastic cytotrophoblasts and syncytiotrophoblasts without chorionic villi. Some intermediate trophoblasts may also be seen. The important risk factor for choriocarcinoma is hydatidiform mole, especially following complete mole. The risk of developing choriocarcinoma after partial mole is rare. Choriocarcinoma can develop after normal pregnancy, abortion, and ectopic pregnancy. In some cases there is no known antecedent pregnancy, and it is postulated that choriocarcinoma may develop from a conceptus ab initio [17]. It stimulates virtually no stromal reaction and is therefore essentially a mixture of hemorrhage and necrosis with tumor cells scattered within the mass. On microscopic examination, viable tumor is usually confined to the rim of the neoplasm as choriocarcinoma lacks an intrinsic vasculature; the tumor cells derive nutrition by invasion of maternal blood vessels. Widespread intravascular dissemination to lungs, brain, and other sites is common. The metastatic sites have a tendency to rapidly outgrow their blood supply resulting in necrosis and hemorrhage. Extensive necrosis, hemorrhage, and vascular invasion are common. The commonest sites for metastasis are lung, brain, liver, pelvis, vagina, spleen, intestine, and kidney (Figs. 21.6, 21.8, and 21.9).

## Placental Site Trophoblastic Tumor (PSTT)

In 1981, Scully and others proposed placental site trophoblastic tumor (PSTT) to describe a variant of gestational trophoblastic tumor [18]. It is a rare type of GTN and is composed mainly of intermediate cytotrophoblastic cells arising from the placental implantation site. These tumors can result from any type of antecedent pregnancy and are locally invasive and less widely metastatic. Placental site trophoblastic tumor produces more of hPL than hCG as it contains less syncytiotrophoblast, and hence hCG may not serve as a reliable tumor marker for follow-up. However clinically the diagnosis should be suspected when hCG levels are low relative to the tumor burden. It is a slow-growing tumor with late metastasis and involvement of lymph nodes and produces low levels of free β-hCG.

PSTT is generally seen as a proliferation of extravillous or intermediate trophoblast in the myometrium or endomyometrium. Chorionic villi are rarely found and the typical dimorphic pattern of choriocarcinoma is absent. Instead,

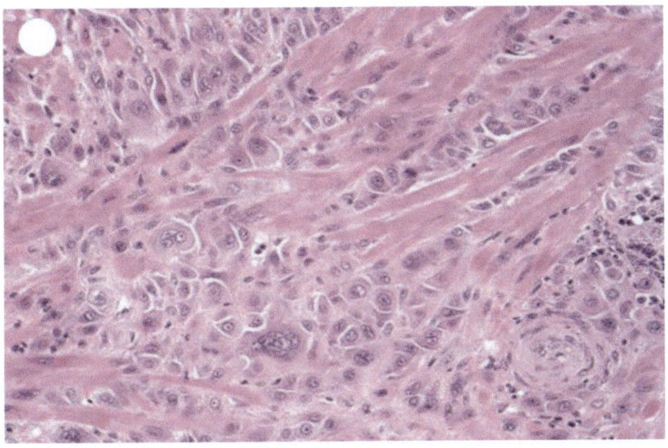

**Fig. 21.10** PSTT showing proliferation with atypia of extravillous trophoblast splitting apart muscle fibers

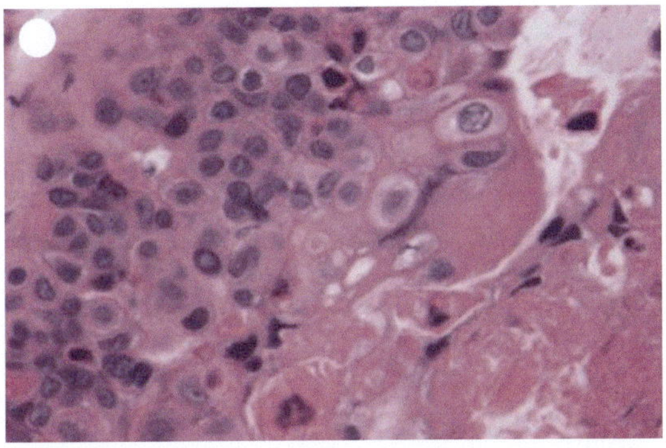

**Fig. 21.11** ETT – showing epithelioid intermediate trophoblastic tumor cells and eosinophilic hyalinization (keratin-like material) within tumor nests, simulating invasive squamous cell carcinoma

there is a characteristic pattern consisting of a relatively monomorphic population of predominantly mononuclear trophoblastic cells infiltrating the myometrium and splitting apart the muscle fibers. Necrosis is more prominent in PSTT as opposed to hemorrhage in choriocarcinoma and vascular invasion is not as common as in choriocarcinoma. Immunohistochemical staining for human placental lactogen (hPL), CD146 (MEL-CAM), and placental alkaline phosphatase (PLAP) are additional diagnostic tests for PSTT that have a specificity of approximately 60 % [19]. PSTT usually presents with amenorrhea or irregular vaginal bleeding months or years after a normal pregnancy, an abortion, or, rarely, a hydatidiform mole [20]. Origin from both moles and normal pregnancy has been demonstrated genetically [21, 22]· Response to chemotherapy is poor in PSTT and stage one disease is better treated with hysterectomy. Metastatic disease is started on with multi-agent chemotherapy.

## Epithelioid Trophoblastic Tumor (ETT)

Epithelioid trophoblastic tumor is a rare neoplasm and is the most recent addition to the gestational trophoblastic tumor category [23]. Most of the patients reported in the literature were women of reproductive age, and the antecedent pregnancy event was full-term deliveries, spontaneous abortions, and molar gestations. The average interval between the antecedent gestation and the development of the tumor is 5–6 years.

Only 52 cases were reported till 2008 [24]. It is composed of chorionic-type intermediate trophoblast and is distinct from choriocarcinoma and PSTT. The tumor is composed of sheets and nests of mononuclear trophoblast with clear, eosinophilic, and vacuolated cytoplasm resembling "chorionic-type" intermediate trophoblast. Histologically, epithelioid trophoblastic tumor is a distinct neoplasm whose cytological features and growth patterns mimic squamous cell carcinoma. Gross inspection of ETT shows a solid to cystic, fleshy, and well-defined mass in the uterine wall, lower uterine segment, or endocervix. It can be confused with squamous cell carcinoma because of its frequent involvement of the lower uterine segment or endocervix and its epithelioid histologic appearance and expression of p63 and cytokeratins (Figs. 21.10 and 21.11).

## Clinical Presentation of Molar Pregnancy

Patients with molar pregnancy may present with excessive nausea and vomiting in early weeks. Vomiting may be severe enough requiring hospitalization for correction of fluid and electrolyte imbalance. Most patients with hydatidiform mole will have vaginal bleeding, which may be sudden and profuse. Previously reported features such as anemia, uterine enlargement more than for the period of amenorrhea, preeclampsia, hyperemesis, hyperthyroidism, and respiratory distress are rarely seen nowadays due to early termination of failing pregnancy due to routine use of ultrasonography. The symptoms in partial mole are very mild and late to start, and may be diagnosed as missed abortion. The routine use of ultrasonography in first trimester will diagnose cases of hydatidiform mole as blighted ovum or failed pregnancy and may be terminated without a diagnosis. Even today, patients without proper antenatal care may report at a more advanced gestational age with excessive uterine size, large theca lutein cysts, and symptoms of hyperthyroidism, early onset preeclampsia, and anemia.

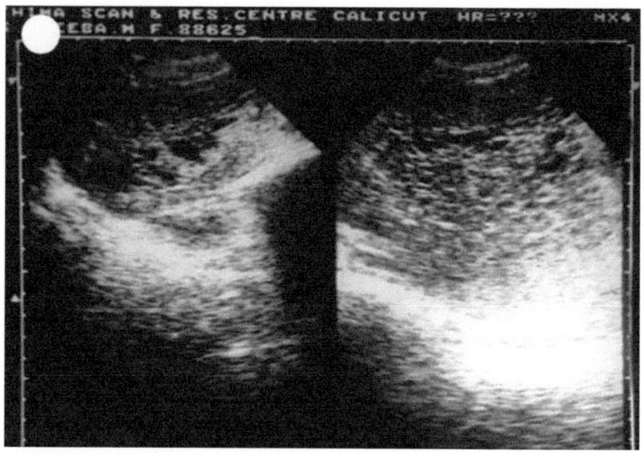

**Fig. 21.12** USG showing complete mole

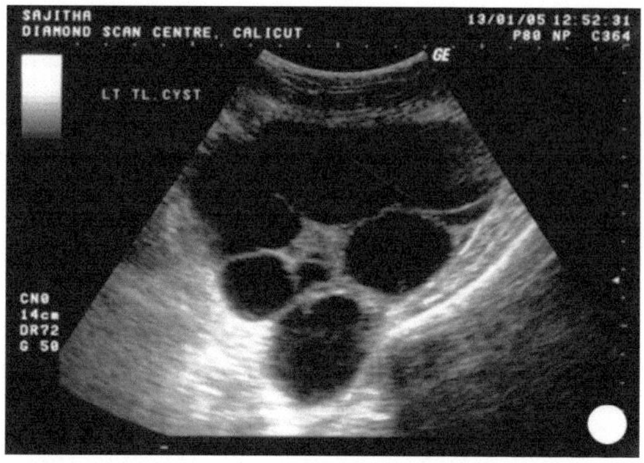


**Fig. 21.13** USG showing theca lutein cyst in complete mole

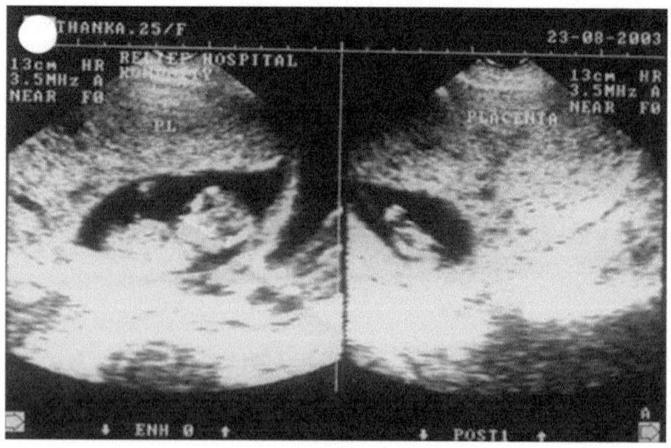


**Fig. 21.14** USG showing partial mole

## Ultrasound in Diagnosis of H. Mole

Characteristic ultrasonographic scans of complete mole show a uterine cavity filled with a heterogeneous mass with anechoic spaces of varying size and shape, a snowstorm-like appearance without any fetal parts. Theca lutein ovarian cysts secondary to high hCG level may be present in about 30 % of cases, where the pregnancy has reached 14–18 weeks. With early detection and termination of failing pregnancy, these classic sonographic findings will be absent. However, the majority of first trimester complete moles still demonstrate a typical ultrasound appearance of a complex, echogenic intrauterine mass containing multiple small cystic spaces [25]· In about 30 % of partial moles, the sonographic diagnosis will be possible; the rest may be diagnosed as missed abortion. The ultrasound findings observed in partial mole are an excessively enlarged placenta, cystic spaces within the placenta, gestational sac which is either empty or containing amorphous echoes, or a growth retarded fetus.

Ancillary techniques are needed in some cases to differentiate non-molar miscarriage from hydatidiform mole, including immunostaining for P57kip2, the product of CDKN1C. P57kip2 is expressed by the maternal allele and is visible on histology as nuclear staining of cytotrophoblast and villous mesenchyme in placenta of all gestations apart from androgenetic complete mole [26] (Figs. 21.12, 21.13, and 21.14).

In cases of a coexisting normal fetus in a twin pregnancy with mole and in cases of placental mesenchymal dysplasia, a mistaken diagnosis of partial mole is possible and in both cases the careful repeated examination and use of 3-D ultrasound will help to make a correct diagnosis. Amniocentesis and fetal karyotyping will confirm the diagnosis as in partial mole, the baby

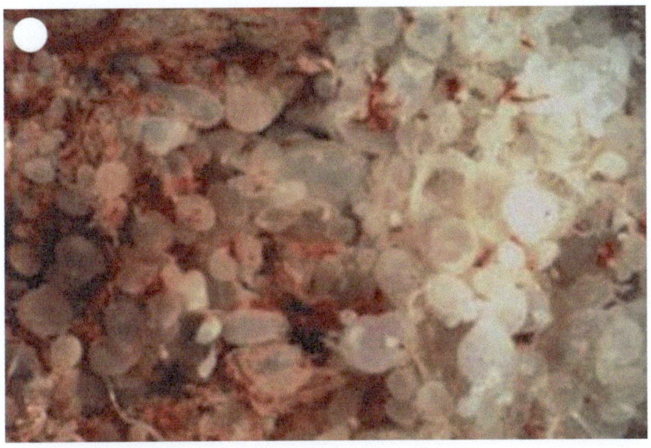

**Fig. 21.15** Moles evacuated by suction

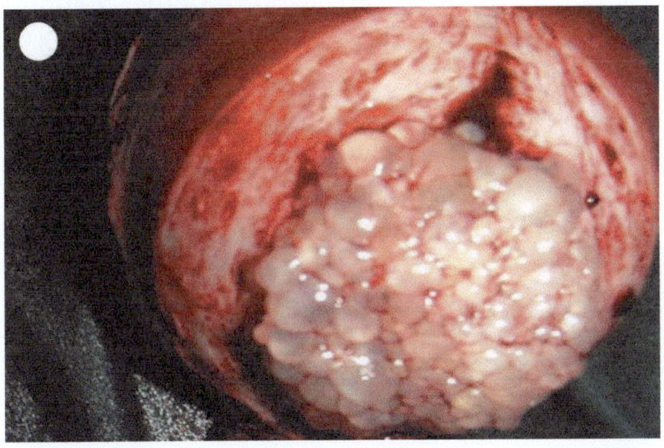

**Fig. 21.16** Hysterectomy with mole in situ

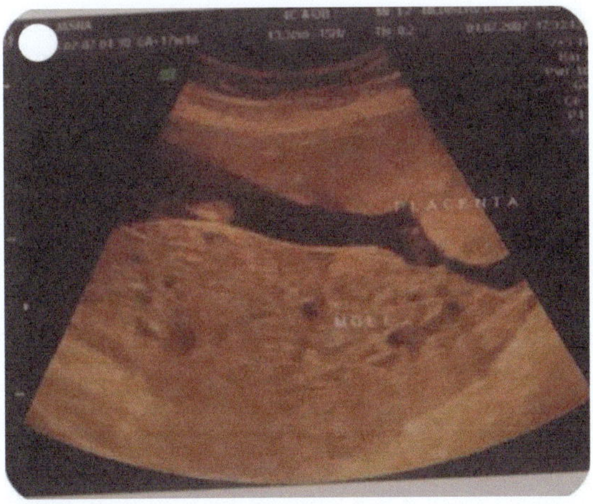


**Fig. 21.17** 3-D ultrasound showing molar tissue and normal placenta in a case of twin with one mole

will be triploid (Figs. 21.6, 21.15, 21.16, and 21.17).

All products of conception from nonviable pregnancies should undergo histological examination irrespective of ultrasonographic findings, and all patients after medical termination of pregnancy should have urine hCG tested after 4–6 weeks to rule out any persistent trophoblastic activity.

## Management of Hydatidiform Mole

When a diagnosis of complete or partial molar pregnancy is made, the most appropriate method of evacuation should be decided. Assessment of the patient for the presence of medical complications, including anemia, preeclampsia, hyperthyroidism, and respiratory insufficiency, is essential. It is appropriate to have a baseline pre-evacuation hCG, and a chest X-ray may be taken in addition to routine blood and urinalysis. The primary management of hydatidiform mole is evacuation of the mole. Crossmatched blood for transfusion and appropriate fluid resuscitation measures should be kept ready at the time of evacuation.

Suction evacuation under anesthesia is the preferred method of evacuation of the mole irrespective of the size of the uterus. The cervix can be made favorable by per vaginal application of PGE1 analogues 4–6 h prior to evacuation. Intravenous oxytocin may be started at the end of the procedure, and uterine cavity is gently curetted to ensure complete evacuation. Evacuation can be done under ultrasound guidance especially in cases of big uterus, and large lutein cysts present can be aspirated to avoid torsion later. It may take 6–8 weeks for the resolution of the lutein cysts. An ultrasound evaluation is done 1 week later to make sure the evacuation is complete, and a second curettage is done only if there is evidence of incomplete evacuation.

Hysterectomy with mole in situ is an option for patients who are above 40 years and who desire no further childbearing. Hysterectomy reduces the risk of subsequent development of choriocarcinoma and completely eliminates the risk of invasive mole [27]. It does not eliminate the potential for malignant squeal and monitoring with β-hCG levels is mandatory. Theca lutein cysts if present are left alone after reducing the size with multiple needle pricks. Hysterotomy is not to be considered as a method of evacuation of the mole. Patients who are Rh negative should receive Rh immune globulin at the time of evacuation as the

Rh D factor is expressed on trophoblast and also due to the reported presence of fetal RBCs in complete mole [12].

## Chemoprophylaxis

The use of chemoprophylaxis during evacuation of hydatidiform mole remains controversial. However, several investigators have reported that chemoprophylaxis can reduce the incidence of post-molar tumor [28, 29]. In a prospective randomized trial, Kim et al. observed that in patients with high-risk complete mole, prophylactic chemotherapy reduced the incidence of post-molar tumor from 47 to 14 %, and among patients with low-risk complete mole, prophylactic chemotherapy did not influence the incidence of persistent disease (7.7 % versus 5.6 %) [29]. However, patients who developed persistent tumor after prophylactic chemotherapy required more courses of chemotherapy. Prophylactic chemotherapy may be useful in patients with high-risk complete mole when hormonal follow-up is either unavailable or unreliable. The main objection to exposing all patients with molar pregnancy to chemotherapeutic agents is that only about 15 % are at risk for developing persistent disease and can be readily identified by proper follow-up. If any patient is started on prophylactic chemotherapy, it is not just one injection at the time of evacuation, but the full course to be continued till the hCG becomes negative.

## Follow-Up

Following evacuation of hydatidiform mole, all patients should have regular follow-up with serial estimation of hCG till they achieve complete sustained remission and should be registered at regional centers/tertiary care hospitals for further care. The expected fall in serum β-hCG per week follows a log-linear fashion (fall by one log per week). Patients must be encouraged to use reliable contraception during the period of follow-up. There is no conclusive evidence to suggest that oral contraceptives increase the risk of development of choriocarcinoma [30]. Present-day low-dose oral contraceptive pills may be safely prescribed without increasing the risk of persistent disease. With the controversy surrounding this issue, it may be prudent to advise them on barrier contraceptives till the hCG is normal and then to start on OC pills. Intrauterine devices are avoided due to the risk of perforation.

Follow-up requires serial quantitative serum hCG measurements every 1–2 weeks until at least two consecutive values are normal and thereafter monthly up to 6 months. Patients whose hCG values normalize within 8 weeks of primary evacuation have a reduced risk of developing GTN and are monitored for 6 months, and those requiring more than 8 weeks are followed up for 12 months.

## Diagnosis of Gestational Trophoblastic Neoplasia

Diagnosis of gestational trophoblastic neoplasia (GTN)/persistent trophoblastic disease is made by a rise in serum β-hCG of three values (10 % increases) over a 2-week period, a plateauing of serum β-hCG of four values over a period of 3 weeks (fall less than 10 %), persistence of hCG after 6 months of evacuation, and/or histological evidence of choriocarcinoma. Serum β-hCG value of more than 20,000 IU/L, after 4 weeks of evacuation, is considered an indication for chemotherapy.

On an average 20 % of patients undergoing evacuation of complete hydatidiform mole may develop post-molar GTD, with a range of 6–36 % as reported by various authors [31–33]. In our own series of 1569 cases of hydatidiform moles diagnosed and treated over a period of 15 years from June 1990, the incidence of gestational trophoblastic neoplasia (GTN) was 20.5 % [34]; 60 % of GTN develops after hydatidiform mole, 30 % following abortions, and 10 % following normal pregnancy or ectopic.

## FIGO Staging and Risk Factor Scoring

In 2002 the International Federation of Obstetrics and Gynecology (FIGO), following the recommendation of its cancer committee, ratified a revised classification system for trophoblastic disease and promulgated a combined FIGO anatomic staging with a revised World Health Organization (WHO) risk factor scoring system for gestational trophoblastic neoplasia [35, 36].

## FIGO Staging of GTN (2002)

| | |
|---|---|
| Stage I | GTN strictly confined to the uterine corpus. |
| Stage II | GTN extends to the adnexa or to the vagina but is limited to the genital structures (adnexa, vagina, broad ligament). |
| Stage III | GTN extends to the lungs with or without genital tract involvement. |
| Stage IV | All other metastatic sites. |

Placental site trophoblastic tumor will be categorized separately from other gestational trophoblastic neoplasia. The staging is as for GTN but no risk scoring is done.

## FIGO Risk Factor Scoring Values

In order to stage and allot a risk factor score, a patient's diagnosis is allocated to a stage as represented by Roman numerals I, II, III, and IV. This is then separated by a colon from the actual risk factor score expressed in Arabic numerals. For purposes of reporting, patients are divided into low-risk (score 0–6) and high-risk (score ≥7) groups. Bagshawe's risk scoring system [37] which was modified and adopted by WHO [38] was further modified in the FIGO risk scoring system. From the WHO scoring, ABO blood grouping has been omitted and liver metastasis has been given a score of 4. Placental site trophoblastic tumor has been classed separately. There is no intermediate risk group.

## FIGO Risk Factor Scoring System

| FIGO scoring | 0 | 1 | 2 | 4 |
|---|---|---|---|---|
| Age | <40 | >40 | | |
| Antecedent pregnancy | Mole | Abortion | Term | |
| Months from index pregnancy | <4 | 4 – <7 | 7 – <13 | ≥13 |
| Pretreatment serum hCG (IU/L) | $<10^3$ | $10^3 - <10^4$ | $10^4 - <10^5$ | $\geq 10^5$ |
| Largest tumor size (cm) | <3 | 3 – <5 | ≥5 | |
| Site of metastasis | Lung | Spleen, kidney | GIT | Liver, brain |
| Number of metastasis | – | 1–4 | 5–8 | >8 |
| Previous failed chemotherapy | – | – | Single drug | Two or more drugs |

Management of GTN depends on the stage and risk scoring:

(a) Low-risk GTN
Stage I, II, and, III risk score ≤ 6 – single-agent chemotherapy
(b) High-risk GTN
Stage I, II, and III with risk score ≥7 and stage IV – combination chemotherapy

## Low-risk GTN

Patients in FIGO stage I, II, or III with risk score of 6 and below are grouped as low-risk GTN and can be started on single-agent chemotherapy. A sustained remission can be achieved in these patients after primary treatment with single-agent chemotherapy. Methotrexate and actinomycin D are the primary drugs used in the management of low-risk GTN in various dose schedules.

## Methotrexate

Methotrexate has been used in the management of malignant GTD since the 1950s and achieves up to 100 % cure rates in nonmetastatic disease. Pretreatment evaluation of liver function and renal function tests along with complete hemogram should be done. Total WBC count and platelet count are monitored twice a week. Toxicity includes ulceration of the GI tract, bone marrow depression, alopecia, and photosensitivity reaction of the skin. Presence of anemia and infections increase the risk of toxicity. Methotrexate should not be given if there is impairment of liver or renal function as the drug is detoxified in the liver and partially excreted by the kidney.

## Methotrexate-Folinic Acid Regimen (MTX-FA)

Bagshawe and Wilde proposed the use of folinic acid along with methotrexate to rescue normal tissues from the dihydrofolate reductase block of methotrexate, allowing safe use of higher dose of methotrexate [39, 40]. The regimen used is inj. methotrexate 1 mg/kg weight on days 1, 3, 5, and 7 and inj. folinic acid 0.1 mg/kg body weight on days 2, 4, 6, and 8. Inj. folinic acid is started 30 h after the methotrexate. The cycle is repeated every 2 weeks to achieve complete remission in nonmetastatic and low-risk metastatic GTN. Patients who develop resistance to methotrexate with folinic acid rescue can be started on actinomycin D when hCG concentrations are less than or equal to 100 IU/L. Patients showing resistance and if the hCG level is more than 100 IU/L are started on multidrug chemotherapy, which will cure nearly all patients [41, 42]. The UK gestational trophoblastic disease service has increased the hCG concentration at which combination chemotherapy is started to more than 300 IU/L, to reduce the need for multi-agent chemotherapy [42]. Repeat CBC, LFT, and RFT at the beginning of every course. Chemotherapy should be continued till hCG comes to the normal range and then one to two more courses to eliminate the residual tumor cells to prevent recurrence.

## Other Single-Agent Chemotherapy Schedule for Low-Risk GTN

(a) Methotrexate 0.4 mg/kg IM for 5 days repeated every 2 weeks. About 10 % of low-risk cases may need further treatment.
(b) Methotrexate 50 mg/m$^2$ IM given weekly. The failure rate may be higher than the daily dose schedule and may be started on actinomycin D 9–12 μgm/kg for 5 days to achieve complete remission.
(c) Actinomycin D 9–12 μgm/kg IV daily for 5 days, repeated every 2 weeks. Actinomycin causes severe slough if extravasated and must be injected via a new free-running intravenous infusion. If any extravasation does occur, the area should be infiltrated with 100 mg hydrocortisone and 2 ml of 1 % Xylocaine.

In a series of 321 cases of nonmetastatic disease treated by the author using MTX-FA regimen, complete remission could be achieved in 92 % of cases. Remission could be achieved in 3 % cases with alternating course of actinomycin D and 3.6 % required multi-agent chemotherapy (MAC, EMA-CO) [34].

## High-Risk Gestational Trophoblastic Neoplasia

Most high-risk patients present with signs and symptoms of metastases at different organs, months or years after the antecedent pregnancy. Patients with brain metastases may present with seizures, headaches, or hemiparesis, whereas those with lung metastasis might have a combination of hemoptysis, breathlessness, or pleuritic chest pain. Patients may not have any menstrual irregularities and until and unless the possibility of GTN is thought of and measurement of hCG is made, the diagnosis may be missed. Along with hCG measurement, imaging by CT abdomen, MRI of brain, and Doppler ultrasonography should be done to stage the disease and to calculate the risk score.

FIGO stages I, II, and III with WHO score of 7 or greater or stage IV are high-risk GTN, and these patients should be treated initially with multi-agent chemotherapy with or without adjuvant radiotherapy or surgery. Until the mid-1980s, the primary multi-agent regimen used was MAC, methotrexate, actinomycin D, and cyclophosphamide, and reported cure rates ranged from 63 to 71 % [43, 44]. Bagshawe and colleagues at Charing Cross Hospital, London, developed the seven-drug CHAMOCA protocol in the mid-1970s employing cyclophosphamide, hydroxyurea, actinomycin D, methotrexate with folinic acid, vincristine, and doxorubicin and reported a primary remission rate of 82 % [45].

After the discovery of etoposide in the late 1970s as a very effective chemotherapeutic agent for gestational trophoblastic tumors, Newlands et al. formulated the EMA-CO regimen employing etoposide, high-dose methotrexate with folinic acid, actinomycin D, cyclophosphamide, and vincristine with a complete clinical response of 80 % [46].

## EMA-CO Regimen for High-Risk GTN

| Day | Drug | Dose |
|---|---|---|
| 1 | Etoposide | 100 mg/m$^2$ IV over 30 min |
| | Actinomycin D | 0.5 mg IV bolus |
| | Methotrexate | 100 mg/m$^2$ bolus and 200 mg/m$^2$ IV infusion 1000 ml 5 % dextrose over 12 h |
| 2 | Etoposide | 100 mg/m$^2$ IV infusion over 30 min |
| | Actinomycin D | 0.5 mg IV bolus |
| | Folinic acid | 15 mg IM every 12 h, for four doses beginning 24 h after start of methotrexate |
| 8 | Cyclophosphamide | 600 mg/m$^2$ IV |
| | Vincristine | 1 mg/m$^2$ IV bolus |

Repeat cycles on days 15, 16, and 22 (every 2 weeks)

Patients are advised not to become pregnant until 12 months after completion of chemotherapy to reduce the risk of teratogenicity.

The EMA-EP regimen, substituting etoposide and cisplatin for cyclophosphamide and vincristine in the EMA-CO regimen, seems to be the most appropriate therapy for patients showing incomplete remission. The BEP (bleomycin, etoposide, cisplatin), VIP (etoposide, ifosfamide, cisplatin), and ICE (ifosfamide, carboplatin, etoposide) protocols were also successful in a patient who failed to respond to EMA-CO regimen.

## Twin Pregnancy with One CHM and Coexisting Normal Fetus

This is a rare condition with an estimated incidence of one per 22,000 to 100,000 pregnancies [47]. Patients present with what appears to be hydatidiform mole or twin gestation with rapid enlargement of uterus. Careful ultrasound examination will reveal a normal fetus, amniotic sac, and placenta with separate molar tissue elsewhere. Partial moles may have a fetus but have diffuse molar changes throughout the single placenta. However the diagnostic accuracy of this condition is only 70 %. 3-D ultrasound examination may delineate the normal placenta of the twin having the amniotic sac and normal baby from the molar tissue seen separately. For continuation of the pregnancy, it is necessary to confirm the normalcy of the baby, and this could be made sure by amniocentesis and karyotype. The twin with one normal baby will have 46XX or 46XY, while partial mole will have 69XXX or 69XXY, and baby of the partial mole will have congenital anomalies as it is triploid and should be terminated. The twin with one complete mole and the other normal baby can have 30–40 % live birth rate, though they are at a higher risk of developing preeclampsia and hemorrhage [48]. The subsequent need for chemotherapy for persistent disease is greater than other molar pregnancies [49, 50]. The present policy is to allow the pregnancy to go to term depending on the patient's choice. Patients are counseled regarding a substantial risk of fetal loss and the need for operative interventions and the need for follow-up after delivery. Conservative management of these patients allowing the pregnancy to go ahead

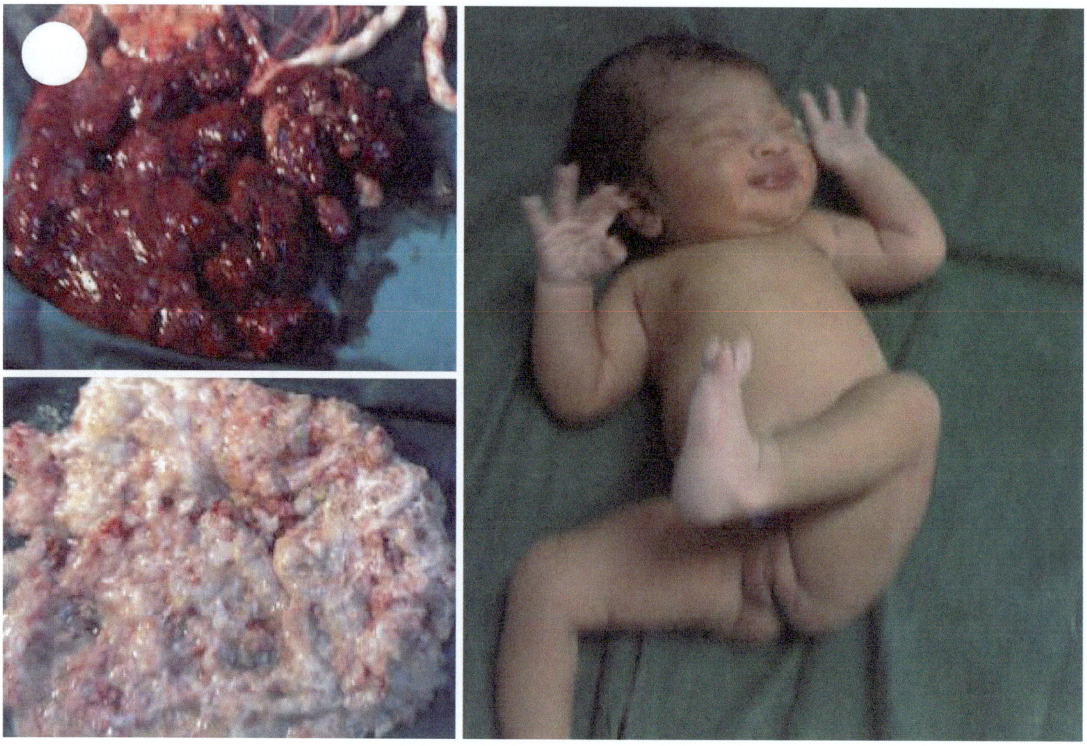

**Fig. 21.18** Twin – one CHM and the other normal baby (46XX) and placenta

unless there are clear-cut medical grounds for termination such as preeclampsia or hemorrhage appears to be the treatment of choice (Fig. 21.18).

## Quiescent Gestational Trophoblastic Disease

Quiescent gestational trophoblastic disease appears to be due to the presence of inactive, non-invasive trophoblastic cells. Highly differentiated syncytiotrophoblast cells are the predominant cell line. This is slow-growing tissue and does not respond to chemotherapy. The majority of cases follow complete hydatidiform mole, but quiescent gestational trophoblastic disease has also occurred after treatment of choriocarcinoma, invasive mole, and partial mole. These cases should be followed up as they may become active and metastatic disease may develop later. Presence of hyperglycosylated hCG (hCG-H) is an indication to start treatment. Low levels of hCG are seen in PSTT. An increase in free β-subunit is associated with PSTT. One of the fascinating aspects of gestational trophoblastic neoplasia is the ability of the disease to exist in a quiescent form without producing clinical problems for long periods of time. Clearly there must be a small amount of abnormal tissue present but not producing enough hCG to be detected by currently available assays. These rests of GTN are important since they can be reactivated by the hormonal surge of subsequent pregnancies. The dilemma of false positive hCG vs. low persistent levels of real hCG has to be addressed by refining the hCG assay methods [51, 52]

**Conclusion**

The outcome of gestational trophoblastic disease depends on the early detection of persistent disease by regular follow-up of patients after evacuation of hydatidiform mole. The regional and national referral centers for management of GTN in the UK and USA have resulted in very high cure rates and elimination of fatality from GTN. In developing countries including India, there is no such program. It is up to the practicing physicians to organize such follow-up clinics in regional tertiary care centers and start a trophoblastic disease registry for scientific analysis. We at Calicut in the northern region of Kerala in South India have started such a center 15 years ago and so far have followed up more than 1500 cases with excellent results.

## References


1. Vassilakos P, Riotton G, Kajii T. Hydatidiform mole: two entities. A morphological and cytogenetic study with some clinical considerations. Am J Obstet Gynecol. 1977;127:167–70.
2. Szulman AE, Surti U. The syndromes of hydatidiform mole. I. Cytogenetic and morphologic correlations. Am J Obstet Gynecol. 1978;131:665–71.
3. Szulman AE, Surti U. The syndromes of hydatidiform mole. II. Morphologic evolution of the complete and partial mole. Am J Obstet Gynecol. 1978;132:20–7.
4. Surti U, Szulman AE, O'Brien S. Dispermic origin and clinical outcome of three complete hydatidiform moles with 46, XY karyotype. Am J Obstet Gynecol. 1982;144:84–7.
5. Lawler SD, Pickthall VJ, Fisher RA, Povey S, Evans MW, Szulman AE. Genetic studies of complete and partial hydatidiform moles. Lancet. 1979;2:58.
6. Azuma C, Saji F, Tokugawa Y, Kimura T, Nobunaga T, Takemura M, Kameda T, Tanizawa O. Application of gene amplification by polymerase chain reaction to genetic analysis of molar mitochondrial DNA: the detection of anuclear empty ovum as the cause of complete mole. Gynecol Oncol. 1991;40:29–33.
7. Wake N, Fujino T, Hoshi S, et al. The propensity to malignancy of dispermic heterozygous moles. Placenta. 1987;8:319–26.
8. Moglabey YB, Kircheisen R, Seoud M, El Mogharbel N, Van den Veyver I, Slim R. Genetic mapping of a maternal locus responsible for familial hydatidiform moles. Hum Mol Genet. 1999;8:667–71.
9. Murdoch S, Djuric U, Mazhar B, et al. Mutations in NALP7 cause recurrent hydatidiform moles and reproductive wastage in humans. Nat Genet. 2006;38:300–2.
10. Deveault C, Qian JH, Chebaro W, et al. NLRP7 mutations in women with diploid androgenetic and triploid moles: a proposed mechanism for mole formation. Hum Mol Genet. 2009;18:888–97.
11. Sebire NJ, Foskett M, Fisher RA, Rees H, Newlands E, Seckl M. Risk of partial and complete hydatidiform molar pregnancy in relation to maternal age. BJOG. 2002;109:99–102.
12. Fisher RA, Newlands ES, et al. Diploid hydatidiform moles with foetal blood cells in molar villi. 2—genetics. J Pathol. 1997;181(2):189–95.
13. Seckl MJ, Fishjer RA, Newlands ES, et al. Choriocarcinoma and partial hydatidiform mole. Lancet. 2000;356:36–9.
14. Szulman AE, Surti U, Berman M. Patient with partial mole requiring chemotherapy. Lancet. 1978;ii:1099.
15. Loi LM, Sivanesaratnam V. Malignant evolution with fatal outcome in a patient with partial hydatidiform mole. Aust N Z J Obstet Gynaecol. 1981;21:51–2.
16. Szulman AE, Wong LC, Hsu C. Residual trophoblastic disease in association with partial hydatidiform mole. Obstet Gynecol. 1981;57:392–4.
17. Acosta-Sison H. Ab initio choriocarcinoma: two unusual cases. Obstet Gynecol. 1959;13:350–2.
18. Scully R, Young R. Trophoblastic pseudotumour: a reappraisal. Am J Surg Pathol. 1981;5:75–6.
19. Vardar MA, Altintas A. Placental-site trophoblastic tumor. Principles of diagnosis, clinical behaviour and treatment. Eur J Gynaecol Oncol. 1995;16(4):290.
20. Eckstein RP, Paradinas FJ, Bagshawe KD. Placental site trophoblastic tumour (trophoblastic pseudotumour): a study of four cases requiring hysterectomy including one fatal case. Histopathology. 1982;6:211–26.
21. Fisher RA, Paradinas FJ, Newlands ES, Boxer GM. Genetic evidence that placental site trophoblastic tumours can originate from a hydatidiform mole or a normal conceptus. Br J Cancer. 1992;65:355–8.
22. Bower M, Paradinas FJ, Fisher RA, et al. Placental site tropho- blastic tumour: molecular analysis and clinical experience. Clin Cancer Res. 1996;2:897–902.
23. Shih IM, Kurman RJ. Epithelioid trophoblastic tumor: a neoplasm distinct from choriocarcinoma and placental site trophoblastic tumor simulating carcinoma. Am J Surg Pathol. 1998;22(11):1393.
24. Palmer JE, Macdonald M, Wells M, Hancock BW, Tidy JA. Epithelioid trophoblastic tumor: a review of the literature. J Reprod Med. 2008;53(7):465.
25. Benson CB, Genest DR, Bernstein MR, Soto-Wright V, Berkowitz RS. Sonographic appearance of first trimester complete hydatidiform moles. Ultrasound Obstet Gynecol. 2000;16:188–91.
26. Fisher RA, Hodges MD, Rees HC, et al. The maternally transcribed gene p57(KIP2) (CDNK1C) is abnormally expressed in both androgenetic and biparental complete hydatidiform moles. Hum Mol Genet. 2002;11:3267–72.
27. Bahar AM, et al. Hydatidiform in the elderly: hysterectomy or evacuation. Int J Obstet Gynecol. 1989;29:233.
28. Kohorn EI. hydatidiform mole and gestational Trophoblastic disease in Southern Connecticut. Obstet Gynecol. 1982;59:78–84.
29. Kim O, Moon I, Kim KT, et al. Effects of prophylactic chemotherapy for persistent trophoblastic disease in patients with complete hydatidiform mole. Obstet Gynecol. 1986;67(5):690–4.
30. Berkowitz RS, Goldstien DP, et al. Oral contraceptives and postmolar trophoblastic disease. Obstet Gynecol. 1981;58:474.

31. Bagshawe KD. Trophoblastic neoplasia. In: Holland Frei III JF, Bast Jr R, et al., editors. Cancer medicine. 3rd ed. Baltimore: Williams & Wilkins; 1993. p. 169–968.
32. Lurain JR, Brewer JI, Torok FE, Halpern B. Natural history of hydatidiform mole after primary evacuation. Am J Obstet Gynecol. 1983;145:591–5.
33. Morrow CP, Kletzky OA, DiSaia PT, et al. Clinical and laboratory correlates of molar pregnancy and trophoblastic disease. Am J Obstet Gynecol. 1977;128:424–30.
34. Sekharan PK, Sreedevi NS, Rasheedabeegam O, Radhadevi VP, Jayandhiraghavan T, Guhan B. Management of postmolar gestational trophoblastic diseases with methotrexate and folinic acid: 15 years of experience. J Reprod Med. 2006;51:835–40.
35. Kohorn EI, Goldstein DP, Hancock BW, et al. Combining the staging system of the International Federation of Gynecology and Obstetrics with the scoring system of the World Health Organization for trophoblastic neoplasia. Report of the Working Committee of the International Society for the Study of Trophoblastic Disease and the International Gynecologic Cancer Society. Int J Gynecol Cancer. 2000;10:84–8.
36. Ngan HY. The FIGO staging for gestational trophoblastic neoplasia 2000, FIGO Committee Report. Int J Gynecol Obstet. 2002;77:285–7.
37. Bagshawe KD. Risk and prognostic factors in trophoblastic neoplasia. Cancer. 1976;38:1373–85.
38. WHO. Scientific Group: gestational trophoblastic diseases technical report series no. 692. Geneva; 1983.
39. Bagshawe KD, Newlands ES, et al. The role of low dose Methotrexate and Folinic acid in gestational trophoblastic tumours. Br J Obstet Gynecol. 1989;96:795.
40. Berkowitz RS, Goldstein DP, Bernstein MR. Ten years experience with methotrexate and Folinic acid as primary therapy for gestational trophoblastic disease. Gynecol Oncol. 1986;23(1):111–8.
41. McNeish IA, Strickland S, Holden L, et al. Low risk persistent gestational trophoblastic disease: outcome following initial treatment with low-dose methotrexate and folinic acid, 1992–2000. J Clin Oncol. 2002; 20:1838–44.
42. Seckl MJ, Sebire NJ, Berkowitz RS. Gestational trophoblastic disease. 2010. www.thelancet.com. Published online July 28, 2010. doi:10.1016/S0140-6736(10)60280-2.
43. Berkowitz RS, Goldstein DP, Bernstein MR. Modified triple therapy in the management of high-risk metastatic gestational trophoblastic tumours. Gynecol Oncol. 1984;19(2):173–81.
44. Lurain JR, Brewer JI. Treatment of high-risk gestational trophoblastic disease with methotrexate, actinomycin D and cyclophosphamide chemotherapy. Obstet Gynecol. 1985;65:8304.
45. Bagshawe KD, Begent RHJ. The management of high-risk choriocarcinoma. Semin Oncol. 1982;9: 198–203.
46. Newlands ES, Bagshawe KD, Begent RHJ, et al. Results with EMA-CO REGIMEN in high-risk gestational trophoblastic tumors. Br J Obstet Gynecol. 1991;98:550–7.
47. Vejerslev LO. Clinical management and diagnostic possibilities in hydatidiform mole with co-existent fetus. Obstet Gynecol Surv. 1991;46:577–88.
48. Newlands ES. Opinion: twin gestation comprising mole in concert with normal foetus: test, treat, abort or let go to term. J Int Soc Troph Dis. 1999;3:3–5.
49. Goldstien DP, Berkowitz RS. Malignant potential of Twin with one mole and one normal fetus. J Int Soc Troph Dis. 1999;3:5–7.
50. Steller MA, Genest DR, Bernstein MR. Clinical features of multiple conception with partial or complete molar pregnancy and coexisting foetus. J Reprod Med. 1994;39:147–54.
51. Cole LA. Choosing a test for monitoring gestational trophoblastic disease. In: Proceedings of the XIII World congress on gestational trophoblastic disease, Hongkong. Abstract # 10.3; 2005.
52. Cole LA. Choosing a test for monitoring gestational trophoblastic disease. In: Proceedings of the XIII World congress on gestational trophoblastic disease, Hongkong. Abstract # 12.4; 2005.

# 22 Peripartum Cardiomyopathy

Vidya A. Thobbi and Abhijit V. Kulkarni

## Introduction

Peripartum cardiomyopathy (PPCM) is a type of dilated cardiomyopathy of unknown origin. It is seen in healthy women in the final month of pregnancy and up to 5 months after delivery in absence of cardiac disease prior to pregnancy. Even if heart failure has its onset out of the historical definition, the process is similar and is designated as pregnancy-associated cardiomyopathy [1, 44]. Incidence is less than 0.1 %. Morbidity and mortality ranges from 5 to 32 %. In some, the cardiac status may improve and return to normal, but in others it may progress to severe cardiac failure and even death due to cardiac arrhythmias, heart failure, and thromboembolism. The lesser the ejection fraction at diagnosis, the worse the outcome is [14].

## Epidemiology

The reported frequency of this condition varies from 1 in 300 to 1 in 4000 live births. The incidence varies by race and is more common in black women in whom the incidence reported is 1 in 1400. This wide variation is due to geographic distribution and overestimation by echocardiography [5].

The exact etiology is not very clear. The following are the implicated factors in the pathogenesis [30, 35]:

## Etiology

It occurs during pregnancy [20].

1. Viral myocarditis
2. Abnormal immune response
3. Abnormal hemodynamic response
4. Apoptosis and inflammation
5. Prolactin
6. Prolonged tocolysis
7. Malnutrition
8. Familial predisposition [37]

1. Viral myocarditis is the main postulated mechanism for PPCM. The biopsy specimen revealed dense lymphocytic infiltration with variable amount of myocytic edema, necrosis, and fibrosis. Outcome does not differ in women with or without myocarditis.
2. Abnormal immune response to fetal cells in maternal circulation (fetal microchimerism). Due to natural immunosuppression during pregnancy, these fetal cells are not

V.A. Thobbi (✉)
Department of OBG, Al-Ameen Medical College, Bijapur, India
e-mail: thobbividya86@yahoo.com

A.V. Kulkarni
Consultant Cardiologist, Department of Cardiology, Apollo Group of Hospitals, Bangalore, India


A. Gandhi et al. (eds.), *Principles of Critical Care in Obstetrics: Volume II*,
DOI 10.1007/978-81-322-2686-4_22

rejected. After delivery immune response is initiated, and if fetal cells reside in cardiac tissue, it initiates a pathological autoimmune response [2].
3. Abnormal hemodynamic response. Due to hemodynamic changes during pregnancy, there is reversible hypertrophy of the left ventricle, which resolves shortly after delivery. PPCM may occur because of exaggerated decrease in the left ventricular function.
4. Apoptosis and inflammation increased levels of tumor necrosis factor alpha, C-reactive protein, and Fas/Apo-1 levels (marker for programed cell death). Fas/Apo-1 levels are higher in women who died of PPCM than who lived. However, ejection fraction is the strongest predictor of outcome.
5. Prolactin. Excessive prolactin production is a new mechanism for PPCM. In women with PPCM, STAT3 protein levels were low in the heart, and serum levels of activated cathepsin D and 16-kD prolactin were elevated. The deletion of STAT3 led to enhanced expression of cardiac cathepsin D, promoting the formation of a 16-kD form of prolactin [23].
6. Prolonged tocolysis – use of beta-sympathomimetic drugs for more than 4 weeks. These women develop pulmonary edema and hence PPCM [27].
7. Selenium and nutrition – Deficiency of selenium increases the cardiovascular risk of viral infection, hypertension, and hypocalcemia. Cena et al. concluded that the low level of selenium or any micronutrients doesn't play any role in PPCM [7, 18].

## Pathogenesis and Pathological Changes in Myocardium

Alterations in the cellular immunity have been observed in PPCM patients compared to normal postpartum women. An increase in the activation of regulatory T cells and innate immunity is a necessary part of all pregnancies [10, 45]. But in PPCM patients, it has been observed that in the ratio of increased T cells compared to NK cells, the NK cell fraction is grossly reduced [22–31, 46–52].

The pathology is that it is an inflammatory cardiomyopathy. The process may be either cellular or molecular or both. Mean levels of inflammatory cytokines is elevated. Multiple proinflammatory cytokines involved in the pathogenesis of PPCM include Fas, HsCRP, interferon gamma, IL-6, TGF-beta, TNF-alpha, and others in the process of evaluation [6, 16, 53, 54].

## Risk Factors

- Non-Caucasian ethnicity, advanced maternal age, multiparity, poor socioeconomic status, multiple pregnancy, and prolonged tocolytic use are some of the associations for increased risk of PPCM [5].
- Up to 50 % of PPCM patients have experienced some form of hypertension during their index pregnancy. This hypertension includes gestational hypertension, toxemia, and essential hypertension.
- This hypertension includes gestational hypertension, toxemia, and essential hypertension.
- The take-home message is that there should be enhanced screening in pregnancy for PPCM in those having hypertension.

| Variables | Traditional ($N$ = 100) | Early ($N$ = 23) | $P$ value |
|---|---|---|---|
| Age (years) | 31 ± 6 | 30 ± 6 | 0.67 |
| Parity | 2.1 ± 1.7 | 1.9 ± 1.5 | 0.64 |
| Hx of gestational HTN | 43 % | 30 % | 0.56 |
| Twin pregnancy | 13 % | 26 % | 0.009 |
| LVEF at diagnosis | 31 ± 12 % | 30 ± 12 % | 0.72 |
| LVEF at last F/U | 46 ± 14 % | 44 ± 16 % | 0.54 |
| Duration of F/U (months) | 6 ± 7 | 7 ± 9 | 0.52 |
| Mortality | 9 % | 13 % | 0.7 |

## Clinical Manifestations

Onset of PPCM can be masked and missed as features of normal pregnancy mimic those of mild heart failure.

- These patients present with dyspnea, dizziness, chest pain, cough, neck vein distension, fatigue, and peripheral edema [33].

- Left ventricular dysfunction causes dilatation of left ventricle in turn causing arrhythmias and embolic events.
- They also can have other features of heart failure – hypoxia, jugular venous distension, $S_3$ and $S_4$ gallop, hepatomegaly, and rales [32].
- They have tachycardia, but blood pressure is normal or decreased.
- Features of pregnancy like edema, tachycardia, JV distension, and S3 can be normal also.. Closer look at cardiac profile is necessary in order not to miss the diagnosis of heart failure [14].

## Diagnosis

PPCM is a diagnosis of exclusion. Hence, other causes of heart failure are to be excluded such as pulmonary embolism, sepsis, myocardial infarction, valvular disease, severe preeclampsia, and other forms of cardiomyopathy [15].

- Chest radiographs – cardiomegaly, pleural effusion, and pulmonary congestion may be seen [40].

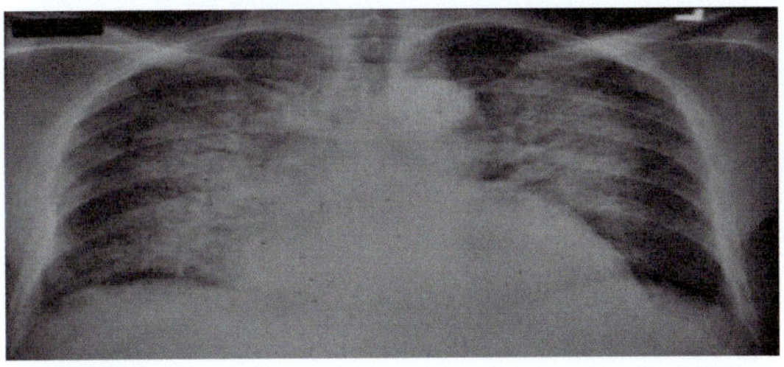

- Electrocardiogram may be normal or shows changes of left ventricular hypertrophy, ST-T wave abnormalities, dysrhythmias, Q waves in the anteroseptal precordial leads, and prolonged PR and QRS intervals [34].

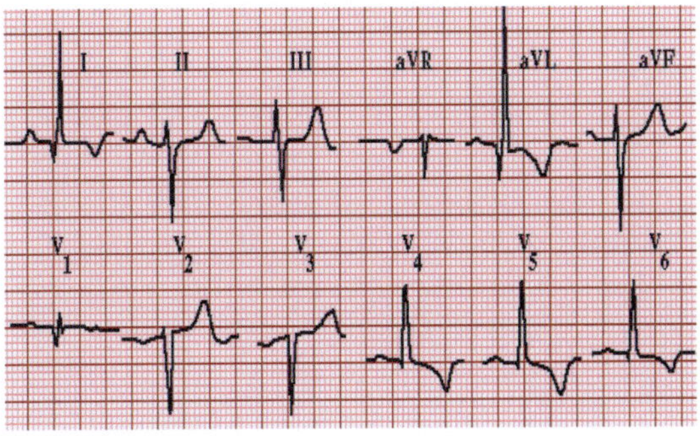


- Laboratory tests – complete blood picture, blood urea, serum creatinine, serum electrolytes, and serum troponin levels (to rule out myocardial infarction, but may be raised in acute phase of PPCM). Levels of B-type natriuretic peptide and N-terminal pro-B-type natriuretic peptide can help in confirming the diagnosis [3].
- Echocardiography and Doppler imaging – it is the most validated and practical tool for establishing the diagnosis. Evaluate ventricular function, valvular structure and function, pathological pericardial changes, and mechanical complications. Features suggestive of PPCM are decreased ejection fraction, global dilatation, and thinned out cardiac walls [9].

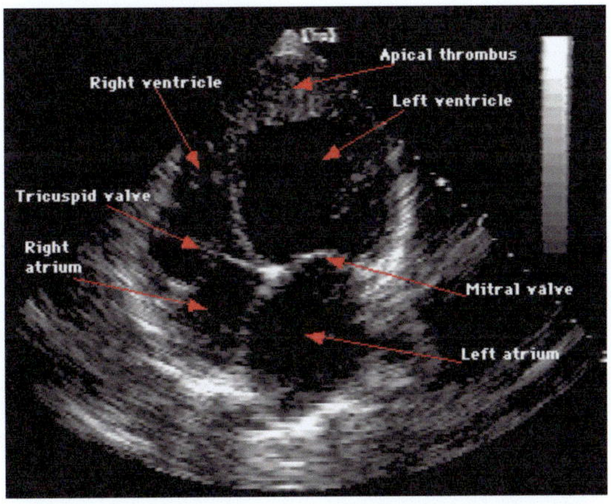


- Cardiac MRI measures global and segmental myocardial contraction [4, 34].

## Diagnostic Criteria for Peripartum Cardiomyopathy

All four of the following:

*Classic*

1. Development of cardiac failure in the last month of pregnancy or within 5 months postpartum
2. No identifiable cause for the cardiac failure
3. No recognizable heart disease before the last month of pregnancy

*Additional*

1. Strict echocardiographic indication of left ventricular dysfunction:
   (a) Ejection fraction <45 %
   And/or:
   (b) Fractional shortening <30 %
   (c) End-diastolic dimension >2.7 cm/m$^2$

## Differential Diagnosis

- Idiopathic dilated cardiomyopathy – seen at a younger age. It occurs postpartum (78–93 %). Higher incidence of myocarditis is seen in PPCM. PPCM leads to rapid worsening of clinical course and poor outcome, but heart size returns to normal in more number of patients soon after delivery [17].
- Occult valvular heart disease can be ruled out by transthoracic echocardiography. Finding of normal systolic function rules out PPCM [41].
- Ischemic heart disease is uncommon, but women with type 1 diabetes mellitus should have noninvasive assessment of coronary ischemia.
- Pulmonary thromboembolism.
- Severe eclampsia.
- Pneumonia.

## Management

Compensated heart failure:

- The goal is to improve hemodynamic status and minimize signs and symptoms and to reduce preload and afterload and increasing cardiac inotropy [39, 40].
- For preload reduction, nitrates are used which are safe in pregnancy and lactation.
- Restriction of dietary sodium is helpful.
- Loop diuretics are used in management of signs and symptoms of preload reduction, but it causes decrease in blood supply to uterus and fetus [41].
- Exercise such as walking can be advised once stable.
- During the intrapartum period, hydralazine, digoxin, nitrates, and diuretics can be used.
- Angiotensin-converting enzyme inhibitors are contraindicated in pregnancy [40].
- Beta-adrenergic antagonist (carvedilol and metoprolol) has been approved and improves the survival in PPCM. Carvedilol can be continued in the postpartum period in whom symptoms of heart failure persists and have left ventricular compromise more than 2 weeks after therapy [42].
- Digoxin can be used in women whose ejection fraction is <40 % and who have signs and symptoms of heart failure [3].

## Guidelines for Management of Compensated Heart Failure

### Nonpharmaceutical Therapies [8]

Low sodium diet: limit of 2 g sodium per day
Fluid restriction: 2 L/day
Light daily activity: if tolerated (e.g., walking)

### Oral Pharmaceutical Therapies [8]

**Antepartum Management of Peripartum Cardiomyopathy**

*Beta-blocker*

Carvedilol (starting dosage, 3.125 mg twice a day; target dosage, 25 mg twice a day)

Extended-release metoprolol (starting dosage, 0.125 mg daily; target dosage, 0.25 mg daily)

*Vasodilator*

Hydralazine (starting dosage, 10 mg 3 times a day; target dosage, 40 mg 3 times a day)

Digoxin (starting dosage, 0.125 mg daily; target dosage, 0.25 mg daily). Monitor serum levels.

Thiazide diuretic (with caution)

Hydrochlorothiazide (12.5–50 mg daily)

May also consider loop diuretic with caution

Low molecular weight heparin if ejection fraction <35 %

**Postpartum Management of Peripartum Cardiomyopathy**

*Angiotensin-converting enzyme (ACE) inhibitor*

Captopril (starting dosage, 6.25–12.5 mg 3 times a day; target dosage, 25–50 mg 3 times a day)

Enalapril (starting dosage, 1.25–2.5 mg 2 times a day; target dosage, 10 mg 2 times a day)

Ramipril (starting dosage, 1.25–2.5 mg 2 times a day; target dosage, 5 mg 2 times a day)

Lisinopril (starting dosage, 2.5–5 mg daily; target dosage, 25–40 mg daily)

Angiotensin receptor blocker (if ACE inhibitor is not tolerated)

Candesartan (starting dosage, 2 mg daily; target dosage, 32 mg daily)

Valsartan (starting dosage, 40 mg twice a day; target dosage, 160 mg twice a day)

Consider nitrates or hydralazine if woman is intolerant to ACE inhibitor and angiotensin receptor blocker.

*Loop diuretic*

Furosemide intravenously or by mouth. Dosing considerations should be made on the basis of creatinine clearance.

Glomerular filtration rate >60 mL/min per 1.73 $m^2$: furosemide 20–40 mg every12–24 h

Glomerular filtration rate <60 mL/min per 1.73 $m^2$: furosemide 20–80 mg every 12–24 h

*Vasodilator*

Hydralazine (starting dosage, 37.5 mg 3 or 4 times a day; target dosage, 40 mg 3 times a day)

Isosorbide dinitrate (starting dosage, 20 mg 3 times a day; target dosage, 40 mg 3 times a day)

*Aldosterone antagonist*

Spironolactone (starting dosage, 12.5 mg daily; target dosage, 25–50 mg daily)

Eplerenone (starting dosage, 12.5 mg daily; target dosage, 25–50 mg daily)

*Warfarin* if ejection fraction is <35 %

## Decompensated Heart Failure [28]

- Establish airway, breathing, and circulation. Pregnancy results in third spacing of intravascular volume which can result in suboptimal airway [41].
- ST segment monitoring with cardiac monitor.
- Blood pressure monitoring with noninvasive blood pressure cuffs until cardiac catheters are placed [42].
- Venous and arterial access.
- In acute heart failure, administer intravenous positive inotropic agents such as milrinone and dobutamine. These agents facilitate diuresis, improve cardiac performance, and preserve end-organ function [40].
- If systolic blood pressure is less than 90 mmHg, dobutamine is preferred over milrinone. Nitroglycerin and nitroprusside also may be used. Nitroprusside can cause toxic effects of thiocyanate which can be harmful to the fetus [40].
- Warfarin is given in postpartum period and heparin or low molecular weight heparin is given in pregnancy in patients with ejection fraction <35 % as it causes left ventricular thrombus and continued until left ventricular function becomes normal on echocardiography.
- If medical therapy fails, intra-aortic balloon pump or left ventricular assist device may be used [19].

- In persistent pulmonary edema with hypoxemia, extracorporeal membrane oxygenation can be done [36, 43].
- Heart transplantation is a practical therapeutic option for women with PPCM who have advanced heart failure and signs and symptoms unresponsive to medical therapies [38].

## Summary for Management of Decompensated Heart Failure [21]

*Airway*

Intubate promptly upon distress for increased work of breathing to prevent complications with difficult airway later in treatment.

*Breathing*

Provide supplemental oxygen.

Maintain continuous pulse oximetry to monitor $SaO_2$.

Measure arterial blood gases (if available) every 4–6 h until breathing is stable.

*Circulation*

Start cardiac and blood pressure monitoring.

Insert arterial catheter for accurate blood pressure monitoring and blood sampling.

Obtain central venous access with central venous pressure monitoring.

In antepartum women, obtain fetal monitoring.

*Pharmacological management of acute heart failure in peripartum cardiomyopathy*

*Intravenous loop diuretic (caution is advised in antepartum women)*

Furosemide: dosing considerations should be made on the basis of creatinine clearance.

Glomerular filtration rate <60 mL/min per 1.73 $m^2$

Furosemide 20–40 mg intravenously every 12–24 h

Glomerular filtration rate >60 mL/min per 1.73 $m^2$

Furosemide 20–80 mg intravenous every12–24 h

In severe fluid overload, consider furosemide infusion or ultrafiltration.

*Vasodilator*

Nitroglycerin infusion 5–10 μg/min, titrate to clinical status and blood pressure.

Nitroprusside 0.1–5 μg/kg/min is used with caution in antepartum women.

*Positive inotropic agents*

Milrinone 0.125–0.5 μg/kg/min

Dobutamine 2.5–10 μg/kg/min

Avoid beta-blockers in the acute phase, as they can decrease perfusion.

Heparin sodium, alone or with oral warfarin (Coumadin) therapy

Monitor oxygenation with arterial blood gases every 4–6 h until patient's condition is stable.

Consider endomyocardial biopsy; if proven as viral myocarditis, consider immunosuppressive medications (e.g., azathioprine, corticosteroids).

Every effort should be made to devise an oral regimen that can maintain symptomatic improvement and reduce the subsequent risk of worsening clinical status.

If no improvement clinically:

Consider cardiac magnetic resonance imaging.

Perform endomyocardial biopsy to detect viral myocarditis (if not previously completed).

Assist devices:

Intra-aortic balloon pump [19]

Left ventricular assist devices

Extracorporeal membrane oxygenation

Transplantation

If a woman remains refractory to therapy, consult your institution's guidelines for bromocriptine or cabergoline administration for suppression of prolactin production [11].

## Management During Pregnancy

- Welfare of the fetus should always be considered along with that of the mother.
- Patients with severe forms of heart failure will require ICCU management, with monitoring of arterial blood pressure (ABP), central venous pressure (CVP), and sometimes pulmonary artery catheter (PAC).
- Coordinated management with specialist's team is essential.
- Angiotensin-converting enzyme (ACE) inhibitors and angiotensin receptor blockers are contraindicated in pregnancy because these can cause birth defects, while remaining the main treatment option for postpartum women with heart failure [40].
- The teratogenic effects occur particularly in the second and third trimester, characterized by fetal hypotension, pulmonary hypoplasia, oligohydramnios, anuria, and renal tubular dysplasia [44].
- Digoxin, loop diuretics, sodium restriction, and drugs which reduce afterload such as hydralazine and nitrates have been proven to be safe.
- Amlodipine has been found to improve survival in nonischemic cardiomyopathy patients.
- Beta-blockers have been used in pregnant women with hypertension without any known adverse effects on the fetus, and patients taking these agents prior to diagnosis can continue to use them safely.

## Management during Postpartum Period

- Treatment is identical as for nonpregnant women with dilated cardiomyopathy.
- Angiotensin-converting enzyme inhibitors and angiotensin receptor blockers are useful. The dosage is one half the maximum antihypertensive doses.
- Diuretics are given for symptomatic relief (spironolactone or digoxin) and are used in patients who have New York Heart Association class III or IV symptoms. The dosage of spironolactone is 25 mg/day after dosing of other drugs is maximized. The goal with digoxin therapy is the lowest daily dose to obtain a detectable serum digoxin level, which should be kept at less than 1.0 ng/ml [42].
- Beta-blockers are recommended as they improve symptoms, ejection fraction, and survival. Nonselective beta-blockers such as carvedilol and selective ones such as metoprolol have shown benefit. The dosage of carvedilol is 25 mg twice a day or metoprolol 100 mg once a day [41].

## Newer Treatment Modalities

*Pentoxifylline*: treatment with pentoxifylline, a xanthine derivative known to inhibit the production of tumor necrosis factor alpha, improves functional class and left ventricular function in patients with idiopathic dilated cardiomyopathy.

*Bromocriptine and cabergoline:* prolactin secretion can be reduced with bromocriptine and with use of cabergoline which is a strong and long-lasting antagonist of prolactin, significant improvement in left ventricular functions was seen [11].

*Immunomodulating therapy*: in patients with myocarditis on endomyocardial biopsy, immunosuppressive and immunomodulatory therapy has been utilized. Intravenous immunoglobulin improved the ejection. Plasmapheresis has also been utilized effectively for this purpose and may be an alternative to immune globulin. Immunoadsorption therapy in idiopathic dilated cardiomyopathy demonstrated significant improvements in left ventricular function. Other therapies such as calcium channel antagonists, statins, monoclonal antibodies, and interferon beta are also used [29].

Interventional cardiology options:

- Class II and class III HF despite optimal medical management is at high risk for sudden cardiac deaths. They are appropriate candidates for prevention of arrhythmic deaths by implantation of automated implantable cardiac defibrillator (AICD).

- Patients having LBBB on ECG with severe LV dysfunction and significant symptoms are candidates for cardiac resynchronization therapy (CRT).

## Follow-Up

- Echocardiographic evaluation at rest or with low-dose dobutamine stress test can be allowed to taper and then discontinue heart failure treatment in 6–12 months.
- Aerobic activities and heavy lifting are discouraged for at least the first 6 months postpartum.
- Breastfeeding is strongly discouraged in more symptomatic patients as some drugs are secreted in breast milk. If breastfeeding is considered in these women, it has to be with careful monitoring of the baby.
- Echocardiogram should be repeated at 6 months post delivery. For those patients with persistent cardiomyopathy, beta-blockers may be added at this point if not already on therapy.

## Outcome

- A fractional shortening less than 20 % and a left ventricular diastolic dimension of 6 cm or greater at the time of diagnosis are associated with a more than threefold higher risk for persistent cardiac dysfunction [26].
- Future pregnancies are not recommended in women with persistent heart failure, because the heart most likely would not be able to tolerate the increased cardiovascular workload associated with the pregnancy [12].
- Because multiparity has been associated with PPCM, subsequent pregnancies can increase the risk for recurrent episodes of PPCM, irreversible cardiac damage and decreased left ventricular function, worsening of a woman's clinical condition, and even death.
- The majority of PPCM mothers who experience full recovery with LVEF >50 % will not experience a relapse of heart failure with a subsequent pregnancy.
- Ninety percent of those who begin the post PPCM pregnancy with LVEF >50 % will recover to their presubsequent pregnancy cardiac function despite relapse.
- The subset of women with persistent left ventricular systolic dysfunction LVEF <40 % at the start of pregnancy should be counseled against subsequent pregnancies; the risks are 19 % higher for maternal death than among women with PPCM whose heart failure has resolved.

## Prognosis

- An important distinction is that women with this disorder have a much higher rate of spontaneous recovery of left ventricular function on echocardiography in postpartum period; nearly half of the women will normalize their ejection fraction during follow-up within 6 months.
- Prognosis is directly correlated to recovery of left ventricular function. For those women whose LVEF normalizes during follow-up, the prognosis is excellent as without the stimulus of a subsequent pregnancy, the chance of development of heart failure or future LV dysfunction is minimal.
- For those women whose left ventricular function does not recover, prognosis remains guarded, and mortality rates as high as 10–50 % have been reported.
- Left ventricular size is an important predictor, women without significant LV dilatation have a greater chance of spontaneous recovery during follow-up, but women with marked LV dilatation at presentation appeared to have a greater likelihood of developing into a chronic cardiomyopathy [12].
- A fractional shortening on echocardiogram less than 20 % and an LV end-diastolic dimension greater than or equal to 6 cm were associated with a threefold increase in persistent LV dysfunction.

Recovery of left ventricular function in PPCM (Amos et al. *AHJ* 2006;15:509–513)

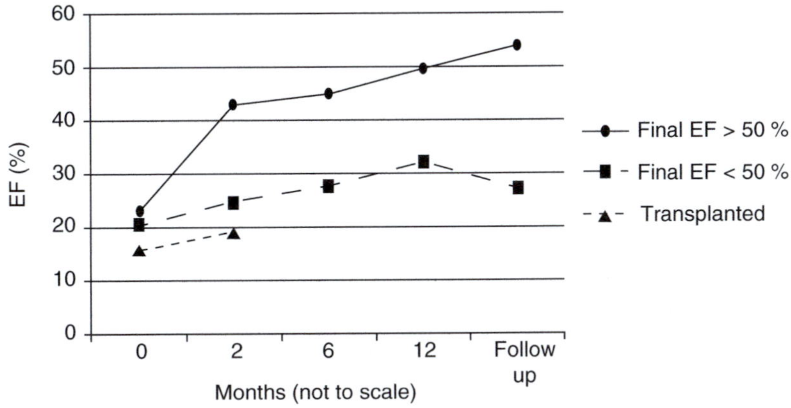


## Risk in Subsequent Pregnancies

- In patients whose left ventricular function does not normalize during follow-up, subsequent pregnancies carry a high risk of left ventricular deterioration and progressive heart failure, and hence, pregnancy is strongly discouraged given the possible risk to the life of the mother. Mortality was reported to be in the range of 8–17 % compared to 0–2 % in patients with normal left ventricular ejection fraction before the subsequent pregnancy [13].

## Outcome in Subsequent Pregnancies (Elkayam et al. *NEJM* 2001;344:1567)

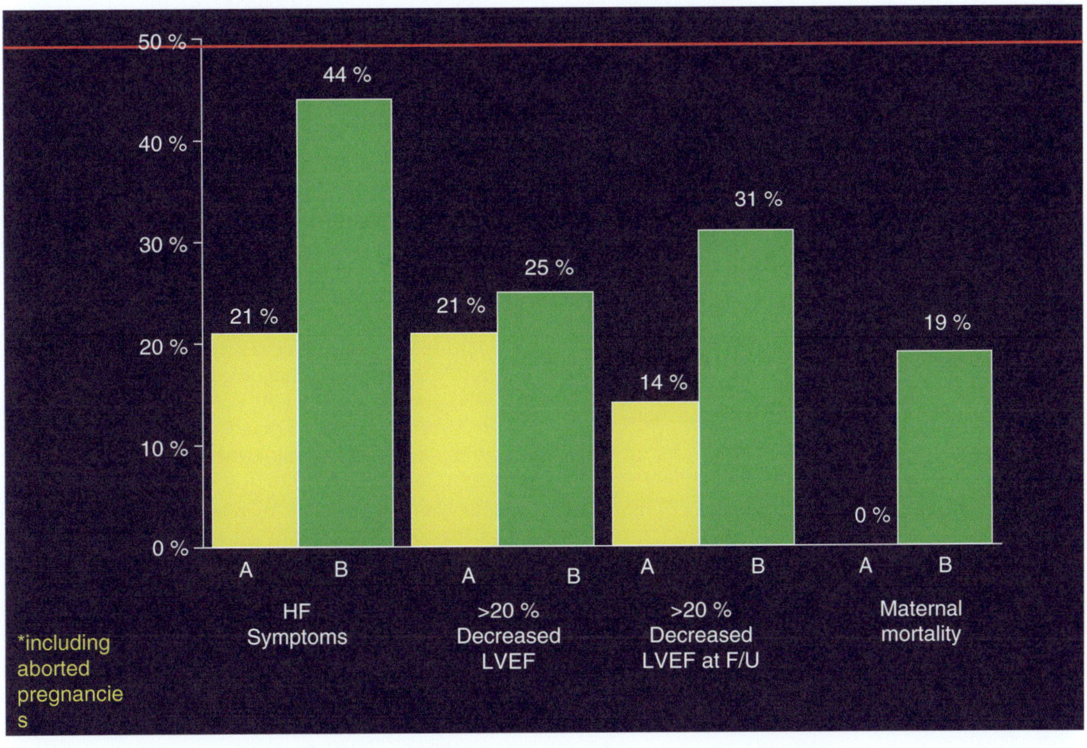


Maternal complications associated subsequent pregnancies (Elkayam U, *Eur Heart J* 2002)

## Conclusions

Peripartum cardiomyopathy is a pregnancy-related immune cardiomyopathy. The manifestations are dependent on the severity (ejection fraction at diagnosis). The presentation is like dilated cardiomyopathy with manifestations ranging from dyspnea on exertion to florid heart failure. Hypertension is a significant risk factor for PPCM apart from multiparity. Early diagnosis and treatment is directly related to prognosis. It is a form of cardiomyopathy with better prognosis. More than half of the patients depending on the baseline EF recover completely with normal ejection fractions. A small fraction do not recover on their EF and are the ones in whom subsequent pregnancies are not encouraged.

| What do we know about PPCM? | What remains unknown about PPCM? |
|---|---|
| Awareness is important for making an earlier diagnosis with less dysfunction<br>Hypertension in pregnancy increases risk for development of PPCM<br>Most serious complications can be decreased or avoided | Actual "triggers" that initiate the process<br>Role of virus in pathogenesis<br>Why higher incidence and more severe disease in those with African heritage |
| Full recovery occurs more frequently than with any other cardiomyopathy | How important the role of cardiac autoantibodies play in pathogenesis |
| Autoimmunity (or immune system dysfunction) a part of pathogenesis<br>Inflammatory cardiomyopathy is common | The extent and details of genetic factors<br>Importance of the role of prolactin and prolactin inhibition treatment |
| Higher incidence and more severe disease in those of African heritage<br>There can be a genetic predisposition | Importance of the role of sFLT1 in pathogenesis<br>Why do some who have recovered have a relapse of heart failure with subsequent pregnancy |
| Effective evidence-based treatment guidelines available<br>Most recovered do not have a relapse of heart failure in subsequent pregnancy<br>Occurs globally but with geographic variations for incidence and unique characteristics | Role of micronutrients and trace metals in pathogenesis |

## References


1. Abboud J, Murad Y, Chen-Scarabelli C, Saravolatz L, Scarabelli TM. Peripartum cardiomyopathy: a comprehensive review. Int J Cardiol. 2007;118(3):295–303.
2. Ansari AA, Fett JD, Carraway RE, Mayne AE, Onlamoon N, Sundstrom JB. Autoimmune mechanisms as the basis for human peripartum cardiomyopathy. Clin Rev Allergy Immunol. 2002;23:301–24 [PMID: 12402414].
3. Arnold JM, Liu P, Demers C, et al. Canadian Cardiovascular Society. Canadian Cardiovascular Society consensus conference recommendation on heart failure 2006: diagnosis and management. Can J Cardiol. 2006;22(1):23–45.
4. Baruteau AE, Leurent G, Martins R, et al. Peripartum cardiomyopathy in the era of cardiac magnetic resonance imaging: first results and perspectives. Int J Cardiol. 2010;144(1):143–5.
5. Brar SS, Khan SS, Sandhu GK, et al. Incidence, mortality, and racial differences in peripartum cardiomyopathy. Am J Cardiol. 2007;100(2):302–4.
6. Burkett EL, Hershberger RE. Clinical and genetic issues in familial dilated cardiomyopathy. J Am Coll Cardiol. 2005;45(7):969–81.
7. Cénac A, Simonoff M, Moretto P, Djibo A. A low plasma selenium is a risk factor for peripartum cardiomyopathy: a comparative study in Sahelian Africa. Int J Cardiol. 1992;36(1):57–9.
8. Carlin AJ, Alfirevic Z, Gyte ML. Interventions for treating peripartum cardiomyopathy to improve outcomes for women and babies. Cochrane Database Syst Rev. 2010;(9):CD008589, p 216.
9. Chapa JB, Heiberger HB, Weinert L, Decara J, Lang RM, Hibbard JU. Prognostic value of echocardiography in peripartum cardiomyopathy. Obstet Gynecol. 2005;105(6):1303–8.
10. Demakis JG, Rahimtoola S, Sutton GC, et al. Natural course of peripartum cardiomyopathy. Circulation. 1971;44(6):1053–61.
11. de Jong JS, Rietveld K, van Lochem LT, Bouma BJ. Rapid left ventricular recovery after cabergoline treatment in a patient with peripartum cardiomyopathy. Eur J Heart Fail. 2009;1(2):220–2.
12. Egan DJ, Bisanzo MC, Hutson HR. Emergency department evaluation and management of peripartum cardiomyopathy. J Emerg Med. 2009;36(2):141–7.
13. Elkayam U, Tummala PP, Rao K, et al. Maternal and fetal outcomes of subsequent pregnancies in women with peripartum cardiomyopathy. N Engl J Med. 2001;344(21):1567–71.
14. Elkayam U, Akhter MW, Singh H, Khan S, Bitar F, Hameed A, et al. Pregnancy associated cardiomyopathy: clinical characteristics and a comparison between early and late presentation. Circulation. 2005;111(16):2050–5 [PMID: 15851613].
15. Elliott P, Andersson B, Arbustini E, et al. Classification of the cardiomyopathies: a position statement from the European Society of Cardiology Working Group on Myocardial and Pericardial Disease. Eur Heart J. 2008;29(2):270–6.

16. Felker GM, Jaeger CJ, Klodas E, Thiemann DR, Hare JM, Hruban RH, et al. Myocarditis and long-term survival in peripartum cardiomyopathy. Am Heart J. 2000;140(5):785–91 [PMID: 11054626].
17. Fett JD, Christie LG, Carraway RD, Murphy JG. Five-year prospective study of the incidence and prognosis of peripartum cardiomyopathy at a single institution. Mayo Clin Proc. 2005;80(12):1602–6 [PMID: 16342653].
18. Fett J, Ansara A, Sundstrom J, Combs Jr G. Peripartum cardiomyopathy: a selenium disconnection and an autoimmune connection. Int J Cardiol. 2002; 86(2):311–6.
19. Gavaert S, van Belleghem Y, Bouchez S, et al. Acute and critically ill peripartum cardiomyopathy and "bridge to" therapeutic options: a single center experience with intra-aortic balloon pump, extra-corporeal membrane oxygenation and continuous-flow left ventricular assist devices. Crit Care. 2011;15(2):R93.
20. Goulet B, McMillan T, Bellet S. Idiopathic myocardial degeneration associated with pregnancy and especially the puerperium. Am J Med Sci. 1937; 194(2):185–99.
21. Heart Failure Society of America. Executive summary: HFSA 2006 comprehensive heart failure practice guideline. J Card Fail. 2006;12(1):10–38.
22. Hilfiker-Kleiner D, Sliwa K, Drexler H. Peripartum cardiomyopathy: recent insights in its pathophysiology. Trends Cardiovasc Med. 2008;18(5):173–9.
23. Hilfiker-Kleiner D, Kaminski K, Podewski E, et al. A cathepsin D-cleaved 16 kDa form of prolactin mediates postpartum cardiomyopathy. Cell. 2007;128(3): 589–600.
24. Jahns BG, Stein W, Hilfiker-Kleiner D, Pieske B, Emons G. Peripartum cardiomyopathy—a new treatment option by inhibition of prolactin secretion. Am J Obstet Gynecol. 2008;199(4):e5–6.
25. James P. A review of peripartum cardiomyopathy. Int J Clin Pract. 2004;58(4):363–5.
26. Keogh A, Macdonald P, Spratt P, Marshman D, Larbalestier R, Kaan A. Outcome in peripartum cardiomyopathy after heart transplantation. J Heart Lung Transplant. 1994;13(2):202–7.
27. Lampert MB, Hibbard J, Weinert L, Briller J, Lindheimer M, Lang RM. Peripartum heart failure associated with prolonged tocolytic therapy. Am J Obstet Gynecol. 1992;168(2):493–5.
28. Lata I, Gupta R, Sahu S, Singh H. Emergency management of decompensated peripartum cardiomyopathy. J Emerg Trauma Shock. 2009;2(2):124–8.
29. McNamara DM, Holubkov R, Starling RC, et al. Controlled trial of intravenous immune globulins in recent-onset dilated cardiomyopathy. Circulation. 2001;103:2254–9.
30. Melvin KR, Richardson PJ, Olsen EG, Daly K, Jackson G. Peripartum cardiomyopathy due to myocarditis. N Engl J Med. 1982;307(12):731–4.
31. Midei MG, DeMent SH, Feldman AM, Hutchins GM, Baughman KL. Peripartum myocarditis and cardiomyopathy. Circulation. 1990;81:922–8.
32. Mielniczuk LM, Williams K, Davis DR, et al. Frequency of peripartum cardiomyopathy. Am J Cardiol. 2006;97(12):1765–8.
33. Moioli M, Menada MV, Bentivoglio G, Ferrero S. Peripartum cardiomyopathy. Arch Gynecol Obstet. 2010;281(2):183–8. doi:10.1007/s00404-009-1170-5.
34. Ntusi NB, Chin A. Characterisation of peripartum cardiomyopathy by cardiac magnetic resonance imaging. Eur Radiol. 2009;19(6):1324–5.
35. Ntusi NB, Mayosi BM. Aetiology and risk factors of peripartum cardiomyopathy: a systematic review. Int J Cardiol. 2009;131(2):168–79.
36. Palanzo DA, Baer LD, El-Banayosy A, et al. Successful treatment of peripartum cardiomyopathy with extracorporeal membrane oxygenation. Perfusion. 2009;24(2):75–9.
37. Pearl W. Familial occurrence of peripartum cardiomyopathy. Am Heart J. 1995;129(2):421–2.
38. Pearson G, Veille J, Rahimtoola S, et al. Peripartum cardiomyopathy: National Heart, Lung, and Blood Institute and Office of Rare Diseases (National Institutes of Health) workshop recommendations and review. JAMA. 2000;283(9):1183–8.
39. Pyatt JR, Dubey G. Peripartum cardiomyopathy: current understanding, comprehensive management review and new developments. Postgrad Med J. 2011;87(1023):34–9.
40. Ramaraj R, Sorrell VL. Peripartum cardiomyopathy: causes, diagnosis, and treatment. Cleve Clin J Med. 2009;76(5):289–96.
41. Rasmusson K, de Jong M, Doering L. Update on heart failure management. Current understanding of peripartum cardiomyopathy. Prog Cardiovasc Nurs. 2007;22(4):214–6.
42. Sliwa K, Hilfiker-Kleiner D, Petrie MC, et al. Heart Failure Association of the European Society of Cardiology Working Group on Peripartum Cardiomyopathy. Current state of knowledge on aetiology, diagnosis, management, and therapy of peripartum cardiomyopathy: a position statement from the Heart Failure Association of the European Society of Cardiology Working Group on Peripartum Cardiomyopathy. Eur J Heart Fail. 2010;12(8):767–78.
43. Smith IJ, Gillham MJ. Fulminant peripartum cardiomyopathy rescue with extracorporeal membranous oxygenation. Int J Obstet Anesth. 2009;18(2):186–8.
44. Williams J, Mozurkewich E, Chilimigras J, Van De Ven C. Critical care in obstetrics: pregnancy-specific conditions. Best Pract Res Clin Obstet Gynaecol. 2008;22(5):825–46.
45. Fett JD. Earlier detection can help avoid many serious complications of peripartum cardiomyopathy. Future Cardiol. 2013;9:809–16. PMID: 24180539. doi:10.2217/fca.13.63.
46. Kamiya CA, Kitakaze M, Ishibashi-Ueda H, Nakatani S, Murohara T, Tomoike H, Ikeda T. Different characteristics of peripartum cardiomyopathy between patients complicated with and without hypertensive disorders. results from the Japanese Nationwide survey of peripartum cardiomyopathy. Circ J. 2011;75:1975–81 [PMID: 21617320].

47. Okamoto H, Takenaka T, Saitoh Y. Is hypertensive disorder a unique risk factor for peripartum cardiomyopathy and pregnancy-associated cardiomyopathy? Circ J. 2011;75:1827–8 [PMID: 21727752].
48. Harper MA, Meyer RE, Berg CJ. Peripartum cardiomyopathy: population-based birth prevalence and 7-year mortality. Obstet Gynecol. 2012;120:1013–9 [PMID: 23090517].
49. Fuster V, American Heart Association, editors. The AHA guidelines and scientific statements handbook. Oxford: Wiley- Black-well; 2009.
50. McTiernan C, Hanley-Yanez K, Pisarcik JE, Morel PA, Cooper LT, Elkayam E, Fett JD, McNamara DM. Activation of cellular immunity in peripartum cardiomyopathy: results of the multicenter IPAC Registry. Circulation. 2011;124:A14173, Supplement vol 124.
51. Cooper LT, Mather PJ, Alexis JD, Pauly DF, Torre-Amione G, Wittstein IS, Dec GW, Zucker M, Narula J, Kip K, McNamara DM. Myocardial recovery in peripartum cardiomyopathy: prospective comparison with recent onset cardiomyopathy in men and nonperipartum women. J Card Fail. 2012;18:28–33 [PMID: 22196838. doi: 10.1016/j.cardfail.2011.09.009].
52. McTiernan C, Hanley-Yanez K, Cooper LT, Rajagopalan N, Thohan V, Zucker M, Boehmer J, Bozkurt B, Mather P, Thornton J, Ghali J, Pisarcik J, Fett JD, Morel J, McNamara D. Racial differences in circulating Natural Killer cells in peripartum cardiomyopathy: results of the NHLBI-sponsored IPAC investigation. Circulation. 2013;128 (Suppl 22): Abstract 16587.
53. Sliwa K, Förster O, Libhaber E, Fett JD, Sundstrom JB, Hilfiker-Kleiner D, Ansari AA. Peripartum cardiomyopathy: inflammatory markers as predictors of outcome in 100 prospectively studied patients. Eur Heart J. 2006;27:441–6 [PMID: 16143707].
54. Ellis JE, Ansari AA, Fett JD, Carraway RD, Randall HW, Mosunjac MI, Sundstrom JB. Inhibition of progenitor dendritic cell maturation by plasma from patients with peripartum cardiomyopathy: role in pregnancy-associated heart disease. Clin Dev Immunol. 2005;12:265–73 [PMID: 16584112].

# Cerebral Venous Thrombosis in Pregnancy

23

Shobha N. Gudi

## Introduction

Cerebral venous thrombosis (CVT) is encountered during later weeks of pregnancy and more commonly during the second or third week of puerperium. The global incidence is about 1:2500–10,000 deliveries [1, 2]. It is a cerebrovascular disorder of considerable morbidity and can be fatal when care is delayed. Although rare in the developed world (1 in 11,000 to 1 in 45,000 pregnancies) [3], it remains the commonest cause of stroke in young women in the developing countries. In a 10-centre study in the United States, 7 % of all cases of CVT were associated with pregnancy [4], whereas an incidence of CVT of 1 in 273 obstetric admissions has been reported by two groups of investigators in a study of 40 years in India [5].

## Aetiology and Predispositions

Pregnancy has long been recognised as an acquired, transient, prothrombotic risk factor. The physiological changes of increase in procoagulation and decrease in anticoagulation factors are marked in the late second and third trimesters and resolve to normal levels only 2–3 weeks after delivery [6]. Increased levels of fibrinogen and factor VII, VIII, and X and decreased natural anticoagulant proteins S and C in pregnancy and puerperium are strong predisposing factors. The mutations of factor V Leiden and prothrombin gene [7] are important predisposing factors in post-oral contraceptive thrombosis. These defects can also cause pregnancy-related CVT.

Traditional beliefs about birthing care practised by elders in the family involves restriction of water intake. The post natal mother becomes dehydrated. This dehydration along with the enforced bed rest become a risk factor for thrombosis. Cerebrovenous thrombosis has also been associated with local or systemic infection and anaemia, conditions which are prevalent in obstetric population of the developing countries. Rarely, associated causes for the clinical presentation have been reported, e.g. hemoglobinopathies (sickle cell anaemia), hyperviscosity syndromes (polycythaemia), leukaemia and other malignancies, collagen vascular diseases, hypercoagulable states such as thrombophilia both APLA [8–10] and inherited thrombophilias [11, 12], AVM (arteriovenous malformation), paroxysmal nocturnal haemoglobinuria etc. In suspected cases, thrombophilia testing should include evaluation for the factor V Leiden mutation, prothrombin gene mutation 20210, lupus anticoagulant, anticardiolipin antibodies, hyperhomocysteinaemia and deficiencies of protein C, S, and antithrombin 3. However, protein C and

S.N. Gudi, Prof. & HOD
Department of OBG, St Philomena's Hospital, Bangalore, India
e-mail: sngudi@yahoo.co.in


A. Gandhi et al. (eds.), *Principles of Critical Care in Obstetrics: Volume II*,
DOI 10.1007/978-81-322-2686-4_23

S, and antithrombin levels may be abnormal in the setting of acute thrombosis, anticoagulation, oral contraceptives or pregnancy and therefore should be interpreted with due care. At least one risk factor can be identified in >85 % of patients with cerebral venous thrombosis (Table 23.1) [13]. In the International Study on Cerebral Vein and Dural Sinus Thrombosis (ISCVT) cohort, a thrombophilia was noted in 34 %, and an inherited thrombophilia was detected in 22 %. Use of oral contraceptives has been identified as an important cause of CVT in developed countries. Prolonged use of oral contraceptives leads to acquired 'activated protein C resistance'. This phenomenon gets aggravated if factor V Leiden and factor II gene mutations are present, increasing the risk of thrombosis by 10 times.

**Table 23.1** Risk factors for cerebral venous thrombosis

| |
|---|
| *Women's health concerns* |
| Pregnancy |
| Post-partum state |
| Hormonal contraceptive or replacement therapy |
| *Thrombophilia*<br>Deficiency of antithrombin 3 and protein C and S<br>Factor V Leiden and prothrombin gene mutation<br>Antiphospholipid antibodies |
| Hyperhomocysteinaemia |
| *Infection* |
| Puerperal sepsis, episiotomy or wound infections<br>Localised infections such as otitis, mastoiditis, sinusitis |
| Meningitis |
| Systemic infectious disorders |
| *Chronic inflammatory diseases* |
| Vasculitis |
| Inflammatory bowel disease |
| *Cancer*<br>Leukaemia |
| *Hematologic disorders* |
| Sickle cell anaemia<br>Polycythaemia |
| Essential thrombocytosis |
| Paroxysmal nocturnal haemoglobinuria |
| *Trauma* |
| Head trauma |
| Local injury to cerebral sinuses or veins |
| Jugular venous cannulation |
| Neurosurgical procedures |
| Lumbar puncture |
| *Nephrotic syndrome* |

## Pathogenesis

The human brain has a unique cerebral venous system. It has sinuses which are lacking in muscular walls or valves and hence do not have the ability to contract. The sagittal sinuses (superior and inferior) drain into transverse, cavernous, right and left sigmoid sinuses and finally into the internal jugular vein. In susceptible patients, blood can pool, clot and obstruct these sinuses, leading to increased intracranial pressure and cytotoxic and vasogenic oedema of variable degree, which can progress to intracerebral bleeding, ischaemia and infarction (Fig. 23.1). Pathological findings observed in central nervous system as a result of CVT are determined by:

(a) Underlying disease pathology
(b) Nature of sinus/cerebral vein involved
(c) Interval between the onset and pathological examination

Cortical vein thrombosis usually presents as a cord-like swelling with minimal or absent haemorrhagic infarction of the brain [14]. This discrepancy has been explained on the presence of frequent intercommunications between various cortical veins and sinuses. In case of superior sagittal sinus thrombosis, the sinus is distended and appears blue. Cortical veins are also swollen and may rupture at some places giving rise to haemorrhagic infarction and even intracerebral haemorrhage. In an occasional case, haemorrhagic infarction may appear on the other side due to occlusion of opposite cortical vein (parasagittal). In deep cerebral vein thrombosis, white matter may be involved, e.g. basal ganglia, thalamus, etc. In due course, thrombosis gets recanalised and organised and may even disappear in majority of cases. Cerebral oedema with or without increased intracranial hypertension is a frequent finding in early stage. It may even lead to transtentorial herniation with notching of uncus of temporal lobe [15]. Microscopy shows typical

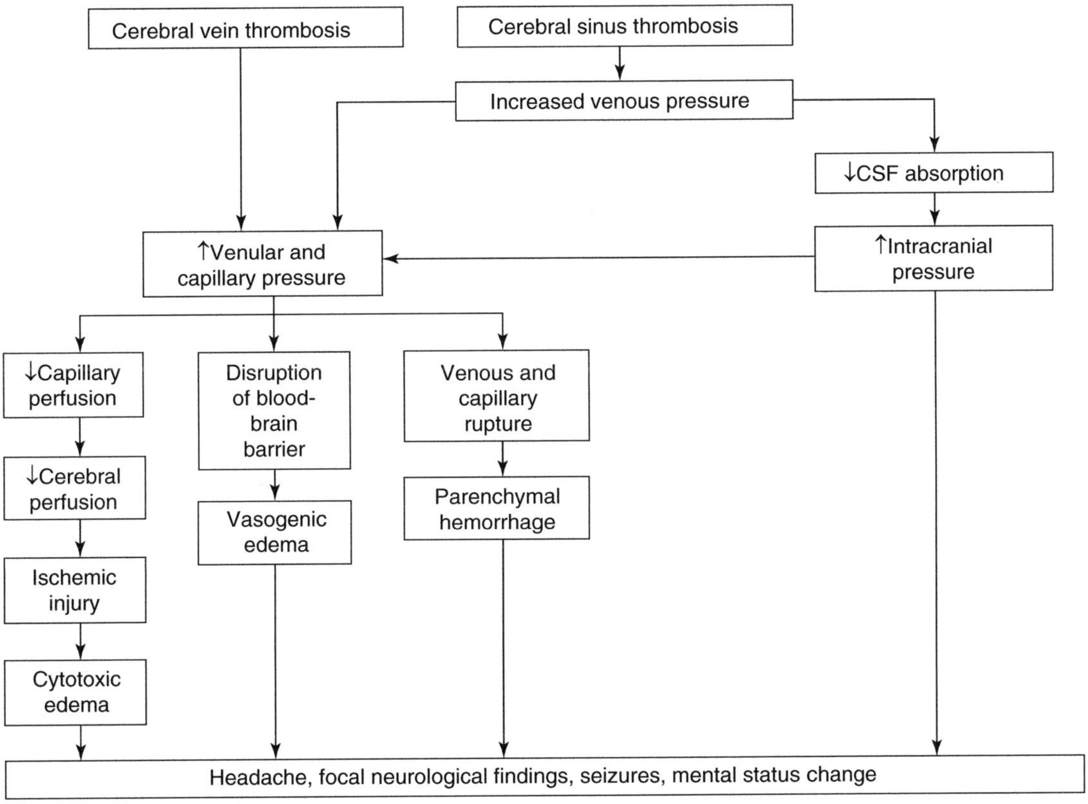


**Fig. 23.1** Pathophysiology of cerebral venous thrombosis. CSF indicates cerebrospinal fluid

changes of haemorrhage, but specific feature appears to be 'profuse leukocyte invasion' because of patent arteries allowing inflow.

The terminology used and the clinical presentation will vary on the location and extent of the thrombosis. In pregnant women, the common sites are thrombosis of the sagittal sinus with extension into the cortical veins or primary thrombosis of a cortical vein [16].

## Clinical Features

Clinical presentation can be varied depending on the site and extent of thrombosis (Fig. 23.2). CVT often has an insidious onset, though rarely it can present as an acute episode of sudden neurological illness. The most consistent symptom is unrelenting headache, not responding to analgesia and may be progressive over several days. It may be accompanied by nausea and vomiting. Neurological signs of focal seizures, focal neurological deficits and generalised seizures are sometimes seen. Visual impairment, blurring of vision, diplopia and blindness can result from very high intracranial pressure and papilloedema [17]. When the deep cerebral venous system of thalami is involved, behavioural symptoms such as lethargy, dementia, amnesia, mutism and coma can develop, undoubtedly reflecting a graver prognosis [18].

The common differential diagnosis is eclampsia. It is differentiated by presence of hypertension and proteinuria, clinical course of pregnancy and delivery, response to treatment and results of brain imaging. The other confusing situation is the postdural puncture headache if spinal anaesthesia is used for delivery [19]. Spinal headache resolves with hydration and posture and has no neurological deficits. Posterior reversible encephalopathy syndrome (PRES), occurring as a squeal to hypertension and eclampsia in recently

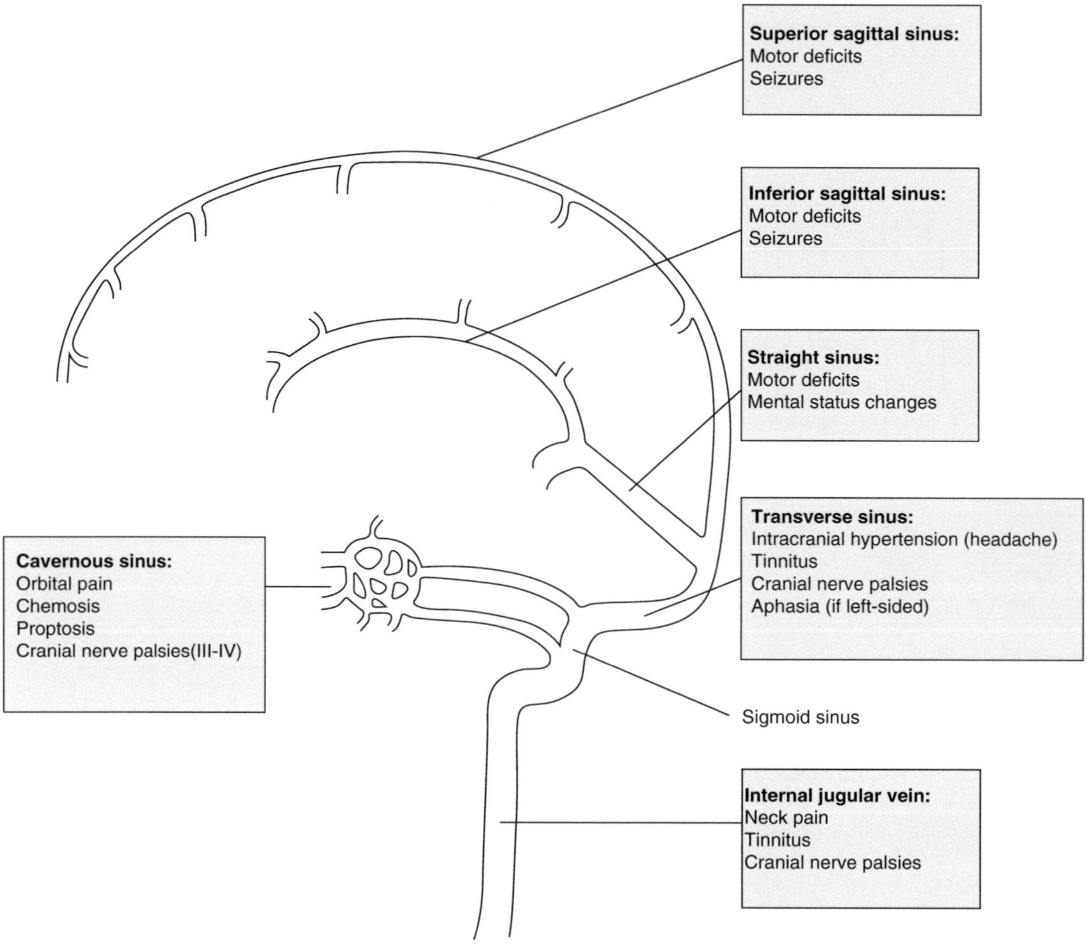


**Fig. 23.2** Major clinical syndromes according to location of cerebral venous thrombosis

delivered women, presents as mental confusion, headache, seizures and visual impairment but no neurological deficits. It is diagnosed on MRI, seen characteristically as hyperintensities on T2-weighted images as distinct from CVT.

## Diagnosis

The confirmation of a diagnosis of dural venous sinus thrombosis is reliant on demonstration of the thrombus by neuroimaging. The initial evaluation during pregnancy begins with a brain computerised tomography (CT) without contrast. Signs of cerebral venous thrombosis on CT include hyperdensity in the area of a sinus or cortical vein (cord sign) and filling defects, especially in the superior sagittal sinus (empty Δ sign), in contrast-enhanced studies [20]. A partially filled posterior segment of the superior sagittal sinus is seen (empty delta sign) (Fig. 23.3), but this is found only in 20 % of cases [2]. It is seen on axial CT images and represents enhancement with i.v. contrast of the wall of the posterior sagittal sinus, outlining the clot within the lumen anteriorly.

Conventional CT can be entirely normal in the presence of CVT and miss the diagnosis in 60 % of cases. The most sensitive non-invasive technique is magnetic resonance imaging (MRI) with MR venography (Fig. 23.4) and is the investigation of choice for demonstrating CVT, as it may exclude significant alternative diagnoses and will also demonstrate cerebral venous infarction complicating cerebral venous occlusion.

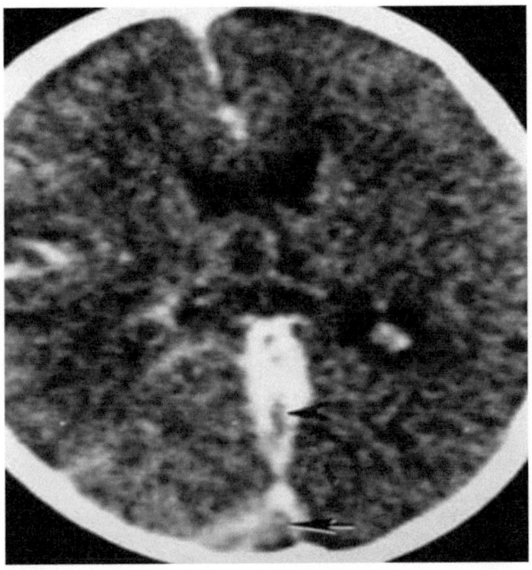

**Fig. 23.3** Axial head CT scan demonstrating cerebrovenous thrombosis of the straight sinus (*arrowhead*) and the empty delta sign (*arrow*)

Difficulties in diagnosis arise due to unusual normal anatomical variants and cases where there is near occlusion of the venous sinus. T1-weighted and T2-weighted images can identify the thrombosed sinuses if done within 5 days of the event and are currently the test of choice [21, 22]. CT venography is the new technique that can provide better details and in experienced hands will show dilated 'corkscrew' veins with thrombosis [23].

## Management

A multidisciplinary approach involving the obstetrician, neurophysician, intensivist, specialised nursing staff and physiotherapist in an intensive care setting is the ideal requirement. General principles of intravenous fluid, nutrition and postural measures for a patient with neurological illness need to be followed. Obstetric assessment and treatment of any coexisting risk factor, e.g. pre-eclampsia and anaemia, should be prompt. The patient should be administered with anticonvulsants for seizures and antimicrobials if septic thrombophlebitis is suspected. The treatment of choice to arrest the thrombotic process and prevent pulmonary embolism is systemic anticoagulation with intravenous heparin [24], despite the potential risk that a venous infarct might become haemorrhagic. This recommendation is based on the results of three small RCTs [25, 26] and a large multicentric observational study [27]. Evidence supports the use of smallest effective dosage of unfractionated heparin of 15,000 units per day in three divided subcutaneous doses, aiming for a target APTT of 2.5 times the normal. This treatment is continued for 3–7 days or till the patient stabilises. Low molecular weight heparin in a fixed high subcutaneous dose is a suitable alternative, but there are no studies to compare its effectiveness against unfractionated heparin. Following the management of acute episode, oral anticoagulant therapy with vitamin K antagonists (coumarin derivatives) should be continued for 6 months or longer in the presence of predisposing factors, with a target international ratio of 2.5 (APTT of 1.4–2.8 times the normal).

## Potential Thrombolytic Therapy

Thrombolytic therapy with tissue plasminogen activator is an emergent therapeutic approach wherein endovascular thrombolytic is attempted by experienced interventional radiologist most often in arterial ischaemic stroke. In contrast to arterial stroke, since the diagnosis of CVT is made several hours after the onset of thrombus and symptoms, potential for thrombolytic therapy probably holds less promise. Some pregnant and parturient women with high risk CVT, with significant neurological deficits, deteriorate despite intensive anticoagulation [11]. In such poor prognosis CVT, catheter-directed endovascular thrombolysis can be attempted using a combination of a thrombolytic enzyme such as r-tPA (recombinant tissue plasminogen activator, e.g. alteplase) infused into the dural sinus and mechanical intervention techniques to aspirate, dislodge and disrupt the thrombus [28]. Although tissue plasminogen activator thrombolysis in pregnancy has been so far regarded as relatively contraindicated, recently published case reports and series have been reassuring regarding maternal safety and efficacy issues in treatment of acute ischaemic stroke in gestation.

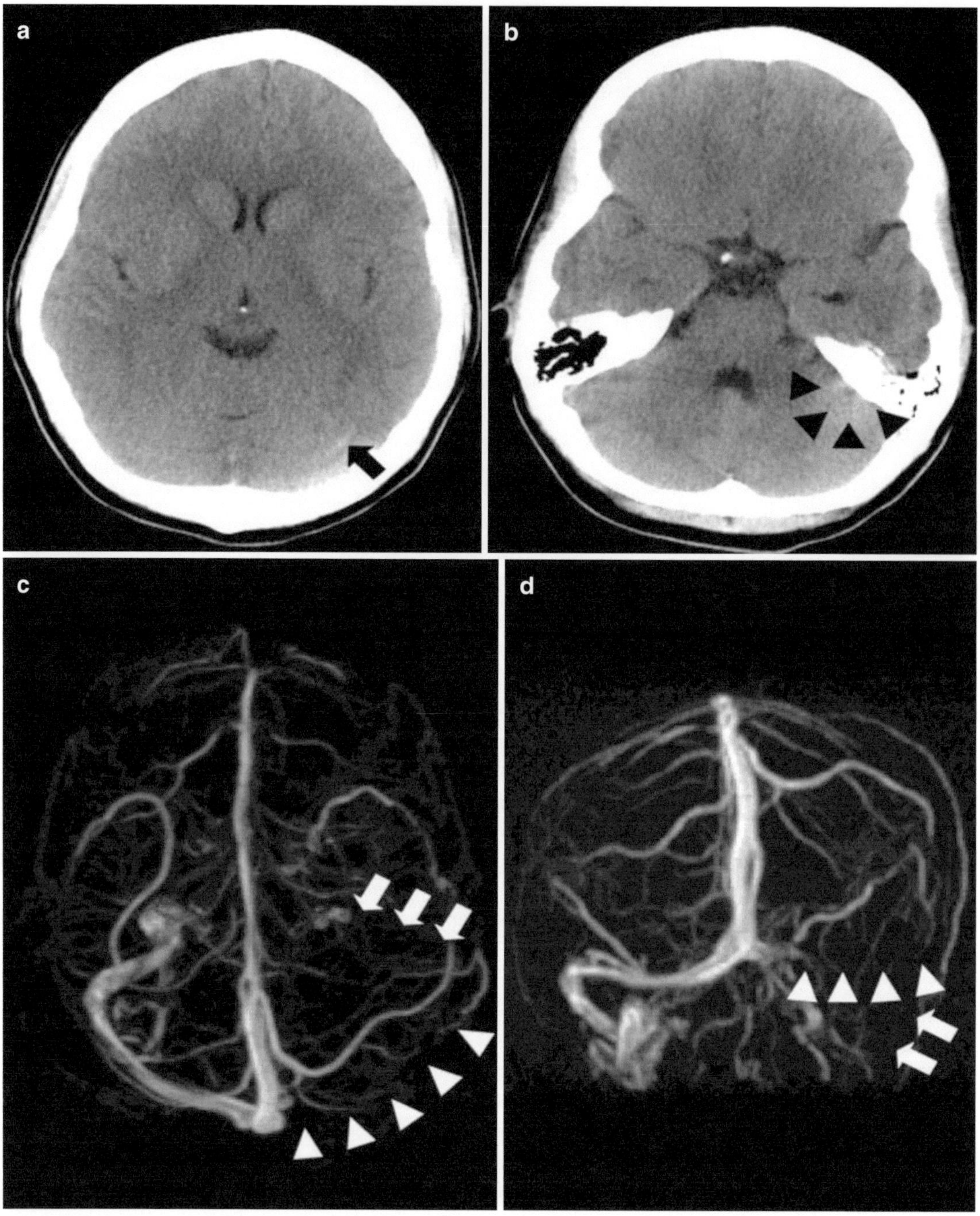


**Fig. 23.4** Computed tomogram (CT) of the head without intravenous contrast demonstrating hyperdensities along the left tentorium (*arrows*, **a**) and involving the left sigmoid sinus (*arrowheads*, **b**) that were concerning for cerebral venous thrombosis. Magnetic resonance (MR) venography demonstrating thrombosis of the left transverse (*arrowheads*) and sigmoid sinus and proximal jugular vein (*arrows*) in the axial (**c**) and coronal (**d**) planes

## Prognosis

Despite remaining a diagnostic challenge and a potentially disabling or lethal disease, CVT associated with pregnancy and the puerperium overall has good prognosis with 90–93 % survival with very few permanent neurological deficits, and so the long-term outcome is generally better than for arterial stroke. The exceptions are patients who are comatose, have recurrent seizures or have rapidly declining neurologic function. In such cases, the clinical course is unpredictable and the prognosis extremely guarded with mortality rates of 15–30 %. The primary cause of death during the acute phase of cerebral venous thrombosis is transtentorial herniation, most frequently from large venous haemorrhage [29]. The majority of patients have a complete or partial recovery, only 10 % is found to have permanent neurological deficits by 12 months of follow-up [15]. Recurrence of cerebral venous thrombosis is rare (2.8 %) [30].

**Conclusions**

CVT is a potentially life-threatening neurological complication in pregnant and parturient women, and early diagnosis by MRI and prompt anticoagulant and supportive therapy in an intensive care set-up by a multidisciplinary team will give excellent outcome. In patients who present late or suffer delay in diagnosis, mortality can be prevented by endovascular thrombolytic therapy, although due to the lack of experience and evidence in pregnant patients, caution should be exercised.

**Key Points**

- In pregnant or puerperal women patients with suspected cerebral venous thrombosis, MR venography is the most sensitive test. If this test is not possible, then CT should be performed.
- Screening for thrombophilias in select patients is important.
- Current evidence recommends heparin anticoagulation as safe and effective treatment for cerebral venous thrombosis.
- Follow-up treatment with oral vitamin K antagonist (after delivery), maintaining an INR – 2.0–3.0 is recommended for 3–6 months in patients with provoked CVT as with pregnancy and puerperium, 6–12 months in those with unprovoked CVT and indefinitely in recurrent CVT with thrombophilia.
- Women who have suffered CVT should be offered non-oestrogen-based methods for contraception.
- After a period of 3–6 months, follow-up imaging to assess for recanalisation is recommended.

## References


1. Srinivasan K. Cerebral venous and arterial thrombosis in pregnancy and puerperium: a study of 135 patients. Angiol J Vasc Dis. 1983;34:731–74.
2. Fehr PR. Sagittal sinus thrombosis in early pregnancy. Obstet Gynecol. 1982;59:7–9.
3. Cross JN, Castro PO, Jennett WB. Cerebral strokes associated with pregnancy and the puerperium. Br Med J. 1968;3(5612):214–8.
4. Wasay M, Bakshi R, Bobustuc G, et al. Cerebral venous thrombosis: analysis of a multicenter cohort from the United States. J Stroke Cerebrovasc Dis. 2008;17:49.
5. Bansal BC, GuptaRR PC. Stroke during pregnancy and puerperium due to CVT. Jpn Heart J. 1980;21:171–83.
6. Matinelli I, Sacchi E, Landi G, et al. High risk of cerebral venous thrombosis in carriers of prothrombotic gene mutation and in users of oral contraceptives. N Engl J Med. 1988;338:1793–7.
7. Bousser MG, Chiras J, Bories J, et al. Cerebral venous thrombosis—a review of 38 cases. Stroke. 1985;16:199–213.
8. Carhuapoma JR, Mitsias P, Levine SR. Cerebral venous thrombosis and anticardiolipin antibodies. Stroke. 1997;28:2363–9.
9. Levine SR, Kieran S, Puzio K, et al. Cerebral venous thrombosis with lupus anticoagulants. Report of two cases. Stroke. 1987;18:801–4.
10. Provenzale JM, Loganbill HA. Dual sinus thrombosis and venous infarction associated with antiphospholipid antibodies: MR findings. J Comput Assist Tomogr. 1994;18:719–23.
11. Deschiens MA, Conard J, Horellou MH, et al. Coagulation studies, factor V Leiden, and anticardiolipin antibodies in 40 cases of cerebral venous thrombosis. Stroke. 1996;27:1724–30.

12. Zuber M, Toulon P, Marnet L, et al. Factor V Leiden mutation in cerebral venous thrombosis. Stroke. 1996;27:1721–3.
13. De Freitas GR, Bogousslavsky J. Risk factors of cerebral vein and sinus thrombosis. Front Neurol Neurosci. 2008;23:23.
14. Banerjee AK, Chopra JS, Sawhney BB. Puerperal cerebral venous thrombosis. Study of autopsy material. Neurol India. 1973;21:19–22.
15. Wilterdink JL, Easton JD. Cerebral ischaemia. In: Devinsky O, Feldmann E, Hainline B, editors. Neurological complications of pregnancy. New York: Raven; 1994. p. 1–11.
16. Piazza G. Clinician Update, Cerebral venous thrombosis, AHA J. Circulation associated with pregnancy and the puerperium. Br Med J. 1968;3:214.
17. Stam J. Thrombosis of the cerebral veins and sinuses. N Engl J Med. 2005;352:1791–8.
18. Kothare SV, Ebb DH, Rosenburger PB, Buonanno F, Scefer PW, Krishnamoorthy KS. Acute confusion and mutism as a presentation of thalamic strokes secondary to deep cerebral venous thrombosis. J Child Neurol. 1998;13:300–3.
19. Kapessidou Y, Vokaer M, Laureys M, Bier JC, Boogaerts JG. Case report: cerebral venous thrombosis after subarachnoid analgesia for labor. Can J Anaesth. 2006;53:1015–9.
20. Carhuapoma JR, Tomlinson MW, Levine SR. High risk pregnancy: management options/David K. James … [et al.].—3rd ed. p. cm. Section V, Ch. 49. Neurologic disorders.
21. Dormont D, Axionnat R, et al. MRI in cerebral venous thrombosis. J Neuroradiol. 1994;21(2):81–99.
22. Ehtisham A, Stern BJ. Cerebral venous thrombosis: a review. Neurologist. 2006;12:32.
23. Veillon EW, Martin JN, Maternal F, et al. Critical care. In: Belfort M, editor. Obstetrics, 5th ed. USA: Wiley – Blackwell; 2010.
24. Einhaupl KM, Villringer A, Meister W, et al. Heparin treatment in sinus venous thrombosis. Lancet. 1991;338:597–600. Erratum, Lancet 1991; 338–958.
25. De Bruijn SF, Stam J. Randomised placebo controlled trial of anticoagulant treatment with low molecular weight heparin in puerperal cerebral venous sinus thrombosis. Stroke. 1999;30:484–8.
26. Nagaraja D, Rao BSS, Taly AB, Subhash MN. Randomised controlled trial of heparin in puerperal cerebral venous /sinus thrombosis. Nimhans J. 1995;13:111–5.
27. Ferro JM, Canhao P, Stam J, Bousser MG, Barinagarrementeria F. Prognosis of cerebral vein and dural sinus thrombosis: results of the International Study on Cerebral Vein and Dural Sinus Thrombosis (ISCVT). Stroke. 2004;35:664–70.
28. Baker MD, Opatowsky MJ, Wilson JA, LGlazier SS, Morris PP. Rheolytic catheter and thrombolysis of dural venous sinus thrombosis: a case series. Neurosurgery. 2001;48:487–93.
29. Chopra JS, Banerjee AK. Primary intracranial sinovenous occlusions in youth and pregnancy. In: Vinken PJBG, Klawans HL, editors. Handbook of clinical neurology. Amsterdam: Elsevier Science Publishers; 1989. p. 425–52.
30. Mehraein S, Ortwein H, Busch M, et al. Risk of recurrence of cerebral venous and sinus thrombosis during subsequent pregnancy and puerperium. J Neurol Neurosurg Psychiatry. 2003;74:814.

# Post-operative Ileus

# 24

Radhakrishna Nayak

## Introduction

Ileus is a Greek word which means "intestinal obstruction". It is a disruption of the normal propulsive ability of the gastrointestinal tract. It may be due to bowel obstruction which is called dynamic ileus or due to intestinal atony or paralysis which is called adynamic ileus.

Intestinal paralysis often termed as paralytic ileus needs not to be a complete paralysis, but it must be sufficient to prohibit the passage of food through the intestine and lead to intestinal blockage which results in accumulation of gas and fluids in the bowel.

## Pathogenesis

Following surgery the return of the small intestine's action begins first, usually 4–8 h post-operatively, and generally becomes complete around 24 h. The colon resumes its function between 48 and 72 h post-operatively. Physiologic ileus spontaneously resolves within 2–3 days. If it persists for >3 days post-operatively, it leads to post-operative adynamic or paralytic ileus. Multiple causes have been suggested in the pathogenesis of post-operative ileus, but exact pathophysiology still remains unclear. Various causes leading to paralytic ileus are sympathetic reflexes, inhibitory humoral agents, release of norepinephrine from the bowel wall, the effects of anaesthesia agents and opiates and inflammation.

*However, the two important aetiologies are:*

- Inhibitory spinal reflex due to spinal anaesthesia, abdominal sympathetectomy and nerve-cutting techniques
- Inflammatory mediators released from the site of injury

## Causes

- Major abdominal and extra-abdominal surgeries, particularly gastrointestinal surgery or other GI procedures – postsurgical ileus
- Electrolyte imbalance
- Sepsis and pneumonia
- Diabetic ketoacidosis (DKA) and other causes of metabolic acidosis
- Endocrine disorders: hypothyroidism, diabetes and adrenal insufficiency
- General anaesthesia
- Drugs (e.g. opiates, antimuscarinics, antacids, warfarin, chlorpromazine, amitriptyline etc.)
- Severe illness (acute pancreatitis and peritonitis)

R. Nayak
Professor at Kasturba Medical College, Mangalore, Karnataka, India
e-mail: laproscope@gmail.com


A. Gandhi et al. (eds.), *Principles of Critical Care in Obstetrics: Volume II*,
DOI 10.1007/978-81-322-2686-4_24

- Spinal cord injury, those above thoracic T5 vertebrae
- Cardiopulmonary failure

**Note** Laparoscopic procedures are associated with shorter periods of ileus than open procedures.

## Symptoms

- Abdominal pain, distension and discomfort
- Nausea
- Vomiting of biliatic fluid or bile
- Flatulence
- Belching
- Constipation

## Signs

- There may be tenderness on palpation and tympanic note on percussion.
- Hypoactive or absent bowel sounds on auscultation in contrast to high-pitched bowel sounds of obstruction.

## Characteristics of Ileus, Pseudo-obstruction and Mechanical Obstruction

| | Ileus | Pseudo-obstruction | Mechanical obstruction |
|---|---|---|---|
| Symptoms | Nausea, vomiting, mild abdominal pain, bloating, obstipation and constipation | Nausea, vomiting, anorexia, crampy abdominal pain, obstipation and constipation | Nausea, vomiting, anorexia, crampy abdominal pain, obstipation and constipation |
| Physical examination | Distension (+), tympanic on percussion, silent abdomen with absent bowel sounds | Distension (+), localised tenderness (+), borborygmi sounds heard. Hypo- or hyperactive bowel sounds heard | Distension (+), localised tenderness (+), borborygmi sounds heard. High-pitched bowel sounds heard |
| Plain radiograph features | Diaphragm elevated, small and large bowel dilatation seen | Diaphragm elevated, isolated large bowel dilatation seen | Diaphragm mildly elevated, bow-shaped loops in ladder pattern, paucity of colonic gas distal to the lesion, air-fluid levels seen |
| Associated risks | Nil | Perforation | Peritonitis due to strangulated obstruction |

## Differential Diagnosis of Paralytic Ileus

1. Pseudo-obstruction/Ogilive syndrome
2. Mechanical bowel obstruction

**Psuedo-obstruction** Acute and marked distension of the large bowel

| Pseudo-obstruction | Paralytic ileus |
|---|---|
| Limited to the colon | Involves both small bowel and colon |
| Occurs in elderly bedridden patients | Any age group particularly in post-operative patients |
| There will be abdominal distension without pain and tenderness | Abdominal distension associated with pain and tenderness |
| Increased risk of perforation if caecum is >12 cm in diameter | No such risks |

**Mechanical Obstruction** Caused by adhesions, volvulus, hernias, intussusception, foreign bodies or neoplasms

## Workup

Laboratory studies should evaluate for infections and electrolyte and metabolic derangements.

**Note** White cell count can differentiate ileus and secondary obstruction.

**Imaging** *By plain abdominal radiographs*

Copious gas dilatation of small bowel and colon is seen in ileus. Contrast medium reaches caecum within 4 h in paralytic ileus. If contrast medium remains stationary for more than 4 h, mechanical obstruction is suggested.

## Management of Ileus

Most cases of post-operative ileus resolve with watchful waiting and supportive treatment. The underlying cause of ileus should be treated like correction of underlying medical conditions and electrolyte and acid base abnormalities. Medications that produce ileus should be discontinued.

Intravenous hydration should be provided. Nasogastric tube may provide symptomatic relief, but no literature supports the use of nasogastric tube for resolution of ileus.

For patient with protracted ileus, mechanical obstruction must be excluded with contrast studies.

The clinician must assess the overall status of patient and evaluate for adequate oral intake and good bowel function.

## Diet

It is advisable to delay oral feeding until ileus resolves completely clinically.

Chewing gum has been advocated as a means of promoting recovery from post-op ileus. Meta-analysis have shown that gum chewing can reduce the time to first flatus and faeces by stimulating gastrointestinal motility through sham feeding.

## Activity

Post-operative ambulation is beneficial in preventing atelectasis, deep vein thrombosis and pneumonia but not treating ileus.

## Medication

1. Bowel movements may be stimulated by lactulose, erythromycin and neostigmine.
2. Thoracic epidural administration is beneficial. Epidural blockade with local anaesthetics may prevent post-operative ileus
3. Peripheral selective opioid antagonists:
   - Methylnaltrexone is indicated for opioid-induced constipation in patient with advanced illness.
   - Alvimopan is also indicated to prevent post-operative ileus following bowel resection.
4. Prokinetic agents have shown mixed results.

In summary management of ileus is a multivariate approach involving minimally invasive surgical procedures, opiate-sparing pain management and fast recovery protocols.

## Note

Traditionally, the routine approach to manage postsurgical ileus consisted of placing a nasogastric (NG) tube to decompress the bowel and delaying feeding until bowel function resumed.

*However, more recent studies indicate a different tactic approach, with a simple 3-step process:*

- Withholding the nasogastric (NG) tube
- Feeding the patient early in the recovery process
- Continuing epidural local anaesthesia post-operatively as it blocks the reflex that causes post-operative ileus

**Acknowledgement** 1. Burt Cagir M.D, FACS, Assistant Professor of Surgery, State University of New York Upstate, Consulting Staff, Director of Medical Research, Robert Packer Hospital, Associate Program Director, Department Of Surgery – Guthrie Clinic.

2. Fransisco Talavera, Adjunct Assistant Professor, University Of Nebraska Medical Center. Editor In Chief, Medscape Drug Reference.

# Trauma and Pregnancy

# 25

Anuradha Khanna, Uma Pandey, and Pooja Singh

## Introduction

Trauma as such is a disaster, and, during pregnancy, it is more dangerous for both the mother and baby and poses a special challenge to emergency department. Trauma during pregnancy may be caused by accidents, homicide, or other violent events

## Epidemiology

Incidence of trauma in pregnant women is 7 % of all pregnancies, and it is the most common cause of nonobstetric morbidity and mortality in pregnancy [4]. In India and also all over the world, it accounts for 46 % of all the maternal deaths. According to ACOG, as many as 10–20 % of pregnant women suffer physical trauma [1].

Motor vehicle accidents contribute 54.6 % of all the injuries sustained by pregnant trauma patient (Rudra et al.). The use of proper restraints directly influences the pregnant patient outcome in motor vehicle collision. Typically only 46 % of the pregnant trauma patients were using seat belts during motor vehicle collision [3]. With the proper use of seat belt, chance of vaginal bleeding is decreased by half and that of intrauterine death is decreased by one fourth.

Next most common cause is domestic abuse and assault accounting for 22.3 % of cases resulting in various injuries to abdomen and genitalia [7]. Most of the cases of abuse go unreported. The abuse is recurrent on 50 % of the women.

Falls are another common mechanism of injury during pregnancy accounting for 21.8 % of all cases. Recurrent falls are seen in 2 % of the patients. Other less common causes like burns, puncture wounds, and animal bites constitute 1.3 % cases [7].

## Anatomical and Physiological Alteration in Pregnancy

The understanding of unique anatomical and physiological changes that takes place in pregnancy is essential for adequate management of trauma victim. The pathophysiology and mechanism of maternal injury may significantly differ from those that commonly occur in nonpregnant state.

A. Khanna (✉) • U. Pandey • P. Singh
Department of Obstetrics & Gynaecology, Institute of Medical Sciences, Banaras Hindu University, Varanasi, Uttar Pradesh, India
e-mail: Dr_anuradhakhanna@yahoo.co.in; Uma.pandey2006@gmail.com; singh8515@gmail.com


A. Gandhi et al. (eds.), *Principles of Critical Care in Obstetrics: Volume II*,
DOI 10.1007/978-81-322-2686-4_25

## Physiological and Physical Changes in Pregnancy

| |
|---|
| *Cardiovascular system:* |
| Plasma volume increases by 50 % which leads to dilutional anemia and reduced oxygen-carrying capacity. Signs of hemorrhagic shock appear late. |
| Heart rate is increased by 15–20 beats and cardiac output by 40 % due to the pressure of gravid uterus on IVC. These lead to increase in CPR demands. |
| Uterine blood flow is about 10 % of the cardiac output at term so there is high chance of massive hemorrhage in uterine injuries. |
| Systemic vascular resistance and arterial blood pressure decrease. |
| Coagulation cascade is in activated state; hence, tendency for thrombosis is increased. |
| Decreased venous return due to the pressure of gravid uterus leads to increased CPR demands. |
| *Respiratory system:* |
| Respiratory rate is increased leading to a state of physiologic hyperventilation. |
| Oxygen consumption increases by 20 %, so hypoxia develops more quickly. |
| Hyperventilation, decreased residual capacity, and arterial $pCo_2$ decrease the buffering capacity, so acidosis is more likely. |
| Mucosal congestion and laryngeal edema lead to difficult airway. |
| *Other changes:* |
| Decreased gastric motility and relaxed lower esophageal sphincter lead to the risk of aspiration. |
| Enlarged uterus causes reduced venous return, supine hypotension, and difficulty in respiration. |
| Increased weight during pregnancy leads to difficult airway management. |
| Hypertrophied pelvic vasculature predisposes for massive retroperitoneal hemorrhage. |
| Bowel and bladder are more susceptible for injury due to the upward displacement by uterus. |
| Placenta: lack of elasticity of placenta predisposes it to abruptio placenta leading to release of placental thromboplastin or plasminogen activator from the myometrium. |
| Musculoskeletal: pelvic ligament laxity, protruding abdomen, and change in the center of gravity lead to pelvic widening, lordosis, gait instability, and tendency of fall. |

## Types of Trauma in Pregnancy

1. *Blunt trauma*
   Automobile accidents
   Physical abuse
   Sexual assault
   Falls
   Aggravated assaults
2. *Penetrating trauma*
   Knife wound
   Gunshot wound
3. *Burn injury*

## Blunt Injury

Besides motor vehicle accidents, assaults, abuse, and falls are frequent causes of serious blunt trauma in pregnancy.

The main concerns are immediate assessment of maternal effects of trauma, emergency treatment, and evaluation of collateral effects on fetus.

Problems in blunt abdominal trauma:

1. The enlarged uterus loses the protection of the bony pelvis.
2. Increased chances of retroperitoneal hemorrhage as the pelvic vessels are engorged.

Amniotic fluid provides some protection to fetus by absorbing the thrust of trauma, dissipating the force of the blow by transmitting it equally in all directions.

## Risks to the Mother

Maternal mortality from blunt trauma is estimated to be about 7 % [2]. It includes placental abruption, preterm labor, massive fetomaternal hemorrhage, uterine rupture and fetal loss, amniotic fluid embolism, and DIC. Splenic hemorrhage is the most common cause of intraperitoneal hemorrhage followed by uterine rupture. Retroperitoneal hemorrhage may occur secondary to rupture of the pelvic venous plexus.

## Risks to the Fetus

Direct fetal injuries occur in less than 1 % of cases of severe blunt abdominal trauma. Fetus is at significant risk, especially if placental abruption, uterine rupture, or maternal shocks occur [5]. Fetal mortality after blunt trauma varies from 3.4 to 38 % [7].

## Factors Associated with Increased Fetal Mortality after Trauma

1. Maternal hypotension
2. High maternal Injury Severity Score
3. Ejection from a motor vehicle
4. Maternal pelvic fracture
5. Automobile versus pedestrian accidents
6. Maternal history of alcohol use
7. Young maternal age
8. Motorcycle crashes

## Assessment of a Pregnant Patient with Blunt Trauma

All pregnant women should be evaluated in a medical setting. The assessment and management of a case of blunt abdominal trauma depends upon the gestational age, degree of maternal injury, and mechanism of injury.

The physical examination may be unreliable and difficult due to the displacement of abdominal content by gravid uterus and stretching of peritoneum, diminishing the response to peritoneal irritation.

## Penetrating Trauma

With the progress of pregnancy, there are changes in intra-abdominal organs in position with important implications. Penetrating injury to the upper part of the abdomen is more likely to be associated with multiple gastrointestinal injuries due to upward pushing of bowel by enlarged uterus. Organs involved are small bowel, liver, colon, and stomach in decreasing frequency. Injuries to the lower quadrants of the abdomen during the third trimester almost exclusively involve the uterus which may be advantageous to the mother due to the protective effect of the uterus and amniotic fluid resulting in less destruction to other organs. It is rare for a projectile to clear the posterior wall of the uterus so the maternal viscera are often spared. If the uterus is involved in penetrating trauma, fetal injury may occur in 70 % [3] of cases. Gunshot wounds to the uterus carry a maternal mortality of 7–9 % [2]. In case of injury before 37 weeks, fetal mortality is higher [2].

In cases of trauma in the upper abdomen, surgical exploration is generally recommended. In trauma involving lower abdomen, a more conservative approach, including observation, wound exploration, and laparoscopy, remains an option if maternal and fetal status is reassuring [4].

Stab wounds which do not appear to penetrate beyond the abdominal wall have been managed nonoperatively, whereas laparotomy is usually indicated with evidence of peritoneal penetration, particularly if intraperitoneal hemorrhage or bowel perforation is suspected.

## Severity of Injuries

All patients with major injuries require hospitalization where surgical and obstetric facilities are available due to high rate of mortality. Even minor injuries are associated with complications as feto-maternal hemorrhage, so it needs careful attention.

## Classification of Major Trauma in Pregnancy

Table 1 shows criteria for major trauma in pregnancy. If any one criterion (except systolic BP*) is present from any category (vital signs, injury pattern, or mechanism of injury), trauma is considered "major."

## Minor Trauma

Any trauma injury that does not meet the criteria for defining major trauma.

**Vital signs criteria**

| | |
|---|---|
| Conscious state | Altered level of consciousness |
| Respiratory rate | <10 or >30 breaths/min |
| $SpO_2$ (room air) | <95 % |
| Heart rate | >120 bpm |
| [a]Systolic BP | <90 mmHg |

*[a]Interpret BP in conjunction with gestation, other vital signs, injury pattern, and mechanism of injury*

**Injury pattern criteria**

| |
|---|
| Penetrating or blast injury to the head, neck, chest, abdomen, pelvis, axilla, or groin |
| Significant blunt injury to a single region of head, neck, chest, abdomen, pelvis, or axilla |
| Injury to any two or more body regions of the head, neck, chest, abdomen, pelvis, or axilla |
| Limb amputation above the wrist or ankle |
| Suspected spinal cord injuries |
| Burns >20 % or other complicated burn injury to the hand, face, genitals, and airway and respiratory tract |
| Serious crush injury |
| Major compound fracture or open dislocation with vascular compromise |
| Fractured pelvis |
| Fractures involving two or more of the following: femur, tibia, humerus |

**Mechanism of injury criteria**

| |
|---|
| Ejected from vehicle |
| Fall from height >3 m |
| Involved in an explosion |
| Involved in a high impact motor vehicle crash with incursion into the occupants compartment |
| Involved in a vehicle rollover |
| Involved in a road traffic collision in which there was a fatality in the same vehicle |
| Entrapped for >30 min |
| Pedestrian impact |
| Motorcyclist impact >30 kph |

## Traumatic Complications in Pregnancy

- Vaginal bleeding.
- Preterm rupture of membranes.
- Placental abruption.
- Maternal pelvic fractures.
- Fetal death.
- Fetal fractures, especially skull, clavicles, and long bones.
- Intracranial hemorrhage.
- Indirect injury is generally due to fetal hypoxia secondary to maternal hypotension, fetal hemorrhage, placental abruption, cord injury, uterine injury, or other injury.
- Other: spontaneous abortion, preterm delivery, and Rh isoimmunization.

## Uterine Contractions and Preterm Labor

The most common obstetric problem during trauma is uterine contractions. Myometrial and decidual cells, damaged by contusion or placental separation, release prostaglandins that stimulate uterine contractions. Progression to labor depends upon the size of uterine damage, the amount of prostaglandins released, and the gestational age of the pregnancy. Occasional uterine contractions, the most common finding after trauma in pregnant women, are not associated with adverse fetal outcomes and resolve within a few hours in 90 % of cases.

The occurrence of eight or more uterine contractions per hour for more than four hours is associated with placental abruption. Uterine contractions, which occur in 39 % [8] of pregnant trauma patients, may progress into preterm labor.

Risk factors, outside of trauma, associated with preterm labor include cardiovascular disease, hypertension, preeclampsia, eclampsia, diabetes, smoking, placenta previa, abruptio placenta, infection, and physical abnormalities. The diagnosis of preterm labor is made by the presence of 3 contractions in 20 min plus cervical change or a cervix that is 2 cm dilated and less than 1 cm in length which can be done by serial cervical examinations [8].

## Spontaneous Abortion

Traumatic injuries may result in spontaneous abortion before the 20th week of gestation. The most common signs and symptoms include abdominal pain or cramping and vaginal bleeding.

## Placental Abruption

Placental abruption results as the inelastic placenta shears away from the elastic uterus during sudden deformation of the uterus. It is one of the most common injuries, usually associated with blunt trauma, and accounts for 50–70 % of fetal losses [8]. Incidence of abruption increased with the severity of injury, from 8.5 % in non-injured pregnant women involved in car accidents to 13 % in women with severe injuries [6]. Maternal mortality from abruption is less than 1 %, but fetal death ranges from 20 to 35 %.

Diagnosis is based on the presence of abdominal pain, vaginal bleeding, uterine tenderness, amniotic fluid leakage, maternal hypovolemia, a uterus larger than normal for the gestational age, or a change in the fetal heart rate, but it can also be present in asymptomatic mothers.

Ultrasound is also not sensitive enough to rule out abruption, necessitating the use of routine posttraumatic fetal cardiotocographic monitoring.

## Uterine Rupture

The risk of uterine rupture is 1 % in pregnant trauma patients (Schwaitzberg 2014). The most common cause of uterine rupture is severe blunt trauma to the abdomen, from a vehicular crash when the pelvis strikes the uterus, leading to rupture. Some uterine rupture also involves penetrating trauma.

Such an injury may result in serosal hemorrhage or abrasions; avulsion of the uterine vasculature with hemorrhage; complete disruption of the myometrial wall with extrusion of the fetus, placenta, or umbilical cord into the abdominal cavity; or complete uterine avulsion.

In spite of adequate counseling about the proper use of seat belts, inappropriate seat belt placement can result in significant force directed directly on the uterus. There is more risk of uterine rupture in intentional penetrating trauma which is often directed at the uterus.

Although 75 % of cases of uterine rupture involve the uterine fundus, rare injuries such as a cornual myometrial defect following blunt trauma had been reported. Clinical presentation can vary from subtle findings (e.g., uterine tenderness, nonreassuring fetal heart rate patterns) to a rapid onset of maternal hypovolemic shock. Typical signs of peritoneal irritation can be identified but are not always evident.

## Fetomaternal Hemorrhage

Fetomaternal hemorrhage (FMH) occurs in approximately 10–30 % of pregnant trauma patients and should be considered as early as the fourth week of gestation when the fetal circulation develops.

*Clinical presentation of FMH is variable and can be nonspecific.*

1. Decreased or absent fetal movements.
2. Fetal distress – especially if the fetal heart tracing is sinusoidal (indicating fetal anemia).
3. Massive FMH is a rare but severe complication which can result in fetal anemia, fetal hypoxia, intrauterine death, or neonatal neurologic damage.
4. Transfusion reaction (nausea, edema, fever, and chills) in the mother.

May occur more commonly with anteriorly located placenta and in women who experience uterine tenderness, contractions, vaginal bleeding, and fetal distress.

*Assessment of fetomaternal hemorrhage:* Kleihauer-Betke test.

- Used to detect and quantify FMH.
- Commonly to determine dose of Rh D immunoglobulin for Rh D-negative women.
- Results are reported quantitatively in mL of fetal blood within maternal circulation.
- A "negative" result is commonly understood to be less than 1 mL of fetal blood.
- It is not a test for placental abruption.

The evidence is limited about the usefulness of a positive Kleihauer test for predicting outcomes and guiding clinical management (beyond determining the dose of Rh D immunoglobulin for Rh D-negative women). This test cannot be used to detect FMH in

Rh-positive mothers or in Rh-negative mothers carrying an Rh-negative fetus. A positive Kleihauer-Betke test along with other parameters, such as third trimester trauma, abdominal trauma, and an Injury Severity Score greater than 2, identifies those at risk for adverse perinatal outcomes. Currently antifetal hemoglobin flow cytometry is used for detecting FMH more accurately.

## Pelvic Fractures

Pelvic fractures, most frequently resulting from blunt trauma to the abdomen, are another concern. Along with significant retroperitoneal hemorrhage, mother may sustain bladder, urethral, or intestinal injuries. Maternal pelvic fractures significantly increase fetal susceptibility to head injury, which accounts for 25 % fetal mortality. Patients with pelvic injuries may present with pelvic pain and signs and symptoms of hypovolemia. Pelvic and acetabular fractures are rare during pregnancy.

Diagnosis is made by physical examination supplemented by radiological studies. Plain X-ray along with uterine shield generally exposes the fetus to very small amounts of radiation. The estimated fetal exposure from a single view hip film is 200 milli Rads which is greater than the estimated exposure from chest X-rays and abdominal films, which are 0.02–0.07 milli Rads and 100 milli Rads, respectively. Yet, these values are much lower than 5 Rad, below which the risks of congenital anomalies, growth restriction, or abortions are not increased [4].

Pelvic fractures are characterized by significant morbidity and mortality rates in both the mother and fetus as they can be associated with hypovolemic shock, particularly in the setting of intraperitoneal bleeding. There is a higher maternal and fetal mortality in automobile-pedestrian collisions when compared with falls. Both maternal and fetal outcomes depend on the degree of injury, although the fracture class (simple versus complex) and type (acetabular versus pelvic), and trimester of pregnancy, did not influence mortality rates.

Pelvic fractures can also be associated with bladder or urethral trauma resulting in hematuria and difficult placement of a urinary catheter. According to the ACOG educational bulletin, a pelvic fracture is not a definite contraindication for vaginal delivery even in the presence of a slightly displaced pelvic fracture [4].

## Hemorrhage and Shock

Hemorrhage should be suspected and assessed after any trauma to a pregnant patient. Cardiovascular changes during pregnancy may make it difficult to detect signs and symptoms associated with maternal hypotension and shock. Acute blood loss resulting in hypovolemia is masked by maternal vasoconstriction and tachycardia. Vasoconstriction severely impacts uterine blood flow by about 30 %, commonly resulting in fetal hypoxia and bradycardia [8].

Shock is a frequent cause of death to both the fetus and mother. It is important that the emergency medical services practitioner anticipate shock and maternal hypotension and not rely solely on vital sign changes to aggressively manage the patient. If the traditional signs and symptoms of hypovolemic shock are exhibited, fetal mortality can be as high as 85 % (Swaitzberg 2010).

## Cardiorespiratory Arrest

Cardiorespiratory arrest in a pregnant female poses a significant threat to the viability of the fetus. About 41 % of fetuses die when the mother suffers a life-threatening injury and more deaths occur with cardiac arrest (Swaitzberg 2010). Aggressive management of the mother is necessary to increase fetal survival. Although the chance of the fetus surviving maternal cardiopulmonary arrest due to trauma is poor, resuscitative attempts should be provided for patients who are more than 24 weeks' pregnant. The receiving facility should be notified in advance so staff can prepare for an emergency Caesarean section. The efficiency of CPR is significantly reduced by aortocaval compression. There is limited evidence about the degree of tilt required to achieve IVC decompression and the effectiveness of chest compressions performed in the left lateral position.

> **Key Points in Management of Cardiorespiratory Arrest**
> 1. Position the woman to reduce IVC compression.
> 2. Defibrillate as for the nonpregnant trauma patient – no significant shock is delivered to the fetus.
> 3. Remove CTG leads prior to defibrillation.
> 4. Administer advanced cardiac life support drugs as would be indicated for the nonpregnant patient.

## Amniotic Fluid Embolism

Exposure of the amniotic fluid to the maternal circulation may cause amniotic fluid embolism and DIC. It may present with maternal respiratory distress, seizure, cardiac arrest, fetal distress, massive hemorrhage, and coagulopathy/DIC. Management is supportive; there is no proven effective treatment. Blood product replacement is done including fresh frozen plasma (FFP), platelets, and cryoprecipitate.

## Disseminated Intravascular Coagulation (DIC)

DIC may arise following placental abruption, fetal demise, and amniotic fluid embolism. Early delivery protects against severe DIC – which is partly due to the massive release of thromboplastins from the damaged uterus.

Clinical presentation may vary from detectable microvascular bleeding as well as abnormal blood coagulation tests including:

Various abnormal blood coagulation tests may be:

1. Platelet count less than 50 × 109/L
2. Prothrombin time (PT) greater than 1.5 × normal
3. International normalized ratio (INR) greater than 1.5
4. Activated partial thromboplastin time (aPTT) greater than 1.5 × normal
5. Fibrinogen level less than 2.5 g/L

## The Initial Evaluation and Management of Pregnant Trauma Patients

### Primary Survey

The primary survey of the injured pregnant patient addresses the airway and cervical spine, breathing, and circulation (ABC; volume replacement/hemorrhage control), with the mother receiving treatment priority.

Severe trauma stimulates maternal catecholamine release, which causes uteroplacental vasoconstriction and compromised fetal circulation. Prevention of aortocaval compression is also essential to optimize maternal and fetal hemodynamics.

### Positioning

After 20 weeks' gestation, aortocaval compression by the uterus impedes resuscitation by decreasing venous return causing supine hypotension, reducing stroke volume and cardiac output, and decreasing the effectiveness of thoracic compressions.

*Position the woman to minimize inferior vena cava (IVC) compression:* consider gestation and the ability to provide effective care (e.g., intubation) when determining positioning requirements:

- Left lateral tilt 15–30°.
- Place a firm wedge under the right buttock/hip to achieve tilt.
- In cases of major trauma, place the wedge under the spinal board (Figs. 25.1 and 25.2).

If lateral tilt is not feasible, manual uterine displacement to minimize IVC compressions is done by standing on the woman's left; the clinician places two hands around the uterus and gently pulls the uterus towards themselves (Fig. 25.3).

Rapid maternal respiratory support is critical; anoxia occurs more quickly in advanced pregnancy because of the changes that occur in

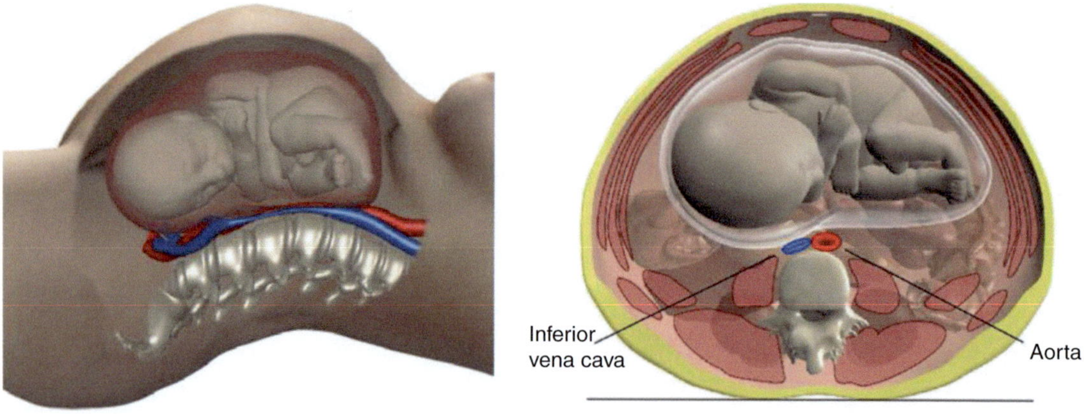


**Fig. 25.1** Inferior vena cava compression when positioned supine. Queensland Clinical Guidelines, Trauma in pregnancy, guideline no MN14.31-V1-R19, Queensland Health. Feb 2014

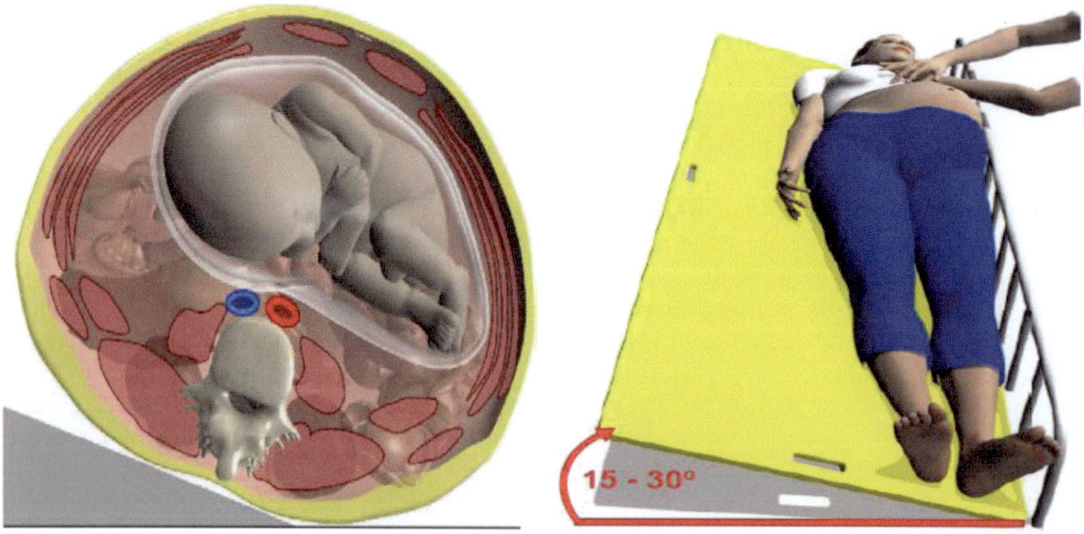


**Fig. 25.2** Left lateral tilt (*right side up*) 15–30° to relieve compression. Queensland Clinical Guidelines, Trauma in pregnancy, guideline no MN14.31-V1-R19, Queensland Health. Feb 2014

respiratory physiology during pregnancy. Supplemental oxygen is essential to prevent maternal and fetal hypoxia.

## Airway and C-Spine

There is increased risk of failed intubation due to laryngeal edema from water retention, lingual and nasal mucosa swelling from capillary engorgement, increased facial adipose tissue affecting space for maneuvering laryngoscope handle, increased abdominal contents elevating diaphragm with anterior shifting larynx, and morbid obesity (heavier than 300 lb). Mask ventilation may also be difficult due to increased intra-abdominal pressure and low chest compliance. Due to these, earlier intubation of nonpregnant patients is considered. Use short handle laryngoscope, cricoid pressure, and a smaller endotracheal tube (ETT) due to laryngeal edema. Factors increasing the risk of aspiration associated with pregnancy include gravid uterus, progesterone mediated lower oesophageal sphincter relaxation, lower gastric pH and delayed gastric emptying during labour. Due to this, consider insertion of an orogastric tube if intubated and nasogastric tube if not intubated. Cervical spine collar should be applied.

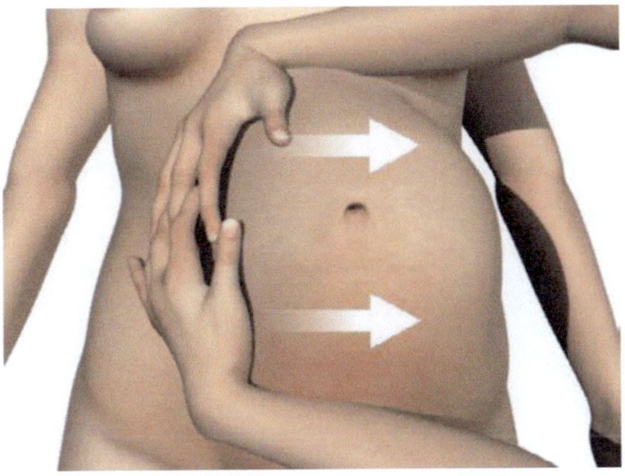

**Fig. 25.3** Manual displacement of the uterus to relieve compression (*arrows*). Queensland Clinical Guidelines, Trauma in pregnancy, guideline no MN14.31-V1-R19, Queensland Health. Feb 2014

## Breathing and Ventilation

Supplemental high flow 100 % oxygen is routinely administered provided by nasal cannula, mask, or endotracheal intubation as deemed appropriate for the situation. Ventilation volumes may need to be reduced because of elevated diaphragm. If safe to do so, raise the head of the bed to reduce weight of uterus on the diaphragm and facilitate breathing. If a chest tube is indicated, place tube 1–2 intercostal spaces above usual fifth intercostal space landmark due to raised diaphragm.

## Circulation and Hemorrhage Control

Hypovolemia should be suspected before it becomes apparent because of the relative pregnancy-induced hypervolemia and hemodilution that may mask significant blood losses. Additionally, the mother's blood pressure may be maintained by shunting blood away from the uterus. Up to 25 % of maternal intravascular blood volume may be lost without change in maternal vital signs. Aggressive volume resuscitation is encouraged even for normotensive patients.

1. Obvious external hemorrhage should be controlled.
2. Position with left lateral tilt 15–30°.
3. Obtain large-bore intravenous (IV) access.
4. Avoid femoral lines due to compression by gravid uterus.
5. Commence crystalloid IV.
6. Assess response – maintain an awareness of pregnancy-related physiological parameters.
7. Aim to avoid large volumes of crystalloids (greater than 2 L) which may lead to pulmonary edema due to the relatively low oncotic pressure in pregnancy.
8. Avoid vasopressors to restore maternal BP as they may compromise uteroplacental flow.
9. Maintain a high index of suspicion for bleeding and an awareness of the limitations of clinical signs.
10. Perform a thorough search for occult bleeding as maternal blood flow is maintained at expense of fetus.
11. Conduct focused abdominal sonography for trauma (FAST) to assess for intra-abdominal hemorrhage.
12. If hypovolemia is suspected, initiate fluid resuscitation to ensure adequate maternal and uteroplacental perfusion.
13. Consider Massive Transfusion Protocol (MTP) activation if nonresponsive to crystalloids.
14. Rapid transfer to operating theatre as indicated.
15. Evaluate fetal heart rate but do not delay resuscitation for fetal assessments.

## Disability

Rapid neurological evaluation utilizing the Glasgow Coma Scale. The examination should be a focused assessment of the patient's level of consciousness using the Glasgow Coma Scale and also an evaluation of their pupillary size, gross motor function, and sensation in each limb. If signs, symptoms, or suspicion of spinal cord injury is present, it is especially important to note any lateralizing signs and the level of intact sensation.

The pneumatic antishock garment (PASG) may be used to stabilize lower extremity fractures and perhaps control hemorrhage. In the pregnant patient, inflation of the abdominal compartment of the PASG should be avoided because it compromises uteroplacental blood flow.

**Flow Chart: Initial assessment and management of the pregnant trauma patient**

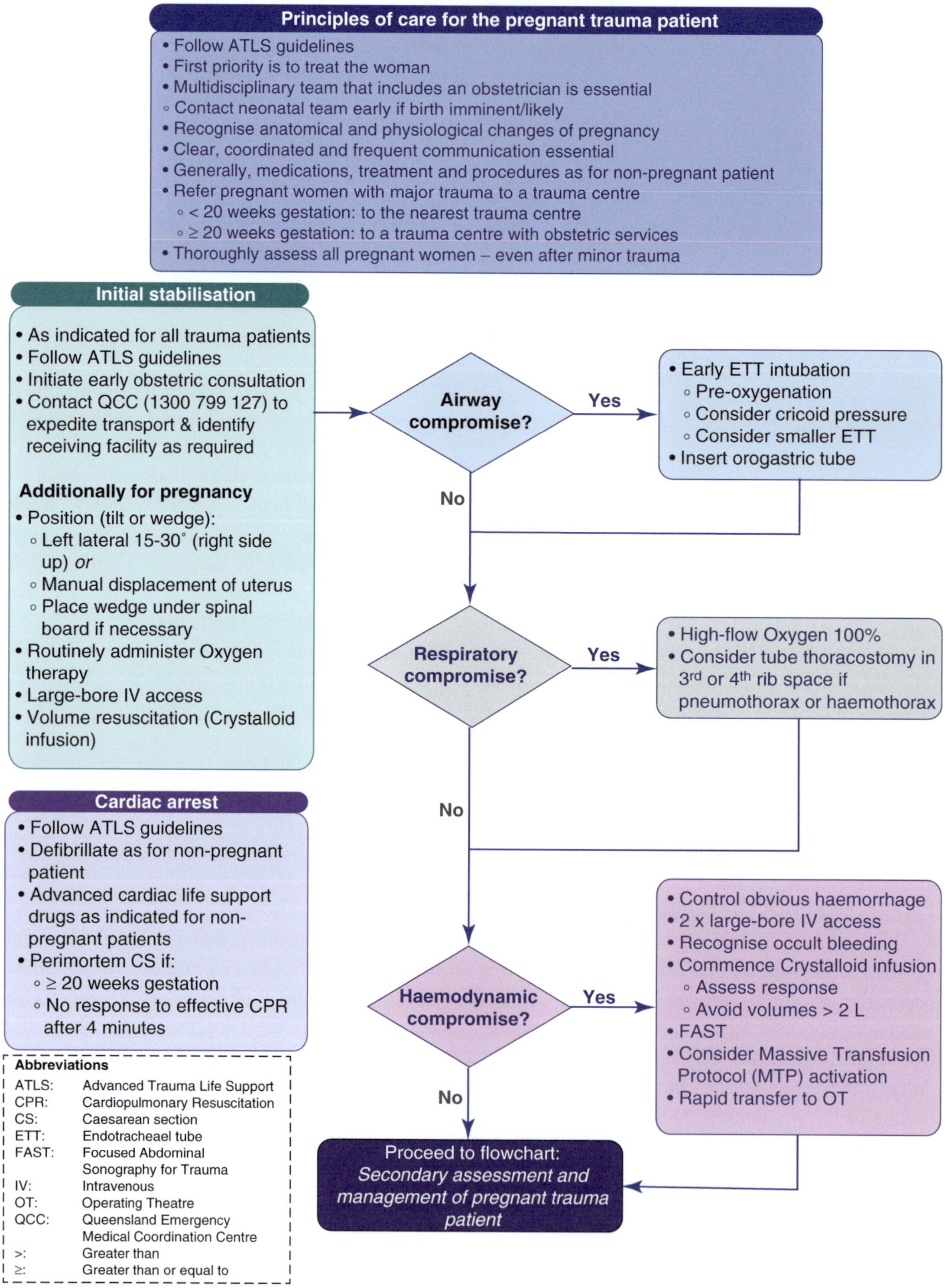


Queensland Clinical Guideline: Trauma in pregnancy. Guideline No: MN14.31-V1-R19

## Secondary Survey

The secondary survey consists of obtaining a complete history, including an obstetrical history, performing a physical examination, and evaluating and monitoring the fetus. The obstetrical history is important because the identification of comorbid factors may alter management decisions

## Obstetric History

The obstetrical history should include the date of the last menstruation, expected date of delivery and any problems or complications of the current and previous pregnancies, prenatal care, and history of vaginal bleeding.

## Physical Examination

The findings of the physical examination in the pregnant woman with blunt trauma are not reliable in predicting adverse obstetric outcomes. Head-to-toe examination as for nonpregnant trauma patients is done. Abdomen is inspected for ecchymosis or asymmetry.

Compared with nonpregnant persons, pregnant women have a higher incidence of serious abdominal injury but a lower incidence of chest and head injuries. Maternal pelvic fractures, particularly in late pregnancy, are associated with bladder injury, urethral injury, retroperitoneal bleeding, and fetal skull fracture. After 12 weeks of gestation, the maternal uterus and bladder are no longer exclusively pelvic organs and are more susceptible to direct injury.

Skull fracture is the most common direct fetal injury, with a mortality rate of 42 %. Altered mental status or severe head injury after trauma in a pregnant woman is associated with increased adverse fetal outcomes.

In cases of motor vehicle accident, incorrect positioning of the seat belt across the gravid uterus may cause marked bruising of the abdomen, increase the risk of placental abruption, and increase the risk of uterine rupture. Assess uterine tone, contractions, rigidity, tenderness, and palpable fetal parts. The gravid abdomen may be relatively insensate to peritoneal irritation.

### Estimation of Gestational Age

Gestational age can be estimated by measuring fundal height and the vertical distance in the midline from the symphysis pubis to the top of the fundus in centimeters. The top of the fundus is marked to evaluate the possibility of concealed abruption as noted by increasing fundal height.

### Fetal Heart Rate Monitoring

Normal FHR 110–160 bpm. FHR can be assessed using standard stethoscope from about 20 weeks and Doppler from about 12 weeks. Maternal and FHR should be differentiated as maternal tachycardia may cause confusion.

For gestations greater than 24 weeks (major trauma), continuous cardiotocography (CTG) should be initiated as soon as possible. It has a good sensitivity for immediate adverse outcome. It detects uterine irritability and abnormal fetal heart rate patterns. Abnormal CTG may be the only indication of injury or compromise to the fetus. Persistent fetal bradycardia more than 5 min, loss of baseline variability or recurrent complex variable, or late decelerations indicate fetal compromise. Sinusoidal trace indicates fetal anemia.

Physiological control of FHR and resultant CTG trace interpretation differs in the preterm fetus compared to the term fetus, especially at gestations less than 28 weeks. Four hours of continuous monitoring is sufficient in the absence of vaginal bleeding and abdominal pain, uterine contractions more frequent than 1 in 10 min, and non-reassuring fetal heart rate tracing. Additional monitoring up to 24 h is warranted with any evidence of more frequent uterine contractions, non-reassuring fetal heart testing, vaginal bleeding, significant uterine tenderness or irritability, serious maternal injury, or rupture of the amniotic membranes

Staff and equipment should be moved to the woman's location rather than transporting a women to an obstetric unit for monitoring.

## Pelvic/Vaginal Examination

In case of major trauma, a rectal examination should be performed to assess for spinal cord damage or local trauma. Sterile speculum vaginal examination should be performed as clinically indicated. Evaluation for ruptured membranes, vaginal bleeding, cord prolapse, cervical effacement, and dilation in labor and fetal presentation should be done. Vaginal bleeding may indicate preterm labor, abruption, pelvic fracture, or uterine rupture. Urinary catheter insertion may be done if required.

## Diagnostic Imaging

The fetus is most vulnerable to radiation during the first 15 weeks of gestation. The risks of radiation to the fetus are small compared with the risk of missed or delayed diagnosis of trauma. Increased risks to the embryo or fetus have not been observed for intellectual disability, birth defects, growth restriction, neurobehavioral effects, impaired school performance, convulsive disorders, or embryonic or fetal death below an effective dose of 100 millisievert (mSv) [5].

Although iodinated contrast agents cross the placenta and may be taken up by the fetal thyroid, no cases of fetal goiter or abnormal neonatal thyroid function have been reported in connection with in utero contrast exposure. Gadolinium used in MRI has known teratogenic effects on animals and is not recommended unless benefits clearly outweigh the risks.

X-ray examinations of the extremities, head, and skull, mammography, and computerized tomography (CT) examinations of the head and neck can be undertaken on pregnant or possibly pregnant women without concern. Other X-ray examinations may also be undertaken if the radiation dose to the embryo or fetus is likely to be less than 1 mSv [5].

Risk benefit ratio should be assessed where a procedure on a pregnant woman may result in a radiation dose of more than 1 mSv to an embryo or fetus.

Personal protective equipment, (e.g., lead gown) is advised for pregnant women only when the position of the uterus is in the direct X-ray beam (and not if it interferes with imaging). It is preferable to perform a single CT scan with iodinated contrast rather than perform multiple suboptimal studies without contrast. Information and counseling to women exposed to radiation during diagnosis and care should be done.

## Ultrasound

Ultrasound (US) can assess solid organ injury, intraperitoneal fluid, gestational age, FHR, fetal activity, fetal presentation, extent of fetal injury, placental location, amniotic fluid volume, and biophysical profile. US is not a reliable indicator of recent placental abruption. FAST (focused assessment with sonography for trauma) scan is as accurate as in nonpregnant patients for intra-abdominal free fluid. Formal obstetric US following FAST should be done if required. It helps identify intra-abdominal fluid, thus increasing the index of suspicion for an intraperitoneal hemorrhage.

## CT Scan

Another imaging modality that may be indicated during evaluation of a trauma patient during pregnancy is computed tomography (CT), which generally exposes the fetus to 3.5 rad. Although a CT scan is indicated in cases where its benefits to the mother outweigh its associated fetal risks, proper counseling, when possible, remains warranted.

## Open Peritoneal Lavage

Open peritoneal lavage may be necessary if an intraperitoneal hemorrhage is suspected on the basis of abdominal signs or symptoms suggestive of intraperitoneal bleeding, altered sensorium, unexplained shock, major thoracic injuries, and multiple major orthopedic injuries. Open peritoneal lavage, usually periumbilical, with sharp dissection and opening of the anterior abdominal peritoneum under direct vision is the preferred technique in pregnancy as this is less likely to injure the uterus or other organs compared with blind needle insertion. It is important to emphasize that, if intraperitoneal bleeding is clinically evident, a lavage is not indicated.

**Flow Chart: Secondary assessment and management of the pregnant trauma patient**

**Secondary survey**

**As for non-pregnant patient AND**

- Consult obstetric team
- Maintain high index of suspicion for occult shock and abdominal injury
- Maintain position (tilt or wedge) left lateral 15-30˚ (right side up) *or*
  - Manual displacement of uterus
  - Wedge spinal board if required
- Obtain obstetric history
  - Gestation
  - Estimated date of delivery
  - Pregnancy complications
- Physical examination
- Assess uterus
  - Tone, rigidity, tenderness
  - Contractions
- Estimate gestational age
  - Fundal height
  - US
  - If uncertain (i.e. severe trauma, no prior US or lack of accurate records) presume viability
- Assess and record FHR
  - Stethoscope *or*
  - Doppler

**Consider - especially for major trauma**

- Rectal examination
- Pelvic exam (obstetric team)
  - Sterile speculum
  - Assess for rupture of membranes, vaginal bleeding, cervical effacement and dilation, cord prolapse, fetal presentation
- Imaging
  - FAST ultrasound
  - Formal obstetric ultrasound
  - Other radiographs
- Blood tests
  - Standard trauma bloods
  - Group and Antibody screen
  - Kleihauer Test if Rh D negative and all women if major trauma (EDTA tube)
  - Consider Coag Profile (major trauma)
- If Rh D negative and ≥ 12 weeks gestation, administer Rh D immunoglobulin (but do not delay definitive care to do so)

→ **Gestation > 24 weeks?**

- **Yes or uncertain** →
  - CTG
    - Application and interpretation by experienced obstetric team member
    - Interpret with caution at < 28 weeks
  - Monitor uterine activity
- **No** → (and following CTG) → **Maternal or fetal compromise?**

**Maternal or fetal compromise?**

- **Yes** → Admit
- **No** → Consider discharge criteria

**Consider discharge criteria**

- Obstetric team consulted/agree for discharge
- Reassuring maternal status
- No vaginal loss/bleeding
- Normal CTG/FHR (minimum 4 hours CTG)
  - Interpret CTG with caution at < 28 weeks
- No contractions
- Blood results reviewed
- Rh immunoglobulin given if required
- Social worker referral offered

→ **Discharge criteria met?**

- **Yes** → Discharge
- **No** → Admit

**Discharge**

- Advise to seek medical advice if:
  - Signs of preterm labour
  - Abdominal pain
  - Vaginal bleeding or discharge
  - Change in fetal movements
- Advise to inform usual maternity care provider of trauma event

**Admit**

- Assess for:
  - Placental abruption
  - Feto-maternal haemorrhage
  - Uterine rupture
  - Preterm labour
  - DIC
- Continuous CTG if > 24 weeks gestation
- Intervene as appropriate
- Consider emergency CS

**Abbreviations**

| | |
|---|---|
| CS: | Caesarean section |
| CTG: | Cardiotocograph |
| DIC: | Disseminated intravascular coagulopathy |
| FAST: | Focused Abdominal Sonography for trauma |
| FHR: | Fetal heart rate |
| US: | Ultrasound scan |
| <: | Less than |
| >: | Greater than |
| ≥: | Greater than or equal to |

Queensland Clinical Guideline: Trauma in pregnancy. Guideline No: MN14.31-V1-R19

## Perimortem Caesarean Section

It is a Caesarean section (CS) that is initiated after CPR has commenced. It may improve survival of either or both the woman and fetus but should be considered a resuscitative procedure performed primarily in the interests of maternal survival. It improved maternal condition/survival from the increase in venous return after removal of the gravid uterus from the IVC.

Survival and neurologic outcome of the viable fetus is related to time between maternal death and birth. Best fetal survival occurs when birth is within 4–6 min of the maternal cardiac arrest. Intact fetal survival has not been demonstrated beyond 30 min of cardiac arrest. Delay in initiating a perimortem CS has been linked to adverse outcomes.

### Management

Where gestation is greater than 20 weeks, perimortem CS is performed 4 min after commencement of nonresponse to effective CPR. CS is performed at the point of resuscitation. CPR is continued during and after the procedure.

## Prevention Strategies

Prenatal care is essential for optimal outcomes for the pregnant patient and the infant. Part of prenatal care is appropriate education regarding prevention of injury, particularly blunt trauma, although proper seat belt use.

### Social Violence

Interpersonal violence has been emphasized as an etiology of trauma only during the past few decades. Sexual or physical abuse occurs in up to 17–32 % of pregnancies, and 60 % of those abused reported multiple episodes of abuse. Abuse often begins or escalates during pregnancy or the immediate postpartum period. Most often the abuser is known to the patient, frequently her husband or partner. Such interpersonal violence is not a function of marital status, race, age, or economic status. All healthcare workers must be aware of this epidemic and must aid in reduction of such abuse, especially during pregnancy.

### Use of Illegal Drugs during Pregnancy

Unfortunately, significant numbers of pregnant women who are injured have elevated blood levels of alcohol or other drugs. These substances contribute to automobile accidents as well as low birth weights.

### Automobile Restraint Systems and Patient Education

Ejection from a moving automobile results in great injury to anyone in an accident. Restraint systems, both air bags and appropriately worn lap belts, decrease the incidence of injury and are considered to be safe for pregnant females. Education about how these lap belts should be worn low at the pelvic brim and not on top of the gravid uterus will aid in decreasing lap belt-associated injury.

*Correct positioning of the seat belt includes:*

- Lap belt over hips below uterus
- Sash between breasts above uterus

*Correct application of the seat belt:*

- Reduces maternal/fetal injuries
- Reduces ejection mortalities
- Improves fetal survival

The use of a lap belt only is not recommended. It increases uterine flexion and may increase placental abruption (Fig. 25.4).

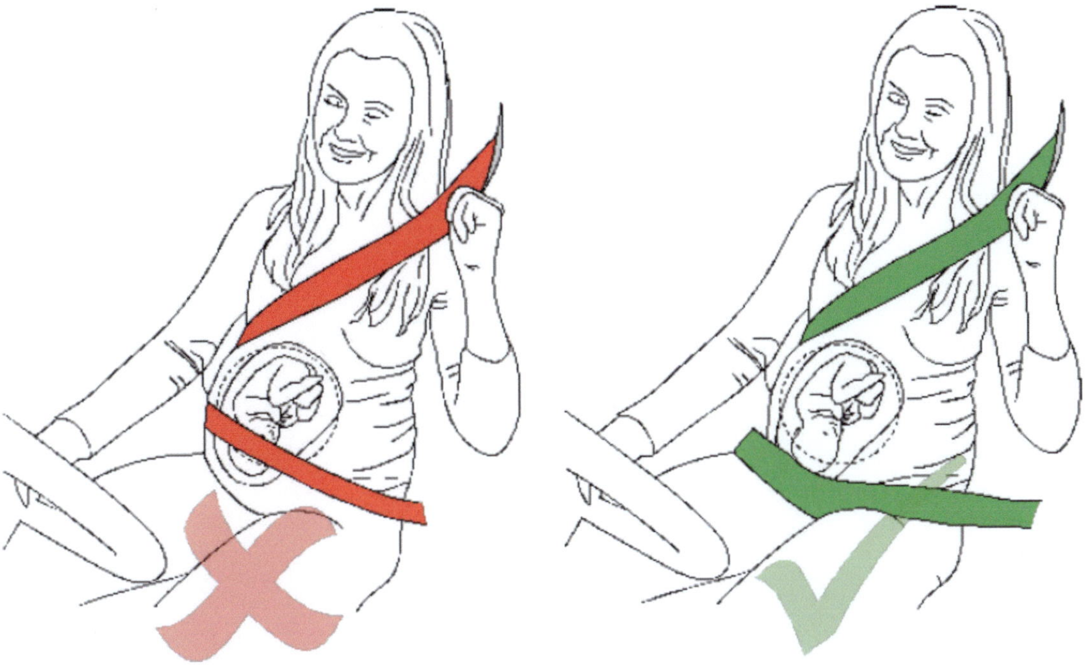

**Fig. 25.4** Queensland Clinical Guidelines, Trauma in pregnancy, guideline no MN14.31-V1-R19, Queensland Health. Feb 2014

## References


1. Chapter 42. Critical care and trauma. In: Cunningham F, Leveno K, Bloom S, Hauth J, Rouse D, Spong C, editors. Williams obstetrics. 23rd ed. 2010. p. 926–45.
2. Desjardins G. Management of the injured pregnant patient. 2014. http://www.trauma.org/archive/resus/pregnancytrauma.html.
3. Mattox KL, Goetzl L. Trauma in pregnancy. Crit Care Med. 2005;33(10 (Suppl)):S385–9.
4. Mirza FG, Devine PC, Gaddipati S. Trauma in pregnancy: a systematic approach. Am J Perinatol. 2010;27(7):579–86.
5. Queensland Clinical Guidelines, Trauma in pregnancy. guideline no MN14.31-V1-R19, Queensland Health. Feb 2014. Available from: http://www.health.qld.gov.au/qcg/.
6. Raja AS, Zabbo CP. Trauma in pregnancy. Emerg Med Clin North Am. 2012;30:937–48.
7. Rudra A, Ray A, Chatterjee S, et al. Trauma in pregnancy. Indian J Anaesth. 2007;51(2):100–5.
8. Schwaitzberg SD. Trauma and pregnancy. 2013. http://emedicine.medscape.com/article/796979-overview.


## Suggested Reading


Barraco RD, et al. Diagnosis and management of injury in the pregnant patient: the East Practice Management Guideline Work Group. 2005. Copyright the eastern association of surgery for trauma.

Brown HL. Trauma in pregnancy. Obstet Gynecol. 2009;114(1):147–60.

Bryan CA, et al. Beyond the basics: trauma during pregnancy. EMS Mag. 2009;38(2):52–5. EMS World.com.

Hill CC, Pickinpaugh J. Trauma and surgical emergencies in the obstetric patient. Surg Clin North Am. 2008;88(2):421–40.

Roemer, Katz, Becerra, Ogburn, Bowes, Roemer B. Trauma in the obstetric patient: a bedside tool. 2014. Americal College of Emergency Physicians. www.acep.org.

Royal College of Obstetricians and Gynecologists. Maternal collapse in pregnancy and puerperium. 2011. www.rcog.org.uk. Green-top Guideline No. 56.

Shah AJ, Kilcline BA. Trauma in pregnancy. Emerg Med Clin North Am. 2003;21:615–29.

South Australian Perinatal Practice Guidelines Trauma in pregnancy (abdominal). Department of Health, Government of South Australia; 2010. ISBN no. 948-1-74242-164–2.

State trauma guidelines for the management of injured pregnant women. Govt. of Western Australia Department of Health; 2012.

Women and newborn health service, King Edward Memorial Hospital, Clinical guidelines. DPMS Ref: 8864. 2014.

# Burns in Pregnancy

# 26

Reeti Mehra and Sanjay Gupta

## Introduction

Thermal injury during pregnancy requires special consideration. The presence of foetus leads to a number of maternal physiological changes, and burn wounds pose additional stress on body systems that are already modified. This compromises body's ability to respond to burns and the reserve required for foetal well-being, thus increasing the risk to both the mother and foetus. It is rarely reported from developed nations, and most of the available data is from developing countries. The incidence in reproductive age group varies from 0.6 to 15 % in different series with highest being reported from India (Table 26.1) [1–8]. Flame burn involving kerosene oil is the most common type of burn seen in these countries. Illiteracy, unsafe cooking habits and social custom of dowry are some of the factors responsible for this high prevalence. In contrast, in developed countries, burns are accidental in nature and are usually scalds or industry-related flame burns [8].

The paucity of data has made it difficult to frame the standard management guidelines of such patients. This chapter aims to describe the management of pregnant female with thermal injuries on the basis of limited available literature.

## Classification and Estimation of Burn Wounds

### Burn Depth

It is classified on the basis of degree of injury to the epidermis, dermis, subcutaneous fat and underlying structures.

*First-degree burns* are confined to the epidermis. These burns are painful, erythematous and blanch to the touch with an intact epidermal barrier. These burns do not result in scarring.

*Second-degree burns* are divided into two types: superficial and deep. This division is based on the depth of injury into the dermis. Superficial dermal burns are erythematous, painful and blanch to touch and often lead to blister formation. These wounds re-epithelialize spontaneously from retained epidermal structures in the rete ridges, hair follicles and sweat glands in 7–14 days. Deep dermal burns that extend

R. Mehra (✉)
Department of Obstetrics and Gynecology, Govt. Medical College and Hospital, Chandigarh 160030, India
e-mail: drreetidatta@yahoo.co.in

S. Gupta
Department of Surgery, Govt. Medical College and Hospital, Chandigarh 160030, India
e-mail: sandiv99@me.com


A. Gandhi et al. (eds.), *Principles of Critical Care in Obstetrics: Volume II*,
DOI 10.1007/978-81-322-2686-4_26

**Table 26.1** Case series reported from India

| Author (year) | Incidence in reproductive age group (%) | Number of cases | Maternal mortality (%) | Foetal mortality (%) |
|---|---|---|---|---|
| Bhattt (1974) [1] | NA | 28 | 71.4 | 82.1 |
| Jain (1993) [2] | 13.3 | 25 | 20 | 36 |
| Akhtar(1994) [3] | 7.1 | 50 | 70 | 72 |
| Sarkar(1996) [4] | NA | 20 | 0 | 60 |
| Prassana (1996) [5] | 15 | 6 | 16.6 | 16.6 |
| Gaffar (2007) [6] | 14.9 | 32 | 71.8 | 81.2 |
| Zalquarnain (2012) [7] | 12.7 | 87 | 21.8 | 54.02 |
| Aggarwal (2014) [8] | 12.2 | 49 | 67.3 | 69.3 |

*NA* not available

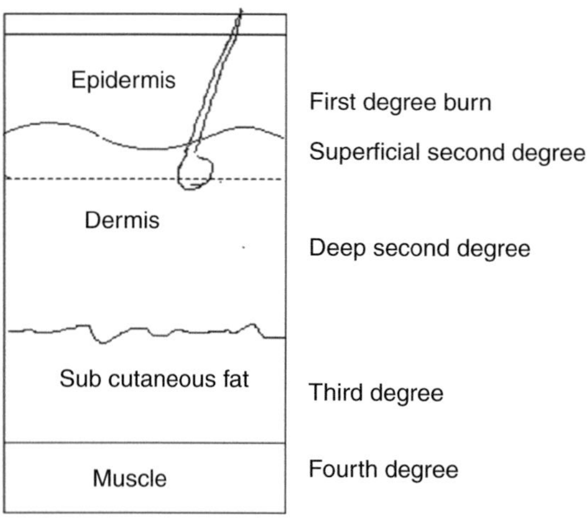


**Fig. 26.1** Burn depth

into the reticular dermis, appear more pale and mottled, and do not blanch to touch but remain painful to pinprick. These burns heal in 14–35 days by re-epithelialization from hair follicles and sweat gland keratinocytes, often with severe scarring.

*Third-degree burns* are full thickness through the epidermis and dermis and are characterized by a hard, leathery eschar that is painless and black, white or cherry red. These wounds heal by re-epithelialization from the wound edges. Deep dermal and full-thickness burns usually require excision with skin grafting.

*Fourth-degree burns* involve other organs beneath the skin, such as the muscle and bone (Fig. 26.1).

## Burn Size

Burn size is generally assessed by the 'rule of nines' (Fig. 26.2). In adults, each upper extremity and the head and neck are 9 % of the total body surface area (TBSA), the lower extremities and the anterior and posterior trunk are 18 % each, and the perineum and genitalia are considered to be 1 % of the TBSA. For smaller burns, the area of the open hand (including the palm and the extended fingers) of the patient is taken as 1 % TBSA.

## Management

In addition to preterm labour and intrauterine foetal death, the pregnant woman with major burns is at risk of all the serious complications that can occur in a nonpregnant woman like cardiovascular instability, respiratory distress, sepsis, liver failure and renal failure. Therefore, a multidisciplinary approach involving a plastic surgeon, obstetrician and intensivist is required for the management of burned pregnant patient. Going by the high incidence of burns in reproductive age group (up to 15 %), all female burned patients of child-bearing age should be tested for pregnancy unless the pregnancy is obvious. Early diagnosis of pregnancy helps in avoiding teratogenic drugs and ionizing imaging studies and at the same time helps in initiating optimal therapy for better outcome [9].

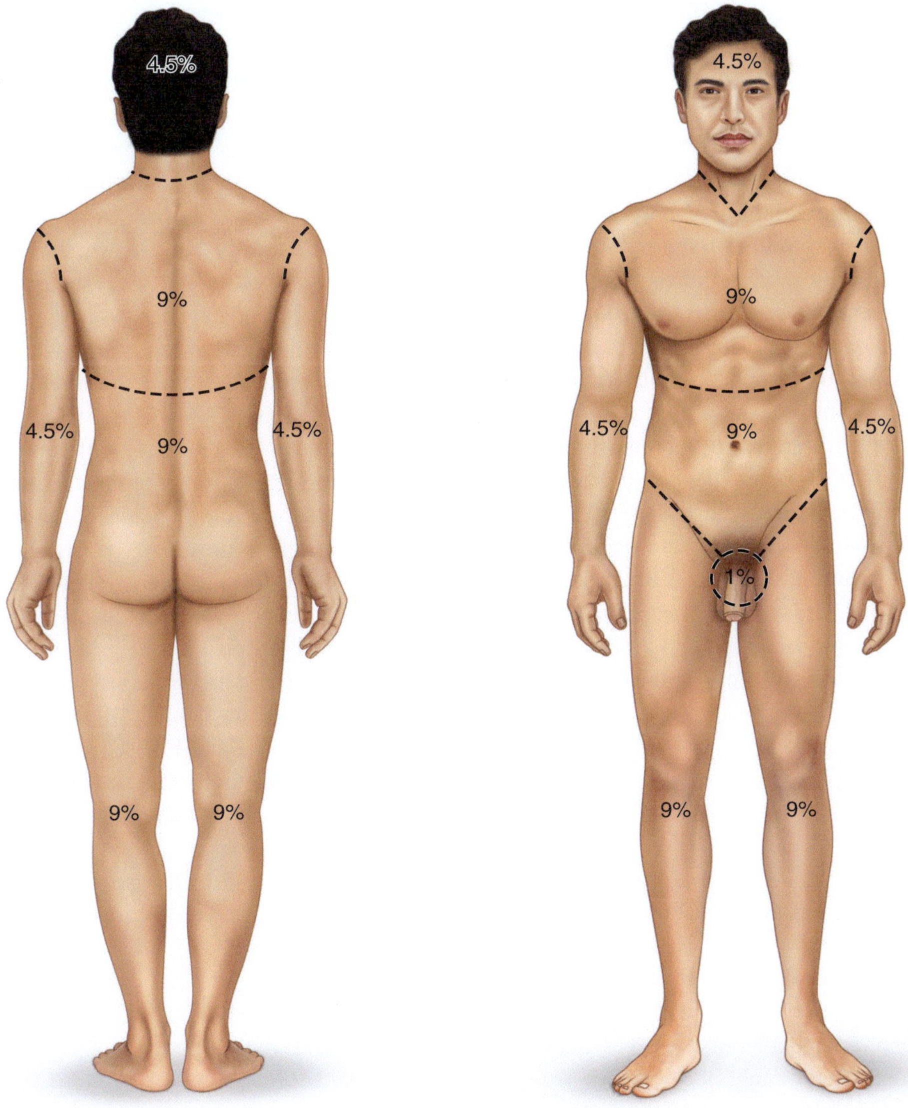


**Fig. 26.2** Burn size

## Fluid Therapy

Proper fluid management is critical to survival following major thermal injury. One of the principal causes of multiple organ failure system (MOFS) is found to be inadequate fluid resuscitation. The primary goal of fluid resuscitation is to ensure end-organ perfusion by replacing fluid that is sequestrated as a result of the thermal injury. Pregnancy is associated with hyperdynamic circulation. As pregnancy progresses, there is also progressive fall in colloid osmotic pressure. These changes, along with an increase capillary permeability in burned patient, predispose the burned pregnant patient to additional fluid loss beyond the amount as seen in nonpregnant individuals. Because uterus has little capacity for autoregulation, early and aggressive fluid resuscitation is vital to avoid maternal hypotension and resultant utero-placental hypoperfusion and foetal hypoxia in these patients [10, 11].

In nonpregnant patients, the fluid requirement in early postburn is estimated using *Parkland formula*. According to this, the fluid requirement in the first 24-h postburn period is 4 ml/kg body weight per percent of burned body surface area. One half of this fluid is to be given in the first 8 h and the rest in the next 16 h. However, it has been found that this formula underestimates the fluid requirement in pregnant patients by almost 50 %. Therefore, it is suggested that volume resuscitation should be titrated to other parameters like urine output (30–60 ml/h), mean arterial pressure, central venous pressure (CVP) and maternal and foetal heart rate, rather than by Parkland formula. As far as the choice of fluid is concerned, crystalloid, i.e. lactated Ringer solution, should be preferred as normal saline invariably leads to hyperchloremic metabolic acidosis [12].

### Ventilation

Thermal injury to the respiratory tract is usually manifests as mucosal and submucosal erythema, oedema and ulceration. It is usually limited to upper airway because of reflex closure of vocal cords to hot air. The presence of significant intraoral and pharyngeal injury is an indication for early endotracheal intubation.

Supplemental oxygen and nursing in semi-sitting posture is recommended for all patients even in the absence of smoke inhalation injury. This improves tissue oxygenation, especially in third trimester when there is reduced functional residual capacity and end-expiratory volume. Inhalation injury must be suspected in patients who sustain burns in closed space or have facial burns. Inhaled carbon monoxide crosses placental barrier, binds to foetal Hb and can result in foetal hypoxemia. Supplementing 100% oxygen helps in reversing this by reducing half-life of carboxyhemoglobin. Ventilatory support should only be initiated when maternal $pO_2$ is less than 60 mmHg [13].

## Wound Management

### Burn Wound Excision

For deeper wounds (deep partial thickness and full thickness), rather than waiting for spontaneous healing, the eschar is surgically removed and wound is closed by split skin graft or by flap. This approach is known as early excision and grafting (E&G). Any burn wound projected to take longer than 3 weeks to heal is a candidate for E&G within the first postburn week. Early tangential excision of burn wound and grafting improves maternal and foetal outcome by reducing septic complications. Removal of burn eschar also reduces the circulating level of prostaglandin E2 (PGE2) and a burn toxin-A lipoprotein complex released form damaged cell membranes, which are responsible for uterine stimulation [5, 14]. Early excision and grafting also minimizes excessive scar formation which is associated with secondary healing of wounds. Wounds over the abdomen and breasts should be treated first. This helps in pain-free stretching of abdominal wall as pregnancy develops, better supervision of growing foetus and easy performance of caesarean section if need arises. Better healing of breast wound prevents infection and sloughing of nipples and subsequent breastfeed. Early excision is recommended not only in patients who sustain minor burns but also in patients who has full-thickness major burns ranging from 25 to 65 % [10, 15].

### Wound Infection

All burn wounds become colonized by 72 h after the injury. Bacteria colonize on the surface of the wound or may penetrate the eschar. This colonization is of no clinical significance; hence, routine wound cultures are not recommended. Bacterial colonization beneath the eschar at the viable nonviable interface rather helps in eschar separation in cases where early E&G is not done. Wound sepsis occurs only if microorganisms invade the deeper viable tissue. This can be diagnosed by biopsy or quantitative tissue culture demonstrating greater than $10^5$ organisms per gram of tissue. Once the diagnosis of wound sepsis is confirmed, suitable antibiotics should be given along with wound excision.

## Use of Topical and Systemic Antibiotics

Chloramphenicol, either in powder form or ointment form, is absolutely contraindicated in pregnancy. It has teratogenic effect if used in the first trimester and can lead to grey baby syndrome in newborns if used in the final trimester. Gentamicin, if used after 14th week of pregnancy, can cause ototoxicity and nephrotoxicity. Most commonly used topical ointment silver sulfadiazine is found to be teratogenic if applied before 14th week of pregnancy and can cause growth retardation if used subsequently. Povidone-iodine, one of the widely used agents for cleaning burn wounds, is not recommended if TBSA increases by more than 20 %. The iodine absorbed through burn wound will cross the placental barrier and can cause thyroid dysfunction and metabolic acidosis. Vancomycin, one of the most commonly used anti-staphylococcal drug, is considered as teratogenic, and ciprofloxacin can damage the articular cartilages [15].

The choice of antibiotics is therefore very limited in burned pregnant patient. The need of antibiotics can be minimized by early wound excision and split skin grafting as this significantly reduces the chances of wound infection. Penicillins and cephalosporins are antibiotics that are considered to be safe in pregnancy.

## Nutritional Support

The hypermetabolic response to burns is associated with exaggerated energy expenditure and massive nitrogen loss. The aim of nutritional support therefore is to provide adequate calories to match energy expenditure and to provide enough nitrogen to replace or support body protein stores. To achieve a positive nitrogen balance, 36 kcal/kg/day with a protein of 1.5–2.0 g/kg/day is recommended. The route of nutritional support directly influences the outcome in burned patients. Total enteral nutrition (TEN) is preferred over total parenteral nutrition (TPN). TPN is indicated only if enteral nutrition fails as TPN is associated with increased mortality due to septic complications [16].

## Obstetric Management

The most common complication for the foetus is intrauterine foetal distress followed by spontaneous abortion and premature labour. In case of maternal hypovolemia, blood is diverted from the gravid uterus to the maternal circulation. Thermal injuries also increase prostaglandin levels and oxytocin release. These actions along with hypovolemia decrease uteroplancetal circulation leading to foetal hypoxia and acidosis thus increasing risk of preterm labour or spontaneous abortion [17].

Foetal survival depends gestational age and extent of maternal injury. Foetal loss is usually high in the first trimester. In the second trimester, the survival is dependent on maternal survival. Therefore, in the second trimester in case preterm labour occurs, tocolytic therapy should be initiated provided the condition of mother permits. Parenteral magnesium sulphate is a better choice than β-mimetic agent as it has got less vasodilatory and metabolic effect. Electronic foetal heart monitoring and ultrasonography should be regularly done to confirm foetal well-being during conservative therapy. However, in the presence of maternal distress, emergency caesarean section is indicated. In the third trimester, conservative approach or urgent delivery (induction/caesarean section) should be considered depending on the extent of injury. Modern neonatal intensive care units have improved the survival for neonates delivered in the third trimester. Therefore, elective obstetrical intervention is indicated in severely burned only if the patient is in the third trimester or if there are features of hypoxia or sepsis. The manner of delivery (vaginal or caesarean section) should be decided on the basis of obstetric considerations, and caesarean section is not a contraindication even when the lower abdominal wall is burned [8].

The general scheme regarding obstetric management of burned pregnant patients as proposed by Gang et al. [18] in 1992 is still being followed (Table 26.2).

## Thromboprophylaxis

Burns aggravates the hypercoagulable state of pregnancy by activation of coagulation system with the release of cytokines. The hemoconcentration associated with fluid loss may further increase the risk thrombosis. The use of prophylactic doses of unfractionated heparin or low-molecular-weight heparin is therefore strongly recommended to prevent deep vein thrombosis and associated complications [15].

## Anaesthetic Considerations

Similar general anaesthesia techniques can be applied for both burn wound excision and for caesarean section. Prevention of hypoxia and hypotension during anaesthesia is vital during any surgical procedure. Intraoperatively, 1 ml/kg/h of urine output and 100 % oxygen saturation should be maintained. In use of difficult intubation due to airway oedema, uses of GlideScope, cricoid pressure and small diameter endotracheal tube (6.5 mm) are other options. Among drugs, ketamine should be avoided as it triggers myometrium excitability and can induce premature labour. Succinylcholine can be safely used within 12–24 h of thermal injury, but beyond this, there is a risk of hyperkalaemia. Non-depolarizing muscle relaxants like curare and pancuronium are found to be safer options [12, 19, 20].

## Psychosocial Care

Psychosocial care should begin immediately. The patient and family members must be made comfortable, and a realistic assessment regarding the prognosis of the burns must be given. At the same time, because of high incidence of homicidal and suicidal burns especially in a developing country

**Table 26.2** Obstetric management of burned pregnant patient

| Burn area (%) | Gestational age | | Management |
|---|---|---|---|
| <30 | First trimester | | No obstetric interference |
| | Second trimester | | No obstetric interference |
| | Third trimester | >36 weeks | Induce labour/caesarean section |
| | | <36 weeks | Conservative approach and monitoring of heart rate |
| 30–50 | First trimester | | Foetal monitoring by ultrasound every 3–4 weeks |
| | Second trimester | | Foetal monitoring every 3–4 weeks. Tocolytic therapy |
| | Third trimester | >36 weeks | Deliver foetus within 48 h |
| | | <36 weeks | Careful foetal monitoring |
| 50–70 | First trimester | | Terminate pregnancy |
| | Second trimester | | Terminate pregnancy |
| | Third trimester | If baby is viable | Induce labour/caesarean section within 24 h |
| | | Intrauterine death | No active intervention up to 4 weeks/monitoring of foetus of haemo coagulation factors |
| >70 | First trimester | | No treatment |
| | Second trimester | | No treatment |
| | Third trimester | | Caesarean section as an emergency procedure at the earliest |

like India, all cases must be reported to the local law enforcing agencies.

## Tetanus Prophylaxis

All burn wounds are tetanus prone. The need for tetanus prophylaxis should be determined by the patient's immune status.

## Rehabilitation

Burns rehabilitation includes care of physical, psychological and social aspects of burn patient. It is same for burn pregnant patient as it is for any other burn patient. It starts on day one of burns and may continue for several years. Burns can leave a patient with severely debilitating and deforming contractures, which can lead to significant disability if left untreated. The aim of burn rehabilitation is to minimize contracture development and impact of scarring on functional ability. Early phase of rehabilitation include proper positioning, splinting, stretching and early mobilization whereas late phase include management of contractures and hypertrophic scars, if these develop. A dedicated multidisciplinary team of professionals and the full participation of the patient is must to achieve maximum outcome.

## Outcome

Maternal and foetal outcome is directly related to burn percentage of TBSA. A mortality rate of (mother or foetus) more than 60 % has been reported for both if burn is 25–50 % of TBSA. Foetal mortality may reach 100 % if burn surface exceeds 50 %. However, it is found that foetal outcome largely depends on maternal outcome and most of the foetuses survive if mother survives and remain free of complications like hypoxia and sepsis. Most common foetal complication is intrauterine foetal death followed by abortion.

## Chemical Burns

Chemical burns occur as a result of industrial accidents, assaults or by improper use of harsh household cleaners. These burns can cause progressive damage to the skin and underlying tissues until the chemical is inactivated or diluted. Acids creates an impermeable barrier of coagulation necrosis at leading edge and thus limits further penetration, whereas alkalis creates soap with cutaneous lipids and continue to spread until they are neutralized.

Initial management includes irrigation under running stream of tepid water for at least 15 min. This will decrease the severity of the burns. The use of neutralizing agents is usually contraindicated (except for hydrofluoric acid burns where calcium is used as an antidote) as neutralization leads to production of substantial heat causing thermal burns. Most of these burns are deep partial or full thickness in nature and early E&G after full demarcation of injury gives best results.

### Conclusion

Burns during pregnancy is associated with significant maternal and foetal mortality. However, adequate fluid resuscitation, wound management and intensive care involving multidisciplinary approach have been found to be associated with better outcome. Early delivery of a viable pregnancy (>32 weeks) must be attempted after resuscitation if burn area is 30–50 % of TBSA, and termination of pregnancy should be done irrespective of gestational age if burned area exceeds 50 %.

## References

1. Bhat RV, Vyas KD. Burns in pregnancy. Obstet Gynecol Ind. 1974;24:264–6.
2. Jain ML, Garg AK. Burns with pregnancy – a review of 25 cases. Burns. 1993;19:166–7.
3. Akhtar MA, Mulawkar PM, Kulkami HR. Bums in pregnancy: effect on maternal and fetal outcomes. Bums. 1994;20:351–5.
4. Sarkar T, Roychowdury S. Plasma 17-beta oestradiol estimation in burns during pregnancy. Indian J Burns. 1996;4:49–52.

5. Prasanna M, Singh K. Early burn wound excision in "major" burns with "pregnancy": a preliminary report. Burns. 1996;22:234–7.
6. Gaffar UB, Akhtar N, Faruqui TH, Rizvi JS. Burns during pregnancy: a socio cultural disease. J Indian Acad Forensic Med. 2007;32:31–3.
7. Masoodi Z, Ahmad I, Khurram F, Ansarul H. Pregnancy in burns: maternal and fetal outcome. Indian J Burns. 2012;20:36–41.
8. Agarwal P. Thermal injury in pregnancy: predicting maternal and fetal outcome. Indian J Plast Surg. 2005; 38:95–9.
9. Guo SS, Greenspoon JS, Kahn AM. Management of burn injuries during pregnancy. Burns. 2001; 27:394–7.
10. Bartle EJ, Sun JH, Wang XW. Burns in pregnancy. J Burn Care Rehabil. 1988;9:485–7.
11. Taylor JW, Plunkett GD, McManus WF, Pruitt BA. Thermal injury during pregnancy. Obstet Gynecol. 1976;47:434–8.
12. Radosevich MA, Finegold H, Goldfarb W, Troianos C. Anesthetic management of the pregnant burn patient: excision and grafting to emergency Cesarean section. J Clin Anesth. 2013;25:582–6.
13. Polko LE, McMahon MJ. Burns in pregnancy. Obstet Gynecol Survey. 1998;53:50–6.
14. Mabrouk AR, el-Feky AE. Burns during pregnancy: a gloomy outcome. Burns. 1997;23:596–600.
15. Napoli B, D'Arpa N, Masellis M, Graziano R. Burns in pregnancy. Ann Burns Fire Disast. 2000;13:18–24.
16. Pacheco LD, Gei AF, VanHook JW, Saade GR, Hankins GD. Burns in pregnancy. Obstet Gynecol. 2005;106:1210–2.
17. Karimi H, Momeni M, Rahbar H. Burn injuries during pregnancy in Iran. Int J Gynaecol Obstet. 2009; 104:132–4.
18. Gang RK, Bajec J, Tahboub M. Management of thermal injury in pregnancy – an analysis of 16 patients. Burns. 1992;18:317–20.
19. MacLennon N, Heimbach DM, Cullen BF. Anesthesia for major thermal injury. Anesthesiology. 1998;89:749–70.
20. Velasco I, Haro LH, Decker WW. Burns. In: Wolfson AB, editor. Harwood-Nuss' clinical practice of emergency medicine. 5th ed. Philadelphia: Lippincott, Williams & Wilkins; 2010. p. 310–4.

# Poisoning in Pregnancy

27

Pushpa Junghare and Sayali Jahagirdar

## Introduction

Poisoning in pregnancy is a rare but possible event due to which the woman may be brought to the hospital in a serious condition, necessitating critical care. Critical care is possible only with critical thinking. Like any other obstetric emergency, poisoning in pregnancy may be life-threatening. Responding to emergency by providing rapid and appropriate care is vital. Certain other things that need to be pondered upon are that the history is often unreliable Even if the woman is in the state of giving history, she may not be aware of her pregnant state or she may have ingested the drug/substance with the purpose of terminating the pregnancy.

Prevalence or incidence in India is not known but is quite infrequent.

Poisoning in pregnancy may be accidental or intentional (suicidal or rarely homicidal)

P. Junghare (✉)
Prof. and HOD, Department of OBGY,
Dr. P. D. M. Medical College, Amravati,
Maharashtra, India
e-mail: pushpasj4@rediffmail.com

S. Jahagirdar
Asst. Prof., Department of OBGY,
Dr. P. D. M. Medical College, Amravati,
Maharashtra, India
e-mail: rupasi2001@yahoo.co.in

## Pathophysiology

A poison is a substance which when administered, inhaled, or ingested can cause deleterious effect on the human body. Poisoning denotes the morbid state produced by the exposure of a toxic agent (poison) that, because of its chemical action, causes a functional disturbance (e.g., renal failure or hepatitis) and/or structural damage (e.g., chemical burn) [1]. Overdose or overdosage refers to a state produced by the excess or abuse of a drug or substance [1]. Envenomations are a particular type of toxic exposure resulting from the human contact with biologic substances (venoms or toxins) produced in specialized glands or tissues from animals, usually by cutaneous or transdermal (parenteral) injection (bee and scorpion stings, snake bites, etc.) [2].

The physiologic changes of pregnancy may influence the absorption, distribution, and metabolic disposition of different potentially toxic agents [3].

In pregnancy not only the woman but also her fetus is likely to be affected. The toxic agent can cross the placental barrier to directly affect the fetus or it can be adversely affected because the mother lands in complications, in which she develops profound delirium, hypotension, renal/hepatic failure, convulsions, or other life-threatening problems. The woman


A. Gandhi et al. (eds.), *Principles of Critical Care in Obstetrics: Volume II*,
DOI 10.1007/978-81-322-2686-4_27

may recover without any long-term effects, but the fetus in utero may suffer for weeks or years due to teratogenic or other effects of the toxic substance.

## Evaluation

The poisoning and the pregnancy can be concealed or unknown at the time of presentation or initial consultation by the patient or her family members [2].

The patient is brought in outpatient department or casualty. The problem can vary from very straight forward with no consequences to a life-threatening and complex situation.

The initial assessment should rapidly determine whether the patient is conscious or unconscious and whether she is in cardiac or respiratory arrest.

In an unconscious patient with a history of suspected toxic exposure, differential diagnosis of trauma, especially to the cervical spine, should be kept in mind and patient stabilized accordingly. One has to see whether she is hemodynamically stable. She may be conscious but disoriented. With such altered mental status, hypoxemia and hypoglycemia should be considered, and she should be treated with oxygen by mask and parental glucose infusion. Oral intake and sedation should be delayed till secondary evaluation.

Thereafter detailed history should be obtained from all possible sources. In addition to general and obstetric history, specific questions should be asked regarding time, route, duration, and circumstances of exposure, location, surrounding events, and intent. The woman might be confused, stimulated, depressed, comatose, discordant, or normal. Rarely, she may be unaware of an exposure. She may be unable or more commonly unwilling to admit to one [4].

## Toxicological Evaluation

- The name and amount of each drug, chemical, or ingredient involved
- Ingestion of food, drink, or medications
- The time of onset, nature, and severity of symptoms
- The time and type of first aid measures provided
- The medical and psychiatric history
- Psychiatric problem like depression
- Family/relationship issues

## Examination

Thorough physical examination should be carried out.

Vital signs.

Cardiorespiratory status.

Neurologic status: dyskinesia, dystonia, fasciculations, myoclonus, rigidity, and tremors.

Evidence of trauma.

Underlying illnesses.

Focal neurological findings (goes more in favor of CNS lesion than poisoning).

Eyes: nystagmus, pupil size, reactivity.

Abdomen: bowel activity, bladder, and obstetrical examination.

Skin: burns, bullae, color, warmth, moisture, pressure sores, and puncture marks [4].

## Investigations

Routine and specific to assess the condition of the patient and fetus: CBC, blood group and Rh type, LFT, KFT, blood sugar, USG, NST.

For identification of toxin/drug causing the poisoning: the collection of sample for toxicology is of utmost importance in the identification of the toxic agent(s) causing the exposure to predict the severity and to implement and monitor specific treatment/antidotes. These will include blood, urine, saliva, vomit, gastric lavage fluid, feces, cerebrospinal fluid, amniotic fluid if collected, and meconium if the patient delivers soon after admission. Occasionally, the analysis of an arterial blood gas and basic chemistry will detect an anion gap or osmolar gap which will assist in the differential diagnosis of acidosis and suggest the possibility of a poisoning or overdose [5–7].

## Management

### General Principles

1. Knowledge of the offending agents, their pharmacokinetics, and pharmacodynamics is helpful.
2. Prior to onset of poisoning, decontamination is the highest priority and treatment is based solely on history.
3. Intravenous access should be obtained along with cardiac monitoring at the earliest. Most patients who remain or become asymptomatic 4–6 h after ingestion will not develop subsequent toxicity and can be discharged.
4. Effects after an overdose begin sooner, peak later, and last longer than they do after a therapeutic dose.
5. Symptomatic patients should have an intravenous line, oxygen saturation determination, cardiac monitoring, and continuous observation. Baseline laboratory, ECG, and X-ray evaluation may also be appropriate. Intravenous glucose (unless the serum level is documented to be normal), naloxone, and thiamine should be considered in patients with altered mental status, particularly those with coma or seizures [4].

*Treatment withheld from women because of their gravid condition will have catastrophic results for both mother and fetus.*

Pelvic tilt or wedge to lift and/or the manual displacement of the uterus off the midline to the left is recommended to relieve aortocaval compression by the gravid uterus and improve the venous return. Perimortem caesarean section should be considered in exceptional cases to save the fetus of moribund mother.

I. *Supportive therapy:* The goal of supportive therapy is to maintain physiologic homeostasis until detoxification is accomplished and to prevent and treat secondary complications such as aspiration, bedsores, cerebral and pulmonary edema, pneumonia, rhabdomyolysis, renal failure, sepsis, thromboembolic disease, coagulopathy, and generalized organ dysfunction due to hypoxia or shock.
   - Airway protection
   - Oxygenation/ventilation
   - Hemodynamic support
   - Treatment of seizures
   - Treatment of arrhythmias
   - Correction of temperature abnormality
   - Correction of metabolic derangement
   - Prevention of secondary abnormalities

#### Indications for ICU Admission

- Patients with severe poisoning (coma, respiratory depression, hypotension, cardiac arrhythmias, hypothermia, hyperthermia, seizures)
- Those needing close monitoring, antidotes, or enhanced elimination therapy
- Those showing progressive clinical deterioration
- Those with significant underlying medical problems
- Those having suicidal tendencies

II. *Prevention of further poison absorption*

Decontamination of skin, eyes, body cavities and GIT (includes induced emesis, gastric lavage, whole bowel irrigation, catharsis, dilution, giving activated charcoal, and rarely endoscopic or surgical removal.)

The skin should be flushed thoroughly with warm soapy water. Eyes should be irrigated with saline.

Inhalational exposures should be treated with fresh air or oxygen.

*GIT:* The efficacy of forced emesis, gastric lavage, and activated charcoal decreases with time, and their beneficial effect is doubtful when they are used 1 h after ingestion. Hence, they should be performed selectively [4].

*Activated charcoal* is the preferred method of gastrointestinal decontamination in most situations. Activated charcoal suspension is given orally via a cup, straw, or small bore nasogatric tube. Charcoal adsorbs ingested poisons within the gut lumen, allowing the charcoal toxin complex to be evacuated with stools.

*Emesis* can be brought about by giving 30 ml of ipepac with water and repeated if vomiting is not induced in 30–90 min of toxin/drug ingestion. It is contraindicated in caustic ingestion, altered mental status, inability to protect airway, seizures, hemorrhagic diathesis, and hematemesis or when patient has rapidly deteriorated [8–11]

*Gastric lavage* is appropriate when emesis is inappropriate or contraindicated, the patient is comatose or mentally altered, the substance ingested has the potential for seizures, or when the substance ingested is lethal and/or rapidly absorbed. It is contraindicated in ingestion of caustics and hemorrhagic diathesis.

It can be performed rapidly and immediately on admission. It also facilitates charcoal administration.

*Dilution:* In case of caustic ingestions, 200–300 ml of milk may be given orally.

*Whole bowel irrigation:* Is carried out by administration of polyethylene glycol at a rate of 50–2000 ml/h orally or through a nasogastric tube to clean the bowel of whole or undissolved pills. It is contraindicated in patients with bowel obstruction, ileus, hemodynamic instability, and compromised unprotected airways.

III. *Enhancement of poison elimination:*
- Multiple dose activated charcoal
- Forced diuresis
- Peritoneal dialysis
- Hemodialysis
- Hemoperfusion
- Hemofiltration
- Plasmapheresis
- Exchange transfusion

IV. *Administration of antidotes* which can counteract the effect of poisons by neutralizing them or by antagonizing their physiologic effects. Antidotes can significantly reduce morbidity and mortality, but most are potentially toxic. Hence, these should be used cautiously after correct identification of a specific poisoning or syndrome in consultation with physician and intensivist. Prevention of reexposure is important so also psychiatric referral [4].

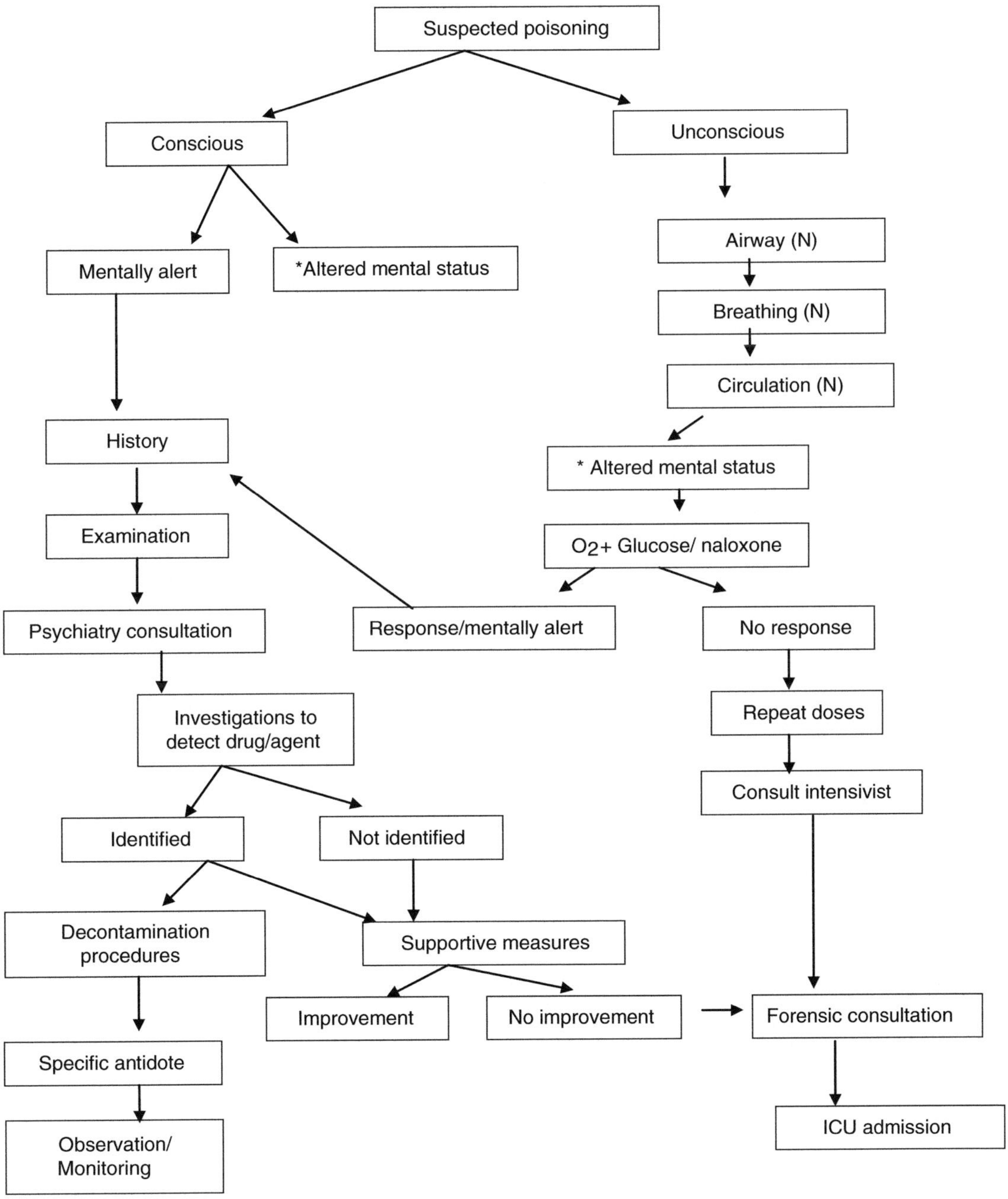


Guidelines for evaluation and management of pregnant patients with a known or suspected toxic exposure [2]

Suspected Poisoning in Unconscious Patient

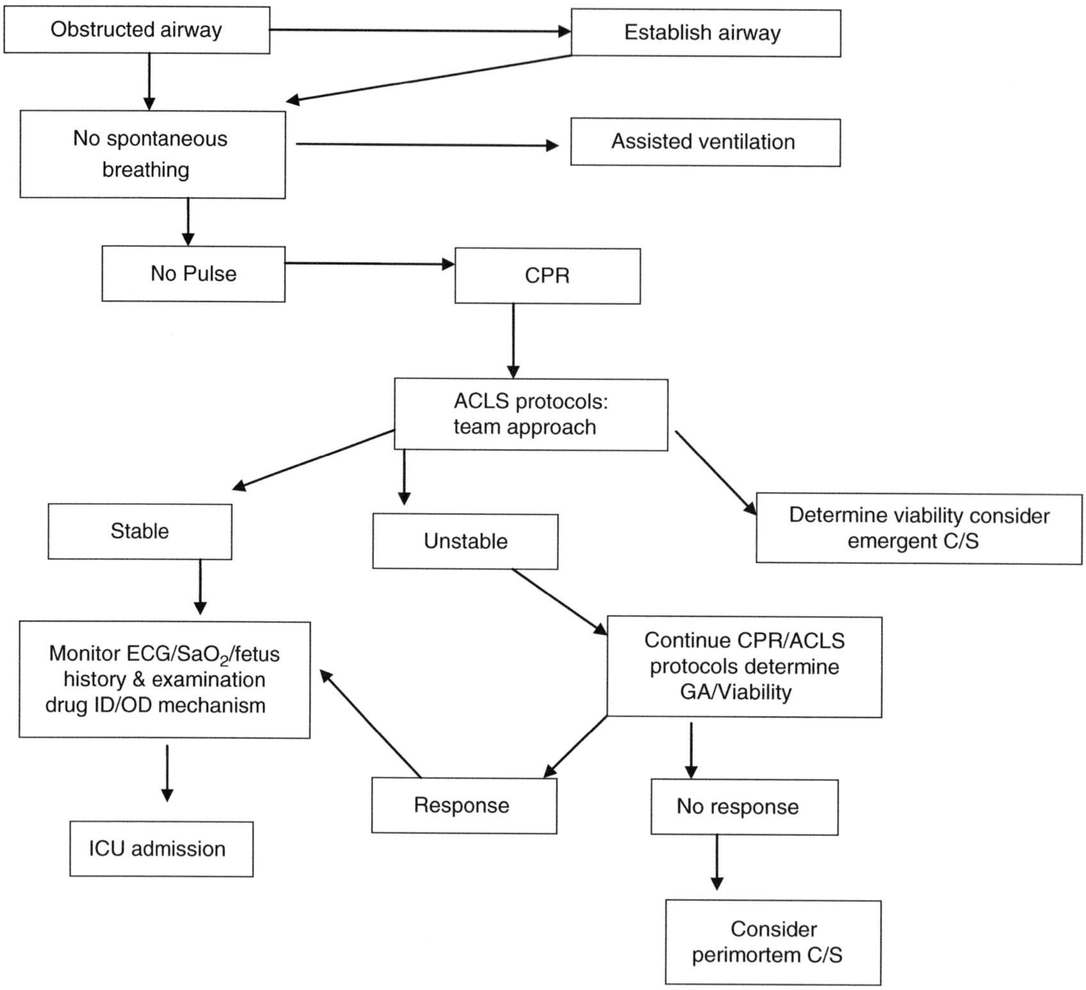


Guidelines for evaluation and management of pregnant patients with a known or suspected toxic exposure [2]

| Drug | Clinical features and Diagnosis | Maternal and fetal effects | Management and antidotes |
|---|---|---|---|
| Acetaminophen<br>Paracetamol<br>Calpol<br>Pacimol | Nausea, vomiting, anorexia; right upper quadrant pain. Icterus, right upper quadrant abdominal tenderness; lethargy; evidence of bleeding<br>Elevated transaminases LDH, amylase, lipase, creatinine, prolonged PTT | *Maternal*: oliguria, pancreatitis, hypotension, myocardial ischemia, and necrosis. Premature contractions, potential for premature delivery<br>Diffuse hepatic necrosis<br>*Fetal*: decreased fetal movements, poor beat to beat variability, nonreactive NST, bradycardia<br>Increased risks of spontaneous abortion and stillbirth<br>Neonatal hyperbilirubinemia | Gastric lavage<br>Activated charcoal (1 g/kg in water or sorbitol).<br>Induced emesis<br>N-acetylcysteine<br>150 mg/kg in 200 ml of 5 % dextrose over 15 min or 100 mg/kg in 1000 ml 5 % dextrose over 16 h<br>*Oral*: methionine (2.5 g every 4 h × 4 doses)<br>N – acetylcysteine(140 mg/kg stat, then half dose every 4 h × 17 doses)<br>ICU admission if hepatic failure or encephalopathy |
| Antidepressants<br>Imipramine<br>Amitriptyline<br>Doxepin<br>Trimipramine<br>Fluoxetine<br>Trazodone | Blurred vision, dysarthria, visual hallucinations, delirium, sedation, coma<br>Tachycardia, dry skin and mucous membranes, blisters, mydriasis, divergent strabismus, decreased bowel sounds, urinary retention, increased muscular tone, hyperreflexia, myoclonic activity, rapid loss of consciousness, seizures, cardiac dysrhythmias, hypotension, pulmonary edema<br>Sinus tachycardia with prolonged PR, QRS and QT intervals, AV block, and ventricular tachycardia on ECG | 3 major toxidromes: anticholinergic crisis, cardiovascular failure, or seizure activity<br>Cardiac dysrhythmias, seizures, urinary retention, GI hypomotility, aspiration pneumonitis and ARDS<br>Rhabdomyolysis, brain damage, and multisystem failure<br>Fetal: abnormal fetal heart rate [12].<br>Rarely congenital malformations like anencephaly, craniosynostosis, and omphalocele [13, 14]<br>In neonate tachypnea, cyanosis, irritability, urinary retention, paralytic ileus, seizures as withdrawal syndrome | Maintain airway if necessary with mechanical ventilation. Treatment of agitation, seizures, hyperthermia, hypotension, and arrhythmias<br>Decontamination with activated charcoal, cathartic, and gastric lavage<br>IV sodium bicarbonate is indicated, if the patient manifests coma, seizures, QRS greater than 0.1 s, ventricular arrhythmias, or hypotension<br>Phenytoin 100 mg over 3 min if perfusion is compromised. Norepinephrine or phenylephrine for refractory hypotension |

(continued)

(continued)

| Drug | Clinical features and Diagnosis | Maternal and fetal effects | Management and antidotes |
|---|---|---|---|
| Aspirin | None. Nausea, vomiting, abdominal pain, tinnitus, decreased audition, dyspnea<br>Hyperventilation; altered mental status, flushing, diaphoresis, hyperpyrexia, GI bleeding, petechiae, bruising, hypovolemia, pulmonary edema, seizures; ARDS, coma<br>ABGs: respiratory alkalosis, compensated metabolic acidosis or metabolic acidosis, increased anion gap, salicylate levels, creatinine, BUN, electrolytes, glucose, CBC, PT and PTT, urinalysis, specific gravity, volume and ferric chloride test. (Add 1 ml of 10 % $FeCl_3$ to 1 ml of urine change of color from purple to purple brown indicates salicylate presence) Chest x ray: pulmonary edema | Volume depletion, shock, hemorrhage, seizures, prolonged pregnancy, prolonged labor, higher risk of peripartum hemorrhage.<br>Fetal: constriction of ductus arteriosus, growth restriction<br>Neonatal: hyperbilirubinemia, clinical evidence of thrombocytopenia | Generous IV fluid replacement (glucose-containing solutions); if hypotension is refractory, may use plasma or blood<br>Gastric lavage<br>Forced alkaline diuresis (3 ampules of 40 % sodium bicarbonate) (50 ml/43 MEq of sodium) in 1 l of 5 % dextrose plus 40 mEQ of KCl at 2–3 ml/kg/h; goal: 5–10 ml/min of urine with pH of 7.5<br>Administer vitamin K 10 mg IV pH of 7.5 or IM<br>Hemodialysis may be indicated in severe acidosis, hypotension, seizures, pulmonary edema or renal failure |
| Barbiturates FDA class: D | Weakness fatigue, sleepiness. slurred speech, ataxia<br>Sedation, altered mental status, miosis, bradypnea, respiratory depression, ataxia, nystagmus, extraocular muscle palsies, dysarthria, hyperreflexia, incoordination, decreased bowel sounds, hypothermia, hypotension, cardiovascular collapse<br>CBC, electrolytes, blood glucose, creatinine and BUN, PT, PTT | Extraocular motor palsies, absent corneal reflexes, sluggish pupillary reaction, mydriasis, absent deep tendon reflexes, absent Babinski sign and coma, a flatline EEG has been reported<br>Respiratory depression atelectasis, pulmonary edema, bronchopneumonia, hypotension, direct myocardial depression, hypothermia, cutaneous bullae, decreased GI motility. Renal failure<br>Withdrawal syndrome<br>Fetal: abnormal BPP, decreased beat to beat variability, bradycardia<br>Fetal compromise<br>Fetal and neonatal addiction and neonatal withdrawal complications [15, 16]. Hemorrhagic disease of newborn [17] | Stabilization of maternal cardiopulmonary status. Gradual withdrawal to prevent abrupt withdrawal complications<br>Respiratory support<br>$O_2$ supplementation.<br>Endotracheal intubation and mechanical ventilation.<br>Adequate volume expansion and diuresis is critical<br>Dopamine or norepinephrine for severe hypotension<br>Gastric emptying followed by charcoal and cathartic agents<br>Forced alkaline diuresis<br>Hemoperfusion<br>Hemodialysis<br>Folate supplementation and vitamin K administration to mother |

| | | | |
|---|---|---|---|
| Benzodiazepines<br>Lorazepam<br>Oxazepam<br>Clonazepam<br>Diazepam<br>Chlordiazepoxide<br>Librium<br>Restoril | Drowsiness, ataxia, nystagmus, dysarthria, dizziness, weakness and confusion, paradoxical irritability, excitation, or delirium [18]<br>Lethargy altered mental status, slurred speech, ataxia, brady- or tachycardia, decreased bowel sounds, respiratory depression, hypotension, dyskinesia, acute dystonic reactions. Respiratory and/or circulatory depression. Coma<br>CBC, serum electrolytes, blood glucose, toxicology screen | Respiratory depression, hypotension and anoxic encephalopathy<br>Withdrawal syndrome (anxiety, insomnia, dysphoria, nausea, palpitations, fatigue, confusion, delirium, muscle twitching, seizures, psychosis)<br>Fetus: decreased beat to beat variability, bradycardia, abnormal biophysical profile<br>Neonatal hypotonia, impaired temperature regulation, lethargy, and apnea needing resuscitation measures [19] | Respiratory assistance<br>Crystalloid infusion<br>Dopamine and norepinephrine infusion for refractory hypotension<br>Gastric emptying followed by activated charcoal and cathartics repeated every 4 h (the sorbitol added only every 12 h). Induced emesis not recommended<br>Flumazenil 0.2 mg IV over 30 s dose can be repeated at 1 min interval up to 3–5 mg<br>Investigate chronic use/abuse of benzodiazepines. Consider drug counselor, psychiatry, and social worker evaluations |
| Carbon monoxide:<br>Is a by-product of cigarette smoking automobile exhaust, open fires, kerosene stoves, and heating systems in improperly ventilated areas | Headache, shortness of breath, nausea, dizziness, dim vision, chest pain, weakness<br>Vasodilation, disturbed judgement, collapse, coma, convulsions, Cheyne-Stokes respiration<br>ECG changes: sinus tachycardia, ST depression, atrial fibrillation, prolonged PR and QT intervals, AV or bundle branch block. Metabolic acidosis and %COHb on ABG | Myocardial ischemia, infarction, rhabdomyolysis, renal failure, pulmonary edema, blindness, and hearing loss<br>Delayed CNS toxicity (perivascular infarction, demyelination of basal ganglia) in comatose or acidotic patients on arrival [20–22]<br>Fetal: decreased variability, decelerations [23]<br>Fetal brain damage, developmental delays.<br>Premature birth, neurological deficits, and anomalies (CNS, skeletal, clefts) [21, 23–25]<br>Increased risk of fetal demise with chronic exposure.<br>Fetal death or permanent neurological damage | 100 % $O_2$ for prolonged duration. Hyperbaric oxygen is indicated if COHb is >15 %, presence of signs of non reassuring fetal condition, any neurologic signs in the mother (altered mental status, coma, focal neurologic deficits, seizures) or history of loss of consciousness |

(continued)

(continued)

| Drug | Clinical features and Diagnosis | Maternal and fetal effects | Management and antidotes |
|---|---|---|---|
| Ethanol: most frequently ingested toxin in the world [26] | Acute alcohol overdosage: euphoria, incoordination, impaired judgement, and altered mental status. Social inhibitions are loosened<br>Aggressive or boisterous behavior is commonly seen<br>Flushed facies, diaphoresis, tachycardia, hypotension, hypothermia, ataxia, abnormal reflexes, nystagmus, altered mental status, mydriasis, impaired judgement and reflexes, and a characteristic breath smell<br>CBC, blood glucose, electrolytes, BUN, creatinine, transaminase, lipase, PT, magnesium, calcium, ketones, acetone, ammonia and alcohol level<br>ABG, drug screen, chest X – ray | Respiratory depression, pulmonary aspiration, hypoglycemia, and coma. GI bleeding, atrial arrhythmias, or rhabdomyolysis are encountered<br>Organic problems include pancreatitis, hepatitis, cirrhosis, hepatic encephalopathy, portal hypertension, GI Bleeding, anemia, thiamine deficiency, alcoholic ketoacidosis, systemic hypertension, decreased resistance to infection, hypomagnesemia, hypokalemia, and hypophosphotemia. Intracerebral hemorrhage [27], nonischemic cardiomyopathy, malnutrition, isolation, depression, or suicide attempts [28]<br>Fetal: Nonreactive NST [29]<br>Poor BPP<br>Fetal alcohol syndrome [30] | Protection of the airway. Treatment of coma and seizures, hypoxemia, hypoglycemia, and opioid intoxication<br>Supplemental oxygen, intravenous dextrose (0.5-1 mg/kg); thiamine (100 mg) should be given routinely. Naloxone should be administered<br>Decontamination, gastric lavage.<br>Hemodialysis considered in respiratory failure or coma |
| Iron:<br>Ferrous gluconate | Indigestion, abdominal pain, nausea, vomiting, hematemesis, diarrhea, hematochezia<br>Bloody stools, tachycardia, fever, lethargy, shock and acidosis in severe cases. Rarely icterus, hypoglycemic symptoms coagulopathy<br>Leukocytosis, anemia or hemoconcentration<br>Serum electrolytes (anion gap metabolic acidosis)<br>Blood glucose, LFT, KFT, coagulation profile, ABG | Direct corrosive insult to the intestinal mucosa; systemic organ failure, GI hemorrhage, cardiovascular collapse, severe metabolic acidosis, intestinal scarring [31, 32]<br>Shock, hemorrhage, hepatic failure, pulmonary edema/hemorrhage, DIC<br>GI scarring, small intestine infraction, hepatic necrosis achlorhydria<br>Fetal: uterine contractions may be associated to maternal hypovolemia and shock | Oxygen supplementation, airway assessment, IV access for vigorous hydration<br>Orogastic intubation<br>Gastric lavage<br>Ipecac emesis<br>Whole bowel irrigation. Endoscopy or surgery to remove iron tablets adherent to the gastric mucosa [33]<br>Correction of hypovolemia with crystalloids before initiation of chelation with deferoxamine. (15 mg/kg/h as in intravenous infusion for up to 24 h.) [34]<br>Hemodialysis for toxic renal failure |

| | | | |
|---|---|---|---|
| Organophosphates/ carbamates | Muscarinic manifestations<br>D = Diarrhea<br>U = Urination<br>M = Miosis<br>B = Bronchospasm, bradycardia<br>E = Emesis<br>L = Lacrimation<br>S = Salivation<br>Nicotinic manifestations<br>M = Muscle weakness<br>A = Adrenal medulla activity increases<br>T = Tachycardia<br>C = Cramps in muscle<br>H = Hypertension [39]<br>CNS effects<br>Irritability<br>Apprehension<br>Restlessness<br>Convulsions<br>Coma<br>Depression of respiratory and circulatory centers<br>Leukocytosis, hypokalemia, hyperglycemia, elevated amylase, reduced erythrocyte cholinesterase, tachycardia/bradycardia, AV block, QT prolongation, asystole on ECG | Bronchorrhea, bronchospasm and respiratory failure, aspiration pneumonia, ventricular arrhythmias, pancreatitis, ARDS<br>Hepatic failure, peripheral neuropathy, personality change, acute cholinergic crisis, muscular paralysis, polyneuropathy<br>Fetal: Preterm delivery [35], fetotoxicity and fetal death [36]. Organic brain dysfunction [37] | 100 % oxygenation<br>Endotracheal intubation. (Only non-depolarizing neuromuscular blockers should be used.)<br>Decontamination: clothing and footwear should be removed and discarded [38].<br>Aspiration of gastric contents (within 1 h of ingestion)<br>Activated charcoal if not contraindicated.<br>Patient should be washed with soap and water.<br>Shaving of head in case of oily insecticides<br>*Atropine* 2 mg IV in repeated doses to control muscarinic effects<br>Continuous infusion of atropine (0.05 mg/kg/h) can be started<br>*Pralidoxime chloride* WHO recommended dose 30 mg/kg stat and 8 mg/kg/h maintenance infusion for 7 days |
| Phenol (carbolic acid) [39] | Local: burning pain, numbness, tingling and anesthesia when applied to skin or mucosa<br>GIT: burning pain followed b tingling numbness, and anesthesia. Nausea and vomiting<br>RS: Respiration is slow and labored<br>CNS: Headache, giddiness, unconsciousness, convulsions, coma<br>Oliguria and hepatic failure. Carboluria (urine color turns to green after exposure to air)<br>Ochronosis. (pigmentation in the cornea and various cartilages) | Convulsions, coma.<br>Oliguria and hepatic failure<br>Fetal: Not known | Skin: wash with undiluted polyethylene glycol<br>Oxygen/ventilatory support<br>Intravenous fluids and vasopressors to support blood pressure<br>Ingestion: Cautious stomach wash with sodium or magnesium sulfate solution<br>Lidocaine for ventricular arrhythmias<br>Benzodiazepines for seizures. |

Details of specific agents/drugs, clinical features and diagnosis of overdosage/poisoning, maternal and fetal effects, management and antidotes

| Drug | Clinical features and diagnosis | Maternal and fetal effects | Management and antidotes |
|---|---|---|---|
| Castor oil:<br>Accidental ingestion<br>Used to procure criminal abortion | Abdominal pain<br>Vomiting and diarrhea<br>Dehydration<br>Convulsions<br>Drowsiness<br>Delirium | Oliguria<br>Hepatic failure<br>Uremia<br>Multiorgan failure, cardiovascular collapse, dermatitis, rhinitis, asthma, conjunctivitis | Supportive treatment<br>Gastric lavage<br>Activated charcoal<br>Sodium bicarbonate to prevent precipitation of hemoglobin in renal tubules |
| Marking Nut: Biba<br>Accidental<br>Used to procure criminal abortion | Dermal: irritation, inflammation, vesication formation, pain, and itching. Ulceration and sloughing of skin<br>Ingestion: Blister formation in and around oral cavity, vomiting, diarrhea, abdominal pain, hypotension/shock, delirium, and coma | Hypotension/shock, delirium and coma | Supportive measures<br>Gastric lavage<br>Activated charcoal |
| Ergot:<br>Accidental<br>Used to procure criminal abortion | Acute: nausea, vomiting, diarrhea, giddiness, breathlessness, muscular weakness, tingling and numbness in hands and feet, paresthesia, cramps in muscle, bleeding from nose and other mucosal surface<br>Chronic (ergotism): Burning of extremities, hemorrhagic vesication, pruritis, formication, nausea, vomiting, bradycardia, headache, miosis, delirium, hallucinations | Peripheral ischemia leading to gangrene of fingers and toes, convulsions, ischemia of cerebral, mesenteric, coronary and renal vessels. | Gastric lavage with activated charcoal<br>For Hypertension or cerebral/mesenteric/cardiac ischemia – IV nitroglycerin or nitroprusside<br>Peripheral ischemia – oral parazosin, captopril, or nifedipine; convulsions and hallucinations: diazepam or lorazepam<br>Hypercoagulable state – heparin or dettran |
| Cow dung:<br>Dried cow dung powder | Nausea, vomiting, | GI irritation, yellow green discoloration of skin and mucous membranes | Gastric lavage<br>Hydration<br>Symptomatic treatment<br>No specific antidote available |

Common organic poisons, clinical features and diagnosis of poisoning, maternal and fetal effects, management and antidotes [39]

## Envenomations During Pregnancy

### Animal Bites and Stings [40]

Common animals which are poisonous include snakes, scorpions, bees, wasps, ants, spiders, and centipedes.

### Snake Bite

Cobra, krait, vipers, and sea snakes are common poisonous snakes encountered in India (Table 27.1).

## Management of Snake Bite

Reassurance.
Limit systemic spread of venom by immobilizing the affected part.
For viperid bites, the bitten limb should be splinted if possible and kept at approximately heart level.
For elapid or sea snake bites, the Australian pressure immobilization technique is beneficial. In this method, the entire bitten limb is wrapped with an elastic or crepe bandage and then splinted.
Tourniquet – a proximal lymphatic – occlusion constriction band or tourniquet may limit the spread of venom if applied within 30 min. The tourniquet should be applied such that it does not prevent arterial flow of blood and the distal pulsation should be appreciated.

### Specific Management

Monitor vital signs, cardiac rhythm, oxygen saturation, and urine output.
Measure the circumference of affected limb every 15 min.
Intravenous fluids and vasopressors as required.
Care of bite site – dry sterile dressings, splint.
Tetanus immunization. Antivenom therapy Fasciotomy for compartment syndrome
Laboratory investigations CBC, KFT, LFT, coagulation studies, blood group/cross matching, urine for blood, myoglobin, ECG, ABG, X-ray chest.

### Indications of Antivenom Therapy

Deranged coagulation profile.
Spontaneous bleeding.
Rapidly progressive and severe local swelling.
Persistent hypotension.
Neurotoxic or myotoxic features.
Depressed consciousness.
Antivenoms are of equine origin and carry risk of anaphylaxis or delayed hypersensitivity reactions.

### Prior to Giving Antivenom Therapy

Keep oxygen and ventilatory support ready; load patient with intravenous antihistaminics; arrange blood and FFP; keep neostigmine ready for neurotoxicity (give atropine prior to neostigmine); keep treatment for anaphylaxis ready.

## Scorpion Bite

Scorpion venom contains phospholipase, acetyl cholinesterase, hyaluronidase, serotonin, and neurotoxin, all of which are toxic [40].

**Table 27.1** Clinical features of snake bite

| Poisonous Snakes | Venom | Clinical features: Local | Clinical features: Systemic |
|---|---|---|---|
| Cobra, banded krait, common krait | Nuerotoxic | Fang marks<br>Burning pain<br>Swelling and discoloration, serosanguinous discharge | Preparalytic stage – vomiting, headache, giddiness, weakness, and lethargy,<br>Paralytic stage – ptosis, opthalmoplegia, drowsiness, dysarthria, convulsions, bulbar paralysis, respiratory failure, and death |
| Saw scaled viper<br>Russell's viper | Vasculotoxic<br>Hemotoxic | Pain, rapid swelling and discoloration, blister formation, bleeding from bite site | Generalized bleeding shock, renal failure |
| Sea snakes | Myotoxic | Local swelling, pain | Myalgia, muscle stiffness, myoglobinaria, renal failure |

## Mechanism of Scorpion Envenomation

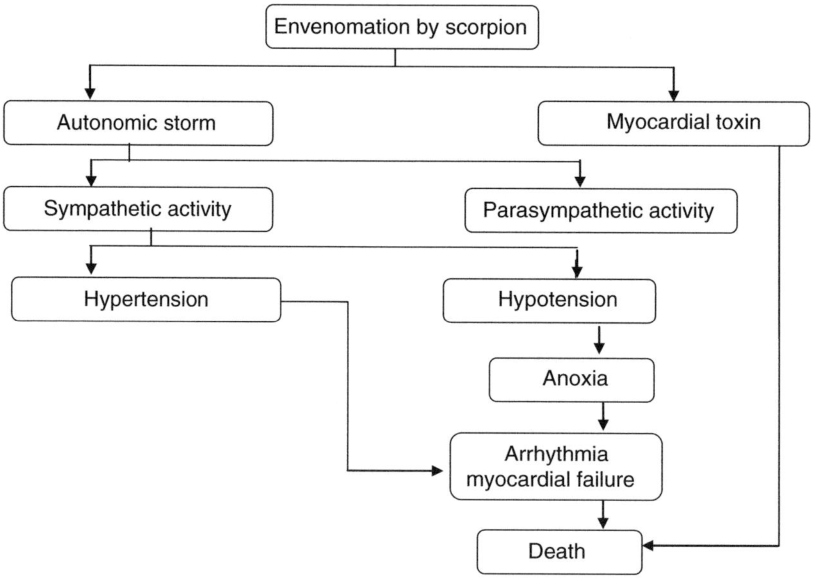


| | Local features | Systemic features | Lab findings | Management |
|---|---|---|---|---|
| Scorpion bite | Burning and excruciating pain at bite site, swelling, redness, itching ecchymosis | Sweating, urticaria, salivation, vomiting, breathlessness, cough, hemoptysis, priaprism, hypertension, bradyarrhythmias, pulmonary edema and myocarditis, myocardial ischemia, giddiness, convulsion, intracerebral hemorrhage | ECG shows changes mimicking acute MI, ST seg depression/elevation inverted and T waves left anterior hemiblock Q waves, elevated CPK | Immobilize affected limb, oxygen administration, Prazosin – $\alpha+\beta$ blocker reverses inotropic, hypokinetic, and metabolic effects. Inotropic support, sodium nitroprusside for massive pulmonary edema, antivenom therapy in life-threatening complications |
| Bee sting | Pain, redness, swelling, pruritus, airway obstruction, and dysphagia | Anaphylaxis, tingling sensation, flushing, dizziness, visual disturbances, syncope, vomiting and diarrhea, wheezing, urticaria, angioedema, glotis edema, coma, renal failure, hemolysis with hematoglobinuria, rhabdomyolysis | Hemoglobin and myoglobin estimation | Parenteral epinephrine for anaphylactic reaction, observation for delayed manifestation, antihistaminics, treatment of renal failure, dialysis may be required |

Clinical features, lab findings, and management of scorpion bite and bee sting

## Summary

1. Poisoning in pregnancy is rare but an important and challenging problem.
2. It may be simple and straight forward or may be complex and life-threatening.
3. The emergency treatment and stabilization of the mother should take priority over the monitoring and treatment of the fetus.
4. The obstetrician should assess the fetal viability and if the fetus can be salvaged should decide about emergency and/or perimortem caesarean section if the patient is moribund.
5. Supportive therapy is the mainstay of treatment. Specific therapy is indicated but will vary according to the poison/drug which the woman has consumed or is exposed to. Hence, basic knowledge about common poisons and overdosages of drugs and their antidotes is desirable.
6. Poisoning/overdosages might be accidental, but it can be intentional suggesting some severe social, emotional, and/or psychiatric pathology which will also require active intervention.
7. Insect and arthropod exposures are not uncommon during pregnancy. The majority of these envenomations result in minor or no effects. Moderate effects are more likely when the cause of the exposure is a spider bite than with other arthropod exposures, including scorpion and bee stings.

## References

1. Clark RF, Wethern-Kestner S, Vance MV, et al. Clinical presentation and treatment of black widow spider envenomation: a review of 163 cases. Ann Emerg Med. 1992;21:782–7.
2. Gci AF, Suarez VR. Overdose, poisoning and evenomation during Pregnancy. In: Belort M, Saade G, Foley M, editors. Critical care obstetrics. 5th ed. Phelan and G. Dildy © 2010 Blackwell Publishing Ltd.
3. Gei AF, Saade G. Poisoning during pregnancy and lactation. In: Yankowitx J, Niebyl JR, editors. Drug therapy in pregnancy. Philadelphia: Lippincott, Williams & Wilkins; 2001. p. 271.
4. Linden CH, Burn MJ. Poisoning and drug overdosage. In: Harrison's principles of Medicine 16th ed. vol II; 2005. p. 2580–93. McGrraw-Hill, Medical Publishing Division.
5. Borak J. Chapter 12: Anion and osmolar gaps. In: Viccellio P, editor. Emergency toxicology. 2nd ed. Philadelphia: Lippincott-Raven Publishers; 1998.
6. Eldridge DL, Dobson T, Brady W, Holstage CP. Utilizing diagnostic investigations in the poisoned patient. Med Clin North Am. 2005;89:1079–105.
7. Akbari A, Wilkes P, Lindheimer M, et al. reference intervals for anion gap and strong ion difference in pregnancy: a pilot study. Hypertens Pregnancy. 2007;26:111–9.
8. Kulig K. Gastrointestinal decontamination. In: Ford MD, Delaney KA, Ling JF, editors. Clinical toxicology. Philadelphia: WB Saunders; 2001.
9. Heard K. Gastrointestinal decontamination. Med Clin North Am. 2005;89:1067–78.
10. Christophersen AJ, Hoegberg LC. Techniques used to prevent gastrointestinal absorption. In: Goldfrank's toxicology emergencies. 8th ed. New York: McGraw Hill; 2006. p. 109.
11. Olson KR. Poisoning and drug overdose. 5th ed. New York: Appleton and Lange; 2007.
12. Gimovsky ML. Fetal heart rate monitoring casebook. J Perinatol. 1995;15:246–9.
13. Berard A, Ramos E, Rey E, et al. First trimester exposure to paroxetine and risk of cardiac malformations in infants: the importance of dosages. Birth Defects Res B Dev Reprod Toxicol. 2007;80:18–27.
14. Reprotox. Paroxetine. Last updated: June 2007. www.reprotox.org.Accessed June 2007.
15. Desmond MM, Schwanecke PP, Wilson GS, et al. Maternal barbiturate utilization and neonatal withdrawal symptomatology. J Pediatr. 1972;80:190–7.
16. Coupey SM. Barbiturates. Pediatr Rev. 1997;18:260–4.
17. Bleyer WA, Skinner AL. Fatal neonatal hemorrhage after maternal anticonvulsant therapy. JAMA. 1976;235:826–7.
18. MacGregor SN, Keith LG. Drug abuse during pregnancy. In: Rayburn RF, Zuspan FP, editors. Drug therapy in obstetrics and gynecology. 3rd ed. St. Louis: Mosby Year Book; 1992. p. 164–89.
19. Malgorn G, Leboucher B, Harry P, et al. Benzodiazepine poisoning in a neonate: clinical and toxicokinetic evaluation following enterodialysis with activated charcoal. Arch Pediatr. 2004;11:819–21.
20. Chale SN. Carbon monoxide poisoning. In: Viccellio P, editor. Emergency toxicology. 2nd ed. Philadelphia: Lippincott – Raven Publishers; 1998. p. 979.
21. Tomaszewski C. Carbon monoxide poisoning. In: Ford MD, Delaney KA, Ling LJ, et al., editors. Clinical toxicology. 1st ed. Philadelphia: W. B. Saunders Company; 2001. p. 657.
22. Kao LW, Nanagas KA. Carbon monoide poisoning. Med Clin North Am. 2005;89:1161–94.
23. Aubard Y, Magne I. Carbon monoxide poisoning in pregnancy. Br J Bostet Gynaecol. 2000;107(7):833–8.
24. Reprotox. Carbon monoxide. Last updated: April 2007. www.reprotox.org. Accessed May 2007.
25. Koren G, Sharav T, Pastuzak A. A multicenter, prospective study of fetal outcome following accidental carbon monoxide poisoning in pregnancy. Reprod Toxicol. 1991;5:397–403.

26. Otten EJ, Prybys KM, Gesell LB. Ethanol. In: Ford MD, Delaney KA, Ling LJ, et al., editors. Clinical toxicology. 1st ed. Philadelphia: W. B. Saunders Company; 2001. p. 605.
27. O'Connor AD, Rusyniak DE, Bruno A. Cerebrovascular and cardiovascular complications of alcohol and sympathomimetic drug abuse. Med Clin North Am. 2005;89:1343–58.
28. Briggs GG, Freeman RK, Yaffe SJ, editors. Drugs in pregnancy and lactation. 6th ed. Philadelphia: Lippincott Willams and Wilkins; 2002.
29. Halmesmaki E, Ylikorkala O. The effect of maternal ethanol intoxication on fetal cardiotocography: a report of four cases. Br J Obstet Gynaeco. 1986;93:203–5.
30. Brien JF, Smith GN. Effects of alcohol (ethanol) on the fetus. J Dev Physiol. 1991;15:21.
31. Schiavone FM. Metals: iron intoxication. In: Viccellio P, editor. Emergency toxicology. 2nd ed. Philadelphia: Lippincott – Reven Publishers; 1998. p. 391.
32. Tran T, Wax JR, Philput C, et al. International iron overdose in pregnancy – management and outcome. J Emerg Med. 2000;18:225–8.
33. Perrone J, Hoffman RS. Toxic ingestions in pregnancy: abortifacient use in a case series of pregnant overdose patients. Acad Emerg Med. 1997;4:206–9.
34. Schiavone FM. Metals: iron intoxication. In: Viccellio P, editor. Emergency toxicology. 2nd ed. Philadelphia: Lippincott – Reven Publishers; 1998. p. 391.
35. Solomon GM, Moodley J. Acute chlorpyrifos poisoning in pregnancy: a case report. Clin Toxicol (Phila). 2007;45(4):416–9.
36. Sebe A, Saatar S, Alpay R, et al. Organophosphate poisoning associated to fetal death: a case study. Mt Sinai J Med. 2005;72:354–456.
37. Reprotox. Malathion. Last updated: February 2007. www.reprotox.org. Accessed May 2007.
38. Aaron CK. Organophosphates and carbamates. In: Ford MD, Delaney KA, Ling T, Erickson LI, editors. Clinical toxicology. 1st ed. Philadelphia: W. B. Saunders Company; 2001. p. 819.
39. Bardale R. Chp 34: Corrosive Poisons In: Principles of Forensic Medicine and Toxicology, p. 439–441. First ed, 2011: Jaypee Brothers Medical Publishers, New Delhi, India.
40. Bardale R, Chapter no 38 Organic irritants In: Principles of Forensic Medicine and Toxicology, p 477–87: First ed, 2011, Jaypee Brothers and Medical Publishers, New Delhi, India.

# 28 Electric Injury in Pregnancy

Alok Sharnma and Rohini Rao

## Introduction

Electric injury in pregnancy is not common; rather, it is a very rare presentation in the emergency department. Even after extensive research, the electric injury with pregnancy is rare and uncommon.

The artificial electricity injury has been reported almost 300 years back, and first death was reported in 1879 in Lyons, France, when a carpenter inadvertently contacted a 250 watt alternating current (AC) generator current [1].

In pregnancy, patients with electrical injuries can present with a wide spectrum of presentations from trivial to fatal injuries. It could range from a mild transient unpleasant sensation having no effect on the mother or the foetus to mortality of either or both due to cardiac arrest (2007) [2]. The foetal outcome is not predicted by the severity of the maternal injury as it requires less current to produce injury to the foetus.

A. Sharnma, MD (OBG), MICOG, DHA (✉)
R. Rao, MD (OBG)
Registrar, Department of Obstetrics and Gynecology, Kamla Nehru State Hospital for Mother and Child, Indira Gandhi Medical College, Shimla, Himachal Pradesh 171001, India
e-mail: md.alok@gmail.com; rohinirao76@yahoo.com

## Epidemiology

The electrical burn injuries account for 3–4 % of all admissions to burn unit [3]. Most of the electrical injuries are occupation related. Children have a predisposition to low-voltage injuries as they are confined to a particular environment [4]. However, in adolescents the injuries are more grievous and can lead to burn death as they explore the environment more actively.

Deaths most often occur in young males (male/female = 9:1). Most of the deaths occur in spring and summer season. Water contact increases the severity.

## Pathophysiology

- The nature and severity of electrical burn injury are directly proportional to the current strength, resistance and duration of current flow.
- Electrical current causes damage through:
  - (a) Direct change in physiology by altering resting cell membrane potential
  - (b) Electrical energy conversion into thermal energy which in turn causes massive tissue destruction and coagulative necrosis
  - (c) Secondary damage after fall or strong muscular contractions


A. Gandhi et al. (eds.), *Principles of Critical Care in Obstetrics: Volume II*,
DOI 10.1007/978-81-322-2686-4_28

## Factors Determining Electrical Injury

- Type of circuit
- Duration of exposure
- Resistance of tissues
- Voltage
- Amperage (strength of current in amperes)
- The pathway of current

## Type of Circuit

The circuit may be:

- Direct current (DC)
- Alternating current (AC)

The high-voltage DC causes a single muscle spasm and often throws the victim away from source, whereas the AC current is 4–5 times as dangerous as an equal voltage of DC. The AC current has its frequency of 50 cycles per second, and it is very dangerous as it corresponds to the frequency of the fibrillation of myocardium. The AC exposure can cause continuous muscle contraction or tetany and can occur when the muscle fibres are stimulated at between 40 and 110 times per second.

## Duration of Exposure

The current greater than the "let-go threshold" (6–9 mA) can prevent the victim from releasing the current source, which prolongs the duration of exposure to electrical current. The longer the duration of contact with high-voltage current, the greater the degree of electrothermal heating and tissue destruction.

## Resistance of Tissues

Resistance is the tendency of a material to resist the flow of electrical current. It is specific for a given tissue depending on the moisture content, temperature and other physical properties. If the resistance of a tissue to the flow of the current is higher, then there is great potential for transformation of electrical energy into thermal energy [5].

Nerves carry electrical energy signals. Muscles and blood vessels have low resistance and good conductance due to high electrolyte and water content. Bones, tendons and fat contain a large amount of inert matrix, thus have a high resistance and tend to heat up and coagulate rather than transmitting current [5].

The amniotic fluid having high level of water content has a low resistance and is a good conductor of current.

Resistance of body tissues [6]:

| | |
|---|---|
| Least resistance | Nerves, blood, mucous membranes, muscles, amniotic fluid |
| Intermediate resistance | Dry skin |
| Most resistance | Tendons, fat, bones |

## Voltage

Voltage is the measure of difference in electrical potential between two points and is determined by the electrical source. Electrical injuries are divided into high or low voltage using 500 or 1000 V as dividing lines. No death is recorded from contact with low-voltage telephone line (65 V).

## Amperage (Strength of Current in Amperes)

Current is expressed in amperes, which is a measure of amount of energy that flows through an object.

Physical effects of different amperage levels at 50–60 Hz:

| Physical effect | Milliamperes (mA) |
|---|---|
| Tingling sensation | 1–4 |
| Let-go current (muscular tetany preventing release of grip from current source) | |

| Physical effect | Milliamperes (mA) |
|---|---|
| (a) Children | 4 |
| (b) Women | 7 |
| (c) Men | 9 |
| Freezing to circuit | 10–20 |
| Respiratory arrest from thoracic muscle tetany | 20–50 |
| Ventricular fibrillation | 60–120 |
| Asystole | >2 A |

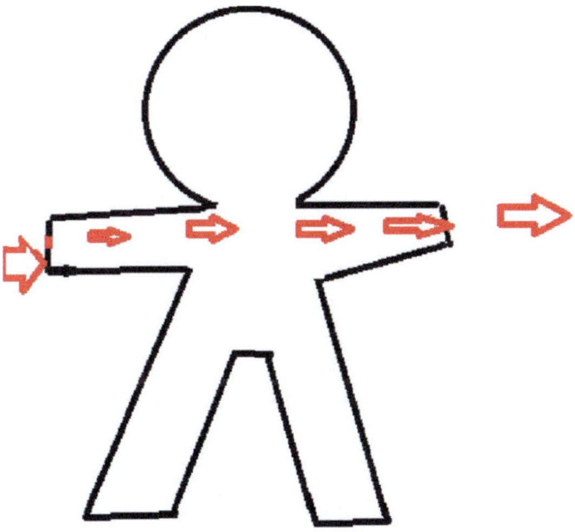

**Fig. 28.1** Hand to hand

## The Pathway of Current

In most of the cases, the current passes from hand to hand (Figs. 28.1 and 28.2), and it does not have effect on the foetus if the duration and strength of current is less. From hand to foot (Fig. 28.3) transmission, the current passes through the uterus and is associated with high incidence of foetal mortality and morbidity [2].

Hands are commonest site for contact with an AC electrical source, and the contractions of the wrist can pull the AC source closer to body [6]. Current passing through the thorax or heart can cause cardiac dysrhythmias or direct myocardial damage. Current passing through the brain can result in respiratory arrest, seizures and paralysis (Fig. 28.4).

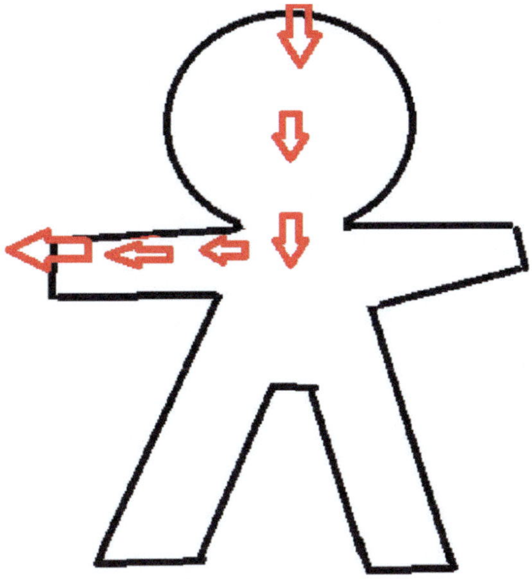

**Fig. 28.2** Head to hand

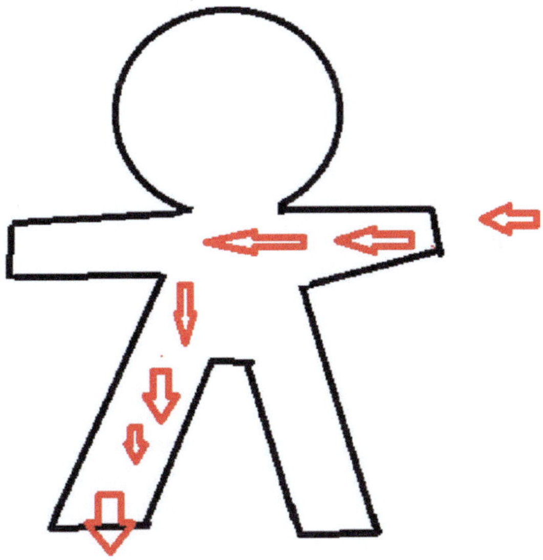

**Fig. 28.3** Hand to foot

## Electrical Shock in Pregnancy

The amount of current which will cause minimal injury to the mother may cause grievous injury to the foetus as the foetal skin is 200 times less resistant than the skin postnatal. So less current is more lethal to the foetus. The pathway of current is also very important; if the pathway is through the uterus, the foetus is seriously injured [7].

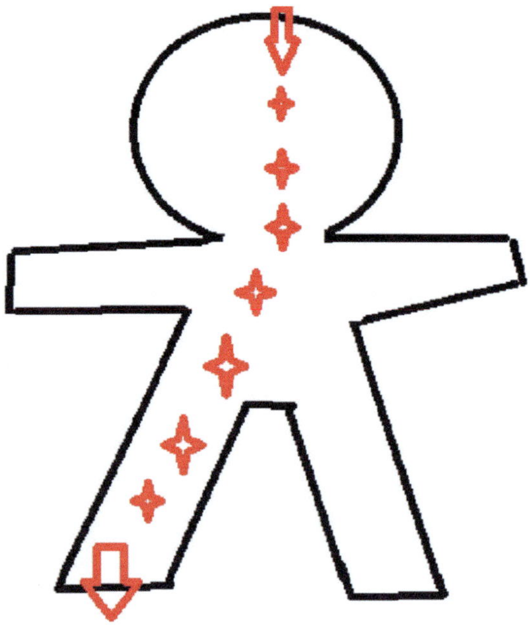

**Fig. 28.4** Head to foot

## Foetal Outcome

The foetus can have cardiac arrest, foetal complications like intrauterine growth retardation, oligohydramnios and reduced foetal movements to spontaneous abortions [7].

## Lightning

Flash or bolt of lightning is due to an electrical discharge from a cloud to the earth. The electric current is direct with a potential of 1000 million volts or more. Lightning is neither a direct current nor an alternating current. It is best regarded as unidirectional massive current impulse; thus, it is classed as a phenomenon of current. A lightning bolt may injure or kill a person by a direct strike, a side flash or conduction through another object (ground current or step voltage) and last but not the least by blunt trauma. After lightning meets the body, current is initially transmitted internally, and then there is skin breakdown, and ultimately external flashover occurs.

Thus, burns and myoglobinuric renal failure are not common injuries in lightning. The injuries which occur are cardiac or respiratory arrest, vascular spasm, neurologic damage and autonomic instability. Lightning causes asystole rather than ventricular fibrillation.

## Prehospital Management

- Immediately turn off the electrical supply, if possible, and separate the patient from the source using non-conducting instrument (e.g. rubber, wood). It should be made a principle to not to touch the patient before the power is turned off.
- Start with cardiopulmonary resuscitation immediately.
- As the most common cause is arrhythmia, start early defibrillation.
- Basic trauma care is also mandatory because these patients often suffer blunt injuries and burns.
- All patients with conductive injury should have at least one large-bore intravenous (IV) line established.
- An electrical injury should be treated like a crush injury rather than like a thermal burn.

## Management

Once the pregnant woman is received in the hospital, trauma team must emphasise on the assessment and resuscitation of mother. A short history should be asked regarding:

1. Source of shock
2. Voltage
3. Environment
4. Presence of tetany
5. Loss of consciousness
6. Burns
7. Pathway (entry or exit signs)

## Physical Examination

Look for injuries including tympanic membrane injury, peripheral nerve injury and vascular injury.

## Continuous Cardiac Monitoring is Recommended if there is [9]

- Loss of consciousness or altered mental status
- Cardiac dysrhythmias
- Abnormal 12-lead electrocardiogram (ECG)
- Known case of cardiovascular disease
- Physical examination showing burn or tissue damage
- Hypoxia
- Chest pain
- Cardiac arrest

## Investigations

- Complete blood picture including serum myoglobin
- Urine analysis for myoglobinuria
- Electrolytes
- Renal function tests
- ECG
- Ultrasound for foetal well-being and any other intra-abdominal injuries
- If there is severe suspected intra-abdominal injuries, then obtain:
  (a) Pancreatic and hepatic enzyme levels
  (b) Coagulation profile
  (c) Cervical spine, chest and pelvic radiography
- If ventilator support is needed, then obtain:
  (a) ABG (arterial blood gas analysis)
  (b) Creatinine kinase and troponin values

## Treatment

- Minor shock:
  In minor shock, the patient is asymptomatic and has a normal ECG. They can be discharged after the normal USG of foetus with reassurance [7].

**Discharge the minor electrical injury patient if**

- Review after 4 h of initial electronic foetal monitoring.
- Discharge criteria:
  (a) No sign of foetal compromise.
  (b) No uterine activity.
  (c) No ruptured membranes.
  (d) No vaginal bleeding.
  (e) No evidence of foetal maternal haemorrhage.
  (f) Normal ultrasound findings.
  (g) Ensure that all Rh (D)-negative women with abdominal trauma receive anti-D injection.

**Discharge home with instructions to report if the following occur**

(a) Any signs of preterm labour
(b) Abdominal pain/vaginal bleeding
(c) Change in foetal movements

- Mild to moderate shock:
  Arrhythmias and neurological sequelae require simple observation and tend to resolve spontaneously. Analgesics for muscle pain from tetany are given [7].
- Severe shock:
  (a) Stabilise any life-threatening dysrhythmias.
  (b) Transfuse crystalloids; titrate volume against central venous pressure(CVP), pulse and blood pressure.
  (c) Check blood gases, RFTs and coagulation profile.
  (d) Perform ECG.
  (e) Perform cervical spine, chest, pelvic and limb imaging.
  (f) Administer antibiotic prophylaxis as indicated.
  (g) Perform wound and burn care.
  (h) All patients with conductive injury should have large-bore intravenous line established. Hypotensive patients should receive a bolus of 20 ml/kg isotonic fluid.
  (i) In case the patient is having haeme pigments in urine, the patient should be assumed to have myoglobinuria. Alkalise the urine so that the solubility of myoglobin and its clearance rate increases. Urine output should be maintained at 1–1.5 ml/kg/h until all traces of myoglobin is cleared [7].

## Foetal Surveillance

- Confirm presence of foetal heart activity.
- If the gestation is 24 weeks or more, electronic foetal monitoring should be continued for 4 h for all women with minor injury.
- EFM (electronic foetal monitoring) is continued for 24 h if there is:
  (a) Abnormal results of maternal ECG
  (b) History of maternal unconsciousness
  (c) History of maternal cardiovascular disease
  (d) Uterine contraction > 1 every 15 min
  (e) Uterine tenderness
  (f) Signs of foetal compromise
  (g) Evidence of vaginal bleeding and rupture of membranes
  (h) Positive Kleihauer test
  (i) USG showing placental or cord abnormality
  (j) Serious maternal injury
  (k) USG showing oligohydramnios or IUGR

There is a high rate of foetal or neonatal death (about 50 %) even when maternal survival occurs [8].

Patient in first trimester should be informed about the remote complications of spontaneous abortion. Patient can be discharged with instructions for the threatened abortion, and close follow-up is required if they have mild to moderate injury.

Patients in the latter half of pregnancy should receive foetal monitoring even if there is minor blunt trauma and should be considered a high risk for the remaining of pregnancy.

## Complications

- Maternal
  (a) Cardiac dysrhythmias
  (b) Muscle contractions
  (c) Skeletal fractures
  (d) Neurological injury
  (e) Placental abruption
  (f) Conversion of electrical injury to thermal
  (g) Loss of consciousness
  (h) Rhabdomyolysis
  (i) Tissue necrosis
  (j) Tetany
  (k) Respiratory arrest
  (l) Asystole
- Foetal
  (a) Foetal burns
  (b) Reduced foetal movement
  (c) Miscarriage
  (d) Cardiac arrest

According to Indian mythology and traditions, in case of maternal mortality, last rituals of mother and foetus are performed separately. The foetus should be extracted out either by hysterotomy or post-mortem caesarean section and should be buried separately from mother.

**Conclusion**

Every pregnancy after having electric injury should be considered and treated as high-risk pregnancy till delivery of baby.

## References

1. Jex-Blake AJ. The Gulstonian lectures of death from electricity in the late nineteenth century. Med Instrum. 1975;9:26. PUBMED Abstract.
2. Muench MV, Canterino JC. Trauma in pregnancy. Obstet Gynecol Clin North Am. 2007;34:555–83.
3. Price TG, Cooper MA. Electrical and lightning injuries. In: Marx JA, Hockberger RS, Walls RM, editors. Rosen's Emergency Medicine: Concepts and Clinical Practice. Philadelphia, PA: Mosby-Elsevier; 2006. p. 2267–78.
4. Hettiaratchy S, Dziewulski P. ABC of burns: pathophysiology and type of burns. BMJ. 2004;328:1427–9.
5. Baker MD, Chiaviello C. Household electrical injuries in children: epidemiology and identification of avoidable hazards. Am J Dis Child. 1989;143:59. PUBMED Abstract.
6. Cameron P, Jelinek G, Kelley A-M, Murray L, Brown AFT, Heyworth J. Chapter 27.6: Electric shock and lightning injury. In: Textbook of adult emergency medicine. 2nd ed. Churchill Livingstone, UK: Postgraduate textbook; 2004.
7. Cooper MA, Edlich RF. Lightening Injuries. Medscape. March 2010.
8. Price TG, Cooper MA. Electrical and lightning injuries. In: Marx JA, Hockberger RS, Walls RM, editors. Rosen's emergency medicine concepts and clinical practice. Philadelphia: Mosby-Elsevier; 2006. p. 2267–78.
9. Andrews CJ, et al. The pathology of electrical and lightning injuries. In: Wecht CJ, editor. Forensic sciences. New York: Mathew Bender; 1995.

# Acute Psychiatric Crisis in Obstetrics

# 29

Neema Acharya

## Introduction and Etiopathology

Although pregnancy has typically been considered a time of emotional well-being, recent studies suggest that up to 20 % of women suffer from mood or anxiety disorders during pregnancy. It is not rare to present women with the first onset of psychiatric illness while pregnant.

It is likely that biological, psychological, and social factors interact to trigger an episode of a major psychiatric disorder in pregnant and postpartum women.

Estrogen has effects on neurotransmitter systems and has been implicated in major depressive disorder. Studies that support this theory have shown that postpartum estrogen supplementation, which slows the postpartum decline in estrogen levels, leads to resolution of depressive symptoms. Hormones and neurotransmitter systems and neurotransmitters implicated in major depressive disorder such as monoamine oxidases (MAOs), i.e., MAO-A and MAO-B, serotonin, and norepinephrine have been specifically studied in perinatal populations. According to hypothalamo-pituitary-cortico axis theory, the placenta independently produces a number of hormones (e.g., CRH, ACTH, and cortisol) that are regulated in a feed-forward manner, which leads to downregulation of autoreceptors in the hypothalamus and anterior pituitary. This process of receptor downregulation and the transition to a nonpregnant hormonal state has been hypothesized by some to constitute a period of vulnerability for mood disorders.

Immune theory states that pro-inflammatory cytokines produced in peripartum period due to pain in physical exertion and tissue injury are also linked to hypothalamic-pituitary-adrenal axis activity and have been associated with mood disorders in nonpregnant individuals.

## Types of Psychiatric Disorders during Pregnancy

1. Major depression
2. Bipolar disorders
3. Anxiety disorder
4. Psychosis

## Antidepressants and Pregnancy

Rates of major and minor depression during pregnancy are as high as approximating 10 %. About one third of depressed pregnant women experience the first episode of major depression. Pregnant women may have many clinical signs and symptoms like sleep and appetite disturbance and low energy, feelings of guilt and hopelessness,

N. Acharya
Department of Obstetrics and Gynecology, DMIMS(DU), Wardha, India
e-mail: nimaneemadk@hotmail.com


A. Gandhi et al. (eds.), *Principles of Critical Care in Obstetrics: Volume II*,
DOI 10.1007/978-81-322-2686-4_29

and suicidal thoughts. Of all the antidepressants, fluoxetine (Prozac) is the best studied antidepressant. Data collected from over 2500 cases indicate no increase in risk of major congenital malformation in fluoxetine-exposed infants.

## Anxiolytic Therapy during Pregnancy

Pregnancy appears to be a protective period for some anxiety disorders, including panic, while it may precipitate to obsessive compulsive disorder. Some studies, however, have shown an increase in both panic disorder and OCD in pregnant women. Women with anxiety related to pregnancy may be at a greater risk for postnatal depression. Hence, recognition and management of anxiety disorders in pregnant women is important. For these cases, fluoxetine or a TCA is a reasonable treatment option. In patients who do not respond to these antidepressants, benzodiazepine use may be considered. Patients with moderate to severe OCD require maintenance therapy.

## Bipolar Disorder During Pregnancy

Bipolar disorder or manic-depressive disorder affects between 3.9 and 6.4 % of women . Bipolar disorder should always be considered in the differential diagnosis of depression; one quarter of those presenting with depression prove to have bipolar disorder. Women who experience relapse appear to be more likely to have relapse into an episode of depression or mixed mood disorder that is characterized by both manic and depressive symptoms. Rates of postpartum relapse range from 32 to 67 %. Almost 33 % of women with bipolar disorder will experience an episode during pregnancy. Use of lithium in pregnancy may be associated with a small increase in congenital cardiac malformations particularly Ebstein's anomaly, neonatal cardiac arrhythmias, hypoglycemia, nephrogenic diabetes insipidus function, premature delivery, and floppy infant syndrome. Symptoms of neonatal lithium toxicity include flaccidity, lethargy, and poor suck reflexes, which may persist for a week.

## Guidelines for Treatment of Women with Bipolar Illness

Guidelines for women treated with lithium and plan to conceive are as follows:

1. In women who experience mild and infrequent episodes of illness, treatment with lithium should be gradually tapered before conception.
2. In women who have more severe episodes but are only at moderate risk for relapse in short-term, treatment with lithium should be tapered before conception but reinstituted after organogenesis.
3. In women who have especially severe and frequent episodes of illness, treatment with lithium should be continued throughout gestation and the patient counseled regarding reproductive risks.
4. Fetal assessment with fetal echocardiography should be considered in pregnant women exposed to lithium in the first trimester.

Several anticonvulsants, including valproate, carbamazepine, and lamotrigine, currently are also used in the treatment of bipolar disorder. A "fetal valproate syndrome" has been described with features of fetal growth restriction, facial dysmorphology, and limb and heart defects with valproate use. Carbamazepine exposure in pregnancy is associated with a *fetal carbamazepine syndrome* manifest by facial dysmorphism and fingernail hypoplasia. Lamotrigine is proven safer with growing reproductive safety profile relative to alternative mood stabilizers. Folate supplementation of 4 mg/day is recommended preconceptionally and for the first trimester of pregnancy in these patients.

## Antipsychotic Medications

Neuroleptic agents such as haloperidol, perphenazine, and trifluoperazine which are high potency agents are recommended over the lower-potency agents in managing pregnant women with psychiatric illness.

Atypical antipsychotic medications are now being used to treat a spectrum of psychiatric disorders, including psychotic disorders and bipolar disorder, as well as treatment of refractory depression and anxiety disorders. Investigators prospectively followed a group of 151 women taking olanzapine (Zyprexa), risperidone, quetiapine, or clozapine and compared outcomes to controls without exposure to known teratogens. There were no differences between the groups in terms of risk for major malformations or rates of obstetrical or neonatal complications.

Not enough information is available regarding safety of these drugs in pregnancy and lactation; hence, National Pregnancy Registry has been created to prospectively gather information regarding outcomes in infants exposed in utero to these newer atypical antipsychotic medications.

The US Food and Drug Administration (FDA) recently updated labels for the entire class of antipsychotic drugs to include warnings regarding the use of antipsychotic drugs (both the typical and atypical agents) during pregnancy. The new drug labels now contain more details about risk for abnormal muscle movements (extrapyramidal signs or EPS) and withdrawal symptoms in newborns exposed to these drugs during the third trimester of pregnancy.

## Postnatal Care and Antipsychotic Treatment

Postpartum psychosis often constitutes a psychiatric emergency, increasing the risk of both infanticide and suicide. Maintenance treatment in the postpartum period is needed to prevent acute episodes. Communication between treating physicians is critical, and infants should be monitored for adverse effects, including with laboratory tests.

Most medications are transferred through breast milk, although most are found at very low levels and likely are not clinically relevant for the neonate. The American Association of Psychiatrists and the World Health Organization (WHO) Working Group on Drugs and Human Lactation have concluded that use of most of the typical psychotic medications is compatible with breastfeeding. The atypical antipsychotics, such as olanzapine, for which we have less information, appear to be like older antipsychotics and can lead to extrapyramidal side effects in the infants. No adverse effects from the use of carbamazepine, valproate, or lamotrigine have been reported.

## Acute Psychosis: A Medical Emergency

Psychosis is a mental disturbance in which there is a loss of contact with reality evidenced by hallucination, delusions, or thought disorganization. Psychotic episodes are seen most commonly in patients who suffer from schizophrenia/schizoaffective disorder or psychotic episodes of bipolar disorder and major depression. The risk of developing a severe mental illness in pregnancy is estimated to be 7.1 in 10,000 per year.

The risk of women presenting with an acute psychotic episode is more in a preexisting disease which may progress during pregnancy mainly so if the woman has discontinued the medications. Relapse rates are also high for women who have experienced a previous psychosis in pregnancy. Proper history and clinical examination should search for an underlying medical or pharmacologic cause in a new-onset psychosis during pregnancy.

Wernicke's encephalopathy is caused by thiamine (vitamin B1) deficiency and is a known complication of hyperemesis gravidarum. This encephalopathy presents with a classic triad of symptoms: confusion, oculomotor dysfunction, and gait ataxia.

The risk factors associated with acute psychosis in pregnancy are:

1. Previous history of psychosis in pregnancy
2. Preexisting psychotic or mood disorder
3. Family history of psychosis

## History Taking and Examination

A multidisciplinary approach is followed taking the opinion of neurologist and a psychiatrist. A thorough history should help in eliminating medical or pharmacologic causes. Physical examination and more so detailed neurologic examination are an important component of the evaluation. In suspected cases, MRI may be done.

Serum electrolytes, complete blood count, hepatic and renal function, coagulation panel, arterial blood gas, thyroid function, albumin, urinalysis, and serum and urine drug screen are done in laboratory investigations. Serum/plasma testing also can be useful in the diagnostic workup of suspected Wernicke's encephalopathy especially in case of hyperemesis gravidarum (viz., erythrocyte transketolase activity, thiamine pyrophosphate effect, and thiamine pyrophosphate) concentration in plasma or whole blood).

## Emergency Management

Psychosis during pregnancy or the postpartum period owing to any cause is a medical emergency. Whatever may be the cause for psychiatric emergency due care should be taken to look after the newborn. Transfer to an inpatient psychiatric unit is recommended.

If labor and delivery is not evident, then patient can be managed in medical or psychiatry indoor unit. In case of associated obstetric complication or labor, appropriate care should be taken more with continuous close supervision of the gravid mother.

## Medications for Acute Psychotic Episode

1. Atypical antipsychotics: aripiprazole, clozapine, olanzapine, paliperidone, quetiapine, risperidone, ziprasidone
2. Typical antipsychotics: haloperidol and perphenazine

Acute psychosis in pregnancy is a clinical emergency, and prompt hospitalization is necessary. Haloperidol is safest in pregnancy with most extensive reproductive safety data as it was used commonly in the management of hyperemesis gravidarum in the past. Therefore, it is typically used to manage new-onset psychosis during pregnancy.

To manage agitation or combativeness during acute psychosis, lorazepam can be used in conjunction with haloperidol; however, lorazepam does not alleviate psychosis itself, and its indiscriminate use can at times aggravates symptoms of disorganization or disinhibition. Consequently, many such patients will have conceived while taking one of the newer so-called atypical antipsychotics.

Though atypical group of medications are preferred for long-term management owing to reduced risk for tardive dyskinesia and extrapyramidal side effects and greater effectiveness in managing the negative symptoms of schizophrenia, the data remains sparse with regard to the safety and efficacy of atypical antipsychotic drug use in pregnancy. Switching agents after conception only heightens risk by exposing the fetus to yet another psychotropic agent and increases the likelihood of maternal psychiatric decompensation; hence, the patient should receive same group of medication.

## Electroconvulsive Therapy (ECT)

Severely depressed patients having acute suicidality or psychosis may require electroconvulsive therapy which is frequently the treatment of choice. ECT use during pregnancy is found to be safe and efficacious. Care while giving ECT during pregnancy should include a pelvic examination, discontinuation of nonessential anticholinergic medication, cardiotocography, and intravenous hydration.

A variety of medications are available to treat psychiatric illness, though their effects are under research. When the risks to the mother and the fetus are to be weighed, effective treatment should be started at times as emergency with multidisciplinary management.

## Further Reading

1. National Institute of Mental Health (US). The numbers count: mental disorders in America. Bethesda: NIMH/NIH Publication; 2008. Available at: http://www.nimh.nih.gov/publicat/numbers.cfm. Accessed 12 Jan 2012.
2. Chrousos GP, Torpy DJ, Gold PW. Interactions between the hypothalamic-pituitary-adrenal axis and

the female reproductive system: clinical implications. Ann Intern Med. 1998;129:229–40.
3. Yim IS, Glynn LM, Dunkel-Scheter C, et al. Risk of postpartum depressive symptoms with elevated corticotrophin-releasing hormone in human pregnancy. Arch Gen Psychiatry. 2009;66:162–9.
4. Robertson E, Grace S, Wallington T, et al. Antenatal risk factors for postpartum depression: a synthesis of recent literature. Gen Hosp Psychiatry. 2004;26:289–95.
5. Lorenzetti V, Allen NB, Fornito A, et al. Structural brain abnormalities in major depressive disorder: a selective review of recent MRI studies. J Affect Disord. 2009;117:1–17.
6. Belmaker RH, Agam G. Major depressive disorder. N Engl J Med. 2008;358:55–68.
7. Sacher J, Wilson AA, Houle S, et al. Elevated brain monoamine oxidase A binding in the early postpartum period. Arch Gen Psychiatry. 2010;67:468–74.
8. Doornbos B, Fekkes D, Tanke MA, et al. Sequential serotonin and noradrenalin associated processes involved in postpartum blues. Prog Neuropsychopharmacol Biol Psychiatry. 2008;32:1320–5.
9. Practice Bulletin ACOG. Use of psychiatric medications during pregnancy and lactation. Obstet Gynecol. 2008;111:1001–19.

# 30 Cancer in Pregnancy

M. Jayaraman Nambiar and Theincherry Rema

## Introduction

Cancer complicating pregnancy is not common. The incidence is about 1 in 1000 [1, 2]. In a study by Van Calsteren K. et al., the commonest cancer complicating pregnancy is cancer of the breast and haematological malignancies. Carcinoma of the cervix is the commonest gynaecological malignancy which occurs during pregnancy. Cancers which occur less frequently include malignant melanoma, brain tumours, thyroid cancer, ovarian cancer and colon [3].

The treatment of cancer is easy in pregnancy when pregnancy is unwanted or foetus is mature. In these situations, pregnancy can be terminated and treatment of cancer can be undertaken. Dilemmas arise when pregnancy is remote from term. In this situation, a balance should be taken with preservation of pregnancy and treatment of malignancy.

The safety of chemotherapy after the first trimester is being established. Radiotherapy can be used with shielding, and many chemotherapeutic agents are now used with safety after the first trimester [4, 5]. The prognosis of cancer in pregnancy is not different from cancer in non-pregnant women.

M. Jayaraman Nambiar (✉)
Department of OBGYN, KMC,
Manipal 576104, Karnataka, India
e-mail: drramnambiar@gmail.com

T. Rema
Obstetric Ultrasound, Dr TMA Pai Hospital Udupi,
Udupi, Karnataka, India

## Radiotherapy in Pregnancy

Radiotherapy if given to pelvis invariably results in foetal damage. Whenever possible, one should wait for foetal maturity and delivery before radiotherapy. However, radiotherapy can be given to areas other than pelvis with shielding of abdomen [6].

## Chemotherapy in Pregnancy

Most chemotherapeutic agents can be given after 14 weeks of gestation without much foetal damage. Doxorubicin, alkylating agents, cyclophosphamide, cisplatin and carboplatin can be administered after 14 weeks of gestation. The teratogenic effects include ventriculomegaly and cerebral atrophy. However, incidence of these effects were low (<10 %) [7–13].

## Surgery in Pregnancy

Surgery during pregnancy is not associated with increased congenital malformation in foetus. There is a risk of preterm labour during surgery,


A. Gandhi et al. (eds.), *Principles of Critical Care in Obstetrics: Volume II*,
DOI 10.1007/978-81-322-2686-4_30

and prophylactic tocolysis should be used during surgery in pregnancy. Laparoscopy can be used up to 26–28 weeks of gestation. Abdominal entry in laparoscopy is through the left upper abdominal quadrant to reduce risk of injury to the pregnant uterus.

## Breast Cancer

Breast cancer is the commonest cancer diagnosed during pregnancy. Physiological changes in pregnancy make diagnosis difficult and often detected at later stage [14]. Suspicious lump in breast must be biopsied. There is difficulty in interpreting FNAC because of pregnancy changes in breast, and it is not recommended. Chest X-ray, non-contrast MRI and ultrasound can be used in staging. No survival benefit is seen if treatment is delayed after delivery; hence, treatment should not be delayed [15]. Option of termination of pregnancy and treatment should be given to the patient. Termination of pregnancy does not alter the outcome of cancer [16]. Radiotherapy has foetal detrimental effects and is given only after delivery. Surgery is used with relative safety during pregnancy.

Cytotoxic drugs can be given after 14 weeks of gestation though IUGR, foetal death and preterm labour have been reported [4]. Chemotherapeutic agents like fluorouracil and epirubicin or doxorubicin pluscyclophosphamide or epirubicin or doxorubicin pluscyclophosphamide and taxane can be used after 14 weeks of gestation. Tamoxifen alters the hormonal milieu and should not be used in pregnancy. Trastuzumab causes oligoamnios and anhydramnios and should not be used for long periods. If the breast cancer is not locally advanced, patients are taken for surgery followed by chemotherapy. Delivery is considered at 35–37 weeks. For locally advanced cancers, neoadjuvant chemotherapy followed by surgery is done. Delivery is conducted in 35–37 weeks. There should be a delay of 3–4 weeks before delivery and chemotherapy to avoid transient myelosuppression associated with chemotherapy.

## Cancer Cervix

### Preinvasive Lesions of Cervix

Interpretation of Pap smear in pregnancy is difficult to physiological changes [17]. In many countries where there is no regular screening, pregnancy may offer the woman a chance of screening during pregnancy. Abnormal smears should be followed up with colposcopy in pregnancy, and a directed biopsy must be taken. Endocervical curettage is contraindicated during pregnancy. The most common complication during colposcopic-directed biopsy is bleeding. Bleeding can be tackled with pressure, packing or rarely ligation of vessels. The risk of progression of CIN to invasive disease in pregnancy is low. The treatment of preinvasive lesions can be postponed after delivery. If there is microinvasive lesion, a cone biopsy or LEEP must be undertaken. The risk of bleeding PROM and preterm labour is more in higher gestational age than in lower gestational age [18, 19]. Cerclage of the cervix after LEEP or cone biopsy can be done to prevent preterm labour. If the pregnancy is close to maturity, LEEP or cone biopsy may be deferred till foetal maturity is achieved.

### Invasive Cancer of the Cervix

Surgery, neoadjuvant chemotherapy followed by surgery and chemoradiation are treatment available for carcinoma cervix. Seventy per cent of cancer cervix presents at stage 1 in pregnancy. Cervical cancer in pregnancy presents with bleeding, and it is important for physicians to remember that nonpregnancy-related causes can also present with bleeding in pregnancy. Pregnancy changes can underestimate the parametrial involvement. Pregnancy does not alter the prognosis in cervical cancer. A policy of termination of pregnancy and treatment of carcinoma of the cervix was advocated before. But currently the management has changed. Since pregnancy makes clinical staging difficult, MRI is used to stage the disease in pregnancy. MRI is the best modality to stage the disease [20].

However, MRI may not detect all enlarged nodes, and the best way to assess nodes is through lymphadenectomy and histopathological examination. Laparoscopic lymphadenectomy has been successfully used in pregnancy [21]. The management of carcinoma depends on the stage of the disease, lymph node metastasis and period of gestation. For stage IA1 squamous cell carcinoma, cone biopsy with preservation of the foetus can be safely performed between 14 and 20th week of pregnancy. In early-stage carcinoma of the cervix (< stage 1 B), the current policy is to do laparoscopic lymphadenectomy after MRI is used for staging [22, 23]. If the lymph nodes are negative, chemoradiation or definite surgery is done after delivery. In later-stage disease (> stage 1b) or if lymph nodes are involved, neoadjuvant chemotherapy is used and patient is delivered when foetal maturity is obtained. Most studies have used cisplatin for neoadjuvant therapy as weekly dose every 3 weeks [24]. No significant foetal effects have been observed. Definitive therapy can be undertaken once the patient is delivered.

If the patient presents in pregnancy and the patient is not keen, continuation of pregnancy chemoradiation can be started. Patient usually aborts in 3 weeks. If the patient is close to term, caesarean delivery followed by chemoradiation can be undertaken. Radical hysterectomy can be done along with caesarean section in early-stage disease.

## Cancer Ovary

Most ovarian masses discovered during pregnancy are benign. Adnexal masses are usually diagnosed during routine scan during pregnancy. Some may present with features of torsion or bleeding. Malignancy is suspected when the mass is >6 cm and morphological appearance is suggestive of malignancy and in the presence of extra-ovarian disease [25]. Tumour markers are unreliable in pregnancy as they may be normally elevated. However, LDH is unaffected by pregnancy. Though elevated in pregnancy, extremely high values of alpha-fetoprotein are suggestive of endodermal sinus tumour. Ovarian cysts less than 6 cm are unlikely to be malignant. Ovarian masses that persist into second trimester and complex echogenic pattern need exploration. CT scan is contraindicated in pregnancy, but MRI can be used in pregnancy to differentiate between benign and malignant tumours. The commonest malignancy that occurs in pregnancy is germ cell tumours followed by borderline epithelial tumours and malignant epithelial tumours [26]. Laparoscopy can be done with standard precautions in pregnancy. The affected ovary is removed and the specimen is sent for frozen section. Further management depends on frozen report.

### Tumours of Low Malignant Potential

Resection of affected ovary and removal of macroscopic deposit should be done. If the tumour is of mucinous type, appendicectomy also should be done. There is no need for postoperative chemotherapy and can be observed full staging if not performed during pregnancy can be 3 weeks after delivery [27].

### Germ Cell Tumours

Patients with germ cell tumours need full staging. Fertility preservation surgery should be done. Routine lymphadenectomy is not indicated; however, suspicious nodes must be removed. Ninety percent of germ cell tumours are discovered at stage 1 disease. They need postoperative chemotherapy. A combination of bleomycin, etoposide and cisplatin is given to these patients. Indications of postoperative chemotherapy are the same as that of non-pregnant patients [27]. Chemotherapy can be used with relative safety after 14 weeks of gestation.

## Epithelial Ovarian Cancer

Patients with ovarian cancers need chemotherapy. Most ovarian cancers present late in pregnancy. Prognosis is bad in epithelial ovarian cancers. The option of preservation of pregnancy and neoadjuvant chemotherapy should be discussed with the patient. In stage 1 A and B tumours, which are of grade 1 and 2, conservative surgery can be undertaken with preservation of pregnancy. Invasive cancer diagnosed in stage II onwards cancer before 24 weeks of gestation, pregnancy termination and full surgical staging followed by chemotherapy must be undertaken. If the cancer is discovered after 24 weeks of gestation, a policy of neoadjuvant chemotherapy and preservation of pregnancy can be undertaken. Caesarean section can be done at 32–34 weeks of gestation. A gap of 3–4 weeks should be there between chemotherapy and caesarean section. Full surgical staging must be undertaken at caesarean section with the help of a gynaecological oncologist [27].

## Haematological Malignancies in Pregnancy

Hodgkin's lymphoma is the commonest haematological malignancy occurring in pregnancy. Prognosis of Hodgkin's lymphoma diagnosed during pregnancy is similar to that of non-pregnant women [28]. Doxorubicin, bleomycin, vinblastine and dacarbazine (ABVD) is the standard chemotherapy for Hodgkin's lymphoma. However, when used in the first trimester, it can lead to congenital anomalies in foetus. Standard approach in the first trimester is termination of pregnancy and chemotherapy. If Hodgkin's lymphoma is diagnosed beyond the first trimester, ABVD regimen can be used and pregnancy terminated at 34 weeks [29].

## Malignant Melanomas in Pregnancy

Malignant melanoma which occurs in pregnancy carries a poorer prognosis [30]. This poor prognosis may be due to a delay in diagnosis in pregnancy. Malignant melanomas in pregnancy tend to be thicker and have a poorer prognosis. Standard treatment of melanoma during pregnancy is surgery. Patients with advanced disease may be given systemic chemotherapy in pregnancy beyond the first trimester. However, systemic chemotherapy is not very effective in disseminated melanomas. Women who have melanoma should not become pregnant as 50 % of melanomas recur within 3 years [31]. Melanomas can metastasise to the foetus and placenta.

### Conclusion

Cancer complicating pregnancy is a rare event. Breast cancer if diagnosed in pregnancy can be managed surgically in early stages and with neoadjuvant chemotherapy and surgery in late stages. In carcinoma cervix less than stage 1 B, a laparoscopic lymphadenectomy is done, and if no nodes are found negative, definitive treatment can be done after delivery. In later stages of carcinoma cervix, neoadjuvant chemotherapy and definite chemoradiation are done after delivery. Borderline ovarian malignancies are treated conservatively. Germ call tumours are also treated conservatively followed by chemotherapy. Stage 1 A and 1 B epithelial cancers are treated conservatively in pregnancy. They do not need post-chemotherapy if they are of grade 1 and 2. Malignant epithelial ovarian tumours presenting less than 24 weeks of gestation are treated with termination of pregnancy and surgical staging followed by chemotherapy. If epithelial tumours are detected after 24 weeks of gestation, neoadjuvant chemotherapy can be given and pregnancy terminated at around 34 weeks. Full staging is done after delivery. In Hodgkin's lymphoma, ABVD chemotherapy can used beyond the first trimester preserving pregnancy. Melanomas are treated surgically in pregnancy.

## References

1. Pavlidis NA. Coexistence of pregnancy and malignancy. Oncologist. 2002;7:279–87.
2. Pereg D, Koren G, Lishner M. Cancer in pregnancy: gaps, challenges and solutions. Cancer Treat Rev. 2008;34:302–12.
3. Van Calsteren K, Amant F, De Smet F, Gziri MM, Halaska M, Heyns L, Ottevanger N, Van Eycken L,

Van Gemert W, Vergote I. Cancer during pregnancy: an analysis of 215 patients emphasising the obstetrical and neonatal outcome. J Clin Oncol. 2010;28(4):683–9.
4. Cardonick E, Iacobucci A. Use of chemotherapy during human pregnancy. Lancet Oncol. 2004;5:283–91.
5. Kal HB, Struikmans H. Radiotherapy during pregnancy: fact and fiction. Lancet Oncol. 2005;6:328–33.
6. Woo SY, Cundiff BS, Fredrick B, Fernando C, Swan Jr F, Hagemeister FB, Jackson H, Rodriguez MA, Bondy ML, Fuller LM, McLaughlin P, Alle PK, Carpenter Jr RJ, Velasquez WS. Radiotherapy during pregnancy for clinical stages IA-IIA Hodgkin's disease. Int J Radiat Oncol Biol Phys. 1992;23:407–12.
7. Karimi ZM, Behtash N, Modares GM. Good pregnancy outcome after prenatal exposure to bleomycin, etoposide and cisplatin for ovarian immature teratoma: a case report and literature review. Arch Gynecol Obstet. 2008;277:75–8.
8. Kim DS, Park MI. Maternal and fetal survival following surgery and chemotherapy of endodermal sinus tumor of the ovary during pregnancy: a case report. Obstet Gynecol. 1989;73:503–7.
9. Kim JH, Kim HS, Kim CH, Kim KJ, Lee KY, Sung CW. Docetaxel, gemcitabine, and cisplatin administered for non-small cell lung cancer during the first and second trimester of an unrecognized pregnancy. Lung Cancer. 2008;59:270–3.
10. Machado F, Abad L, Leon J, Parrilla JJ, Perez A, Sanchez R, Vegas C. Ovarian cancer during pregnancy: analysis of 15 cases. Gynecol Oncol. 2007; 105:446–50.
11. Malhotra N, Sood M. Endodermal sinus tumor in pregnancy. Gynecol Oncol. 2000;78:265–6.
12. Otton G, Higgins S, Phillip KA, Quinn M. A case of early-stage epithelial ovarian cancer in pregnancy. Int J Gynecol Cancer. 2001;11:413–7.
13. Palaia I, Bellati F, Graziano M, Panici PB, Pernice M. Neoadjuvant chemotherapy plus radical surgery in locally advanced cervical cancer during pregnancy: a case report. Am J Obstet Gynecol. 2007;197:e5–6.
14. Ulery M, Carter L, Giurgescu C, McFarlin BL. Pregnancy-associated breast cancer: significance of early detection. J Midwifery Womens Health. 2009;54:357–63.
15. Loibl S, Amant F, Kaufmann M. 313 patients with breast cancer during pregnancy—a prospective and retrospective registry (GBG-20/BIG02-03). San Antonio Breast Cancer Symposium, San Antonio, 8–12 Dec 2010. Abstract S6-2.
16. Cardonick E, Dougherty R, Ghaffar S, Gilmandyar D, Grana G, Usmani A. Breast cancer during pregnancy: maternal and fetal outcomes. Cancer J. 2010;16:76–82.
17. Morimura Y, Fujimori K, Hashimoto T, Sato A, Soeda S, Takano Y, Yamada H, Yanagida K. Cervical cytology during pregnancy—comparison with non-pregnant women and management of pregnant women with abnormal cytology Fukushima. J Med Sci. 2002;48:27–37.
18. Robinson WR, Degefu S, O'Quinn AG, Tirpack J, Webb S. Management of cervical intraepithelial neoplasia during pregnancy with LOOP excision. Gynecol Oncol. 1997;64:153–5.
19. Seki N, Kodama J, Hiramatsu Y, Hongo A, Kusumoto T, Nakamura K. Complications and obstetric outcomes after laser conization during pregnancy. Eur J Gynaecol Oncol. 2010;31:399–401.
20. Doyle S, Messiou C, Rutherford JM, Dineen RA. Cancer presenting during pregnancy: radiological perspectives. Clin Radiol. 2009;64:857–71.
21. Alouini S, Mathevet P, Rida K. Cervical cancer complicating pregnancy: implications of laparoscopic lymphadenectomy. Gynecol Oncol. 2008;108:472–7.
22. Ishioka S, Endo T, Ezaka Y, Inoue M, Nagasawa K, Saito T, Sato A, Shimizu A. Outcomes of planned delivery delay in pregnant patients with invasive gynecologic cancer. Int J Clin Oncol. 2009;14: 321–5.
23. Lee JM, Cho CH, Choi HS, Kim KT, Kim YT, Lee KB, Lee KH, Namkoong SE, Ryu HS. Cervical cancer associated with pregnancy: results of a multi center retrospective Korean study(KGOG-1006). Am J Obstet Gynecol. 2008;198:92.e1–6.
24. Caluwaerts S, Amant F, Calsteren K, Hanssens M, Lagae L, Mertens L, Moerman P, VergoteI VAN, Wuyts K. Neoadjuvant chemotherapy followed by radical hysterectomy for invasive cervical cancer diagnosed during pregnancy: report of a case and review of the literature. Int J Gynecol Cancer. 2006; 16:905–8.
25. Pentheroudakis G, Hoekstra HJ, Orecchia R, Pavlidis N, ESMO Guidelines Working Group. Cancer, fertility and pregnancy: ESMO Clinical Practice Guidelines for diagnosis, treatment and follow-up. Ann Oncol. 2010;21 suppl 5:v266–73.
26. Hoover K, Jenkins TR. Evaluation and management of adnexal mass in pregnancy. Am J Obstet Gynecol. 2011;205:97–102.
27. Marret H, Canis M, Golfier F, Lecuru F, Lhommé C, Lévèque J, Morice P. Guidelines for the management of ovarian cancer during pregnancy. Eur J Obstet Gynecol Reprod Biol. 2010;149:18–21.
28. Lishner M, Degendorfer P, Koren G, Panzarella T, Sutcliffe SB, Zemlickis D. Maternal and foetal outcome following Hodgkin's disease in pregnancy. Br J Cancer. 1992;65:114–7.
29. El-Hemaidi I, Robinson SE. Management of haematological malignancy in pregnancy. Best Pract Res Clin Obstet Gynaecol. 2012;26:149–60.
30. Slingluff CL, Reintgen DS, Seigler HF, Vollmer RT. Malignant melanoma arising during pregnancy. A study of 100 patients. Ann Surg. 1990;211:552–7.
31. Mackie RM. Pregnancy and exogenous female sex hormones in melanoma patients. In: Balch CM, Houghton AN, Sober AJ, Soong S-J, editors. Cutaneous melanoma. 3rd ed. St Louis: QMP Publishing; 1998. p. 187–93.

# Life-Threatening Complications of MTP/Abortion

31

Shrinivas Gadappa and Rajendrasing Pardeshi

## Introduction

Unwanted pregnancies and abortion have existed since time immemorial. Chinese, Greek, and Roman cultures all developed systems of dealing with unwanted pregnancies and regulating population growth in their respective societies. The Egyptians were some of the first to create abortion techniques, which were discussed and reported in some of their first, and our oldest, medical texts [1].

The term "abortion" is derived from the Latin word "aboriri," which means "to get detached from the proper site." "Abortion" is the termination of pregnancy when the fetus is not viable or termination prior to 20 weeks of gestation or a fetus born weighing less than 500 g (World Health Organization (WHO), Centers for Disease Control (CDC), National Center for Health Statistics (NCHS)).

*"Miscarriage" or spontaneous abortion* means the premature expulsion of the product of conception (an ovum, embryo, or a fetus) from the uterus, without the application of any deliberate methods to terminate it during the early weeks after conception. *"Induced abortion"* means willful termination of pregnancy before viability. Induced termination of pregnancy whether in hands of skilled or unskilled persons are always fraught with health hazards, leading to increased incidence of "maternal mortality" and "morbidity" especially when performed in "unsafe" and "unhygienic conditions." *Safe abortions* – those done by trained providers in hygienic settings – and early medical abortions (using medication to end a pregnancy) carry few health risks (WHO 2003).

Unsafe abortion is a persistent, but preventable pandemic with grave implications on the life of women and their reproductive career [2]. The World Health Organization (WHO) defines *unsafe abortion* ——as a procedure for terminating an unintended pregnancy carried out either by persons lacking the necessary skills or in an environment that does not conform to minimal medical standards, or both (WHO 2007). The term *"septic abortion"* refers to a spontaneous miscarriage or therapeutic/artificial abortion complicated by a pelvic infection. Unsafe abortion is most often associated with attendant complications of sepsis, hemorrhage requiring blood transfusion, uterine and bowel perforation, pelvic abscess, endotoxic shock, renal failure, and death. Long-term sequelae include ectopic pregnancy, chronic pelvic pain and infertility with grave implications for future reproductive health of the woman. What is particularly worrisome

S. Gadappa (✉)
Department of OBGY, Government Medical College, Aurangabad, India
e-mail: drshrinivasgadappa@yahoo.com; gadappashrinivas@gmail.com

R. Pardeshi
Jijai Maternity and Nursing Home, Food and Drug Committee FOGSI, Aurangabad, India
e-mail: varadsing@yahoo.co.in


A. Gandhi et al. (eds.), *Principles of Critical Care in Obstetrics: Volume II*,
DOI 10.1007/978-81-322-2686-4_31

about the scenario of unsafe abortion is that these deaths or disabilities are occurring in spite of the fact that the world has safe, effective, and affordable means of preventing unwanted pregnancy

Unsafe abortion is one of the leading causes of maternal mortality and morbidity. In developing countries, the risk of death following complications of unsafe abortion procedures is several hundred times higher than that of an abortion performed professionally under safe conditions (WHO 1998).

Before the enactment of MTP Act, 1971, induced abortion was illegal and violation of law (IPC 312 Causing Miscarriage). Abortion was liberalized in India after the Medical Termination of Pregnancy (MTP) Act which came into effect on 1 April 1972, according to which a pregnancy may be terminated within 20 weeks of gestation.

Abortion being a sensitive issue, a large number of women, is not aware of its being legal. In such circumstances, most of these women if they had to go for abortion, they would prefer sources which are not public and go to private clinics where privacy and confidentiality are better maintained [3].

## Incidence

WHO estimates that globally 210 million women become pregnant each year and that around 80 million of these pregnancies are unplanned (WHO 2004) [4]. However, every year, close to 20 million women risk their lives and health by undergoing unsafe abortions. Twenty-five percent of these women will face a complication with permanent consequences and close to 66,500 women will die. The majority of these women live in the developing world, and half of those who die are under the age of 25 years (WHO 2007) [1].

Among all unsafe abortions, 97 % occur in developing countries and more than half (55 %) are in Asia, particularly in south-central Asia. Nearly 13 % of all illegal abortions in the world are carried out in India [4].

Globally, five million women are estimated to be hospitalized because of abortion-related complications (WHO 2007) and 67,900 maternal deaths are the result of unsafe abortions annually, representing 13 % of maternal mortality deaths (Singh 2006; WHO 2007; Fawcus 2008). Every 8 min, a woman dies in the developing world due to complications from unsafe abortion (id21, 2007; cited in Bhandari et al. 2008) [4].

According to the Consortium on National Consensus for Medical Abortion in India (2008), every year, an average of about 11 million abortions take place annually and around 20,000 women die every year due to abortion-related complications. Most abortion-related maternal deaths are attributable to illegal abortions [3].

## Causes for Unsafe Abortion

- Lack of access
- Lack of trained MTP providers
- Lack of equipment
- Lack of facilities
- Lack of information about availability of safe abortion services
- Social causes

## Complications of Abortion

Complications of abortion depend upon gestational age, method employed, or the abortion process. Earlier abortions are definitely safer. Fourfold rise in complications with late abortions (Fig. 31.1 and Table 31.1).

Complications of spontaneous miscarriages and therapeutic abortions include the following:

### Immediate

1. *Injury to the cervix (cervical lacerations):* The cervix is sometimes torn during the procedure. The most common complication after dilatation and evacuation was cervical laceration that required suturing [5], but in

most cases, the tear is minimal and heals quickly on its own without treatment.

2. *Vasovagal shock (cervical shock):* Vasovagal syncope produced by stimulation of the cervical canal during dilatation may occur. Rapid recovery usually follows.
3. *Uterine perforation and/or injury to the bladder/bowel*: Rarely, an instrument may puncture the wall of the uterus. The frequency of this event is about one in one thousand cases. Hospitalization is usually necessary for observation and/or completion of the abortion. To inspect the condition of the uterus in this situation, laparoscopy can be done. If damage is serious, an abdominal operation may be required to repair the damage. This can include hysterectomy.
4. *Postabortion triad* (i.e., pain, bleeding, low-grade fever) due to retained clots or products.

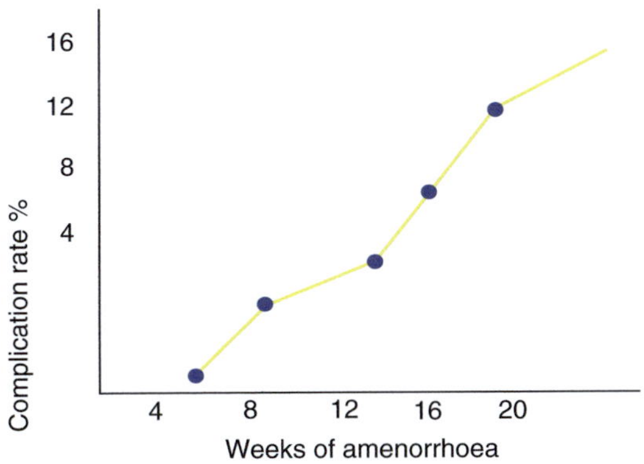


**Fig. 31.1** Relation of rate of abortion complications and gestational age

5. *Thrombosis and embolism.*
6. *Hematometra*: Also known as postabortion syndrome, this is the result of retained products of conception or uterine atony for other causes. The endometrium is distended with blood, and the uterus is unable to contract to expel the contents.
7. *Retained products of conception*: During a nonsurgical abortion, medication will induce the uterus to contract and naturally slough and empty of blood and tissue. Occasionally, however, this process is incomplete and can lead to infection, hemorrhage, or both especially if fetal tissue remains in the uterus. The thickened lining of the uterus is never completely removed during a surgical abortion, and therefore, it is normal for the uterus to naturally shed excess blood and tissue while healing. This process can lead to infection, hemorrhage, or both. To remove remaining tissue, it will be necessary to repeat the misoprostol or perform a uterine aspiration at the office. In rare instances, hospitalization or surgery is required.
8. *Infection*: Infection is caused by germs from the vagina and cervix getting into the uterus, and this can occur when the cervix is dilated to pass the pregnancy. If a woman has gonorrhea, syphilis, or chlamydia, a serious tubal infection can occur. The risk of infection associated with early medical abortion is very low. Such infections usually respond to aspiration and antibiotics, but in some instances, hospitalization can be necessary.

**Table 31.1** Complications of MTP/abortion

| Immediate | Remote | |
|---|---|---|
| 1. Injury to the cervix (cervical lacerations) | A. *Gynecological* | C. *Obstetrical* |
| 2. Vasovagal shock | 1. Menstrual disturbances | 1. Recurrent midtrimester abortion due to cervical incompetence |
| 3. Hemorrhage and shock | 2. PID | 2. Ectopic pregnancy |
| 4. Retained products of conception | 3. Infertility | 3. Preterm labor |
| 5. Infection | 4. Scar endometriosis | 4. Increased perinatal loss |
| 6. Uterine perforation | 5. Incisional hernia | 5. Rupture uterus |
| 7. Injury to bladder/bowel | 6. Uterine synechiae leading to secondary amenorrhea | 6. Rh isoimmunization |
| 8. Postabortion triad with pain | B. *Psychological/emotional trauma* | 7. Abruptio placenta |
| 9. Thrombosis and embolism | | 8. Failed abortion and continued pregnancy |
| 10. Hematometra | | 9. Placenta acreta |

Surgery may also be required in extreme cases. It is very important to observe all follow-up instructions and return for your check up to ensure that your risk of infection is minimized. In severe form, it may cause septic abortion and peritonitis.

9. *Hemorrhage and shock* due to trauma, incomplete abortion, atonic uterus, or coagulation failure (DIC). Bleeding from the uterus heavy enough to require treatment occurs rarely. Hemorrhage, heavy enough to require a blood transfusion, occurs in less than one in one thousand cases. A bleeding problem may require medications to help the uterus contract, a repeat aspiration or dilation and curettage or, rarely, surgery to correct the bleeding
10. *Related to methods employed*
    - (i) *Prostaglandins*
        1. Vomiting
        2. Diarrhea
        3. Fever
        4. Abdominal pain
        5. Cervico-uterine injury
    - (ii) *Oxytocin*
        1. Water intoxication
        2. Convulsions
    - (iii) *Hysterotomy*
        - Hemorrhage and shock
        - Complications of anesthesia
        - Peritonitis
        - Intestinal Obstruction
    - (iv) *Saline*
        - Hypernatremia
        - Pulmonary edema
        - Endotoxic shock
        - DIC
        - Renal failure
        - Cerebral edema

## Remote

(i) *Gynecological*

1. Menstrual disturbances.
2. PID: 5 % of women suffer PID following induced (or surgical) abortion. PID can lead to fever and infertility.
3. Infertility due to cornual block.
4. Scar endometriosis especially in hysterotomy (1 %).
5. Incisional hernia.
6. Uterine synechiae leading to secondary amenorrhea.

(ii) *Obstetrical*

1. *Recurrent midtrimester abortion* due to cervical incompetence.
2. *Ectopic pregnancy*: Studies point out that the risk of an ectopic pregnancy is 30 % higher for women who have had one abortion and up to four times higher for women with two or more abortions. When a woman has an ectopic pregnancy, she has a 12 % risk of dying in a future pregnancy.
3. *Preterm labor.*
4. *Increased perinatal loss.*
5. *Rupture uterus.*
6. *Rh isoimmunization* in Rh-negative women, if not prophylactically protected with immunoglobulin.
7. *Abruptio placenta*: Abruptio placenta can result in extreme and severe life-threatening bleeding. Women who have experienced abortion have a 600 % increase in their risk for abruptio placenta in future pregnancies.
8. *Failed abortion and continued pregnancy.* Failed MTP is defined when there is failure to achieve termination of pregnancy within 48 h. Sometimes, an early abortion does not succeed in terminating the pregnancy. The likelihood of this event is less than one in one thousand cases. In such cases, another abortion procedure is recommended, because the first attempted abortion can adversely affect the normal development of the pregnancy. Alternately, this can also be a sign of a tubal pregnancy, which would require hospitalization and abdominal surgery.
9. *Placenta acreta*

(iii) *Psychological/emotional trauma:* 50 % of women who have had abortions report experiencing emotional and psychological problems lasting for months or years. These emotions include, but aren't limited to:

1. Acute feeling of grief
2. Depression
3. Anger
4. Fear of disclosure
5. Preoccupation with babies or getting pregnant again
6. Nightmares
7. Sexual dysfunction
8. Termination of relationships
9. Emotional coldness
10. Increased alcohol and drug abuse
11. Eating disorders
12. Anxiety
13. Flashbacks of the abortion procedure
14. Suicide

Many of these women go on to report that they regret their choice and would do anything to go back and undo the decision that resulted in so much pain.

Severity of complications is another important measure of effects on health. The proportion of women classified with severe complications if:

- Fever of 38 °C or more
- Organ or system failure
- Generalized peritonitis
- Pulse 120 per min or more
- Shock
- Evidence of a foreign body
- Mechanical injury

Out of the abovementioned life-threatening complications are uterine hemorrhage due to perforation, severe sepsis, peritonitis, visceral injuries, hemorrhagic and septic shock, renal failure, DIC, hepatic failure, and encephalopathy.

## Mortality

Early abortion is one of the safest procedures. Maternal death is lowest (0.6/100,000 procedures) in the first trimester termination while mortality rate increases 5–6 times in midtrimester termination of pregnancy.

## Pathophysiology

Postabortion complications develop as a result of three major mechanisms as follows: incomplete evacuation of the uterus and uterine atony, which leads to hemorrhagic complications; infection; and injury due to instruments used during the procedure.

In septic abortion, infection usually begins as endometritis and involves the endometrium and any retained products of conception. If not treated, the infection may spread further into the myometrium and parametrium. Parametritis may progress into peritonitis. The patient may develop bacteremia and sepsis at any stage of septic abortion. Pelvic inflammatory disease (PID) is the most common complication of septic abortion.

## Prevention of Complications

### Primary Prevention

It includes reduction in the need for unsafe abortion through contraception, legalization of abortion on request, the use of safer techniques, and improvement of provider skills. Access to safe, effective contraception can substantially reduce – but never eliminate – the need for abortion to regulate fertility.

All abortion patients – whether seeking treatment of a complication or an elective induced abortion – should be offered contraceptive counseling and a choice of appropriate methods. Contraceptive counseling and provision at the time of treatment reduced unintended pregnancies and repeat abortions by 50 % over 1 year in Zimbabwe, compared with postabortion patients who did not receive such services.

The advent of vacuum aspiration in the 1960s revolutionized the primary prevention of complications in developing countries. Vacuum aspiration is safer than sharp curettage, and the WHO recommends vacuum aspiration as the preferred method for uterine evacuation before 12 weeks of pregnancy. This method is faster, safer, more comfortable, and associated with shorter hospital stay for induced abortion than sharp curettage.

Additional advantages compared with sharp curettage are its ease of use as an outpatient procedure, the need for less analgesia and anesthesia, and its lower cost per procedure especially if done on an outpatient basis.

The combined use of mifepristone and misoprostol has become the standard WHO-recommended medical regimen for early medication abortion and is better than either drug alone. Regimens with misoprostol alone as an abortifacient have varied widely, with reported success rates ranging between 87 and 97 %. Increased access to misoprostol has been associated with improved women's health in developing countries, and studies are being done to refine the regimen for misoprostol alone to induce abortion.

## Secondary Prevention

Secondary Prevention entails prompt and appropriate treatment of complications. This includes timely evacuation of the uterus after incomplete abortion. WHO has issued technical and clinical guidelines for the provision of safe abortion care and treatment of abortion complications. Misoprostol can be used for the management of incomplete abortion, and vacuum aspiration is better than sharp curettage.

Postabortion care is spreading worldwide. It included postabortion assessment and diagnosis, uterine evacuation procedures and techniques, pain management, infection prevention, management of complications, referral to other sexual and reproductive health services, contraceptive counseling and provision, and follow-up care.

Interventions include clinical training of physicians and midwives, provision of manual vacuum aspiration and other supplies, reorganization of services, supervisory visits to facilities, and improved record-keeping. Critics of postabortion care worldwide complain that the preoccupation with secondary (rather than primary) prevention of unsafe abortion is myopic, tantamount to placing ambulances at the bottom of a cliff instead of erecting a fence at the top.

## Tertiary Prevention

Tertiary prevention mitigates long-term damage. Rapid transfer to a hospital can be lifesaving. Prompt repair of uterine injury could preserve fertility. Acute renal failure and tetanus from unsafe abortions remain important causes of death and lengthy disability. Repair of fistulas in bowel and bladder can end the suffering, stigmatization, and abandonment that these injuries cause.

## Medical/Legal Pitfalls

1. Do not underestimate the amount and rate of bleeding. In the supine position, more than 500 mL of blood may collect in the vagina without severe external bleeding. Always perform a pelvic examination on a postabortion patient who is bleeding.
2. Failure to aggressively treat vaginal bleeding, even if it seems minimal: Stabilize the patient with 2 large-bore IVs and with oxygen. Closely monitor vital signs.
3. Failure to diagnose uterine perforation may lead to life-threatening complications: In postabortion patients with abdominal pain beyond the pelvic area, suspect perforation and evaluate with kidney, ureter, and bladder (KUB)/upright radiographs and pelvic ultrasonography. Consult a gynecologist and, if suspicion is high, insist on laparoscopy.
4. Failure to diagnose ectopic pregnancy: The chance of a missed ectopic pregnancy always exists. Do not presume intrauterine pregnancy in a patient who has just had an abortion; she may have had a missed ectopic pregnancy.
5. Failure to promptly administer broad-spectrum antibiotic therapy may result in complications, including sepsis and septic shock. Do not delay administration of antibiotics if a patient has signs of severe postabortion infection. Administer broad-spectrum antibiotics before completing diagnostic workup.
6. Failure to obtain information about recent termination of pregnancy may lead to a wrong diagnosis or delayed/inappropriate treatment.

7. Failure to evacuate retained products of conception from the uterus leads to treatment failure and possible complications.
8. Failure to diagnose bowel injury may lead to life-threatening complications.

## Diagnosis of Complications

Diagnosis of complications is made by thorough history, physical examination, and investigations.

### History

Presentation depends on the type of complication the patient develops. Intraoperative and early postoperative complications are rarely seen, but some patients develop these types of complications and present to the emergency for treatment. Complications include the following:

1. *Local anesthesia:* Paracervical block is a common method of anesthesia for therapeutic abortion. Accidental intravascular injection of anesthetic is a potentially life-threatening complication of this method that could lead to seizure, cardiopulmonary arrest, and death.
2. *General anesthesia:* Complications with general anesthesia may lead to uterine atony with severe hemorrhage.
3. *Cervical shock:* Vasovagal syncope produced by stimulation of the cervical canal during dilatation may occur. Rapid recovery usually follows.
4. *Postabortion triad:* Pain, bleeding, and low-grade fevers are the most common presenting complaints. Postabortion triad usually is caused by retained products of conception.
5. *Hemorrhage:* Excessive hemorrhage during or after abortion may signify uterine atony, cervical laceration, uterine perforation, cervical pregnancy, a more advanced gestational age than anticipated, or coagulopathy.
6. *Hematometra*: Also known as postabortion syndrome, this is the result of retained products of conception or uterine atony for other causes. The endometrium is distended with blood, and the uterus is unable to contract to expel the contents. Patients usually present with increasing lower midline abdominal pain, absent or decreased vaginal bleeding, and, at times, hemodynamic compromise. This may develop immediately after miscarriage or abortion, or it may develop insidiously.
7. *Perforation:* Patients with uterine perforation missed during the procedure usually present as an emergency with increased abdominal pain, bleeding (possibly ranging from very mild to absent), and fever. If perforation results in injury to major blood vessels, patients may present in hemorrhagic shock.
8. *Bowel injury:* This may accompany uterine perforation. If initially unrecognized, patients present with abdominal pain, fever, blood in the stool, nausea, and vomiting.
9. *Bladder injury:* This occurs as a result of uterine or cervical perforation. Patients present with suprapubic pain and hematuria.
10. *Septic abortion:* This is endometritis. Patients present with fever, chills, abdominal pain, foul-smelling vaginal discharge, vaginal bleeding, and history of recent pregnancy.
11. *Failed abortion* (continued intrauterine or ectopic pregnancy): Failure to terminate the pregnancy is relatively common with very early abortions (<6 weeks gestational age). Such patients may present with symptoms of continuing pregnancy such as hyperemesis, increased abdominal girth, and breast engorgement. In addition, an unrecognized ectopic pregnancy in the postabortion period presents in the usual manner.
12. *Disseminated intravascular coagulation:* Suspect DIC in all patients who present with severe postabortion bleeding, especially after midtrimester abortions.

### Physical Examination

1. Vital signs
   (i) Monitoring of vital signs is essential for patients with postabortion complications.
   (ii) Increasing fever could be a sign of progressing infection.

   (iii) Tachycardia and hypotension may be signs of severe hemorrhage or septic shock.
2. Abdominal examination
   (i) Suprapubic tenderness is common in the postabortion period. Severe tenderness is unusual and may be a sign of hematometra, bladder perforation, or bowel injury.
   (ii) Tenderness in other areas of the abdomen (e.g., rebound tenderness, guarding) strongly indicates instrumental injury complications (e.g., perforation, bowel injury, bladder injury).
   (iii) A tender mass in the suprapubic area suggests hematometra.
   (iv) Diminished or absent bowel sounds are a sign of developing peritonitis.
3. Vaginal examination
   (i) Assess the quantity and rate of hemorrhage.
      - Look for possible vaginal or cervical injury.
      - Identify the source of bleeding (e.g., uterine, cervical os, lesions of the vulva, vagina, or vaginal portion of cervix).
   (ii) Cervical motion tenderness on bimanual examination may be suggestive of pelvic infection or ectopic pregnancy.
   (iii) A large tender uterus may be a sign of hematometra.
   (iv) Adnexal tenderness or masses may suggest ectopic pregnancy, pelvic inflammatory disease (PID), cyst, or hematoma.
4. Rectal examination
   (i) A rectal examination must be performed if bowel injury is suspected.
   (ii) The presence of rectal tenderness and blood (or guaiac-positive stool) makes the diagnosis of bowel injury almost certain.

## Management of Complications of Abortion

### Investigations

A. Laboratory Studies
   1. Complete blood count and platelets: Repeat CBC may be helpful in assessing the degree of ongoing hemorrhage.
   2. Blood grouping and cross-matching.
   3. Complete metabolic panel.LFT, RFT.
   4. Beta-human chorionic gonadotropin level: A quantitative level may provide useful information and a basis for future comparison.
   5. Coagulation profile: PT and aPTT, INR.
   6. Urinalysis.
   7. If DIC is suspected, fibrinogen, fibrin split products, and D-dimer should be obtained.
   8. Erythrocyte sedimentation rate may be helpful in assessing developing infection.
   9. Endocervical cultures (e.g., aerobic, anaerobic, gonorrheal, chlamydial) and Gram stain may be indicated.
   10. Blood cultures should be obtained if the patient is febrile and systemic infection is suspected.

B. Imaging Studies
   1. To exclude free air as a result of bowel perforation, obtain either an *upright chest radiograph or an upright abdominal radiograph*. Both supine and upright radiographs of the abdomen assist in the detection of free air or foreign bodies.
   2. USG: Transvaginal *ultrasonography* to rule out ectopic pregnancy, retained products of conception in the uterus, adnexal masses, free fluid in the cul-de-sac, and hematometra.
   3. *Abdominal and pelvic CT* may be useful in evaluating the acutely tender abdomen and pelvis if pelvic ultrasonography is not diagnostic.

## Treatment

A. Prehospital care
   1. Monitor vital signs.
   2. Stabilize with intravenous fluids (e.g., normal saline, Ringer's lactate), if the patient is hemodynamically unstable.
   3. Administer oxygen.

B. Emergency care
   1. Screen all patients with postabortion complications for Rh factor. Administer Rho(D) immune globulin (RhoGAM) if

results indicate that the patient is Rh negative and unsensitized.

2. Patients with the postabortion triad (i.e., pain, bleeding, low-grade fever) may respond to treatment with oral antibiotics and ergot preparations. Immediately initiate these agents. In most cases, however, blood clots or retained products of conception must be evacuated from the uterus. In these cases, administer medications parenterally, as the patient will undergo anesthesia.
3. Hemorrhage or hematometra
   (i) Monitor vital signs and rate of bleeding. Administer fluids, blood, and blood products as needed.
   (ii) Administer intravenous oxytocin for treatment of uterine atony.
   (iii) Alternative treatments for uterine atony include intracervical vasopressin or carboprost tromethamine and bimanual uterine massage.
   (iv) If bleeding persists, screen for coagulopathy/DIC and obtain immediate gynecologic consultation with the intention of transferring the patient to the operating room (OR) for repeat curettage and, if necessary, hysterectomy.
4. Uterine perforation, bowel injury, and bladder injury: If one or any combination of these complications is suspected or diagnosed treat as follows:
   (i) Hemodynamically stabilize the patient.
   (ii) Insert a Foley catheter.
   (iii) Transfer to the OT for laparoscopy/laparotomy and further treatment.
5. Failed abortion, continued pregnancy, and ectopic pregnancy.
   (i) If the patient is stable, perform ultrasonography and obtain a beta-human chorionic gonadotropin (hCG) level to establish the diagnosis and further treatment.
   (ii) If the patient is unstable, transfer to the OT for dilation and curettage (D&C) and/or laparoscopy/laparotomy.
6. Suspected septic abortion.
   (i) Administer intravenous fluids through a large-bore angiocatheter.
   (ii) For patients who are unstable, administer oxygen and insert a Foley catheter.
   (iii) Early antibiotic treatment may be guided by Gram stain, but broad-spectrum coverage is recommended.
   (iv) Perform evacuation of retained tissues from the uterine cavity, preferably by D&C. If D&C is not immediately available, high doses of oxytocin can be used.
   (v) Laparotomy may be needed if the above measures elicit no response.
   (vi) A hysterectomy may be necessary in cases of uterine perforation, bowel injury, clostridial myometritis, and pelvic abscess.

C. Specialty care
Consult surgery and urology if bowel or bladder injury is diagnosed.

## Medication Summary

- The goals of pharmacotherapy are to eradicate the infection, reduce morbidity, and prevent complications. Aggressive antimicrobial therapy prevents death by eliminating all septic sources during the early stages of the disease.

A. Antibiotics
Immediately administer broad-spectrum antibiotics to patients with severe postabortion infection.

1. Cefoxitin
   Indicated for infections caused by susceptible Gram-positive cocci and Gram-negative bacilli. Many infections caused by Gram-negative bacteria resistant to some cephalosporins and penicillins respond to cefoxitin.
2. Doxycycline
   Treats infections caused by susceptible Gram-negative and Gram-positive organisms, in addition to infections caused by susceptible *Rickettsia, Chlamydia,* and *Mycoplasma* species.
3. Gentamicin sulfate
   Aminoglycoside antibiotic for Gram-negative coverage. Used in combination

with both an agent against Gram-positive organisms and an agent that covers anaerobes. Not the drug of choice. Consider if penicillins or other less toxic drugs are contraindicated, when clinically indicated, and in mixed infections caused by susceptible staphylococci and Gram-negative organisms. Dosing regimens are numerous; adjust dose based on creatine clearance and changes in volume of distribution. May be administered intravenous or intramuscular.

4. Ticarcillin and clavulanate potassium
   Presumptive therapy prior to identification of organism. Inhibits biosynthesis of cell wall mucopeptide; effective during stage of active growth.
5. Ampicillin and sulbactam sodium
   Drug combination of beta-lactamase inhibitor with ampicillin. Covers skin, enteric flora, and anaerobes. Not ideal for nosocomial pathogens.
6. Imipenem and cilastatin sodium
   Treats multiple-organism infections for which other agents lack wide-spectrum coverage or are contraindicated due to potential toxicity.
7. Piperacillin and tazobactam sodium
   Treats septicemia caused by many Gram-positive and Gram-negative pathogens.
8. Clindamycin
   Useful as treatment against aerobic streptococci and most staphylococci. Inhibits bacterial growth, possibly by blocking dissociation of peptidyl tRNA from ribosomes, causing RNA-dependent protein synthesis to arrest.
9. Cefotaxime
   Treats septicemia caused by *Streptococcus* spp., *S. aureus*, *E. coli*, and *Klebsiella* spp. organisms. Used in genitourinary infections such as pelvic inflammatory disease, endometritis, and pelvic cellulitis. Arrests bacterial cell wall synthesis, which, in turn, inhibits bacterial growth.
10. Vancomycin HCL
    Potent antibiotic directed against Gram-positive organisms and active against enterococcal species. Useful in the treatment of septicemia and skin structure infections. Indicated for patients who cannot receive or have failed to respond to penicillins and cephalosporins or who have infections with resistant staphylococci. To avoid toxicity, current recommendation is to assay only vancomycin trough levels after the third dose, drawn 0.5 h before next dosing. Doses and dosing intervals may be adjusted based on creatine clearance.
11. Ceftriaxone
    Third-generation cephalosporin with broad-spectrum Gram-negative activity; lower efficacy against Gram-positive organisms; higher efficacy against resistant organisms. Arrests bacterial growth by binding to one or more penicillin-binding proteins.

B. Synthetic posterior pituitary hormones
   When D&C is not immediately available, these hormones are used to induce contractions to help evacuate retained products of conception from the uterus (carbetocin).
   1. Oxytocin: Produces rhythmic uterine contractions and can stimulate the gravid uterus, as well as antidiuretic effects. Also can control postabortal hemorrhage.
   2. Carbetocin: Carbetocin is a long-acting synthetic octapeptide analogue of oxytocin with agonist properties. It can be administered intravenously to prevent hemorrhage after abortion.

C. Ergot alkaloids
   Ergot derivatives are used for oxytocic effects on uterine muscle. These agents prevent postabortion uterine atony and hemorrhage.
   1. *Methylergometrine (Methergine)*: Acts directly on the smooth muscle of the uterus; induces a rapid and sustained tetanic uterotonic effect that reduces bleeding.

D. *Syntometrine*: Is available in injectable form as combination of oxytocin and methylergometrine.

E. *Prostaglandins*
   1. *PGE1/misoprostol:* Misoprostol is mostly used in cases of retained products of conception per vaginal.

2. *15 Methyl PGF2α/Carboprost:* Is available in injectable form used in cases of retained products of conception and also used to prevent postabortal hemorrhage.

## Further Inpatient Care

1. Inpatient treatment of patients with abortion complications includes repeat D&C, laparoscopy, and laparotomy (for treatment of complicated perforation, bowel and bladder injuries, refractory bleeding).
2. Further inpatient care for patients with septic abortion include the following:
   (i) Perform a prompt evacuation of retained products of conception from the uterus.
   (ii) Administer aggressive antibiotic therapy.
   (iii) Monitor the patient's temperature, vaginal discharge, and bleeding.

## Further Outpatient Care

1. If the patient is discharged, arrange definite follow-up care in 1–2 days with the patient's primary gynecologist.
2. Patient should be counseled about contraception.
3. Patient should be advised to follow up as soon as there is period of amenorrhea and early ANC registration.
4. Advise the patient to observe for menstrual pattern for menstrual disturbances.
5. At the time of discharge, patient should be discharged on oral iron preparation for 3 months.

## Case Report

### Case No. 1

A 21-year-old woman, ABC, G3P2L2, last child birth 10 months back, brought by relatives with referral from private hospital as "uterine perforation" with c/o repeated vomiting and distended abdomen since 2 days, termination of a 10-week pregnancy by an uncertified practitioner 2 days ago. She was dehydrated, pale, having tachycardia, and BP – 90/60 mm of Hg. Outside USG s/o uterine perforation. X-ray erect abdomen s/o intestinal obstruction. So in view of uterine perforation with intestinal obstruction, exploratory laprotomy done.

On laparotomy, there was evidence of posterior uterine wall rent with small bowel loop incarcerated into the uterine cavity which was gangrenous so resection anastomosis with rent repair done. Postop was uneventful and patient discharged on day 8 postop (Figs. 31.2 and 31.3).

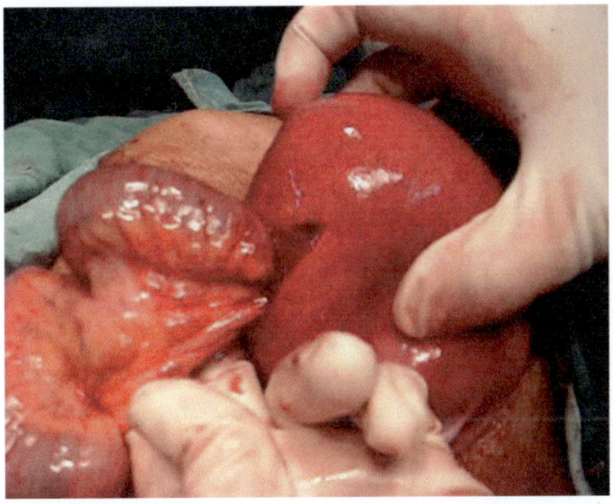

**Fig. 31.2** Postabortal posterior uterine wall rent with bowel incarceration in uterine cavity

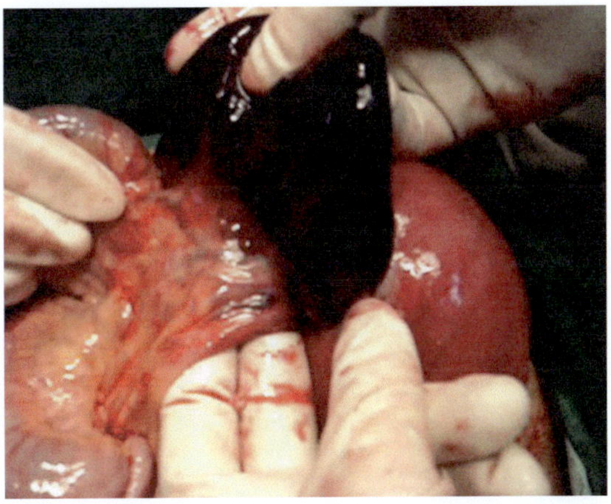

**Fig. 31.3** Gangrenous bowel loop with posterior uterine wall rent

**Case No. 2**

A 24-year-old woman, primigravida, had undergone SE in private hospital at 12 weeks of gestation brought by relatives to emergency department with severe abdominal pain, sweating and giddiness. On examination, patient was pale and had tachycardia, hypotension, guarding, and rigidity over abdomen, Ut 12–14 weeks. On PV examination, tender mass present in anterior fornix. USG done s/o ant uterine wall hematoma measuring 10×10 cm. 2 units PCV given and exploratory laparotomy done, Hematoma drained, there was e/o ant uterine wall peforation, repaired. Postop patient went home uneventfully on day 8 (Figs. 31.4 and 31.5).

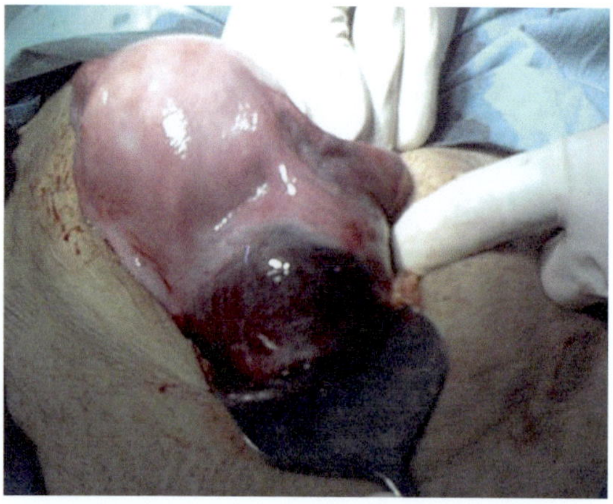

**Fig. 31.4** Anterior uterine wall hematoma following SE

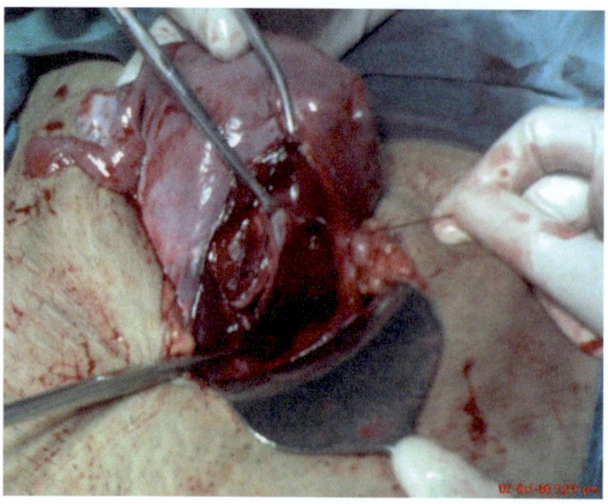

**Fig. 31.5** Anterior uterine wall rent

## Conclusion

1. Legally induced abortion is one of the safest procedures in medicine. Although complications are not completely avoidable, they can be minimized by careful prescreening and sound medical and surgical practices, including the following.
2. Diligent effort to determine gestational age prior to attempting abortion
3. Sound aseptic technique
4. Simple regimens of anesthesia and evacuation of the uterus
5. Confining operative procedures to those with which the surgeon is experienced and comfortable
6. Avoiding vigorous sharp curettage
7. Dilating the cervix adequately to perform a rapid, safe operation
8. Condemn procedures like aspirotomy for gestational age less than 12 weeks.
9. Rational use of uterotonic regimens to prevent and treat hypotonus
10. Maintaining a high index of suspicion for occult injury and insidious medical complications
11. Use of periabortal antibiotic prophylaxis
12. Careful tissue examination and confirmation of products of conception to rule out incomplete abortion or molar pregnancy
13. Assiduous monitoring during and after surgery
14. 24-h telephone access to a clinician knowledgeable about postabortal complications
15. Appropriate emergency consultation and hospital referral when necessary

## References


1. Kumar A, Hessini L, Mitchell EM. Conceptualising abortion stigma. Cult Health Sex. 2009;11(6):625–39.
2. Ibrahim IA, et al. Complicated Unsafe Abortions, Niger Health J. 2011;11(4):112–116.
3. Maharana B. Correlates of Spontaneous and Induced Abortion in India: An Investigation using a Nationwide Large Scale Survey Data.
4. Islam N, Akter Chowdhury S. The impact of imposing time limits on access to safe abortion care in Bangladesh. In: Reproductive laws for the 21st century papers center for women policy studies, July 2012.

5. Berek JS. Berek & Novak's Gynecology South Asian edition. 15th ed. Lippincott Williams and Wilkins. Philadelphia, United States; 2011.

## Suggested Reading

Bhattacharya S. Safe abortion – still a neglected scenario: a study of septic abortions in a tertiary hospital of Rural India. Online J Health Allied Sci. 2010;9(2).

Chaudhary SK. Practice of fertility control. In: A comprehensive manual 7th ed. Elsevier. Philadelphia, Pennsylvania, United States; 2008.

Mentula M. Second trimester medical termination of pregnancy: procedure, immediate complications and the risk of repeat termination. Department of Obstetrics and Gynaecology Helsinki University Central Hospital, University of Helsinki, Finland; 2012.

RCOG. The care of women requesting induced abortion. Evidence-based Clinical Guideline Number 7, November 2011.

WHO. Safe Abortion: technical and policy guidance for health systems. 2nd ed. WHO. Beijing, China; 2012.

# 32 Ovarian Hyperstimulation Syndrome and Pregnancy

Rishma Pai, Hrishikesh Pai, Nandita Palshtetar, and Pritimala Gangurde

Ovarian hyperstimulation syndrome (OHSS) is an iatrogenic complication of ovarian stimulation occurring during the luteal phase or during early pregnancy.

The most common form occurs a few days after the induction of rupture of follicle following the administration of hCG when ovarian stimulation has been medically induced by using either clomiphene citrate or gonadotrophins, along with GnRh agonists or antagonists. OHSS is more frequent and severe in conception cycles and in multiple vs singleton conceptions.

R. Pai, MD, DNB, DGO, FCPS, FICOG (✉)
Lilavati and Jaslok Hospitals, Mumbai, India
e-mail: rishmapai@hotmail.com

H. Pai, MD, FCPS, FICOG, MSc (USA)
Bloom IVF Centre, Mumbai, India

Lilavati Hospital Mumbai, Fortis Hospitals, New Delhi, Gurgaon, Noida, Faridabad, Mohali, Navi Mumbai, India

N. Palshetar, MD, FCPS, MICOG
Lilavati Hospital IVF Centre, Mumbai, India

P. Gangurde
Bloom IVF Centre, Mumbai, India

## Incidence

*The reported prevalence of the severe form of OHSS is ranging from 0.5 to 5 %.*

With the use of clomiphene citrate for ovarian stimulation, Schenker and Weinstgein [1] reported occurrence of OHSS in 13.5 % in a mild form, while moderate and severe OHSS forms were described only sporadically.

When considering IVF cases, the reported incidence of OHSS is $3 \pm 6$ % for the moderate form and $0.1 \pm 2$ % for severe forms (Serour et al. 1998) [2].

ESHRE report on ART in Europe (2004) found an incidence of OHSS of 1.2 % of all stimulated cycles (Nyboe et al. [3]).

## Classification

OHSS is classified as early and late OHSS depending upon the time of appearance of clinical signs and symptoms:

| Early OHSS | Late OHSS |
|---|---|
| Related to an exaggerated ovarian<br>Response to gonadotrophin stimulation | Mainly related to the secretion of placental HCG |
| <10 days after the ovulation triggering injection of HCG | ≥10 days after HCG |

Those cases which constitute a combination of the early form and are followed by pregnancy are serious and long-lasting.


A. Gandhi et al. (eds.), *Principles of Critical Care in Obstetrics: Volume II*,
DOI 10.1007/978-81-322-2686-4_32

Another classification is based on severity of symptoms, clinical presentation and ultrasound findings:

**Mild OHSS**

Abdominal bloating
Mild abdominal pain
Ovarian size usually <8 cm

**Moderate OHSS**

Moderate abdominal pain
Nausea ± vomiting
Ultrasound evidence of ascites; ovarian size usually 8–12 cm

**Severe OHSS**

Clinical ascites (occasionally hydrothorax)
Oliguria Haemoconcentration
Haematocrit >45 %
Hypoproteinaemia; ovarian size usually >12 cm

**Critical OHSS**

Tense ascites or large hydrothorax
Haematocrit >55 %
White cell count >25,000/ml
Oliguria/anuria
Thromboembolism
Acute respiratory distress syndrome

OHSS is more likely to develop in patients with following risk factors [4]:

1. Polycystic ovarian syndrome
2. Elevated baseline AMH
3. Increased ovarian volume
4. High antral follicle count (AFC) on baseline scan
5. Age <30 years
6. Low body mass index (BMI)
7. Previous history of OHSS
8. High doses of FSH used during ovarian stimulation
9. Large number of oocytes collected (>25)
10. rapidly rising and/or high oestradiol levels (>17,000 pmol/l)

## Diagnosis

1. *History*: Nature, duration and severity of symptoms, presence of risk factors if any. Past history of any major medical disorder. Previous history of hyperstimulation
2. Examinations: body weight and body mass index:
   Abdominal circumference
   Heart rate
   Blood pressure
   Cardiovascular system
   Respiratory systems
   Per abdomen

*Pelvic examination should be avoided, as this may induce cyst rupture.*

## Laboratory Investigations

1. Full blood count: white cell count and haematocrit
2. Urea, creatinine and electrolytes (hyponatraemia, hyperkalaemia)
3. Liver function tests: albumin level
4. Coagulation profile: elevated fibrinogen and reduced antithrombin III
5. HCG: if it is 10 days post oocyte retrieval

## Radiology

Ultrasound pelvis: For size of ovaries, ascites if any
Ovarian vessel Doppler studies: if suspected ovarian torsion

## Others

*In particular cases if clinically indicated*
*Arterial blood gases* – to diagnose respiratory failure
*D-dimers* – elevated
*ECG, echocardiogram* – pericardial effusion
*Chest x-ray*
Pleural effusion
Interstitial oedema
*CTPA or V/Q scan* – definitive diagnosis of pulmonary embolism

## OHSS and Complications in Pregnancy

1. In 1st trimester:
   Ovarian torsion (more common between 6 and 10 weeks of pregnancy and with multiple pregnancies)
   Abortion
   Vanishing twin
   Abdominal distention and pain in abdomen
   Respiratory distress because of pleural effusion
   Dehydration and oliguria
2. In 2nd trimester:
   Development of pregnancy-induced hypertension
   Development of glucose intolerance or gestational diabetes mellitus
3. In 3rd trimester:
   Preterm labour
   Abruption of placenta
4. Low birth weight babies with lower Apgar scores

A study by Blandine Courbiere et al. published in 2011 [5] about the outcomes of pregnancy in patients with OHSS showed that the incidence of OHSS requiring hospitalization was 1.14 %.

Early OHSS occurred in 22.5 % of patients and late OHSS in the remaining 77.5 % patients.

In the OHSS group, 10 % had thromboembolic complications.

The miscarriage rate was similar for the OHSS group and the control IVF group.

Incidence of vanishing twin was higher in OHSS group.

There was definitely higher incidence of ovarian torsion and laparoscopy required in OHSS group. Laparoscopy was done in patients with exacerbated abdominal pain and signs of localized peritoneal irritation, and the decision was based on physical examination, clinical judgement and colour Doppler showing decreased or absent venous and/or arterial flow. Incidence was 3.5 times higher in twin pregnancies than singleton pregnancies.

Majority of cases were treated with detorsion of ovary and had an uneventful pregnancy course. Laparoscopic detorsion of ovary is now routinely performed.

Concerning ongoing clinical pregnancies, pregnancy-induced hypertension (PIH) and preterm labour were significantly higher in the OHSS group.

One hypothesis to explain an insufficiency of placentation is a systemic vascular dysfunction with the conjunction between haemoconcentration, hypoxaemia, electrolytic disorder and microthromboembolic events [6].

Kamada et al. observed high concentrations of endothelin-1 (ET-1) in the follicular fluids of women undergoing IVF [7].

ET-1 is a powerful vasoconstrictor agent and may be implicated in the etiopathogeny of vascular diseases like PIH [8].

In the subgroup of singletons, PIH was significantly higher for OHSS pregnancies than for controls.

The incidence of preterm delivery was higher but with biases of uterine malformation and low BMI.

Other studies have reported a high rate of preterm deliveries: 25 % for Mathur and Jenkins [9] and 44.1 % for Abramov et al. [10].

Bastek et al. recently suggested a link between inflammation, placental dysfunction and preterm births [11].

According to a case control study by Haas J in 2014, rates of preterm delivery were significantly increased among patients with severe OHSS as was the rate of smaller babies. However, this was only in singleton pregnancies [12].

The mean birth weights in OHSS multiple pregnancies were lower than in the control group. One hypothesis is that fetal growth restriction could be induced by altered placenta development and PIH due to OHSS.

In this study, GDM was not increased after OHSS, and the rate was similar to the 2.5 % in the general population [13].

In a study by A Wiser et al. published in 2005 [14] on the outcome of pregnancies complicated by severe ovarian hyperstimulation syndrome (OHSS), a follow-up beyond the second trimester showed that in the study population, GDM and PIH were the major complications noted during the second half of pregnancy. The incidence was similar in singleton and twin pregnancies.

The incidence of preterm delivery was more with twin pregnancies as in control group. No significant difference in birth weight as well as Apgar scores.

Two cases of placental abruption noted in control group.

Generally, severity of symptoms dictate the need for admission, and mild cases can usually be treated on an outpatient basis, as long as resolution is reported and review takes place every 2–3 days.

### Outpatient Management Includes

1. Daily fluid balance
2. Daily weight and girth check
3. Regular blood tests and scans

*Analgesia*: Use of paracetamol or codeine; avoiding NSAIDS as these may affect renal function

*Luteal support: use of progesterone not hCG*

*Hydration*: drinking if thirsty, not excess fluid intake

*Activity*: avoidance of strenuous exercise and sexual intercourse, as injury or torsion to enlarged ovaries can occur

*Blood investigations*: at each visit

*Ascites*: if tense ascites is present and expertise exists, tapping should be done. Ultrasound guidance is mandatory.

Transvaginal drainage could be considered.

If symptoms do not resolve and severe OHSS develops, hospital admission should be considered.

### Indications for Hospitalization

Intolerance of oral fluids

Vomiting or diarrhoea

Hypotension

Difficulty breathing and decreased breath sounds

Tense, distended abdomen or peritonism

Thromboembolic event

In cases of suspected ovarian torsion

The management is essentially supportive until the condition resolves spontaneously.

The following parameters should be monitored:

1. Abdominal girth and weight on admission and daily.
2. Blood pressure, pulse and respiratory rate 4 hourly.
3. Input/output balance: indwelling catheter should be kept.
4. Bloods tests daily.
   - Full blood count
   - Coagulation screen
   - Urea and electrolytes
   - Liver function tests
5. Pelvic ultrasound size of ovaries and presence of ascites.
6. Ultrasound for well-being of pregnancy.
7. Screening for glucose intolerance and gestational diabetes.

Supportive management includes:

**Prevention of Thromboembolism (TE)** Thromboembolic deterrent stockings (TEDs) should be used for all patients admitted with OHSS.

Prophylactic anticoagulant therapy with low molecular weight heparin should be commenced (dose to be determined according to patient's weight).

**Hydration** Fluid management in patients with severe OHSS is a challenge due to the porous nature of the vascular bed.

In principle, women that can drink should be encouraged to drink to thirst rather than to excess.

If the woman cannot tolerate oral fluids, intravenous (IV) fluids such as normal saline should be commenced.

The volume should be titrated using the haematocrit as indicator of the state of hydration.

Excess i.v. fluids could make the condition worse.

Constant monitoring of the input/output balance is mandatory.

*Of note, diuretics are contraindicated when haemoconcentration is present as they can precipitate critical OHSS.*

*Diuretics can be used only where renal output is decreased on a background of normal haematocrit.*

Women with severe haemoconcentration (Hb >14 g/dl); Htc >45 %) require a bolus of 500 ml fluids intravenous (i.v.) on admission.

Plasma expanders like HES (hydroxyethyl starch) 6 % solution in isotonic sodium chloride solution can be used at a maximum daily dose of 33 ml/kg in 250–500 cc/day, in very slow administration to avoid lung congestion.

*Albumin administration should be kept for a later stage* [4], once hypoalbuminaemia is proven because of risk of hepatitis, excessive albumin overload, renal function impairment and potential viral contamination.

Administration is mainly important during drainage of ascites.

Daily dose: 25–75 g (100–300 ml) per day according to the severity of hypoalbuminaemia and the total volume of ascitic fluid drained.

**Paracentesis Should Be Considered**

In women with severe abdominal distension

In women with dyspnoea

In women with renal impairment (oliguria persists despite adequate volume replacement)

Paracentesis results in increased venous return, increased cardiac output, improved diuresis and renal function and improved lung function.

The following should be followed:

1. Drainage will take place abdominally or vaginally under ultrasound guidance.
2. Rate of drainage is very slow to prevent cardiovascular collapse (maximum 2 l within 12 h).
3. Blood pressure and pulse need continuous monitoring.
4. Use pigtail catheter and cover patient with antibiotics.

**Pain Relief** Paracetamol or opiates (oral, i.v.) can be routinely used for pain management. Nausea and vomiting are treated with antiemetics.

## Laparoscopy

Laparoscopy should be considered in cases of ovarian torsion. Patients presenting with symptoms of acute and severe abdominal pain should be admitted to hospital. Diagnosis is by clinical examination demonstrating signs of peritoneal irritation as well as by ultrasound with colour Doppler examination. Detorsion is adequate treatment in majority of cases as long as the tissue viability is confirmed. Very rarely oophorectomy may be required in neglected cases with necrosis of ovarian tissue or patients with severe bleeding due to ovarian rupture.

As such, the indications for admission for critical nursing care in ICU in a general hospital are:

1. Renal compromise (oligoanuria) or failure to respond to fluid management or paracentesis as patient may require dialysis.
2. In respiratory compromise not responding to diuresis or paracentesis, patient may require ventilation.
3. Clinical appearance of acute respiratory distress syndrome (ARDS).
4. Thromboembolism.
5. Tense ascites or large hydrothorax.
6. Haematocrit >55 %.
7. WCC >25,000/ml.

## Prevention of OHSS [4]

OHSS today is completely preventable. In patients who show excessive response during ovarian stimulation, preventative measures to be implemented include:

1. Metformin cotreatment in women with PCOD.
2. Lower starting dose of FSH in women with previous OHSS.
3. Cancellation of cycle of treatment and continuation of downregulation with GnRHa or GnRh antagonist.
4. Coasting (withholding the FSH injections) and monitoring follicular development as well as E2 levels. Triggering with a low-dose hCG only is E2 levels' safe zone.
5. Withholding the ovulatory trigger (hCG), if ovarian response is significantly high (number of follicles and oestradiol level).
6. Reducing the dose of the hCG trigger to 5000 IU instead of the standard 10,000 IU.
7. Nowdays, with the use of GnRh antagonist for downregulation, using GnRha for trigger instead of HCG is very safe. This reduces dramatically the risk of OHSS. If the number of follicles is not too many, a small 1500 U HCG dose can be added on day of trigger in order to improve pregnancy outcomes.
8. Cochrane review 2012 has concluded that using cabergoline 0.5 mg daily post oocyte retrieval reduces OHSS and does not affect pregnancy outcome.
9. Using progesterone and not hCG for luteal phase support.
10. Intravenous administration of prophylactic 25 % albumin (20–50 g) at the time of oocyte retrieval in high-risk cases (e.g. where oestradiol levels are markedly elevated or history of previous OHSS episode exists). This however is controversial. Also using recombinant HCG or LH does not reduce OHSS incidence.
11. The practice of cryopreservation of all embryos resulting from the cycle ("freeze all" policy) makes ART treatment safer. It should be routine for all cases where the estimated risk of OHSS is high as it reduces the risk of late (pregnancy-induced) OHSS. Using GnRh agonist trigger instead of HCG and freezing all embryos gives no OHSS. Transferring back embryos in a later cycle gives a cumulative pregnancy rate of 50 %.
12. Infusions of 10 ml 10 % calcium gluconate in 100 ml of 0.9 % saline on the day of ovum pick up and day 1, 2 and 3 after was found to reduce the incidence of OHSS from 23 to 7 % when compared with the placebo group. Severe OHSS reduced from 4 to 0 %+.
13. Using in vitro maturation in patients with PCOS, the problem of OHSS can be avoided completely [15].

With all these measures, it is possible to have 'OHSS' Free Clinics. In view of the morbidity and potential mortality pertaining to OHSS and its progressive nature, it is crucial that women attending an assisted conception unit be provided with written information about OHSS including risks, symptoms and a 24-hour contact number with prompt access to a suitably informed professional with expertise in the diagnosis and management of OHSS. Reassurance is necessary that pregnancy may continue normally despite OHSS, and there is no evidence of an increased risk of congenital abnormalities.

## References

1. Shenker JG, Weinstein D. OHSS. A current survey. Fertil Steril. 1978;30:255–68.
2. Serour GI, Aboulghar M, Mansour R. Complications of medically assisted conception in 3500 cycles. Fertil Steril. 1998;70:638–42.
3. Nyboe A, et al. ESHRE report on ART in Europe found an incidence of OHSS of 1.2 % of all stimulated cycles. Hum Reprod. 2004;23:756–71.
4. Institute Obstetricians & Gynaecologist. Royal College of Physicians of no. 9; rev Ireland. Directorate of Strategy & Clinical Programmes. Health Service Executive; Ovarian hyperstimulation Syndrome Diagnosis & Management; version 1; guideline. Clinical practice guidelines. 2014.
5. Courbiere B, Oborski V, Braunstein D, Desparoir A, Noizet A. Obstetric outcome of women with in vitro fertilization pregnancies hospitalized for ovarian hyperstimulation syndrome: a case-control study. Fertil Steril. 2011;95:1629–32. 2011 by American Society for Reproductive Medicine.

6. Rizk B, Aboulghar M, Smitz J, Ron-El R. The role of vascular endothelial growth factor and interleukins in the pathogenesis of severe ovarian hyperstimulation syndrome. Hum Reprod Update. 1997;3:255–66.
7. Kamada S, Kubota T, Taguchi M, Aso T. High levels of immunoreactive endothelin-1 in human follicular fluids. Hum Reprod. 1993;8:674–7.
8. Rogers RG, Thorp Jr JM. Pregnancy-induced hypertension: genesis of and response to endothelial injury and the role of endothelin 1. Obstet Gynecol Surv. 1997;52:723–7.
9. Mathur RS, Jenkins JM. Is ovarian hyperstimulation syndrome associated with a poor obstetric outcome? Br J Obstet Gynecol. 2000;107:943–6.
10. Abramov Y, Elchalal U, Schenker JG. Obstetric outcome of in vitro fertilized pregnancies complicated by severe ovarian hyperstimulation syndrome: a multicenter study. Fertil Steril. 1998;70:1070–6.
11. Bastek JA, Brown AG, Anton L, Srinivas SK, D'Addio A, Elovitz MA. Biomarkers of inflammation and placental dysfunction are associated with subsequent preterm birth. J Matern Fetal Neonatal Med. 2011;24(4):600–5. doi: 10.3109/14767058.2010.511340. Epub 2010 Sep 7.
12. Hass J, Bavem M, Meridor H. In severe OHSS associated with adverse pregnancy outcomes? Evidence from a case control studies. Reprod Biomed Online. 2004;29(2):216–21.
13. Xiong X, Saunders LD, Wang FL, Demianczuk NN. Gestational diabetes mellitus: prevalence, risk factors, maternal and infant outcomes. Int J Gynaecol Obstet. 2001;75:221–8.
14. Wiser A, Levron J, Kreizer D, Achiron R, Shrim A. Outcome of pregnancies complicated by severe ovarian hyperstimulation syndrome (OHSS): a follow-up beyond the second trimester. Hum Reprod. 2005;20(4):910–4.
15. Das M, Son WY, Bucket W. In vitro maturation versus IVF with GnRH antagonist for women with PCOS, treatment outcome and rates of OG+HSS. Reprod Biomed online. 2014;29(5):545–51.

# 33 Obesity in Obstetric Intensive Care Patient

Narendra Malhotra, Esha Sharma, Jaideep Malhotra, and Neharika Malhotra Bora

Admission of the pregnant or post partum women to the Intensive Care Unit is uncommon but may require specialised knowledge for successful management.

Obstetric patients are generally young and healthy. However, potential for catastrophic event is real, and despite the therapeutic advances of the last few decades, maternal morbidity and mortality continue to occur. This may be related to pregnancy itself, aggravation of a pre-existing illness or complication of delivery. Every year, more than half a million women—most of them living in developing countries—die from pregnancy- or childbirth-related complications.

N. Malhotra, MD, FICOG, FRCOG (✉)
Department of Obstetrics and Gynecology, Global Rainbow Health Care, Agra, India
e-mail: mnhagra3@gmail.com

E. Sharma, MBBS, MS, DNB
Department of Obstetrics and Gynecology, Rainbow IVF, Agra, India
e-mail: eshabaral@gmail.com

J. Malhotra, MD, FICOG
Department of Obstetrics and Gynecology, Rainbow IVF, Agra, India
e-mail: jaideepmalhotraagra@gmail.com

N.M. Bora, MBBS, MD
Department of Obstetrics and Gynecology, Bhartiya Vidya Peeth, Pune, India

## Obesity and Pregnancy

Obesity has become a major health problem of modern society and is increasing globally at nearly epidemic proportion especially in western and European countries [1, 2]. Obesity is often expressed with reference to body mass index (BMI).

Body mass index = weight (in kg)/height (in $m^2$)

Though BMI is a useful measure of prevalence and associated health risks of obesity, it does not account for the wide variation in the distribution of fat and may not correspond to the same degree of fatness in different individuals. WHO classifies obesity primarily based on the association between BMI and mortality (Table 33.1).

**Table 33.1** WHO classification of Obesity

| Classification | Body mass index (kg/$m^2$) | Associated health risks |
|---|---|---|
| Underweight | <18.5 | Low |
| Normal range | 18.5–24.9 | Average |
| Overweight | >25 | |
| Preobese | 25–29.9 | Increased |
| Obese class I | 30–34.9 | Moderately increased |
| Obese class II | 35–39.9 | Severely increased |
| Obese class III | >40 | Very severely increased |


A. Gandhi et al. (eds.), *Principles of Critical Care in Obstetrics: Volume II*,
DOI 10.1007/978-81-322-2686-4_33

**Table 33.2** Physiological effects and risks in the critically ill morbidly obese patient

| | |
|---|---|
| Respiratory | Reduced lung volumes<br>Atelectasis and ventilation–perfusion mismatch<br>Increased work of breathing and oxygen consumption<br>Obstructive airways disease (mechanical and asthma)<br>Obstructive sleep apnoea<br>Obesity hypoventilation syndrome |
| Cardiovascular | Coronary artery disease<br>Hypertension<br>Systolic and diastolic left ventricular dysfunction<br>Pulmonary arterial hypertension<br>Obesity supine death syndrome |
| Other | Diabetes mellitus<br>Increased risk of venous thromboembolism<br>Increased risk of gastric acid aspiration<br>Altered drug pharmacokinetics<br>Difficult venous access<br>Increased risk of renal failure<br>Increased risk of pressure ulcers |

The World Health Organization (WHO) characterised obesity as a pandemic issue whose prevalence is higher in women than in men [3].

Almost all the organ systems are affected by the impact of obesity either directly or indirectly. The degree of obesity and its prolonged duration are the main factors which determine the harmful effect of obesity in the human body. Even moderate overweight is a risk factor for gestational diabetes and hypertensive disorders of pregnancy, and the risk is higher in subjects with overt obesity. Compared with normal weight, maternal overweight is related to a higher risk of Caesarean deliveries and a higher incidence of anaesthetic and postoperative complications in these deliveries (Table 33.2).

## Challenges to Anaesthetist

Adding to the spectrum of medical and surgical pathologies, obesity is also associated with an increased incidence of antenatal disorders. A thorough understanding of physiology, pathophysiology, associated conditions, their complications and the implications for analgesia and anaesthesia should place the anaesthetist in a better position to care for these patients. As a result, increasing number of obese patients is being presented to critical care units for various indications. The attending intensivist has to face numerous challenges during management of such patients. Consequently, the anaesthetist is increasingly confronted with the problems of anaesthetising obese patients, and even more so the obstetric anaesthetist.

## Anaesthetic Considerations

Obesity has been identified as a significant risk factor for anaesthesia-related maternal mortality [4, 5]. The increased incidence of operative procedures, both elective and emergency, and the concurrent medical and antenatal problems may contribute to the risk. Postoperative complications such as wound infection, deep vein thrombosis, atelectasis and chest infection are more prevalent [5–7]. In addition to the associated medical problems, the anaesthetist is challenged by these patients with technical difficulties of airway management and insertion of regional blocks. No anaesthetic technique is without special hazards in grossly obese patients.

## Airway

The incidence of failed tracheal intubation is approximately 1 in 280 in the obstetric population compared to 1 in 2230 in the general surgical population [8–10]. This is in contrast with an incidence of difficult intubation in an obese population as high as 15.5%.

So it is evident that difficult or failed tracheal intubation in obese parturients is very high, and optimal assessment and management of the airway cannot be overemphasised in this population.

Though there are no bony differences between the pregnant and non-pregnant population, obese and nonobese patients, fat deposition in obese and soft tissue changes during pregnancy do influence the airway. Operational factors such as poor head positioning, cricoid pressure and anxiety contribute to the difficulty on occasion [11, 12]. In addition, pregnancy-induced hypertension, upper respiratory tract infection, stridor and voice changes may suggest the presence of airway oedema. Weight gain in excess of 15 kg during pregnancy has been shown to be associated with an increase in suboptimal laryngoscopic views [13].

Anaesthesia for both emergency and elective scenarios should be planned in advance. It is appropriate to involve patients in the decision-making process for safe delivery of the foetus.

## Respiratory System

The likelihood of obstructive sleep apnoea (OSA) has been alluded to, but it is often under-diagnosed in women of childbearing age [14]. It is possible that, in as much as complaints of difficulty in sleeping and daytime fatigue are common, women suffering from OSA are not identified. Careful history taking may help diagnose OSA. Prompt diagnosis by polysomnography and treatment with continuous positive airway pressure may be beneficial. Pulmonary hypertension and right heart failure need to be excluded in parturients with OSA [15, 16]. Measurement of oxygen saturation by pulse oximetry, both in sitting and supine positions, may provide evidence of airway closure during normal tidal volume ventilation, thereby identifying candidates for postoperative oxygen administration.

## Cardiovascular System

Cardiovascular co-morbidities such as hypertension, ischaemic heart disease and heart failure dominate the clinical picture in the obese population, and these can coexist in obese parturients. Nearly 40% of the obese population experience angina without demonstrable coronary artery disease [17]. Hence, routine electrocardiograph recording may be useful. Cardiologists should be involved early in the care of symptomatic morbidly obese parturients to investigate and optimise the disease status wherever appropriate.

## Gastrointestinal and Endocrine Systems

Gastro-oesophageal reflux and diabetes mellitus are the most commonly seen disorders [18]. Any previous laboratory investigations such as fasting blood glucose concentration and liver function tests should be noted. If there is any abnormality of liver function, HELLP syndrome should be ruled out. Though aggressive prophylaxis against acid aspiration is advocated for all obese mothers undergoing Caesarean section [19], there is a lack of conclusive evidence for starvation policies and prophylaxis during labour.

## Postoperative Complications

Obese parturients are at increased risk of postoperative complications such as hypoxaemia, atelectasis and pneumonia, deep vein thrombosis and pulmonary embolism, pulmonary oedema, postpartum cardiomyopathy, postoperative endometritis and wound complications such as infection and dehiscence [6, 7]. Early mobilisation, thromboprophylaxis, aggressive chest physiotherapy and adequate pain control are the key to the success of effective postoperative care.

In the recovery room, critical respiratory events (desaturation, hypoventilation and airway obstruction) occur twice as commonly in the obese compared to nonobese [20]. Computerised tomography has demonstrated that obesity predisposes to the formation of pulmonary atelectasis per se and even more so under general anaesthesia, persisting into the postoperative period [21]. Moreover, even after spinal anaesthesia, there is a BMI-dependent decrease in respiratory function. Hence, these critical respiratory events may not be benign and can lead to postoperative pulmonary morbidity. Nursing in the reclined position and oxygen supplementation can potentially reduce critical respiratory events. Early mobilisation has been shown to improve the respiratory volumes in the immediate postoperative phase [22].

Thromboembolic episodes remain the leading cause of direct maternal deaths in the UK. Obesity is a known independent risk factor for deep vein thrombosis. Both pharmacological and mechanical strategies are used for thromboprophylaxis and an adequate dose of an anticoagulant for an appropriate duration is recommended [23]. Obesity cardiomyopathy is a well-recognised clinical entity, and at least three cases of peripartum cardiomyopathy in obese patients have been reported [24, 25]. Although not established yet, obesity may well be a risk factor for peripartum cardiomyopathy [25]. Wound complications occur more frequently in obese than in nonobese patients and often lead to prolonged recovery. They have been found to be increased with midline abdominal incision compared to a Pfannenstiel incision [26]. An increased incidence of postoperative complications and antepartum medical disease probably contributes significantly to longer hospitalisation for the morbidly obese. Hospital stay and costs have been found to be increased for morbidly obese patients after both vaginal delivery and Caesarean section [27].

**Conclusion**

The critically ill obstetric patient presents a unique clinical challenge to the intensivist because of maternal physiological adaptations to pregnancy, pregnancy-specific conditions which may require critical care management and also the presence of foetus whose well being is linked to the mother. Successful maternal and neonatal outcome for patients admitted to a critical care facility are largely dependent on a multidisciplinary approach to management requiring input from critical care personnel, obstetricians, anaesthetists, neonatologists and midwives.

## References

1. Seidell JC. Epidemiology of obesity. Semin Vasc Med. 2005;5(1):3–14.
2. Garrow JS. Obesity and related diseases. London: Churchill Livingstone; 1988.
3. World Health Organization. Obesity: preventing and managing the global epidemic. Report on a WHO consultation, WHO Technical Report Series 894. Geneva: WHO; 2000.
4. Endler GC, Mariona FG, Sokol RJ, Stevenson LB. Anesthesia related maternal mortality in Michigan, 1972–1984. Am J Obstet Gynecol. 1988; 159:187–93.
5. Cooper GM, McClure JH. Anaesthesia. In: Why Mothers Die, 2000–2. Sixth report on confidential enquiries into maternal deaths in the United Kingdom. London: RCOG press; 2004. p. 122–33.
6. Jordan H, Perlow MD, Mark A, Morgan MD. Massive maternal obesity and perioperative cesarean morbidity. Am J Obstet Gynecol. 1994;170:560–5.
7. Hood DD, Dewan DM. Anesthetic and obstetric outcome in morbidly obese parturients. Anesthesiology. 1993;79:1210–8.
8. Hawthorne L, Wilson R, Lyons G, Dresner M. Failed intubation revisited: a 17-yr experience in a teaching Maternity unit. Br J Anaesth. 1996;76:680–4.
9. Barnardo PD, Jenkins JG. Failed tracheal intubation in obstetrics: a 6 year review in a UK region. Anaesthesia. 2000;55:685–94.
10. Samsoon GL, Young JR. Difficult tracheal intubation: a retrospective study. Anaesthesia. 1987;42:487–90.
11. Juvin P, Lavaut E, Dupont H, et al. Difficult tracheal intubation is more common in obese than lean patients. Anesth Analg. 2003;97:595–600.
12. Noguchi T, Koga K, Shiga Y, Shigematsu A. The gum elastic bougie eases tracheal intubation while applying cricoid pressure compared to a stylet. Can J Anesth. 2003;50:712–7.
13. Sankar KB, Krishna S, Moseley HSL. Airway changes during pregnancy. Anesthesiology. 1997; 87:A895.
14. Lefcourt LA, Rodis JF. Obstructive sleep apnea in pregnancy. Obstet Gynecol Surv. 1996;51:503–6.
15. Lewis DF, Chesson AL, Edwards MS, Weeks JW, Adair CD. Obstructive sleep apnea during pregnancy resulting in pulmonary hypertension. South Med J. 1998;91:761–2.
16. Roush SF, Bell L. Obstructive sleep apnea in pregnancy. J Am Board Fam Pract. 2004;17:292–4.
17. Lean ME. Obesity and cardiovascular disease: the waisted years. Br J Cardiol. 1999;6:269–73.
18. Weiss JL, Malone FD, Emig D, et al. Obesity, obstetric complications and cesarean delivery rate – a population based screening study. Am J Obstet Gynecol. 2004;190:1091–7.
19. Roberts RB, Shirley MA. Reducing the risk of acid aspiration during cesarean section. Anesth Analg. 1974;53:859–68.
20. Ross DK, Cohen MM, Wigglesworth DF, Deboer DP. Critical respiratory events in the postanesthesia care unit. Anesthesiology. 1994;81:410–8.
21. Eichenberger AS, Proietti S, Wicky S, et al. Morbid obesity and postoperative pulmonary atelectasis: an underestimated problem. Anesth Analg. 2002;95:1788–92.
22. von Ungern-Sternberg BS, Regli A, Bucher E, Reber A, Schneider MC. Impact of spinal anaesthesia and obesity on maternal respiratory function during elective caesarean section. Anaesthesia. 2004;59:743–9.

23. Drife J. Thrombosis and thromboembolism. In: Why Mothers Die, 2000–2. Sixth Report on Confidential Enquiries into Maternal Deaths in the United Kingdom. London: RCOG press; 2004. p. 61–78.
24. Kaufman I, Bondy R, Benjamin A. Peripartum cardiomyopathy and thromboembolism; anesthetic management and clinical course of an obese, diabetic patient. Can J Anesth. 2003;50:161–5.
25. Shnaider R, Ezri T, Szmuk P, et al. Combined spinalepidural anesthesia for cesarean section in a patient with peripartum dilated cardiomyopathy. Can J Anesth. 2001;48:681–3.
26. Wall PD, Deucy EE, Glantz JC, Pressman EK. Vertical skin incisions and wound complications in the obese parturient. Obstet Gynecol. 2003;102:952–6.
27. Galtier-Dereure F, Montpeyroux F, Boulot P, Bringer J, Jaffiol C. Weight excess before pregnancy: complications and cost. Int J Obes Relat Metab Disord. 1995;19:443–8.

# Drug-Induced Serious Maternal and Fetal Complications in Pregnancy

34

Rajendrasing Pardeshi and Ajay Mane

## Introduction

A woman starts out with a 3–5 % chance of having a baby with a birth defect. Drugs can have a variety of harmful effects on the fetus and neonate. This chapter briefly elaborates on drugs that can affect pregnancy and the fetus.

## Thalidomide

Thalidomide, an immunomodulatory sedative, reduces the ability of the body to grow new blood vessels and was one of the first drugs recognized to cause birth defects in humans. First-trimester risk is higher in all infants exposed to thalidomide. The fetal and infant death rate is 40 % with maternal thalidomide intake. If the mother consumes thalidomide early in pregnancy, there is a risk of approximately 20 % or more of having a baby with birth defects, such as extremely short stature or missing arms and legs, missing ears, and deafness. Heart defects, kidney abnormalities, missing or small eyes, paralysis of the face, gastrointestinal/genital/urinary tract abnormalities, poor growth, and mental retardation may also occur.

R. Pardeshi (✉)
Food & Drug Committee, FOGSI, Jijai Maternity & Nursing Home, 2-Chaitanya Co-op hsg Society, Near Gajanan Maharaj Temple, Garkheda, Aurangabad, MS, India
e-mail: varadsing@yahoo.co.in

A. Mane
Sexual Medicine Committee, FOGSI, "Yashwant", 228/2, N-4, Opp. V.N.Patil Law College, CIDCO, Aurangabad, MS, India
e-mail: drmaneajay@gmail.com

## Tetracycline

Tetracycline, an antibiotic, and minocycline, doxycycline, oxytetracycline, and from that group only. The risk of major birth defects increases with tetracycline use in the first trimester. There may also be a slightly increased risk of minor birth defects, such as an inguinal hernia. It is possible that the baby's teeth and bones might be affected if tetracycline is consumed in the second and third trimesters of pregnancy. Also, dental discoloration may occur with tetracycline exposure in the fourth month of pregnancy; hence, it should be avoided after 4 months' gestation.

The use of tetracycline may even result in calcification of the bones and teeth and reduced growth. Although the tooth discoloration is permanent, bone growth seems to return to normal after exposure to tetracycline ends.


A. Gandhi et al. (eds.), *Principles of Critical Care in Obstetrics: Volume II*,
DOI 10.1007/978-81-322-2686-4_34

## Valproic Acid

Valproic acid is used to control epileptic seizures and bipolar disorder and migraines. Long-term use is associated with menstrual problems and difficulty getting pregnant.

Major birth defects, such as a heart defect or an opening in the lip (called cleft lip), are observed with exposure to valproic acid. In higher doses, the risks associated with valproic acid are higher or if taken as a combination of more than one seizure medicine. A 1–2 % risk of neural tube defects has been found, which usually occur in the first trimester, the most common being spina bifida.

Minor birth defects such as facial differences, for example, a thin upper lip, a flat face, and an upturned nose, may be observed in some cases of valproic acid exposure.

## Prednisolone

Prednisone, or prednisolone, is a corticosteroid. Long-term use in pregnancy is associated with premature and/or low birth-weight babies.

A slightly increased risk of oral clefts has been observed when used in the first trimester. The risk is usually approximately 1 in 1000. If consumed during the first trimester, the risk of oral clefts is between 3 and 6 in 1000.

## Methotrexate

Methotrexate stops the growth of cells and also interferes with the immune system. It decreases folic acid breakdown and interferes with the metabolism, hence decreasing folic acid levels. Use in early pregnancy increases the risk of miscarriage. Birth defects such as malformations of the infant's head, face, and bones may be more prevalent when methotrexate is administered in the first trimester. Poor growth and developmental delay may even occur in some cases.

## Alcohol

Heavy alcoholism may increase fertility problems among women because of long-term exposure. Hence, women are advised to avoid alcohol to treat fertility problems. Higher rates of miscarriage and stillbirth have been found when alcohol is consumed during pregnancy. This can cause mental retardation and fetal alcohol syndrome, in which a pattern of certain birth defects, such as a small head, small body size, specific facial features, learning/behavioral problems, occurs. This syndrome is severe when alcohol consumption during pregnancy is heavy and takes place on a regular basis.

Fetal alcohol syndrome has been associated with many lifelong challenges. Poor judgment and difficulties with understanding, social relationships, learning, and memory are the lifelong consequences of fetal alcohol syndrome, and even drug abuse, mental health problems, irregularities in the school, and school absenteeism may occur.

## Trimethoprim/Sulfamethoxazole

In combination, these drugs are used to treat bacterial infections and are usually given together in a variety of infections, including urinary tract infections. Birth defects due to their exposure were seen and included heart defects, neural tube defects, cleft lip or palate, and urinary tract defects. It has been reported that trimethoprim may decrease the level of folic acid; hence, the increase in birth defects. Even because of the decrease in folic acid levels in the mother, preeclampsia, placenta abruption, and intrauterine growth restriction occur. Preterm delivery and prematurity are common with exposure to these drugs during pregnancy.

## Benzodiazepines

These drugs are used to treat anxiety, seizures, sleeplessness, muscle spasms, and alcohol withdrawal. Diazepam, alprazolam, clonazepam, temazepam, and lorazepam belong to this group.

A slight increase in the risk of cleft lip and/or cleft palate occurs if exposed to this group during the first trimester. A higher rate of preterm deliveries and low birth weight in infants was observed with these drugs when consumed during pregnancy. Withdrawal symptoms in the baby, such as breathing difficulties, muscle weakness, tremors, irritability, crying, sleep disturbances, and jitteriness, may be seen if the mother consumed benzodiazepine near the time of delivery.

## Carbamazepine

Carbamazepine is used to control epileptic seizures and bipolar disorder, schizophrenia, trigeminal neuralgia, and pain disorders. Its long-term use is associated with menstrual and infertility problems and hormone disturbances. It crosses the placenta; hence, if the mother is exposed during the first trimester, a 1 % risk of neural tube defects has been observed. In some studies infants were found to have deformities of the nasal bone, upper lip, and small fingernails. Even a 2–3 times increased risk of major birth defects, such as heart defects and cleft lips, has been observed. In one study, small head size and an increased frequency of growth retardation have been observed.

## Depot Medroxyprogesterone

This hormone is used to prevent pregnancy and is effective for 90 days, but it has been found to have higher levels in the blood, even after 90 days; hence, its concern while being pregnant in that state as fertility will be their even that will be in blood in higher levels also. Ambiguous genitalia is a severe external genital anomaly that has been observed in individuals exposed to this drug.

## Diphenhydramine

This is an antihistamine commonly used to treat allergy symptoms, nausea, vomiting, insomnia, motion sickness, and the tremors of Parkinson's disease. Higher levels of diphenhydramine may cause uterine hyperstimulation, which may affect the developing baby and possibly lead to serious complications, including a uterine rupture or placental abruption. Withdrawal symptoms in the baby such as difficulty breathing, muscle weakness, tremors, irritability, crying, sleep disturbances, and jitteriness may be seen if the mother consumed diphenhydramine daily throughout pregnancy. The combination of temazepam and diphenhydramine may increase the risk of stillbirth or infant death shortly after birth. Hence, it is advised to avoid benzodiazepines with diphenhydramine during pregnancy.

## Etanercept

Etanercept is a drug for treating autoimmune diseases such as rheumatoid arthritis, ankylosing spondylitis, psoriasis, psoriatic arthritis, and juvenile rheumatoid arthritis. It is known as a tumor necrosis factor (TNF) inhibitor as it binds and blocks TNF. Birth defects reported include the VACTERL association, which is a pattern of birth defects that includes vertebral (spine), anal, cardiac (heart), tracheal–esophageal (structures in the neck), renal (kidney), and limb (arms and legs) defects. If two or more defects are observed in a baby, then it is diagnosed with VACTERL.

## Fluconazole

Fluconazole is an antifungal medicine used to treat various infections. A single dose of fluconazole does not in itself provoke an increase in premature delivery or low birth weight. However, in higher doses a pattern of major malformations of the head, face, bones, and heart have been reported in the five children of four mothers.

## Calcium Carbonate

This is a dietary supplement, needed for healthy bones, nervous system, muscles, and heart. The recommended level of calcium for pregnant and breastfeeding women is 1000 mg. If more is consumed, lower fetal weight may occur. Calcium carbonate has also been associated with milk–alkali syndrome, which is caused by increased levels of calcium in the blood. This may lead to the breakdown of calcium in other body tissues and to kidney failure.

## Carbon Monoxide

Carbon monoxide gas comes from motor vehicles, furnaces, working heaters, or fuel-burning appliances. Carbon monoxide exposure from cigarettes, a fire, or methylene chloride, if in high enough concentrations, can cause the blood to carry less oxygen to organs and lead to the damage of these organs. Headache, nausea, vomiting and dizziness, confusion, chest pain, stumbling or falling, sleepiness, and loss of consciousness are all symptoms of carbon monoxide poisoning. Severe poisoning may lead to death.

Carbon monoxide crosses the placenta; hence, fetal damage or fetal death can occur because of damage to the developing brain. Cigarette smoking leads to low birth-weight babies. As is postulated in several studies, severe hypoxia in the mother finally affects the brain of the fetus and other organs and leads to death in many cases.

## Fluoxetine

This is a drug for treating depression and belongs to the selective serotonin reuptake inhibitors (SSRIs). Increased chances of premature delivery when using fluoxetine in the first trimester have been shown in one study and the chance of having a low birth-weight baby is higher, incurring a longer stay in the NICU. In another study, fluoxetine use in the second trimester was postulated to cause an increased risk of pulmonary hypertension. Exposure to fluoxetine in the third trimester and up to the time of delivery causes the baby to suffer from withdrawal symptoms such as jitteriness, increased muscle tone, breathing problems, irritability, eating difficulties, altered sleep patterns, and tremors.

## Cigarette Smoking

Newborns of mothers who are smokers are at a higher risk of respiratory infections, asthma, and bronchitis during infancy and childhood. Smoking in pregnancy may also lead to a higher risk of sudden infant death syndrome. The occurrence of oral cleft in newborns is slightly increased; this risk increases if this abnormality is already in their family history. One study even suggests a slightly increased risk of a variety of birth defects. Preterm labor and prematurity or low birth-weight babies are associated with mothers who are smokers. Their pregnancy will be associated with complications such as placental abruption, placenta previa, bleeding, and stillbirth.

## Sertraline

Sertraline is a medication used to treat depression, panic disorder, obsessive compulsive disorder (OCD), post-traumatic stress disorder and is also known as a SSRI. Reports of over 2000 pregnancies exposed to sertraline during the first trimester have found associations between sertraline use during pregnancy and particular birth defects, and it suggests that sertraline might increase the risk of birth defects by approximately 3–5 %. Low birth-weight babies and premature delivery were observed in some studies. Others even suggest an increased risk of pulmonary hypertension.

## Ibuprofen

Ibuprofen is a nonsteroidal anti-inflammatory drug (NSAID) used to treat headaches, arthritis, muscle aches, fever, and menstrual cramps. In some studies it has been observed that the use of NSAIDs in early pregnancy produces a low risk of certain birth defects and in the first trimester there is a slightly increased risk of gastroschisis with ibuprofen use. Heart defects have been observed with the use of NSAIDs during the first trimester of pregnancy.

## Iodine

The body needs iodine for the functioning of the thyroid gland. Women with low levels of thyroid hormone may have fertility problems or hormonal disturbances. Lower levels of thyroid hormone during pregnancy carry an increased risk of miscarriage and high levels could result in hyperthyroidism, which can lead to health problems for both mother and baby and has been observed in many studies.

Low iodine levels during pregnancy may result in the premature birth of babies small for gestational age. Learning problems in babies with severe iodine deficiency have been proven.

## Isotretinoin

Isotretinoin is a form of vitamin A. Miscarriage may be as high as 40 % in women taking isotretinoin during the first trimester of pregnancy. Infants with birth defects have small or absent ears and hearing and eyesight problems. Some may have a small jaw, a small head, a cleft palate, and some may be born with a small or missing thymus gland. With isotretinoin, severe heart defects and fluid around the brain are seen in almost 50 % of the exposed infants. Moderate to severe mental retardation in their childhood will be the possible risk in the future.

## Lead

If high levels of lead are present during pregnancy this can cause miscarriage and stillbirth, low birth weight, and premature delivery. High maternal lead levels cause learning and behavioral problems in exposed babies and mild effects on learning may occur in babies exposed to small amounts of lead.

## Lithium

In one study, case reports of lithium use during pregnancy indicate the development of a goiter in the mother, which, if neglected, can lead to a goiter in the baby. There is an increased chance of heart defects if lithium is used in the first trimester, when the heart is forming. A very rare heart defect, Ebstein's anomaly, has been seen, in which there is abnormal placement of one of the valves that controls blood flow into the heart. This rare heart defect with lithium exposure occurs in approximately 1–5 %.

## Methamphetamine

Babies exposed to methamphetamine during pregnancy are premature, very small, and are at risk of lifelong breathing, hearing, vision, and learning problems. Methamphetamine also increases the chance of sudden infant death syndrome (SIDS). High doses can lead to miscarriage, preterm delivery, and problems in the newborn period, such as jitteriness and trouble sleeping and feeding, together with neurological effects, such as tremors and muscle tone problems. Children later face schooling and behavioral problems if their mother was exposed to methamphetamine.

## Metronidazole

This is an antibiotic used to treat different kinds of infections. Previous studies have suggested an increase in various birth defects. However, some sources still state that this drug should not be used during the first trimester or at all in pregnancy.

## Acetaminophen

High doses of acetaminophen may cause liver damage, kidney damage, and anemia in the mother and are hence seen to cause the same problems in the baby.

## Paroxetine

Paroxetine is a drug that is used to treat depression, obsessive compulsive disorder (OCD), social anxiety disorder, and panic disorder. The risk of miscarriage is slightly increased in some studies. A 2 % risk has been observed. An increased risk of pulmonary hypertension has been observed in one study.

## Opioids

Opioids are known as narcotics. Heart and other birth defects have been observed in some studies with exposure in the first trimester. Withdrawal signs are common in babies, including breathing difficulties, extreme drowsiness, irritability, sweating, poor feeding, tremors, vomiting, and diarrhea. Rarely, seizures and death have occurred in severe, untreated cases.

## Pseudoephedrine

An oral decongestant, it has been found that the use of pseudoephedrine during the first trimester was related to an increase in the risk of gastroschisis. One study suggested that pseudoephedrine might slightly increase the risk of some birth defects; hence, it should be avoided during the first trimester of pregnancy. Pseudoephedrine and cigarette smoking can both constrict the blood vessels. Thus, when a mother who smokes cigarettes also consumes pseudoephedrine, the risk of gastroschisis may be greater than if she was exposed to either one alone (Table 34.1).

**Table 34.1** List of contraindicated drugs in pregnancy

| Sr. No. | Name of drug | Drugs type/used for |
|---|---|---|
| 1 | Acitretin | Vitamin A derivative |
| 2 | Amantadine | Antiviral/antiparkinson |
| 3 | Cerivastatin | Antilipemic |
| 4 | Chenodiol | GI agent |
| 5 | Cocaine | Sympathomimetic |
| 6 | Coumarin derivatives | Anticoagulants |
| 7 | Danazol | Androgen |
| 9 | Anisindione | Anticoagulant |
| 10 | Atorvastatin | Antilipemic |
| 11 | Benzphetamine | Anorexiant |
| 12 | Carbarsone | Amebicide |
| 13 | Dienesterol | Estrogenic hormone |
| 14 | Diethylstilbestrol | Estrogenic hormone |
| 15 | Doxycycline | Antibiotic |
| 16 | Ergotamine | Antimigraine |
| 17 | Estazolam | Hypnotic |
| 18 | Estradiol | Estrogenic hormone |
| 19 | Estrogens, conjugated | Estrogenic hormone |
| 20 | Ethanol | Sedative |
| 21 | Ethinyl estradiol | Estrogenic hormone |
| 22 | Ethisterone | Progestogenic hormone |
| 23 | Ethynodiol | Progestogenic hormone |
| 24 | Etretinate | Vitamin/psoralen |
| 25 | Fenfluramine | Anorexiant |
| 26 | Flucytosine | Antifungal |
| 27 | Fluoxymesterone | Androgenic hormone |
| 28 | Fluvastatin | Antilipemic agent |
| 29 | Isotretinoin | Vitamin A isomer |

(continued)

**Table 34.1** (continued)

| Sr. No. | Name of drug | Drugs type/used for |
|---|---|---|
| 30 | Kanamycin | Antibiotic (aminoglycoside) |
| 31 | Leflunomide | Immunologic (antirheumatic) |
| 32 | Lenalidomide | Immunomodulator |
| 33 | Lovastatin | Antilipemic agent |
| 34 | Lynestrenol | Progestogenic hormone |
| 35 | Lysergic acid diethylamide | Hallucinogen |
| 36 | Marijuana | Hallucinogen |
| 37 | Meclofenamate | NSAID |
| 38 | Medroxyprogesterone | Progestogenic hormone |
| 39 | Mestranol | Estrogenic hormone |
| 40 | Methylergonovine maleate | Oxytocic |
| 41 | Mifepristone | Antiprogestogenic |
| 42 | Misoprostol | GI agent (secretary) oral contraindicated, for cervical ripening – low risk |
| 43 | Nonoxynol-9/octoxynol-9 | Vaginal spermicide |
| 44 | Norethisterone | Progestogenic hormone |
| 45 | Norethynodrel | Progestogenic hormone |
| 46 | Norgestrel | Progestogenic hormone |
| 47 | Oral contraceptives | Estrogenic/progestogenic hormones |
| 48 | Paramethadione | Anticonvulsant |
| 48 | Phencyclidine | Hallucinogen |
| 50 | Phentermine | Anorexiant |
| 51 | Podofilox | Keratolytic agent |
| 52 | Pravastatin | Antilipemic agent |
| 53 | Ribavirin | Antiviral |
| 54 | Rosuvastatin | Antilipemic agent |
| 55 | Simvastatin | Antilipemic agent |
| 56 | Sodium iodide | Antithyroid |
| 57 | Tazarotene | Dermatological agent |
| 58 | Terpin hydrate | Expectorant |
| 59 | Testosterone | Androgenic drug |
| 60 | Tetracycline | Antibiotic |
| 61 | Thalidomide | Immunologic agent |
| 62 | Trimethadione | Anticonvulsant |
| 63 | Trimethaphan | Antihypertensive |
| 64 | Measles vaccine | Vaccine |
| 65 | Mumps vaccine | Vaccine |
| 66 | Rubella vaccine | Vaccine |
| 67 | Varicella vaccine | Vaccine |
| 68 | Majority of antineoplastic drugs | |

*NSAID* nonsteroidal anti-inflammatory drug

## Further Reading

1. Patel DA, Patel AR. Clorazepate & congenital malformations. JAMA. 1980;244(2):135–6.
2. Yaffe SJ. Drugs in pregnancy & lactation. London, UK: Elsevier; 2005.
3. Shepard TH. Catalog of teratologic agents. 6th ed. The Johns Hopkins University Press. Philaldelphia, USA: Lippincott Wilinams Wilkins 1989. ISBN 0: 0801838363 / ISBN 13: 9780801838361
4. Game E, Bergman U. Benzodiazepine use in pregnancy and major malformations or oral clefts. BMJ. 1999;319:918.
5. Product information: Prozac. Dista Products; 2000. NDC Code(s): 0777-3104-02, 0777-3105-02, 0777-3105-07, 0777-3105-30
6. Organisation of teratology information specialists. http://www.teratology.org/
7. Shuey DL, Sadler TW, Lauder JM. Serotonin as a regulator of craniofacial morphogenesis. Teratology. 1992;46:367–78.
8. Product Information, GSK; 2004. https://www.gsk.com/media/279898/annual-report-2004.pdf
9. Somers GF. Thalidomide and congenital abnormalities. Proc R Soc Med. 1965;58:491–2; Lancet 1962;1:912–3.

# 35 Anesthesia and Pain Relief in Critically Ill Obstetric Patient

Alka Saraswat

## Perianesthetic Evaluation

- Conduct a focused history and physical examination before providing anesthesia care:
  - Maternal health and anesthetic history
  - Relevant obstetric history
  - Airway and heart and lung examination
  - Baseline blood pressure measurement
  - Back examination when neuraxial anesthesia is planned or placed
- A communication system should be in place to encourage early and ongoing contact between obstetric providers, anesthesiologists, and other members of the multidisciplinary team.
- Order or require a platelet count based on a patient's history, physical examination, and clinical signs; a routine intrapartum platelet count is not necessary in the healthy parturient.
- Order or require an intrapartum blood type and screen or crossmatch based on maternal history, anticipated hemorrhagic complications (e.g., placenta accreta in a patient with placenta previa and previous uterine surgery), and local institutional policies; a routine blood crossmatch is not necessary for *healthy and uncomplicated* parturients.
- The fetal heart rate should be monitored by a qualified individual before and after administration of neuraxial analgesia for labor; *continuous* electronic recording of the fetal heart rate may not be necessary in every clinical setting and may not be possible during initiation of neuraxial anesthesia.

## Aspiration Prophylaxis

- Oral intake of modest amounts of clear liquids may be allowed for uncomplicated laboring patients.
- The uncomplicated patient undergoing elective cesarean delivery may have modest amounts of clear liquids up to 2 h before induction of anesthesia.
- The volume of liquid ingested is less important than the presence of particulate matter in the liquid ingested.
- Patients with additional risk factors for aspiration (e.g., morbid obesity, diabetes, difficult airway) or patients at increased risk for operative delivery (e.g., nonreassuring fetal heart rate pattern) may have further restrictions of oral intake, determined on a case-by-case basis.

A. Saraswat, MS, FICOG,FICMCH, FIAJAGO,FICUMB
Saraswat Nursing Home, Agra, India

Ob/Gyn Moolchand Hospital, Agra, India

ICMCH, Agra, India
e-mail: alka.saraswat@rediffmail.com


A. Gandhi et al. (eds.), *Principles of Critical Care in Obstetrics: Volume II*,
DOI 10.1007/978-81-322-2686-4_35

- Solid foods should be avoided in laboring patients.
- Patients undergoing elective surgery (e.g., scheduled cesarean delivery or postpartum tubal ligation) should undergo a fasting period for solids of 6–8 h depending on the type of food ingested (e.g., fat content).
- Before surgical procedures (i.e., cesarean delivery, postpartum tubal ligation), practitioners should consider timely administration of nonparticulate antacids, $H_2$-receptor antagonists, and/or metoclopramide for aspiration prophylaxis.

## Anesthetic Care for Labor and Delivery

### Neuraxial Techniques: Availability of Resources

- When neuraxial techniques that include local anesthetics are chosen, appropriate resources for the treatment of complications (e.g., hypotension, systemic toxicity, high spinal anesthesia) should be available.
- If an opioid is added, treatments for related complications (e.g., pruritus, nausea, respiratory depression) should be available.
- An intravenous infusion should be established before the initiation of neuraxial analgesia or anesthesia and maintained throughout the duration of the neuraxial analgesic or anesthetic.
- Administration of a fixed volume of intravenous fluid is not required before neuraxial analgesia is initiated.

### Timing of Neuraxial Analgesia and Outcome of Labor

- Neuraxial analgesia should not be withheld on the basis of achieving an arbitrary cervical dilation and should be offered on an individualized basis when this service is available.
- Patients may be reassured that the use of neuraxial analgesia does not increase the incidence of cesarean delivery.

### Neuraxial Analgesia and Trial of Labor after Previous Cesarean Delivery

- Neuraxial techniques should be offered to patients attempting vaginal birth after previous cesarean delivery.
- For these patients, it is also appropriate to consider early placement of a neuraxial catheter that can be used later for labor analgesia or for anesthesia in the event of operative delivery.

### Early Insertion of Spinal or Epidural Catheter for Complicated Parturients

- Early insertion of a spinal or epidural catheter for obstetric (e.g., twin gestation or preeclampsia) or anesthetic indications (e.g., anticipated difficult airway or obesity) should be considered to reduce the need for general anesthesia if an emergent procedure becomes necessary. In these cases, the insertion of a spinal or epidural catheter may precede the onset of labor or a patient's request for labor analgesia.

### Continuous Infusion Epidural (CIE) Analgesia

- The selected analgesic/anesthetic technique should reflect patient needs and preferences, practitioner preferences or skills, and available resources.
- CIE may be used for effective analgesia for labor and delivery.
- When a continuous epidural infusion of local anesthetic is selected, an opioid may be added to reduce the concentration of local anesthetic, improve the quality of analgesia, and minimize motor block.
- Adequate analgesia for uncomplicated labor and delivery should be administered with the secondary goal of producing as little motor block as possible by using dilute concentrations of local anesthetics with opioids.

- The lowest concentration of local anesthetic infusion that provides adequate maternal analgesia and satisfaction should be administered.

## Single-Injection Spinal Opioids With or without Local Anesthetics

- Single-injection spinal opioids with or without local anesthetics may be used to provide effective, although time-limited, analgesia for labor when spontaneous vaginal delivery is anticipated.
- If labor is expected to last longer than the analgesic effects of the spinal drugs chosen or if there is a good possibility of operative delivery, a catheter technique instead of a single-injection technique should be considered.
- A local anesthetic may be added to a spinal opioid to increase duration and improve quality of analgesia.

## Pencil-Point Spinal Needles

- Pencil-point spinal needles should be used instead of cutting-bevel spinal needles to minimize the risk of post-dural puncture headache.

## Combined Spinal–Epidural (CSE) Anesthetics

- CSE techniques may be used to provide effective and rapid analgesia for labor.

## Patient-Controlled Epidural Analgesia (PCEA)

- PCEA may be used to provide an effective and flexible approach for the maintenance of labor analgesia.
- PCEA may be preferable to CIE for providing fewer anesthetic interventions, reduced dosages of local anesthetics, and less motor blockade than fixed-rate continuous epidural infusions.
- PCEA may be used with or without a background infusion.

## Removal of Retained Placenta

- In general, there is no preferred anesthetic technique for the removal of retained placenta.
  - If an epidural catheter is in place and the patient is hemodynamically stable, epidural anesthesia is preferable.
- Hemodynamic status should be assessed before administering neuraxial anesthesia.
- Aspiration prophylaxis should be considered.
- Sedation/analgesia should be titrated carefully due to the potential risks of respiratory depression and pulmonary aspiration during the immediate postpartum period.
- In cases involving major maternal hemorrhage, general anesthesia with an endotracheal tube may be preferable to neuraxial anesthesia.
- Nitroglycerin may be used as an alternative to terbutaline sulfate or general endotracheal anesthesia with halogenated agents for uterine relaxation during removal of retained placental tissue.
  - Initiating treatment with incremental doses of intravenous or sublingual (i.e., metered dose spray) nitroglycerin may relax the uterus sufficiently while minimizing potential complications (e.g., hypotension).

## Anesthetic Choices for Cesarean Delivery

- Equipment, facilities, and support personnel available in the labor and delivery operating suite should be comparable to those available in the main operating suite.
  - Resources for the treatment of potential complications (e.g., failed intubation, inadequate analgesia, hypotension, respiratory depression, pruritus, vomiting) should be available in the labor and delivery operating suite.

  - Appropriate equipment and personnel should be available to care for obstetric patients recovering from major neuraxial or general anesthesia.
- The decision to use a particular anesthetic technique should be individualized based on anesthetic, obstetric, or fetal risk factors (e.g., elective vs. emergency), the preferences of the patient, and the judgment of the anesthesiologist.
  - Neuraxial techniques are preferred to general anesthesia for most cesarean deliveries.
- An indwelling epidural catheter may provide equivalent onset of anesthesia compared with initiation of spinal anesthesia for urgent cesarean delivery.
- If spinal anesthesia is chosen, pencil-point spinal needles should be used instead of cutting-bevel spinal needles.
- General anesthesia may be the most appropriate choice in some circumstances (e.g., profound fetal bradycardia, ruptured uterus, severe hemorrhage, severe placental abruption).
- Uterine displacement (usually left displacement) should be maintained until delivery regardless of the anesthetic technique used.
- Intravenous fluid preloading may be used to reduce the frequency of maternal hypotension after spinal anesthesia for cesarean delivery.
- Initiation of spinal anesthesia should not be delayed to administer a fixed volume of intravenous fluid.
- Intravenous ephedrine and phenylephrine are both acceptable drugs for treating hypotension during neuraxial anesthesia.
  - In the absence of maternal bradycardia, phenylephrine may be preferable because of improved fetal acid–base status in uncomplicated pregnancies.
- For postoperative analgesia after neuraxial anesthesia for cesarean delivery, neuraxial opioids are preferred over intermittent injections of parenteral opioids.

## Management of Obstetric and Anesthetic Emergencies

- Institutions providing obstetric care should have resources available to manage hemorrhagic emergencies.
  - In an emergency, the use of type-specific or O-negative blood is acceptable.
  - In cases of intractable hemorrhage when banked blood is not available or the patient refuses banked blood, intraoperative cell salvage should be considered if available.
  - The decision to perform invasive hemodynamic monitoring should be individualized and based on clinical indications that include the patient's medical history and cardiovascular risk factors.
- Labor and delivery units should have personnel and equipment readily available to manage airway emergencies, to include a pulse oximeter and qualitative carbon dioxide detector.
  - Basic airway management equipment should be immediately available during the provision of neuraxial analgesia.
  - Portable equipment for difficult airway management should be readily available in the operative area of labor and delivery units.
  - The anesthesiologist should have a preformulated strategy for intubation of the difficult airway.
  - When tracheal intubation has failed, ventilation with mask and cricoid pressure or with a laryngeal mask airway or supraglottic airway device (e.g., Combitube®, Intubating LMA [*Fastrach*™]) should be considered for maintaining an airway and ventilating the lungs.
  - If it is not possible to ventilate or awaken the patient, an airway should be created surgically.
- Basic and advanced life-support equipment should be immediately available in the operative area of labor and delivery units.

- If cardiac arrest occurs during labor and delivery, standard resuscitative measures should be initiated.
  - Uterine displacement (usually left displacement) should be maintained.
  - If maternal circulation is not restored within 4 min, cesarean delivery should be performed by the obstetrics team.

# 36 Transport of the Critically Ill Obstetric Patient

Lila Vyas and Rekha Menghani

## Introduction

Transport of critically ill patients places the patient at risk of adverse events, due to absent or small physiological reserves, a medical judgement to be made such that the risk of transport outweighs the potential benefits to the patient at the destination.

A physiological track and trigger system should be used to monitor all antepartum and postpartum admissions [1]. The introduction of a national modified obstetric warning score (MOWS) (Appendix 1) [2] for use in all pregnant and postpartum women who become unwell may aid the more timely recognition, treatment and referral of women who are becoming critically ill.

Approximately 3/4 of obstetrics ICU patients are admitted postpartum. Haemorrhage and hypertension are the most common causes of admission from obstetric services to intensive care [3].

L. Vyas (✉)
OBGY SMS Medical College,
20/199, Kaveri Path, Mansorvar, Jaipur 302020, India
e-mail: Jaipur.lilavyas_149@yahoo.com

R. Menghani
OBGY SMS Medical College,
2/52 Malviya Nagar, Jaipur 302017, India
e-mail: rekha.menghani@gmail.com

## Categories of Transport [4]

Transport of critically ill patients may be required in three circumstances, namely, prehospital, intrahospital and interhospital transport.

*Prehospital transport*: Transport of a critically ill patient from their location (home or any other site) to hospital

*Intrahospital transport*: Transport of critically ill patients from one area of a hospital to another area within the hospital (diagnostic or therapeutic reasons)

*Interhospital transport:* Transport of the critically ill patient, either to a higher level of care or for a specialty service due to either lack of diagnostic facilities, staff, clinical expertise and/or facilities for safe and effective therapy in the referring hospital

## Referring Hospital's Role [5]

Referring doctor should be familiar with the transport team, including how to gain access to and appropriately use its services. The referring doctor is responsible for evaluating the patient's condition and initiating the stabilisation procedure before transport team arrives.


A. Gandhi et al. (eds.), *Principles of Critical Care in Obstetrics: Volume II*,
DOI 10.1007/978-81-322-2686-4_36

If the patient transported is pregnant, pretreatment evaluation also includes:

- Fetal assessment
- Fetal position
- Maternal cervical examination, if uterus is contracting

It may be necessary to stabilise the mother before transport. As in the critically ill non-pregnant patient, initial evaluation and resuscitation of the obstetric patient should focus on airway, breathing and circulation. Obstetric patients have increased oxygen requirements and are more prone to rapid acute oxygen desaturation. Initiation of intravenous fluids, blood pressure medication and anticonvulsants may be done at the referring hospital per the requirements. Fetal monitoring is an essential aspect of the management of the critically ill obstetric patient [6].

The best fluid for resuscitation will depend on the cause of haemodynamic instability. Major haemorrhage generally requires replacement with blood products whilst other causes of shock will require judicious use of either a crystalloid or colloid solution or a combination of both. In general, critically ill obstetric patients are probably better off with a slightly negative volume status given the potential deleterious effects of fluid overload and noncardiogenic pulmonary oedema. They may tolerate a negative volume status better given their lack of significant comorbidities [6].

## Initiation and Response

In all situations requiring transport of the critically ill, rapid response of the transport system and minimal delays are paramount. In emergency interhospital transports, dispatch of the medical transport team to the referring hospital should not be delayed pending the identification of a receiving hospital. In Indian scenario, the transport team will often be arranged by the doctor initiating the transfer. The team may be from the receiving ICU or commercial transport ambulance may be asked to transport the patient.

Ideally, the referring doctor should have to make only one telephone call to initiate retrieval or patient transfer

## Coordination and Communication

Coordination of transport services for the critically ill should be centralised to ensure optimum utilisation of resources [4].

Reliable communications must be available at all times between the transport team and the referring and receiving hospitals [4].

It is important to optimise communication of critical information as an essential component of patient care, safety and risk management: *ISBAR – a tool for improved communication within the team* [7]:

*Identification*: identify yourself and your role to the person you are communicating with in the communication.

*Situation*: describe the specific situation about a particular patient, including name, consultant, patient location, vital signs, resuscitation status and any specific concerns.

*Background*: communicate the patient's background, including date of admission, diagnosis, current medications, allergies, laboratory results, progress during the admission and other relevant information.

*Assessment*: this involves critical assessment of the situation, clinical impression and detailed expression of concerns.

*Recommendation:* this includes the management plan, suggestions for care, detail of investigation requests and expected time frame.

Implementing ISBAR takes considerable training for an individual and the organisation.

## Personnel

The transport team should have the expertise necessary to provide supportive care for a wide variety of emergency conditions that can arise with the women at high risk. Team members may include obstetrician, doctor, nurses, emergency medical technicians and respiratory therapists. The composition of the transport team should be consistent with the expected medical need of the patient being transported.

Transport personnel should be thoroughly familiar with the transport equipment to ensure that any malfunction en route can be handled without the assistance of hospital maintenance staff.

## Staffing

**Intrahospital Transport** [8] The transport team should consist at least of an appropriately qualified nurse, an orderly and a medical practitioner with the specific skills and training required for such transport.

Whilst most intrahospital transports are not done by dedicated teams, the principles of transport are similar to inter hospital retrieval.

Each team must be familiar with the equipment used on the transport and be sufficiently experienced with securing airways, ventilation of the lungs, resuscitation and other anticipated emergency procedures [8].

## Interhospital Transport [8]

Interhospital transport of critically ill patients must be performed by an appropriately qualified retrieval team including an experienced medical practitioner. This team must be familiar with their transport equipment particularly power and oxygen supply limitations. The retrieval team needs to have adequate clinical understanding of the patient's medical condition and potential transport complications. The team must also be aware of the treatment options available to them prior to and during transport of the patient.

Staff safety and protection are the responsibility of the employing authority, who should carry appropriate insurance for all contingencies related to patient transport activities and should also provide personnel with personal protective equipment and instruction.

## Equipment

Transfer equipment should be dedicated solely for transfer.

The transport team generally needs the following items to perform its functions:

- Equipment for monitoring physiological functions (heart rate, blood pressure levels, temperature (skin, axillary), respiratory rate, noninvasive pulse oximetry).
- Resuscitation and support equipments (intravenous pumps, suction apparatus, mechanical ventilators).
- In choosing equipment, attention must be given to size, weight, volume, battery life, oxygen consumption and durability, as well as to suitability for operation under conditions of transport.
- For practical reasons, bag valve ventilation is most commonly employed during intrahospital transport.
- Portable mechanical ventilators are gaining popularity in this arena, as they more reliably administer prescribed minute ventilation and desired $FiO_2$ (fraction of inspired $O_2$).
- It is essential that the battery life of the equipments is appropriate for the anticipated journey time required for the transfer

The necessary equipment includes:

**Respiratory Support Equipment** [8]

- Airways, oxygen, masks and nebuliser
- Self-inflating hand-ventilating assembly with PEEP valve
- The Bain circuit with an attached connector to the oxygen cylinder
- Suction equipment of appropriate standard
- Portable ventilator with disconnect and high-pressure alarms
- Intubation set with appropriate size blades and endotracheal tubes
- Emergency surgical airway set
- Oxygen supply in excess of that estimated for the maximum transport time
- Capnography (for ventilated patients)

### Circulatory Support Equipment

- Noninvasive blood pressure measuring device with appropriate-sized cuffs
- Multipara monitor – maternal pulse, BP, $SO_2$ and ECG/cardiotocography
- ECG
- Defibrillator
- Syringe drivers
- Vascular cannulae (peripheral and central)
- IV fluids and pressure set/syringes and needles
- Infusion pumps
- A sharp's disposal container and a bag for biological refuse oxygen supply in excess of that estimated for the maximum transport time

### Other Equipment

- Portable suction
- Nasogastric tube and bag
- Urinary catheter and bag
- Instruments, sutures, dressings, antiseptic lotions and gloves
- Cutting shears and portable torch
- Gloves and goggles for staff protection

## Checklist

All pieces of equipment must be checked, and notes and imaging films gathered. An example of a checklist is listed below:

- The monitors function properly and the alarm limits are set appropriately.
- The manual resuscitator bag functions properly.
- The ventilator (if used) functions properly; respiratory variables and alarms are set appropriately.
- The suction device functions properly.
- Oxygen (± air) cylinders are full. A spare oxygen cylinder is available.
- Airway and intubation equipment are all available and working.
- Emergency drugs ((iv fluids: crystalloids, colloids) oxytocics, hypertensive emergencies (labetalol, hydralazine), anaphylaxis (hydrocortisone, chlorpheniramine), seizures (magnesium sulphate, calcium carbonate), inotropes (dopamine, adrenaline) and bronchospasm (deriphyllin, analgesics, sedatives and muscle relaxants (if appropriate))) are all available.
- Spare IV fluids; inotropic solutions are available if needed.
- Spare batteries are available for all battery-powered equipment.
- Patient notes, imaging films and necessary forms (especially the informed consent form) are available.

## Patient Status

The patient must be reassessed before transport begins, especially after being placed on monitoring equipment and the transport ventilator (if used). Transport preparations must not overshadow or neglect the patient's fundamental care. An example of a brief check on the patient is listed below:

- Ensuring adequate lateral maternal tilt to avoid aorto-caval compression in pregnant women [9].
- Airway is secured and patent.
- The Bain circuit can be used with an attached connector to the oxygen cylinder if needed. The ventilator may or may not be available in such ambulances.
- Also timely estimation of any respiratory obstruction necessitating urgent suction to remove the secretions. Availability of the foot suction apparatus would work, if there is the failure of the electrical vacuum suction apparatus.
- Ventilation is adequate; respiratory variables are appropriate.
- All equipment alarms are switched on.
- Patient is haemodynamically stable.
- Vital signs are displayed on transport monitors and are clearly visible to transport staff.

- PEEP/CPAP (if set) and $FIO_2$ levels are correct.
- All drains (urinary, wound) are functioning and secured.
- Venous access is adequate and patent: A good IV access is an essential requirement for administration of any emergency drug during transportation, and an emergency tray containing all the life saving drugs should be available in the ambulances.
- IV drips and infusion pumps are functioning properly.
- Patient is safely secured on trolley.

## Departure

At the time of departure, all checklists should be complete. One of the most important communication is to inform the receiving team that the referring team is about to leave. Also to check the exact destination and how to access the ward in the hospital (e.g. via the emergency department or main entrance) is important. The transfer form and checklist provide documentation of adequate preparation, and their completion after handover to the receiving hospital team completes the legal record of the transfer.

The receiving person or staff at the destination must be notified, and the arrival time must be clearly understood.

## During Transit

High-speed journeys should be avoided except where strictly necessary. Blue lights and sirens may be used to aid passage through traffic to deliver a smooth journey.

### Patient Care

- Patient should be observed continuously.
- Vital signs monitored and recorded.
- Uterine activity of maternal patients and fetal heart rates monitored.
- Intravenous fluids should be given, monitored and recorded as required.
- The transport team must be aware whom to contact in an emergency in case of deterioration in the patient's condition.
- Presence of a relative or an acquaintance of the patient alongside ensures not only the transparency of healthcare, but it also helps in making them understand if any eventuality occurs during transportation.

## Arrival Procedures

The transport staff must remain with the patient until the receiving team is fully ready to take over care and a complete hand over is given to the team leader.

Receiving staff should inform family members, as well as the referring doctor about the condition of patient on arrival at the receiving hospital and periodically thereafter.

On completion of the patient transfer, the transport team or other designated personnel should immediately restock and reequip the transport vehicle in anticipation of another call.

The instances when mishaps are most likely are:

- Whilst shifting patient from hospital bed to ambulance trolley
- Shifting patient trolley in to the ambulance
- Shifting trolley from ambulance at the receiving hospital

During these intervals extra vigilance is needed to prevent disconnections, equipment malfunction and dislodgement of indwelling catheters.

## **Documentation** (Appendix 2) [10]

Referring hospital and transport team should document the patient's clinical status before, during and after transport, relevant medical conditions, therapy given and procedures undertaken. For intrahospital transport, this documentation may form part of the inpatient notes.

## Medicolegal Aspects

Informed consent for transfer, transport and admission to and care at the receiving hospital should be obtained before the transport team moves the patient. The completed consent form should be signed by the parent or guardian and witnessed; a copy should be placed in the patient's medical record.

## Challenges

- The shortage of well-equipped ambulances [11] in India and lack of centrally organised government funded medical transport pose the challenge. A majority of the ambulances lack even the basic monitoring gadgets required during transportation, such as pulse oximetry, echocardiogram (ECG), noninvasive blood pressure and so on.
- Increasing workload: We experiencing an increase in the number of high-risk pregnant women on account of a rising birth rate and changes in obstetric demographics including an increase in maternal age and co-morbidities, morbid obesity and assisted conception. The rise in caesarean section rate in many countries has resulted in an increase in the incidence of abnormal placentation (accreta, increta and percreta) and subsequent postpartum haemorrhage.

**Key Message**

- All maternity sites must have the facilities and staff to resuscitate, stabilise and transfer critical care patients.
- The critical care transport system should be developed to ensure a complete and safe critical care service for obstetric patients.
- All staff providing critical care for pregnant women should have appropriate care competencies including the early recognition of critical illness in pregnancy.
- *A multidisciplinary training programme should be rolled out nationally to facilitate this.*

## Appendix-1: Maternity Modified Obstetric Warning System (MOWS)

Each parameter is scored and action taken according to the total.

| | 3 | 2 | 1 | 0 | 1 | 2 | 3 |
|---|---|---|---|---|---|---|---|
| Resp rate | | Less than 8 | | 9–18 | 19–25 | 26–30 | More than 30 |
| Pulse rate | | Less than 40 | 40–50 | 51–100 | 101–110 | 111–129 | More than 129 |
| BP Systolic | Less than 70 | 71–80 | 81–100 | 101–159 | 160–199 | 200 | More than 200 |
| BP Diastolic | | | | Less than 95 | 95–109 | More than 110 | |
| Conscious level | Unresponsive | Responds to pain | Responds to voice | Alert | Irritated | | |
| Urine hourly (ml/h) or in 24-h rate | 0 | Less than 30 (less than 720 ml) | Less than 45 (less than 1000 ml) | More | | | V6.1 Nov 2011 |

Originally adapted from Morgan et al. [12]

*Action to be taken*

| | |
|---|---|
| 0 | Repeat observations when appropriate for clinical scenario - at least daily |
| 1 | Minimum of 4 hourly observations as there is potential for deterioration |
| 2 | Inform midwife in charge, obstetric registrar. Minimum 1 hourly observations |
| 3 | Inform senior midwife, obstetric and anaesthetic staff. Minimum ½ hourly observations |
| 4 or more | As above but the consultant obstetrician and consultant anaesthetist should be informed |
| | If no one is available to review the patient, inform the outreach team |

## Appendix 2: Transport documentation

The following information should be recorded on transport documentation

| |
|---|
| *Transfer details* |
| Patient's name, address, date of birth |
| Next of kin, what information they have been given and by whom |
| Referring hospital, ward/unit and contact telephone number |
| Name of referring doctor and contact telephone number |
| Receiving hospital, ward/unit and contact telephone number |
| Name of receiving doctor and contact telephone number |
| Names and status of the escorting personnel |
| *Medical summary* |
| Primary reason for admission to the referring unit |
| History and past history |
| Dates of admission/delivery/operations/procedures |
| Intubation history, ventilatory support |
| Cardiovascular status including inotrope and vasopressor requirements |
| Other medication and fluids |
| Type of lines inserted and dates of insertion |

## References


1. Singh S, McGlennan AP. Validation of the CEMACH recommended modified early warning system (MEOWS). Int J Obstet Anesth. 2010;19:S11. http://www.oaaanaes.ac.uk/assets/_managed/editor/File/Surveys/2010_IJOAsuppl_Newcastle.pdf.
2. Recognition, high dependency care, and transfer of critically ill maternity patients policy (CG489) NHS. 2013.
3. Guideline summary NGC-7086 AHRQ US. http://f.imd.com/medinfo/material/55c/4eb1368444ae4ffe12a8155c/4eb1369d44ae4ffe12a8155f.pdf.
4. Hong Kong College of Anaesthesiologists HKCA-P9-v3 Guidelines for Transport of the Critically Ill. 2014. http://www.hkca.edu.hk/ANS/standard_publications/guidep09.pdf.
5. Interhospital care of perinatal patient chap. 3 (aap&acog2008). http://www.acog.cl/descargar.php?9cafffa6a93d33b8a8c90a4adc70fcef.
6. Obstetric critical care clinical problems 2013 ESICM. http://pact.esicm.org/media/Obstetric%20critical%20care%2030%20April%202013%20final.pdf.
7. Guidelines for the critically ill woman in obstetrics version 1.1 13th August 2014 obstetric & gynaecology, anaesthetic and critical programmes clinical strategy & programmes division health service executive www.hse.ie. http://www.rcpi.ie/content/docs/000001/2976_5_media.pdf.
8. Guidelines for Transport of Critically Ill Patients ANZCA PS52 2013 /P03 by ACEM and IC-10 by CIC. http://www.anzca.edu.au/resources/professional-documents/pdfs/ps52-2015-guidelines-for-transport-of-critically-ill-patients.pdf.
9. ATOTW 310 – Maternal Critical Care 27/10/2014. https://www.aagbi.org/sites/default/files/310%20Maternal%20Critical%20Care.pdf.
10. Intensive Care Society. Guidelines for the transport of the critically ill adult. 3rd ed. 2011. http://www.ics.ac.uk/EasysiteWeb/getresource.axd?AssetID=482&.
11. Bajwa SK, Bajwa SJ. Delivering obstetrical critical care in developing nations. Int J Crit Illn Inj Sci. 2012;2(1):32–9. http://www.ncbi.nlm.nih.gov/pmc/articles/PMC3354375/.
12. Morgan RJM, Williams F, et al. "An early warning system for detecting developing critical illness." Clin Intensive Care. 1997;8(2):100.

# Part V

# Critically Ill Foetus

# 37 Twin-to-Twin Transfusion Syndrome: As an Obstetric Emergency

Shah Aditi and Radhakrishnan Prathima

## Introduction

Dizygotic twins are the result of two eggs fertilized by two separate sperms. Monozygotic twins are the result of a single fertilized egg splitting within the first 14 days after fertilization. The stage at which the egg cell splits determines how the twins will implant in the uterine lining and whether or not they share an amnion, chorion, and placenta as shown in Fig. 37.1 [1].

Dichorionic diamniotic (DCDA) twins form when splitting takes place by the third day after fertilization, i.e., at the two-cell stage. This occurs in almost all cases of dizygotic twins and in 25 % of monozygotic twins. If the split occurs at the early blastocyst stage between days 4–8, then monochorionic–diamniotic twins (MCDA) are formed, and if splitting occurs between days 8–12, which is the late blastocyst stage, then monochorionic–monoamniotic (MCMA) twins are formed. If the split occurs after day 13, conjoined twins result [1].

## Incidence and Definition

Fifteen percent of spontaneous twin pregnancies and almost 5 % of the medically assisted twin pregnancies are monochorionic–diamniotic (MCDA) [1].

Fifteen to twenty percent of monochorionic–diamniotic twin pregnancies are complicated by twin-to-twin transfusion syndrome (TTTS) [1].

Twin-to-twin transfusion syndrome (TTTS) is a specific complication of monochorionic pregnancy resulting from an imbalance in the blood flow between the twins sharing the placenta, leading to unequal distribution of the blood flow such that one twin is compromised and the other is favored. Blood from one twin (the donor) is "transfused" into the other twin (the recipient) via connecting blood vessels within their common placenta. It has life-threatening effects upon both twins with perinatal mortality approaching 90 % if untreated [2–4].

S. Aditi • R. Prathima (✉)
Bangalore Fetal Medicine Centre,
2E, Rich Homes, 2nd floor, 5/1, Richmond road,
Bangalore 560 025, India
e-mail: drprathima@bangalorefetalmedicine.com


A. Gandhi et al. (eds.), *Principles of Critical Care in Obstetrics: Volume II*,
DOI 10.1007/978-81-322-2686-4_37

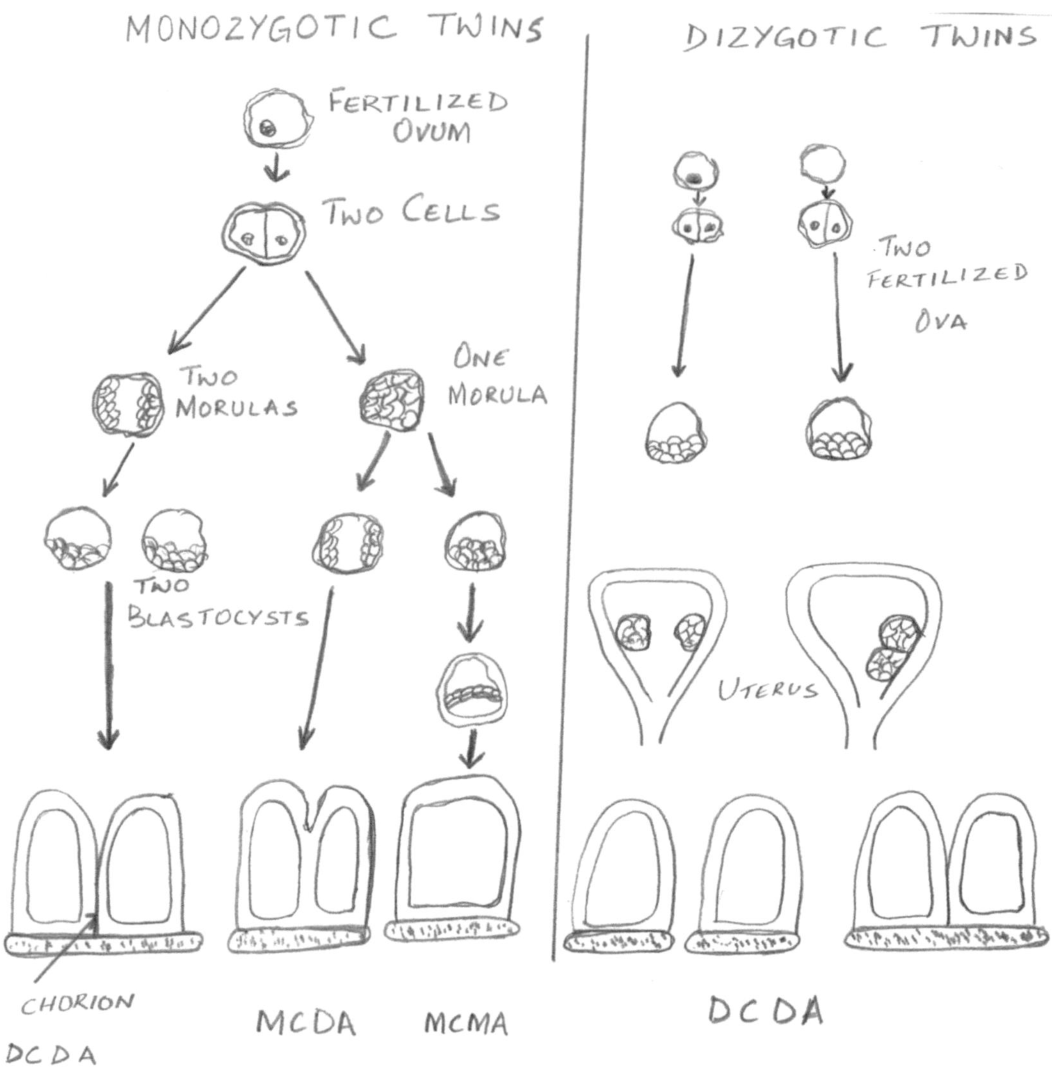


**Fig. 37.1** Insertion of the membrane on the placenta – "T" sign indicated monochorionicity and "λ" sign indicated dichorionicity

## Pathophysiology

Differential cord insertion of the MCDA twins with unequal sharing of the placental disk forms the basis of TTTS. Inter-twin vascular anastomoses as shown in Fig. 37.2 are present in virtually all monochorionic pregnancies. Arteriovenous anastomoses (labeled 1 in Fig. 37.2) with unidirectional flow, arterioarterial (labeled 2 in Fig. 37.2), or venovenous anastomoses with bidirectional flow are seen in the placenta of MCDA twins. Arteriovenous anastomoses are usually

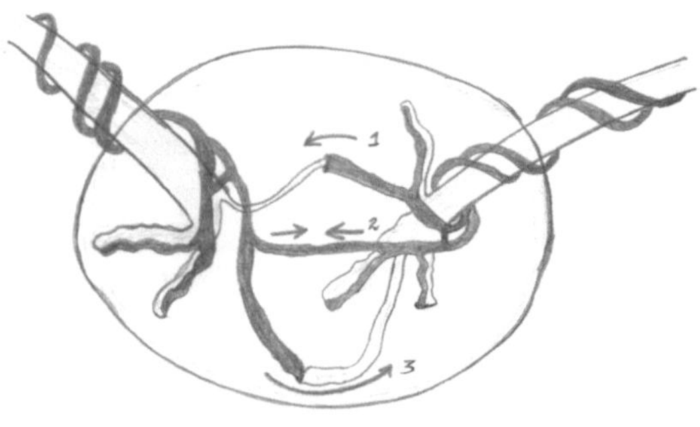


**Fig. 37.2** Dark shaded vessels – veins; light shaded vessels – arteries

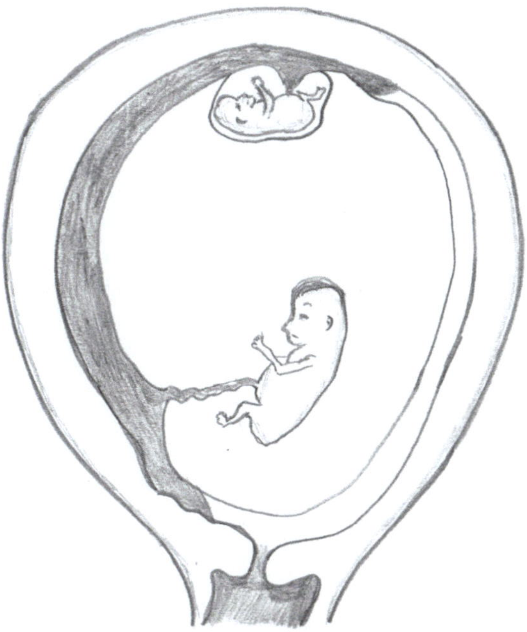

**Fig. 37.3** Twin-to-twin transfusion syndrome (TTTS)

situated deeply in the placenta. Bidirectional anastomoses (arterioarterial, venovenous – both usually located on the placental surface) can assist in regulating unbalanced, unidirectional flow which occurs through the arteriovenous anastomoses and are protective against TTTS. Thrombosis of the superficial vessels may give rise to TTTS [2–4] (Fig. 37.3).

The asymmetric, bidirectional inter-twin exchange of blood and biochemical components that occurs between the donor and recipient twins results in severe hemodynamic, osmotic, and physiologic changes in both twins resulting in renal structural and functional aberrations in the donor twin and cardiovascular compromise in the recipient twin as depicted in the flowchart below [5].

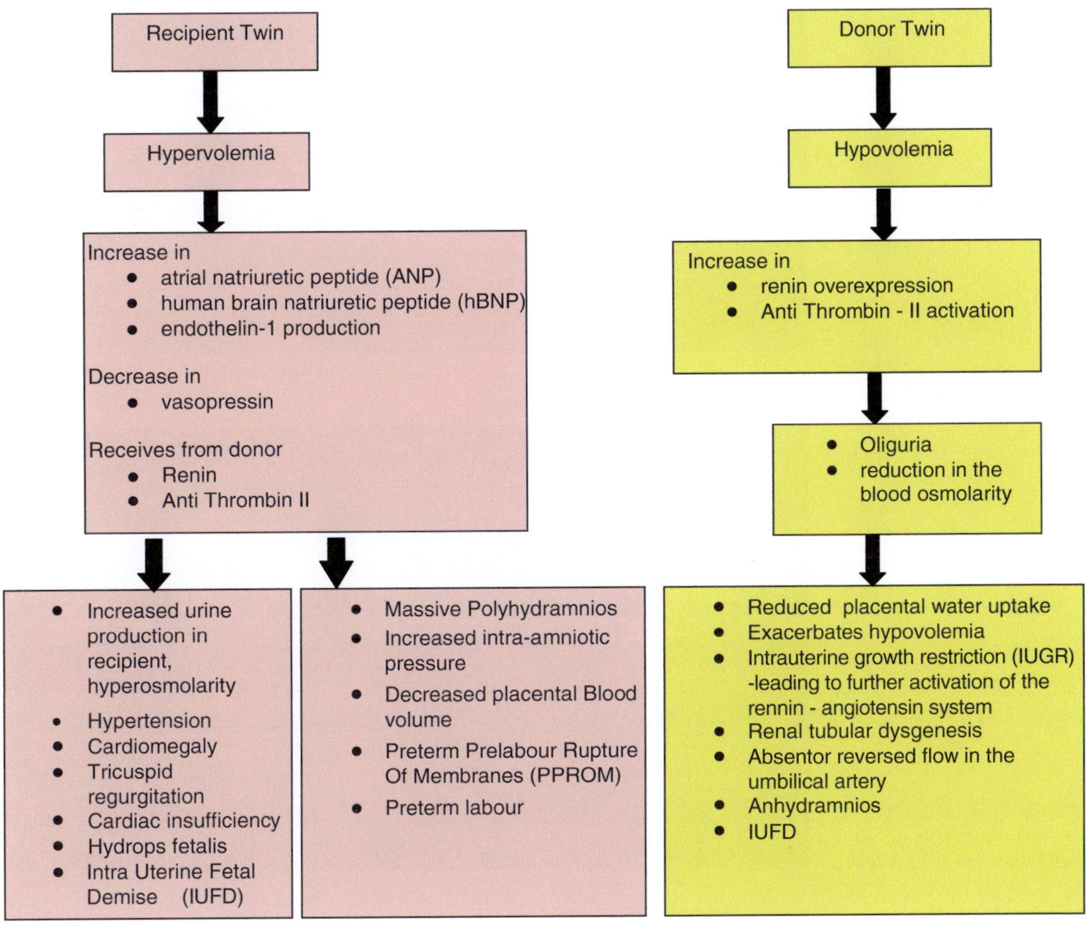

## Prenatal Diagnosis

Characteristic ultrasound findings enable prenatal diagnosis of TTTS. With advances in first trimester ultrasound and the widespread use of first-trimester screening, affected pregnancies are becoming increasingly diagnosed at earlier gestational ages. The first step in prenatal diagnosis is early and accurate determination of chorionicity as shown in ultrasound (USG) Image 37.1.

The diagnostic criteria on ultrasound are:

In the FIRST TRIMESTER

- Nuchal translucency – increased measurement – increased risk of TTTS [6]
- Discordant nuchal translucency measurements (USG Image 37.2) [6]
- Discordant measurements of crown–rump length
- Reversed "a" wave in ductus venosus in either of the twins
- Placental cord insertion – differential – marginal and velamentous (USG Image 37.3)
- Discordant abdominal circumference/amniotic fluid volume/bladder size
- Tricuspid regurgitation in either of the twins

In the SECOND TRIMESTER

- Membrane folding – fluid discordance
- Discrepancy in amniotic fluid volumes – polyhydramnios–oligohydramnios sequence; significant difference in the amniotic fluid

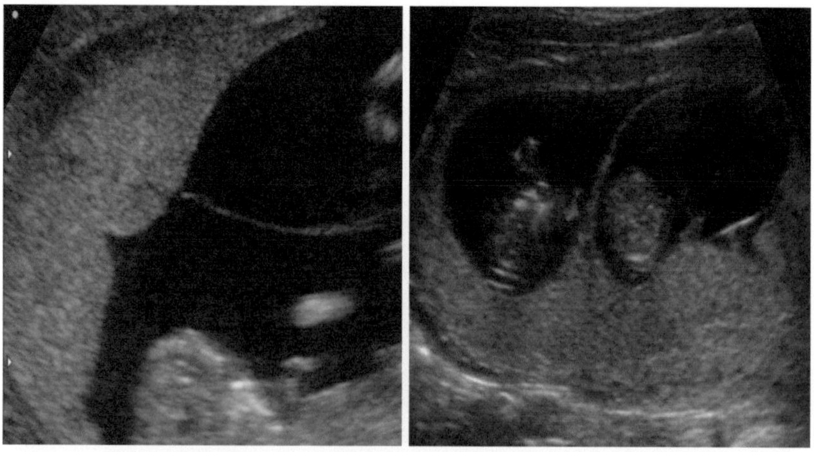

**Image 37.1** Insertion of the membrane on the placenta – "T" sign indicated monochorionicity and "λ" sign indicated dichorionicity

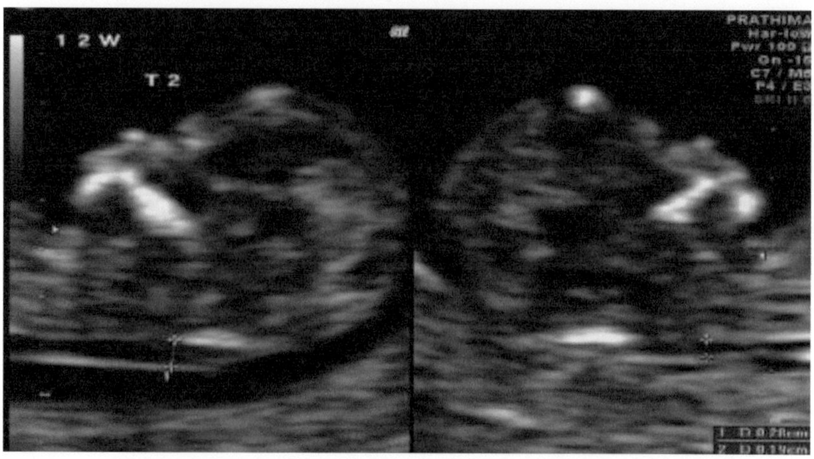


**Image 37.2** Discrepant NT measurements in MCDA twins at 12 weeks

volume – deepest vertical pool (DVP) >8 cm in recipient (USG Image 37.4) and <2 cm in the donor

- Discrepancy in abdominal circumference (AC) measurement (USG Image 37.5)
- Discrepancy in bladder size (USG Image 37.6)
- Doppler – umbilical artery/middle cerebral artery peak systolic velocity/ductus venosus

Though all monochorionic pregnancies are considered "high risk" and need intensive surveillance, Lewi et al. have recommended a method of risk stratification of monochorionic pregnancies based on ultrasound findings.

In the first trimester, if there is discordant amniotic fluid or a discordance in crown–rump length (CRL) of ≥12 mm, these pregnancies are categorized as "high risk." Monochorionic pregnancies with concordant amniotic fluid and difference in CRL of <12 mm are labeled as "low risk" [7].

In the second trimester (after 16 weeks), a high risk of adverse outcome was predicted by the presence of discordant amniotic fluid and discordant cord insertions. Alternatively, for cases with only discordant fluid but concordant cord insertions, adverse outcome was predicted by an inter-twin difference in abdominal circumference of >6 mm and for cases with concordant fluid but discordant cords by a difference in abdominal circumference >13 mm. Finally, in the absence of both discordant fluid and cord insertions, an

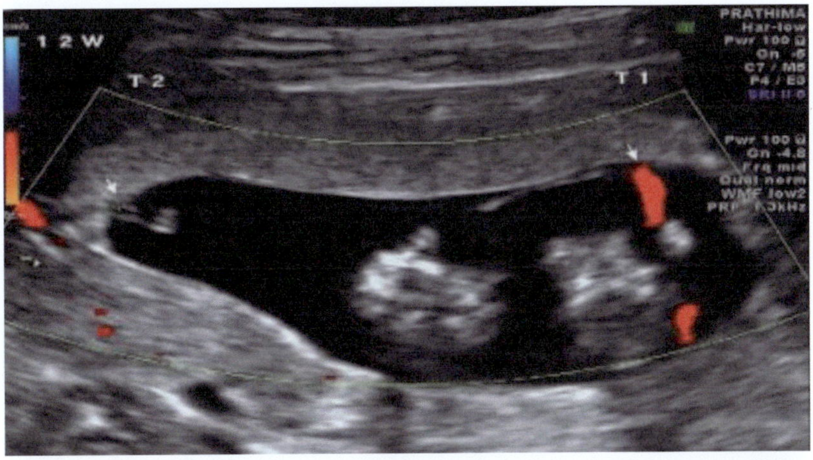


**Image 37.3** Discrepant cord insertions (*arrows*) in MCDA twins at 12 weeks

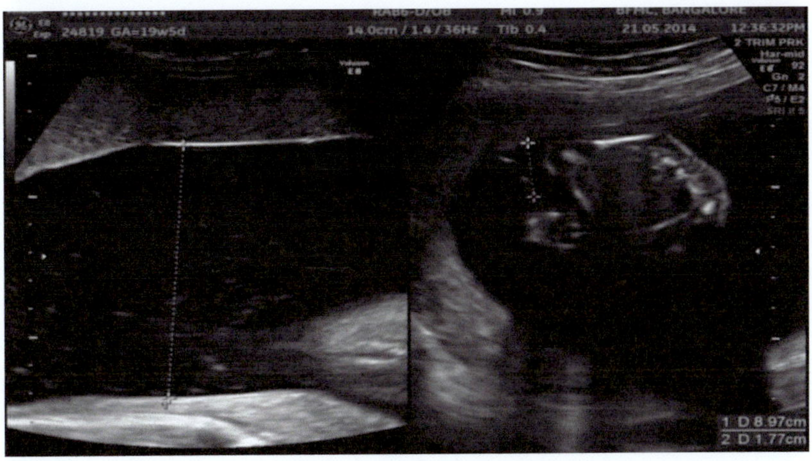


**Image 37.4** Discrepant amniotic fluid in MCDA twins in 2nd trimester

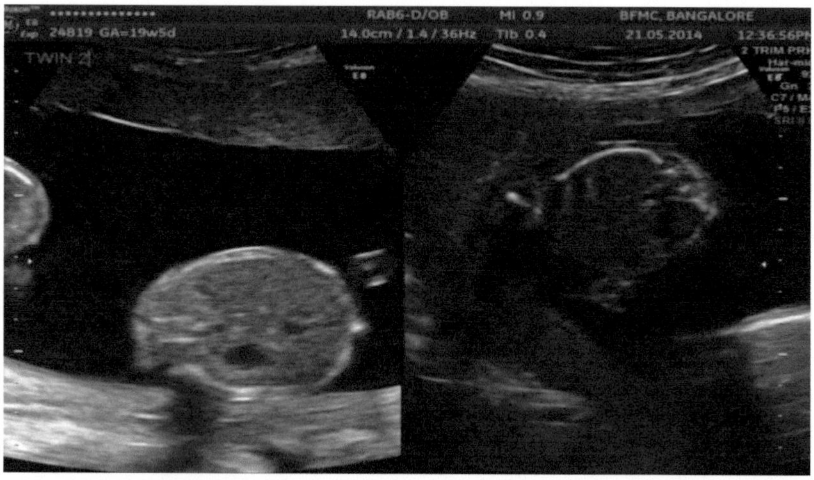


**Image 37.5** Discrepant abdominal circumference in MCDA twins in the second trimester

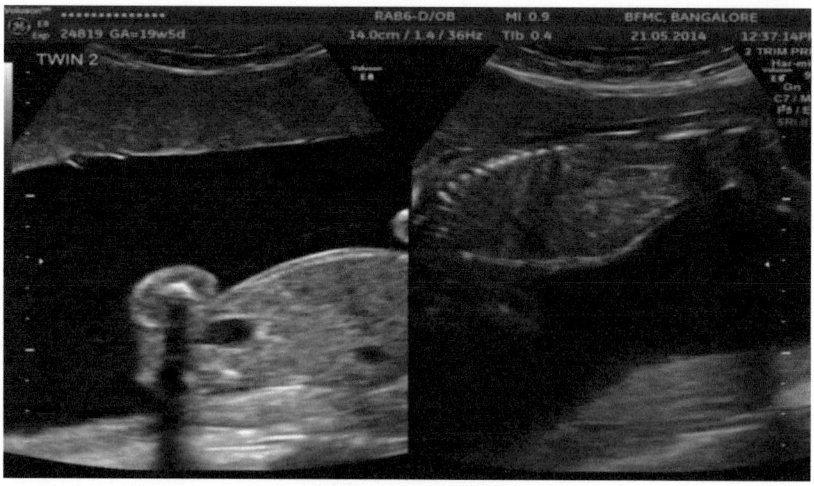


**Image 37.6** Discrepant bladders in MCDA twins in the second trimester

adverse outcome was predicted by a difference in abdominal circumference >24 mm [7].

The "high-risk" pregnancies have >70 % risk of adverse outcome and <70 % survival rate unless treated. They will need weekly surveillance in a tertiary care center and have to be offered invasive fetal therapy [7].

The "low-risk" pregnancies have a 90 % survival rate with <10 % incidence of complications. They are followed up fortnightly in a tertiary care center [7].

TTTS is a dynamic condition which may remain unchanged, progress slowly, or develop quickly with rapid deterioration in fetal well-being hence the importance of serial surveillance of MCDA twin pregnancies, preferably in a maternal fetal medicine unit.

## Staging of TTTS

The Quintero staging for TTTS was proposed in 1999 and is internationally recognized. It helps in early diagnosis and appropriate referral for treatment. The main limitations are in the prediction of progression and outcome. It indirectly considers cardiovascular changes in recipient twin via the ductus venosus Doppler. The staging is as follows:

Stage I – DVP <2 cm donor, DVP >8 cm recipient
Stage II – bladder not visible in donor
Stage III – abnormal umbilical artery (UA), ductus venosus (DV), or umbilical vein (UV) Doppler
  IIIa – absent EDF or reversal of EDF in UA of donor

IIIb – reversal of flow in DV of donor
IIIc – pulsatile flow in UV of recipient
Stage IV – hydrops
Stage V – demise of one or both twins [8]

The newer staging systems [Cincinnati Staging system, Cardiovascular Profile Scoring system (CVPS), Children's Hospital of Philadelphia system (CHOP)] incorporate echocardiographic criteria in order to overcome the limitations of the Quintero staging system, but are more complex and not widely followed in clinical practice currently [9]. Quintero staging system considers the pregnancy as a whole and gives a pregnancy specific risk, whereas the newer classifications offer an individual risk to each fetus. It also minimizes inter- and intraobserver variation. It is important to remember that patients could change from one stage to another rapidly and will not necessarily follow the sequence as specified by Quintero.

## Differential Diagnosis

The differential diagnosis of TTTS includes uteroplacental insufficiency, isolated intrauterine growth retardation of one fetus in a twin pregnancy due to abnormal cord insertions, dichorionic twin pregnancy with fused placentae with growth restriction of one fetus, discordant manifestation of intrauterine infection, preterm premature rupture of membranes of one twin, congenital infections, and discordant chromosomal or structural anomalies of one twin.

## Management of Pregnancy

Once the chorionicity is established on scan, detailed anatomic survey of both fetuses has to be done followed by echocardiography. Deepest vertical pool of amniotic fluid should be measured in both fetuses. Abdominal circumferences and bladder sizes should be compared. Color Doppler studies should be done to note the flow patterns in the umbilical artery, middle cerebral artery, and ductus venosus of the donor and the recipient. Both placental cord insertions must be documented. Invasive testing must be offered to determine fetal karyotype before considering fetal therapy. These pregnancies ideally should be managed in tertiary care centers offering fetal therapeutic options or at least in close liaison with such centers.

After the first trimester scan, all monochorionic pregnancies are monitored by ultrasonography every fortnightly from 16 weeks onward to note the amniotic fluid volume (measured as deepest vertical pool, DVP), free-floating membrane, discrepancy in fetal size – AC, fetal bladder size, and fetal Doppler studies are done in both fetuses [10].

MRI may prove useful in the evaluation of the fetal brain because up to 8 % of cases with TTTS may show signs of ischemic brain injury at the time of presentation. It is usually performed after invasive therapy for TTTS or after death of one twin to document an absence of resultant central nervous system ischemic or hemorrhagic injury [11].

More than three-fourth of fetuses with stage I TTTS remain stable or regress without invasive intervention, with perinatal survival of about 86 %. Advanced stages, i.e., stage ≥III TTTS is bleak, with a reported perinatal loss rate of 70–100 %, when diagnosed at <26 weeks of gestation. Fetoscopic laser photocoagulation is the best available approach for stages II, III, and IV TTTS for continuing pregnancies at <26 weeks of gestation. Steroids for fetal maturation should be considered in pregnancies complicated by stage ≥III TTTS and those undergoing invasive interventions [12].

## Treatment

On diagnosis of TTTS, the fetuses should be closely monitored via periodic scans to evaluate their condition and to look for signs of progression followed by extensive counseling which includes a detailed history of the disease, as well as the management options along with their benefits and risks.

The treatment options include serial amniodrainages, septostomy, cord ligation/coagulation, and fetoscopic laser photocoagulation.

Serial amniodrainages [13] was the mainstay of therapy until the advent of fetoscopic laser ablation of the intercommunicating vessels. It reduced the incidence of extreme preterm birth with TTTS and improved survival in addition to alleviating maternal discomfort. However, evidence shows that though serial amniodrainage does improve survival compared with no treatment, however, it is associated with significant rates of neurological handicap in survivors (20 %). It is no longer used in the treatment of TTTS as a primary option.

Septostomy [13] is associated with a high likelihood of extension thereby creating a monoamniotic state and risk of cord entanglement. In studies to date, there is no apparent advantage to survival compared with serial amniodrainages.

Fetoscopic LASER surgery was first reported by De Lia in 1990 [14]. The main advantage with laser is that underlying pathology of TTTS is treated. The early reports of survival for laser were similar to amniodrainages but showed consistently less neurologic abnormality. The principle of laser therapy is dichorionization whereby fetoscopically directed Nd–YAG laser is used for intrauterine ablation of vascular communications in the placenta after mapping the arteriovenous communications [14].

Prerequisites for laser therapy are polyhydramnios of the recipient DVP >8 cm up to the 20th week of pregnancy or >10 cm as from the 21st week, donor oligohydramnios, i.e., stuck twin syndrome DVP <2 cm, and viability of both fetuses during weeks 16–26 [5].

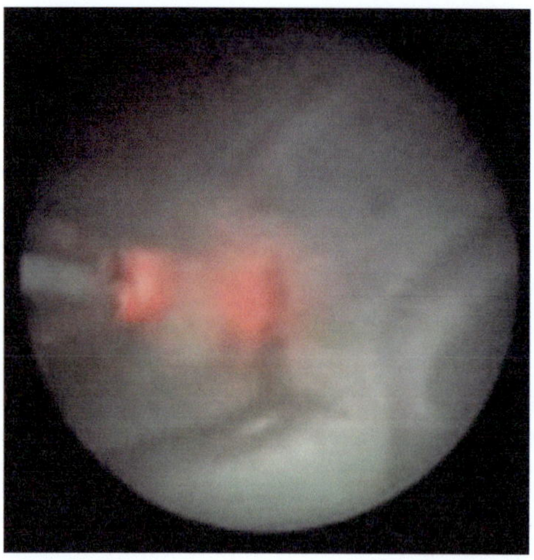

LASER coagulation of the vascular anastomoses on the placental surface

Earlier, nonselective laser coagulation of placental vessels used to be performed, in which all the vessels that crossed the inter-twin membranes ("membranous equator") were coagulated. Subsequently selective laser coagulation of placental vessels was reported, in which vascular anastomoses crossing between the twins ("vascular equator") were first identified and then coagulated. Recently, selective laser coagulation of placental vessels was performed with surface coagulation of the placenta between the ablated anastomotic sites in order to create a physical separation of the donor's and the recipient's vascular territories on the surface of the placenta. This surgical procedure is known as "Solomonization" or the "Solomon technique." This may reduce the recurrence of TTTS and/or the incidence of twin anemia–polycythemia sequence (TAPS) by coagulating microanastomoses that were not coagulated during the selective laser ablation alone [15, 18].

In the Eurofetus trial, the enrolment was halted early after interim analysis showed significantly improved outcomes in the laser group (76 % vs. 56 % of at least one twin surviving). A Cochrane meta-analysis concluded that selective laser surgery is preferred treatment for TTTS when it is available and amniodrainage is preferred when laser surgery is not available. If TTTS is progressive despite an initial amniodrainage, laser surgery should be sought [16, 17].

Indications for laser therapy are:

- Early-onset severe TTTS 16–26 weeks
- Quintero stage II–IV disease
- Echocardiographic evidence of recipient twin-acquired cardiac dysfunction

Placental location influences outcome in laser surgery, the anterior placentae being more technically challenging than the posterior placentae.

Risks of the procedure include:

- Preterm prelabor rupture of membranes (PPROM)
- Preterm labor
- Preterm delivery or pregnancy loss
- Amniotic fluid leakage into the maternal peritoneal cavity
- Abruption

- Intrauterine infection
- Persistent or recurrent TTTS – 14 %
- Reversed TTTS – 13 % of cases
- TAPS – occur spontaneously in MCDA in about 4 %; post-laser therapy about – 13 %
- Known iatrogenic complication of laser

Hence, weekly surveillance is recommended especially after LASER [18, 19] more so in the first few weeks.

There is no contraindication for vaginal delivery. Delivery is usually contemplated at 34 weeks gestation for TTTS. Prenatal steroids should be given, especially when elective cesarean is planned before 36 weeks. Cord hematocrits should be done immediately after delivery. Placental examination should be done after delivery and with vascular dye injection to note the vascular anastomoses. Placenta should also be sent for histopathological examination.

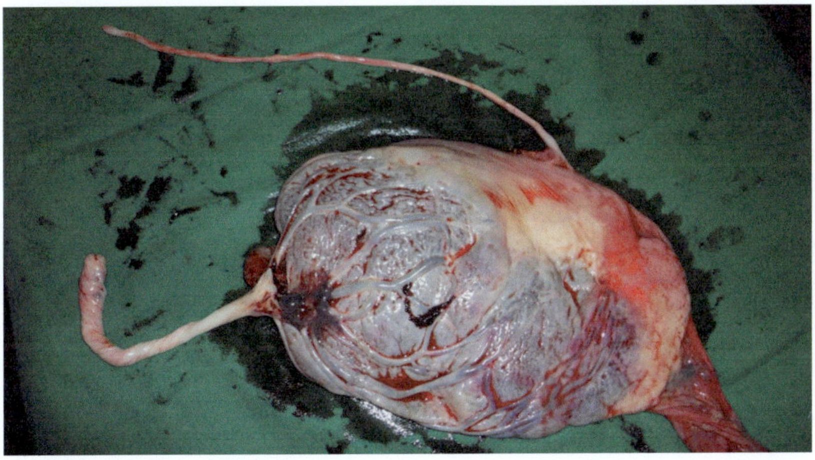

Placental examination

Discordant cord sizes, distantly placed cord insertions, and the imbalance in placental sharing are clearly seen in the above image.

## Recurrence Risk

No recurrence is reported till date.

## Long-Term Outcome

In various studies, the incidence of severe neurodevelopmental abnormalities in MCDA without TTTS was 6 %. The increased likelihood of severe neurodevelopmental abnormalities in MCDA pregnancies complicated by TTTS is largely influenced by prematurity and poor APGAR scores. Studies have shown that post-LASER, 78 % of the babies show normal development at 2 years of age; 11 % have a mild delay in motor milestones, strabismus, mildly abnormal speech; and 11 % have cerebral palsy, hemiparesis, and spastic quadriplegia [16, 17].

**Conclusion**

TTTS may have varied clinical presentation. Early and accurate detection and documentation of chorionicity will ensure a favorable outcome of all twin pregnancies and that of pregnancies with monochorionic placentation in particular. An initial first trimester scan followed by serial fortnightly ultrasound follow-ups from 16 weeks onward ensure early detection and effective management of TTTS. Parental education about the symptoms of TTTS (sudden severe abdominal distension, maternal discomfort, PPROM, preterm labor) may also aid in early detection of

TTTS. The advent of laser has revolutionized the management of TTTS. Selective laser coagulation of placental vessels with surface coagulation of the placenta between the ablated anastomotic sites (Solomon technique) ensures a high double survival rate in MCDA twin pregnancies complicated by severe TTTS.

## Indian Scenario

India presents a unique challenge at every stage, from diagnosis to management. India is still far from making the first trimester mandatory in all pregnancies. The awareness of the importance of the first trimester scan is gradually increasing among the obstetricians, sonologists, and the parents. However, this is true to most urban population but much needs to be achieved in the rural sectors. The reporting of chorionicity is still not done for most pregnancies at the early pregnancy or the first trimester scans. Subsequent to the diagnosis of monochorionicity, most units do not adhere to follow-up protocols from 16 weeks. Following the suspicion of TTTS, many pregnancies are not referred appropriately to the fetal medicine units offering fetal therapy. Late referrals when cervical canal is already compromised lead to relatively lower survival and higher post-procedure miscarriage rates. There are very few centers offering fetal therapy currently and the logistics of travel from their home units to these centers is limited by the stage of the pregnancy and cervical length. At the time of writing this chapter, three centers across the country are offering fetoscopic laser therapy for such twins with reasonably good success. These are at Bangalore, Chennai, and Delhi.

A good protocol-based approach from the time of diagnosis of monochorionicity with liaison with fetal medicine units and early referral for fetal therapy is bound to improve outcome of these pregnancies as majority of these babies are normally formed. This will reduce the unnecessary pregnancy losses, especially before 24 weeks which is the highest risk period for the pregnancies that develop severe TTTS. The development of severe TTTS is considered an obstetric emergency for referral to centers offering fetal therapeutic interventions in order to prevent unnecessary fetal losses.

## References

1. Ohm Kyvik K, Derom C. Data collection on multiple births – establishing twin registers and determining zygosity. Early Hum Dev. 2006;82:357–63.
2. Lewi L, Van Schoubroeck D, Gratacos E, Witters I, Timmerman D, Deprest J. Monochorionic diamniotic twins: complications and management options. Curr Opin Obstet Gynecol. 2003;15:177–94.
3. Fick AL, Feldstein VA, Norton ME, Wassel Fyr C, Caughey AB, Machin GA. Unequal placental sharing and birth weight discordance in monochorionic diamniotic twins. Am J Obstet Gynecol. 2006;195:178–83.
4. Lewi L, Cannie M, Blickstein I, Jani J, Huber A, Hecher K, Dymarkowski S, Gratacós E, Lewi P, Deprest J. Placental sharing, birthweight discordance, and vascular anastomoses in monochorionic diamniotic twin placentas. Am J Obstet Gynecol. 2007;197:587.e1–8.
5. Tchirikov M. Monochorionic twin pregnancy: screening, pathogenesis of complications and management in the era of microinvasive fetal surgery. J Perinat Med. 2010;38:451–9. Copyright by Walter de Gruyter Berlin New York. doi:10.1515/JPM.2010.069.
6. Kagan KO, Gazzoni A, Sepulveda-Gonzalez G, Sotiriadis A, Nicolaides KH. Discordance in nuchal translucency thickness in the prediction of severe twin-to-twin transfusion syndrome. Ultrasound Obstet Gynecol. 2007;5:527–32.
7. Lewi L, et al. Monochorionic diamniotic twin pregnancies: Natural History and Risk Stratification Department of Obstetrics and Gynecology, University Hospital Gasthuisberg, Leuven, Belgium. Fetal Diagn Ther. 2010;27:121–33. doi:10.1159/000313300.
8. Quintero RA, Morales WJ, Allen MH, Bornick PW, Johnson PK, Kruger M. Staging of twin-twin transfusion syndrome. J Perinatol. 1999;19:550–5.
9. Michelfelder E, Gottliebson W, Border W, et al. Early manifestations and spectrum of recipient twin cardiomyopathy in twin to twin transfusion syndrome: relation to Quintero staging. Ultrasound Obstet Gynecol. 2007;30:965–71.
10. Sueters M, Middeldorp JM, Lopriore E, et al. Timely diagnosis of twin-to-twin transfusion syndrome in monochorionic twin pregnancies by biweekly sonography combined with patient instruction to report onset of symptoms. Ultrasound Obstet Gynecol. 2006;28:659–64.
11. Kline-Fath BM, Calvo-Garcia MA, O'Hara SM, et al. Twin to twin transfusion syndrome: cerebral ischemia is not the only MRI finding. Pediatr Radiol. 2007;37:47–56.

12. Molina S, Papanna R, Moise Jr KJ, Johnson A. Management of Stage I twin-to-twin transfusion syndrome: an international survey. Ultrasound Obstet Gynecol. 2010;36:42–7.
13. Malone FD, D'Alton ME. Anomalies peculiar to multiple gestations. Clin Perinatol. 2000;27:1033–46.
14. De Lia JE, Cruikshank DP, et al. Fetoscopic Nd: YAG laser occlusion of placental vessels in severe twin to twin transfusion syndrome. Obstet Gynecol. 1990;75: 1046–53.
15. Ruano R, Rodo C, et al. Fetoscopic laser ablation of placental anastomoses in twin–twin transfusion syndrome using 'Solomon technique'. Ultrasound Obstet Gynecol. 2013;42:434–9.
16. Senat MV, Deprest J, Ville Y, et al. Endoscopic Laser surgery versus serial amnioreduction for severe twin to twin transfusion syndrome. N Engl J Med. 2004; 351:136–44.
17. Rossi AC, D'Addario V. Laser therapy and serial amnioreductions treatment of twin to twin transfusion syndrome: a meta-analysis and review of the literature. Am J Obstet Gynecol. 2008;198:147–52.
18. Chalouhi GE, Essaoui M, Stirnemann J, Quibel T, Deloison B, Salomon L, Ville Y. Laser therapy for twin-to-twin transfusion syndrome (TTTS). Prenat Diagn. 2011;31:637–46.
19. Chalouhi GE, Stirnemann JJ, Salomon LJ, Essaoui M, Quibel T, Ville Y. Specific complications of monochorionic twin pregnancies: twin–twin transfusion syndrome and twin reversed arterial perfusion sequence. Semin Fetal Neonatal Med. 2010;15: 349–56.

# 38 Diagnosis and Management of Fetal Anemia

S. Suresh

Fetal anemia is an inadequate number or quality of red blood cells in the fetal circulatory system. Normal fetal hemoglobin concentration increases linearly during pregnancy: from about 10 to 11 g/dL at 17 weeks to about 14 to 15 g/dL at term, one standard deviation is approximately 1 g/dL [1, 2].

## Causes of Fetal Anemia

The most common causes of fetal anemia are red cell alloimmunization, parvovirus infection, and chronic fetomaternal hemorrhage. The other causes for fetal anemia are inherited red cell abnormalities like alpha thalassemia, tumors like sacrococcygeal teratoma, and placental chorioangioma.

### Rhesus Alloimmunization in Pregnancy

The standard obstetrical nomenclature for designating a pregnant woman's blood type is the ABO type and either Rh positive or Rh negative. These terms are commonly used to describe a woman who has or does not have the Rh(D) antigen on her red blood cells (RBCs). The Rh blood system consists of numerous other antigens, most commonly C, c, E, e, and G.

Maternal Rh(D) alloimmunization develops as a result of maternal immune system exposure to Rh(D)-positive red blood cells (RBCs). Maternal immunization can occur as a result of transplacental fetomaternal hemorrhage during any pregnancy, injection with needles contaminated by Rh(D)-positive blood, or inadvertent transfusion of Rh(D)-positive blood (including during transplantation).

## Minor Red Blood Cell Antibodies during Pregnancy

Minor red blood cell (RBC) antibodies are immunoglobulins associated with RBC antigens other than ABO and Rh (i.e., C, c, D, E, e) like Kell, Duffy, MNS systems, P system, etc.

### Pathogenesis of Fetal Anemia

The pathogenesis of fetal anemia is the same for both major and minor RBC antibodies. The predominant mechanism involves transplacental passage of a maternal IgG antibody directed against a fetal erythrocyte antigen. Red blood cell hemolysis is cell mediated, rather than a complement mediated. In Kell alloimmunization in addition to cell-mediated hemolysis, the erythropoiesis is suppressed at the level of the progenitor cell.

S. Suresh, MB.BS, FRCOG(hon), DSc(hon)
Director MediScan Systems, Chennai, India

Visiting Prof. in Perinatology, Sri Ramachandra University, Chennai, India
e-mail: mediscan@gmail.com


A. Gandhi et al. (eds.), *Principles of Critical Care in Obstetrics: Volume II*,
DOI 10.1007/978-81-322-2686-4_38

Because of this, at the same level of anemia, the fetus with Kell alloimmunization has a lower number of circulating reticulocytes and normoblasts compared with the fetus with Rh(D) alloimmunization [3, 4]. The suppressive effect of anti-Kell antibodies does not extend to fetal granulocyte or megakaryocyte progenitors [5], and hence significant thrombocytopenia is less common than in Rh(D) alloimmunization [6, 7].

## Investigations

The diagnosis of Rh(D) alloimmunization is based upon detection of anti-Rh(D) antibody in maternal serum. In Rh(D)-negative women, the antibody screen may be repeated at 28 weeks of gestation and should be repeated at delivery [8, 9].

A positive anti-D titer means that the fetus is at risk for hemolytic disease, not that it has occurred. Variation in titer results between laboratories is common.

**Critical Titer** A critical titer refers to the titer associated with a risk for fetal hydrops. In most centers, an anti-D titer between 8 and 32 is considered critical.

Minor red blood cell (RBC) antibodies, with the exception of Kell sensitization, are rarely present in pregnant women and usually remain at low titer (≤4).

If the critical titer is reached, the fetus should be evaluated for the presence of anemia.

## Assessment of Fetal Anemia

Over the years, various studies state that Doppler assessment of the fetal middle cerebral artery (MCA) peak systolic velocity is the best noninvasive tool for predicting fetal anemia in at-risk pregnancies [10].

## Middle Cerebral Artery

Doppler assessment of the fetal MCA peak systolic velocity (PSV) in alloimmunized pregnancies was based on the principle that the anemic fetus preserves oxygen delivery to the brain by increasing cerebral flow of low viscosity blood. However, under physiologic circumstances, it appears that the relationship between fetal hemoglobin and viscosity is the primary factor determining MCA-PSV [11].

Middle cerebral artery peak systolic velocity (MCA-PSV) is measured at 1- to 2-week intervals beginning as early as 18 weeks of gestation. MCA-PSV ≥1.5 multiples of the median is predictive of fetal anemia [12].

## Management

Severe fetal anemia can be defined as a hematocrit below 25 % or two standard deviations below the mean hematocrit for the gestational age. Severe fetal anemia is an indication for intervention because it may result in fetal cardiac failure and hydrops.

Intrauterine transfusions (IUTs) are generally done between 18 and 34 weeks. Leukodepleted, irradiated O-negative blood cros-matched to the mother's blood packed to a hematocrit of 75–85 % is used .

The volume of blood for IUT depends upon the initial fetal hematocrit, size of the fetus, the donor hematocrit, and the target hematocrit to be achieved. There are prescribed formulae and charts to calculate the volume for infusion. After 24 weeks of gestation, a target hematocrit of 40–50 % is preferable. The average neonatal survival rate is 80 % [13]. The loss rate from the procedure is approximately 1–3 % per procedure [14, 15].

The packed cells may be given intraperitoneally or by the intravascular route in the umbilical vein either in the cord or intrahepatically. In hydropic cases, the intravascular route is preferred.

The use of intraperitoneal route is on the decline after direct access to the fetal circulation was possible. IPT is effective in non-hydropic cases and is resorted only if vascular access is not available due to fetal position or there is a need to perform a transfusion prior to 20 weeks. The approximate volume of transfusion is calculated by the formula – (gestational age in weeks – 20 × 10).

Vascular access to the fetus can be achieved through the umbilical vein near the insertion into the placenta, in the free loop of the cord, or through the intrahepatic portal vein. The intrahepatic route is what we prefer and use for almost all our transfusions.

### Technique

Fetal paralysis may be achieved by an intramuscular injection of pancuronium in a dose of 0.1–0.3 mg per kg body weight of the fetus is given in the fetal deltoid or gluteal muscle. Intravenous injection of fentanyl (10 μg/kg × 1.25 for placental correction) has been shown to be effective in reducing fetal stress response.

The umbilical vein/portal vein is accessed using a 20 g long spinal needle. Adequate sample of blood is drawn for determining the hematocrit, hemoglobin, grouping and Rh typing, direct Coombs test, and karyotyping. The packed cells are transfused at a rate of 2–4 ml/min. The volume of blood to be transfused depends on the donor hematocrit, fetal hematocrit, and the feto-placental blood volume at this period of gestation [16] Nicolaides et al. [15]. Another guideline proposed by [17] Macgahan et al. [16] is: volume of packed cells = (desired Hct – actual Hct) × estimated fetoplacental blood volume × estimated fetal weight (Kg)/donor hematocrit.

The transfusion is given till a fetal Hct of 45–50 is achieved. Serial 2-week follow-up is performed to decide on the next transfusion which will be typically 2–3 weeks after the first transfusion. The rate of drop of fetal hematocrit will be around 0.8–1.1 per day. Combined with MCA Doppler, this can be used as a guide to time the next transfusion. If the fetus is doing well, there is no need to deliver the babies preterm.

A clear delivery plan with a good neonatal team that is informed well ahead of time is needed to be in place. These babies who have had intrauterine transfusion may need neonatal care including exchange/simple transfusions and management of hyperbilirubinemia.

Complications of intrauterine transfusion include preterm labor, premature rupture of membranes, fetal bradycardia (cord transfusion), and chorioamnionitis. Placental abruption has been reported but is a relatively rare occurrence. In expert hands, the rate of complications are relatively less and the benefits of the procedure far outweigh the risks.

Prior to 18 weeks of gestation, intraperitoneal fetal transfusion is technically easier than intravascular transfusion. When technically possible, the intravascular transfusion is preferred because the therapeutic effects are more rapid and reliable. After 35 weeks, the procedure is generally considered riskier than late preterm delivery for neonatal treatment of severe anemia.

Combined plasmapheresis and intravenous immune globulin therapy to decrease the severity of disease has only been described in case reports and small case series [7, 13–16, 18–20], and the efficacy of this approach is still not proven [17, 18, 21, 22].

## Kell-Sensitized Pregnancies

Management of pregnancies complicated by minor RBC antibodies should be the same as for women with Rh alloimmunization [7, 23]. The efficacy of this approach has been demonstrated in multiple series involving various minor RBC antibodies [19, 24].

## Parvovirus B19 Infection

Parvovirus B19 is a small non-enveloped DNA virus that frequently infects humans, with antibodies to B19 found in 30–60% of adults. The incidence of B19 infection during pregnancy is 3.3–3.8% [20, 21, 25, 26].

Most intrauterine parvovirus infections do not have an adverse outcome. Rarely, it can lead to fetal loss and hydrops fetalis.

### Pathogenesis and Clinical Features

B19 is cytotoxic to fetal red blood cell precursors and may cause anemia and hydrops fetalis and eventually fetal death [22, 23]. B19 can infect myocardial cells, and thus myocardial injury may contribute to the development of hydrops and fetal death in some cases [24, 25].

The risk of developing these complications appears to be greater in women infected during the first half of pregnancy [26, 27].

Maternal parvovirus infection has been associated with transient isolated fetal pleural or pericardial effusions that resolve spontaneously before term. These effusions are thought to result from direct pleural or myocardial inflammation.

Severe thrombocytopenia has been observed in parvovirus-infected fetuses with hydrops [27]. Hence, the platelet count should also be determined and platelets should be available for transfusion at the time of any fetal procedures.

## Investigations

Pregnant women who are suspected to have parvovirus infection should have serologic testing for IgG and IgM antibodies. A positive parvovirus IgM is consistent with acute infection. If both IgG and IgM are negative, PCR testing of maternal plasma for parvovirus B19 DNA may be more sensitive and should be performed [28].

Circulating IgM antibodies can be detected approximately 10 days after exposure and just prior to the onset of symptoms. They may persist for 3 months or longer [38].

Women diagnosed with acute infection should be monitored for serial ultrasounds to evaluate for fetal hydrops. Fetal anemia is diagnosed noninvasively by measuring the peak systolic velocity (PSV) of the middle cerebral artery (MCA) with Doppler ultrasound. A MCA-PSV value ≥1.5 multiples of the median (MoM) correlates strongly with severe fetal anemia.

When severe anemia is suspected on ultrasound findings, the fetus requires close monitoring, and intrauterine transfusion of RBCs is indicated to prevent fetal death from severe anemia.

Polymerase chain reaction (PCR) testing on amniotic fluid is the method of choice to make the fetal diagnosis.

## Management

Intrauterine transfusion of RBCs is indicated to prevent fetal death from severe anemia. Fetal transfusion for hydrops improved the survival rate (82 % vs. 55 % without transfusion) [24, 29, 30].

Immunoglobulin: given the limited available data, the use of IVIG during pregnancy currently is not recommended [31].

Management of the birth of a hydropic infant should be undertaken at a tertiary care center. Drainage of fetal ascites or pleural effusions may be necessary to facilitate resuscitation. Postnatally, these hydropic infants generally require mechanical ventilation.

## Fetomaternal Hemorrhage

Bidirectional passage of minute numbers of cells across the placenta is a physiological event [32, 33]. Small amount (<0.1 ml) of fetal blood is commonly found in maternal circulation. Fetomaternal hemorrhage refers to significant passage of fetal blood into maternal circulation prior to or during delivery. It can be acute or chronic. Absolute thresholds of 10–150 mL have been proposed [34–36]. Massive fetomaternal hemorrhage is suggested as >20 ml of fetal blood volume 960 or >150 ml fetal blood [7]. Massive FMH may occur spontaneously or result from trauma.

### Clinical Features

The mother is usually asymptomatic, but may have symptoms suggestive of a transfusion reaction (e.g., fever, chills, nausea) [37].

Fetal findings associated with massive FMH include absent or persistently decreased movement (most common finding), heart rate abnormality (e.g., sinusoidal fetal heart rate pattern), low biophysical profile score, hydrops fetalis, or fetal death [38, 39].

A heightened index of suspicion is warranted in cases of persistent maternal perception of decreased fetal movements. Evaluation for FMH should be part of the diagnostic evaluation of unexplained fetal anemia.

Fetal anemia is diagnosed noninvasively by measuring the peak systolic velocity (PSV) of the middle cerebral artery (MCA) with Doppler ultrasound. A MCA-PSV value ≥1.5 multiples of the median (MoM) correlates strongly with severe fetal anemia [40].

## Diagnosis

Two maternal assays are available for detecting FMH: the Kleihauer-Betke test and flow cytometry. Both these tests are based on identification of hemoglobin F, the fetal hemoglobin. The volume of fetal blood loss should be calculated as a percentage of the estimated fetoplacental blood volume. Both assays measure the volume of fetal blood in the maternal circulation at a point in time and thus do not necessarily indicate the volume of blood loss over time, if bleeding was chronic or occurred on multiple occasions.

However, adult red blood cells may also contain hemoglobin F (known as F cells). These cells can cause the assay to overestimate the volume of fetomaternal hemorrhage in maternal blood. This is especially important in some hematological disorders, such as sickle cell disease, which can be associated with persistence of hemoglobin F in a large number of cells.

## Kleihauer-Betke Test

This is the main diagnostic test for detection and quantitation of FMH [41]. Red blood cells from the maternal circulation are fixed to a slide that is exposed to an acidic pH solution. Adult red blood cells become "ghost" cells since hemoglobin A is soluble and eluted across membrane defects at a low pH. Fetal red blood cells remain pink because hemoglobin F is stable at pHs in this range.

The volume of fetal whole blood (mL) in the maternal circulation is (% fetal cells) × (maternal hematocrit [%] divided by fetal hematocrit [%]) × (maternal blood volume mL).

In the usual clinical scenario, the maternal blood volume and the fetal hematocrit are not known, and most laboratories do not request the maternal hematocrit for the calculation. The maternal blood volume is often assumed to be 5000 mL, yielding the following formula to calculate the volume of fetal whole blood (mL) in the maternal circulation: (% fetal cells) × 5000 mL. Thus, if the Kleihauer-Betke result is 0.1%, the FMH calculation is (0.001 × 5000) = 5 mL of fetal whole blood.

Flow cytometry: flow cytometry is another assay for detecting and quantitating FMH [42]. A monoclonal antibody to hemoglobin F is conjugated to a fluorochrome and used to detect fetal hemoglobin in permeabilized cells as they pass through the channel of a flow cytometer.

Comparative analysis of flow cytometry and the Kleihauer-Betke test has shown that flow cytometry is more accurate, more reproducible, and less labor intensive [43].

Limitation is the inability to measure the maternal blood volume and interference with persistence of fetal hemoglobin in adult red blood cells (F cells).

Dual-parameter flow cytometry can alleviate the issue with maternal F cells noted in such disease states as hemoglobinopathies and thalassemias.

## Management

Intravascular intrauterine transfusion (IVT) of donor red blood cells can correct fetal anemia. The aim is to prolong the pregnancy to reduce the morbidity and mortality associated with preterm birth. Antenatal corticosteroid therapy is given to enhance fetal lung maturity.

For pregnancies ≥32 weeks of gestation with severe fetal anemia by Doppler, the patient may be delivered after intrauterine transfusion.

Diagnosis of ongoing FMH is challenging after transfusion because the transfused cells contain adult hemoglobin and thus are not detected by Kleihauer-Betke or flow cytometry tests. Continuous monitoring MCA-PSV Doppler ultrasound and fetal heart rate (FHR) monitoring are necessary.

Chronic FMH should be suspected if the percentage of fetal cells in the maternal circulation increases (Kleihauer-Betke testing or flow cytometry) or MCA-PSV increases. Repeated intrauterine transfusions are unlikely to be successful in these cases due to the ongoing FMH [44]. Premature delivery is probably a better option.

Small FMHs with only mild fetal anemia can be followed expectantly with fetal monitoring.

Prognosis: Perinatal prognosis depends upon the volume of the hemorrhage. Some series report neurologic injury in 0–35 % of surviving infants [34, 38], whereas some report no long-term neurologic sequelae related to fetomaternal hemorrhage [45].

## References


1. Nicolaides KH, Soothill PW, Clewell WH, et al. Fetal haemoglobin measurement in the assessment of red cell isoimmunisation. Lancet. 1988;1:1073.
2. Forestier F, Daffos F, Catherine N, et al. Developmental hematopoiesis in normal human fetal blood. Blood. 1991;77:2360.
3. Vaughan JI, Warwick R, Letsky E, et al. Erythropoietic suppression in fetal anemia because of Kell alloimmunization. Am J Obstet Gynecol. 1994;171:247.
4. Weiner CP, Widness JA. Decreased fetal erythropoiesis and hemolysis in Kell hemolytic anemia. Am J Obstet Gynecol. 1996;174:547.
5. Vaughan JI, Manning M, Warwick RM, et al. Inhibition of erythroid progenitor cells by anti-Kell antibodies in fetal alloimmune anemia. N Engl J Med. 1998;338:798.
6. van den Akker ES, de Haan TR, Lopriore E, et al. Severe fetal thrombocytopenia in Rhesus D alloimmunized pregnancies. Am J Obstet Gynecol. 2008;199:387.e1.
7. American College of Obstetricians and Gynecologists. ACOG Practice Bulletin No. 75: Management of alloimmunization during pregnancy. Obstet Gynecol. 2006;108:457.
8. Rodis JF, Quinn DL, Gary Jr GW, et al. Management and outcomes of pregnancies complicated by human B19 parvovirus infection: a prospective study. Am J Obstet Gynecol. 1990;163:1168.
9. Gratacós E, Torres PJ, Vidal J, et al. The incidence of human parvovirus B19 infection during pregnancy and its impact on perinatal outcome. J Infect Dis. 1995;171:1360.
10. Pretlove SJ, Fox CE, Khan KS, Kilby MD. Noninvasive methods of detecting fetal anaemia: a systematic review and meta-analysis. BJOG. 2009;116:1558.
11. Picklesimer AH, Oepkes D, Moise Jr KJ, et al. Determinants of the middle cerebral artery peak systolic velocity in the human fetus. Am J Obstet Gynecol. 2007;197:526.e1.
12. Mari G, Deter RL, Carpenter RL, et al. Noninvasive diagnosis by Doppler ultrasonography of fetal anemia due to maternal red-cell alloimmunization. Collaborative Group for Doppler Assessment of the Blood Velocity in Anemic Fetuses. N Engl J Med. 2000;342:9.
13. Fox C, Martin W, Somerset DA, et al. Early intraperitoneal transfusion and adjuvant maternal immunoglobulin therapy in the treatment of severe red cell alloimmunization prior to fetal intravascular transfusion. Fetal Diagn Ther. 2008;23:159.
14. Ruma MS, Moise Jr KJ, Kim E, et al. Combined plasmapheresis and intravenous immune globulin for the treatment of severe maternal red cell alloimmunization. Am J Obstet Gynecol. 2007;196:138.e1.
15. Isojima S, Hisano M, Suzuki T, et al. Early plasmapheresis followed by high-dose γ-globulin treatment saved a severely Rho-incompatible pregnancy. J Clin Apher. 2011;26:216.
16. Palfi M, Hildén JO, Matthiesen L, et al. A case of severe Rh (D) alloimmunization treated by intensive plasma exchange and high-dose intravenous immunoglobulin. Transfus Apher Sci. 2006;35:131.
17. Wong KS, Connan K, Rowlands S, et al. Antenatal immunoglobulin for fetal red blood cell alloimmunization. Cochrane Database Syst Rev. 2013;5: CD008267.
18. Schwartz J, Winters JL, Padmanabhan A, et al. Guidelines on the use of therapeutic apheresis in clinical practice-evidence-based approach from the Writing Committee of the American Society for Apheresis: the sixth special issue. J Clin Apher. 2013; 28:145.
19. Hughes LH, Rossi KQ, Krugh DW, O'Shaughnessy RW. Management of pregnancies complicated by anti-Fy(a) alloimmunization. Transfusion. 2007;47:1858.
20. Parilla BV, Tamura RK, Ginsberg NA. Association of parvovirus infection with isolated fetal effusions. Am J Perinatol. 1997;14:357.
21. Anand A, Gray ES, Brown T, et al. Human parvovirus infection in pregnancy and hydrops fetalis. N Engl J Med. 1987;316:183.
22. Enders M, Klingel K, Weidner A, et al. Risk of fetal hydrops and non-hydropic late intrauterine fetal death after gestational parvovirus B19 infection. J Clin Virol. 2010;49:163.
23. Puccetti C, Contoli M, Bonvicini F, et al. Parvovirus B19 in pregnancy: possible consequences of vertical transmission. Prenat Diagn. 2012;32:897.
24. De Jong EP, Lindenburg IT, van Klink JM, et al. Intrauterine transfusion for parvovirus B19 infection: long-term neurodevelopmental outcome. Am J Obstet Gynecol. 2012;206:204.e1.
25. Rotbart HA. Human parvovirus infections. Annu Rev Med. 1990;41:25.
26. Marton T, Martin WL, Whittle MJ. Hydrops fetalis and neonatal death from human parvovirus B19: an unusual complication. Prenat Diagn. 2005;25:543.
27. de Haan TR, van den Akker ES, Porcelijn L, et al. Thrombocytopenia in hydropic fetuses with parvovirus B19 infection: incidence, treatment and correlation with fetal B19 viral load. BJOG. 2008;115:76.
28. Török TJ, Wang QY, Gary Jr GW, et al. Prenatal diagnosis of intrauterine infection with parvovirus B19 by the polymerase chain reaction technique. Clin Infect Dis. 1992;14:149.
29. Rodis JF, Borgida AF, Wilson M, et al. Management of parvovirus infection in pregnancy and outcomes of hydrops: a survey of members of the Society of Perinatal Obstetricians. Am J Obstet Gynecol. 1998;179:985.
30. von Kaisenberg CS, Jonat W. Fetal parvovirus B19 infection. Ultrasound Obstet Gynecol. 2001;18:280.
31. Selbing A, Josefsson A, Dahle LO, Lindgren R. Parvovirus B19 infection during pregnancy treated

with high-dose intravenous gammaglobulin. Lancet. 1995;345:660.
32. Bianchi DW, Romero R. Biological implications of bi-directional fetomaternal cell traffic: a summary of a National Institute of Child Health and Human Development-sponsored conference. J Matern Fetal Neonatal Med. 2003;14:123.
33. Lo YM, Lau TK, Chan LY, et al. Quantitative analysis of the bidirectional fetomaternal transfer of nucleated cells and plasma DNA. Clin Chem. 2000;46:1301.
34. de Almeida V, Bowman JM. Massive fetomaternal hemorrhage: Manitoba experience. Obstet Gynecol. 1994;83:323.
35. Leduc L, Moise Jr KJ, Carpenter Jr RJ, Cano LE. Fetoplacental blood volume estimation in pregnancies with Rh alloimmunization. Fetal Diagn Ther. 1990;5:138.
36. Nicolaides KH, Clewell WH, Rodeck CH. Measurement of human fetoplacental blood volume in erythroblastosis fetalis. Am J Obstet Gynecol. 1987;157:50.
37. Murphy KW, Venkatraman N, Stevens J. Limitations of ultrasound in the diagnosis of fetomaternal haemorrhage. BJOG. 2000;107:1317.
38. Christensen RD, Lambert DK, Baer VL, et al. Severe neonatal anemia from fetomaternal hemorrhage: report from a multihospital health-care system. J Perinatol. 2013;33:429.
39. Giacoia GP. Severe fetomaternal hemorrhage: a review. Obstet Gynecol Surv. 1997;52:372.
40. Sueters M, Arabin B, Oepkes D. Doppler sonography for predicting fetal anemia caused by massive fetomaternal hemorrhage. Ultrasound Obstet Gynecol. 2003; 22:186.
41. Kleihauer E, Braun H, Betke K. Demonstration of fetal hemoglobin in erythrocytes of a blood smear. Klin Wochenschr. 1957;35:637.
42. Dziegiel MH, Nielsen LK, Berkowicz A. Detecting fetomaternal hemorrhage by flow cytometry. Curr Opin Hematol. 2006;13:490.
43. Bromilow IM, Duguid JK. Measurement of fetomaternal haemorrhage: a comparative study of three Kleihauer techniques and tow flow cytometry methods. Clin Lab Haematol. 1997;19:137.
44. Sifakis S, Koukoura O, Konstantinidou AE, et al. Sonographic findings in severe fetomaternal transfusion. Arch Gynecol Obstet. 2010;281:241.
45. Rubod C, Deruelle P, Le Goueff F, et al. Long-term prognosis for infants after massive fetomaternal hemorrhage. Obstet Gynecol. 2007;110:256.

# Neonatal Resuscitation "When Baby Does Not Cry"

39

Shruti Sudhir Jadhav, Sushma Malik, and Reena Jatin Wani

## Introduction

The successful transition from fetal to neonatal life is the most complex physiological process, yet in majority (90 %) of the births, babies go through this transition without difficulty. However, certain maternal, placental, mechanical, and fetal factors can jeopardize this smooth transition and signal the need for intervention. A prompt and skilled resuscitation may prevent deaths and avert lifelong adverse sequelae in such babies that had difficulty in breathing or have a weak cry.

WHO has estimated that as many as 10 % of all newborn infants need some intervention at birth and approximately only 1 % need more extensive intervention. The International Liaison Committee on Resuscitation (ILCOR), the American Heart Association (AHA), and the American Academy of Pediatrics (AAP) have established their NRP (Neonatal Resuscitation Program) guidelines of 2010 for newborn resuscitation [1]. These were being followed till 6 months ago till the recent 2015 guidelines based on new scientifically based evidence were released with some changes [2]. This write-up is based on the IAP (Indian Academy of Pediatrics) NRP First Golden Minute (FGM) guidelines and aims to provide with basic steps used for stabilization and resuscitation of the newborn who does not cry [3, 4].

## Overview and Principles of Resuscitation

Birth asphyxia is one of the most important leading causes of neonatal mortality and accounts for about 23 % of the approximately four million neonatal deaths that occur each year worldwide. The outcomes of thousands of these newborns per year can be improved if we use correct and prompt resuscitation techniques [1].

## Fetal Physiology and Normal Transition

In utero, fetus obtains oxygen and nutrients from maternal blood through the placenta. Fetal lungs do not perform gas exchange and are filled with fluids and pulmonary vessels are markedly

S.S. Jadhav, MD (Ped) (✉) • S. Malik, MD (Ped)
Neonatology Division, Department of Pediatrics, T.N. Medical College & BYL Nair Hospital, Mumbai, India
e-mail: mailme_shrutus@rediffmail.com

R.J. Wani, MD (Obs & Gynae)
Department of Obstetrics & Gynaecology, HBT Medical College & Dr R N Cooper Municipal Hospital, Mumbai, India

T.N. Medical College & BYL Nair Hospital, Mumbai, India


A. Gandhi et al. (eds.), *Principles of Critical Care in Obstetrics: Volume II*,
DOI 10.1007/978-81-322-2686-4_39

constricted. Because of which the blood from fetal heart bypasses the lungs and flows to the aorta through the ductus arteriosus. After birth, the baby cries and takes first breath to inhale air into the lungs [1, 4, 5]. Three major changes start as soon as the baby is born.

1. Alveolar fluid clearance: Alveolar fluid *is absorbed and replaced by air.*
2. Increased SVR (systemic vascular resistance): The *umbilical arteries constrict*, and clamping of the umbilical cord results in closure of umbilical arteries and umbilical vein.
3. *Decreased PVR* (pulmonary vascular resistance): Pulmonary vasodilatation in response to increased oxygen level in the lungs.

## In Utero or Perinatal Compromise

Perinatal insult results in an initial period of rapid breathing followed by *primary apnea* (cessation of breathing or gasping). Primary apnea responds to simple measures like drying the baby, flicking the soles, or rubbing the back. During this period of primary apnea if perinatal stress continues, newborn develops gasping respirations followed by *secondary apnea*. Positive pressure ventilation must be provided to reverse the secondary apnea. At birth, it is difficult to differentiate between primary and secondary apnea and therefore every apneic baby is assumed to be in secondary apnea [4].

## Newborn Resuscitation

Anticipation, adequate preparation, accurate evaluation, and prompt initiation of support are critical for successful neonatal resuscitation.

### Anticipation for Need for Resuscitation

The presence of risk factors (Table 39.1) can help identify those who will need resuscitation, but one must always be prepared to resuscitate, as even some of those babies with no risk factors will require resuscitation [1, 3–5].

### Preparation for Resuscitation

**Personnel**

At every delivery, one must ensure that at least one trained NRP personnel is present and his/her primary responsibility is the newly born. For anticipated high-risk deliveries or for those with expected problems, at least two trained people are required. For multiple births, separate team is required for each baby [1, 3, 4].

**Table 39.1** Antepartum and intrapartum risk factors

| Antepartum factors | Postpartum factors |
|---|---|
| Maternal diabetes/gestational diabetes | Premature labor/precipitous labor |
| Chronic medical illness – cardiac, renal, pulmonary, neurologic disease | Emergency caesarean section |
| Gestational hypertension/pre-eclampsia/chronic hypertension | Assisted delivery – forceps/vacuum |
| Age< 16 years or >35 years | Breech or abnormal presentation |
| Primigravida or grand multipara | Macrosomia |
| Maternal infections/TORCH/sexually transmitted diseases/ chorioamnionitis | Abruptio placenta/cord prolapsed/ placenta previa |
| Oligohydraminos/polyhydraminos | Prolonged labor/obstructed labor |
| Bleeding in second or third trimester | Meconium-stained amniotic fluid |
| Previous fetal or neonatal deaths/fetal malformations/diminished fetal activity | Narcotics given to mother within 4 h of delivery |
| Multiple gestations | Use of general anesthesia |
| Fetal anemia/isoimmunization | Altered fetal heart rate changes |
| Premature or prolonged rupture of membranes | Significant intra partum bleeding |

**Equipment**
All the equipment necessary for a complete resuscitation should be regularly checked to ensure that they are available in various sizes and are functional. The equipments needed included in the Table 39.2 below.

## The Resuscitation Flow Diagram (Fig. 39.1)

The above flow diagram describes the steps necessary to determine the need for resuscitation and all the NRP resuscitation procedures [3].

**Initial Assessment**
At the time of birth, as per the IAP -NRP FGM (first golden minute) guidelines one should ask only one question, i.e., *breathing or crying* and then proceed after that as per the response as yes or no.

If the newborn baby is breathing well or crying, then the baby does not need resuscitation and should be kept with the mother and sent for routine care.

**Table 39.2** Equipment required for resuscitation

| |
|---|
| Radiant warmer or other heat source |
| Resuscitation trolley with firm surface |
| Warm blankets/pre-warmed linen or towels, shoulder roll |
| Stethoscope with neonatal head |
| Oxygen source, compressed air source |
| Oxygen blender (for mixing air and oxygen with flow meter) |
| Suction source, suction catheter (5, 6, 8, 10, 12 F) |
| Delee's mucus extractor and meconium aspirator |
| Pulse oximeter and oximeter probe |
| Nasogastric tubes (8 F) |
| Ambu or self-inflating bag, flow inflating bag, T-piece resuscitator |
| Face masks (newborn and premature sizes, cushioned rim masks) |
| Laryngoscopes (handles no. 00,0 and 1 blade; batteries), stylet |
| Endotracheal tubes (2.5, 3, 3.5, 4 mm) |
| Epinephrine (1:10,000 solution) 3 ml or 10 ml ampoules |
| Volume expanders (normal saline, Ringer's lactate, 5 % albumin, O-negative whole blood (cross matched against mother's blood)) |
| Clock (Apgar timer) |
| Syringes, hypodermic needles, and tubes for collection of blood samples |
| Equipment for umbilical cord catheterization |

**Routine Care Involves**

- Provide warmth (skin-to-skin care)
- Cut cord in 1–3 min
- Initiate breastfeeding
- Assess neonate/ongoing evaluation

If any answer is "No" to the question on breathing or crying, then one should continue with initial steps of resuscitation.

## Block A (Airway)

These are initial steps to establish an airway and begin resuscitating newborn. Approximately 60 s ("The Golden Minute") are allotted for completing the initial steps, reevaluating, and beginning ventilation if required (Fig. 39.1) [3].

**Initial Steps of Resuscitation**

1. *Keep baby warm* by wrapping him with towel and placing him on mother's abdomen/chest for skin-to-skin contact with the mother. If the baby has not cried, then place the baby under radiant heat warmer on a resuscitation table.
2. *Open the airway* by slightly extending the neck, thus creating the "sniffing" position.
3. *Clear airway as necessary.* Secretions can be cleared by wiping the nose and mouth with towel or by suctioning with a bulb syringe or suction catheter. Always suction "mouth before nose" by thinking "M" before "N" in the alphabet to prevent aspiration of mouth content. Clearing the airway involves endotracheal suctioning to clear meconium for non-vigorous newborn with meconium-stained fluid [1].

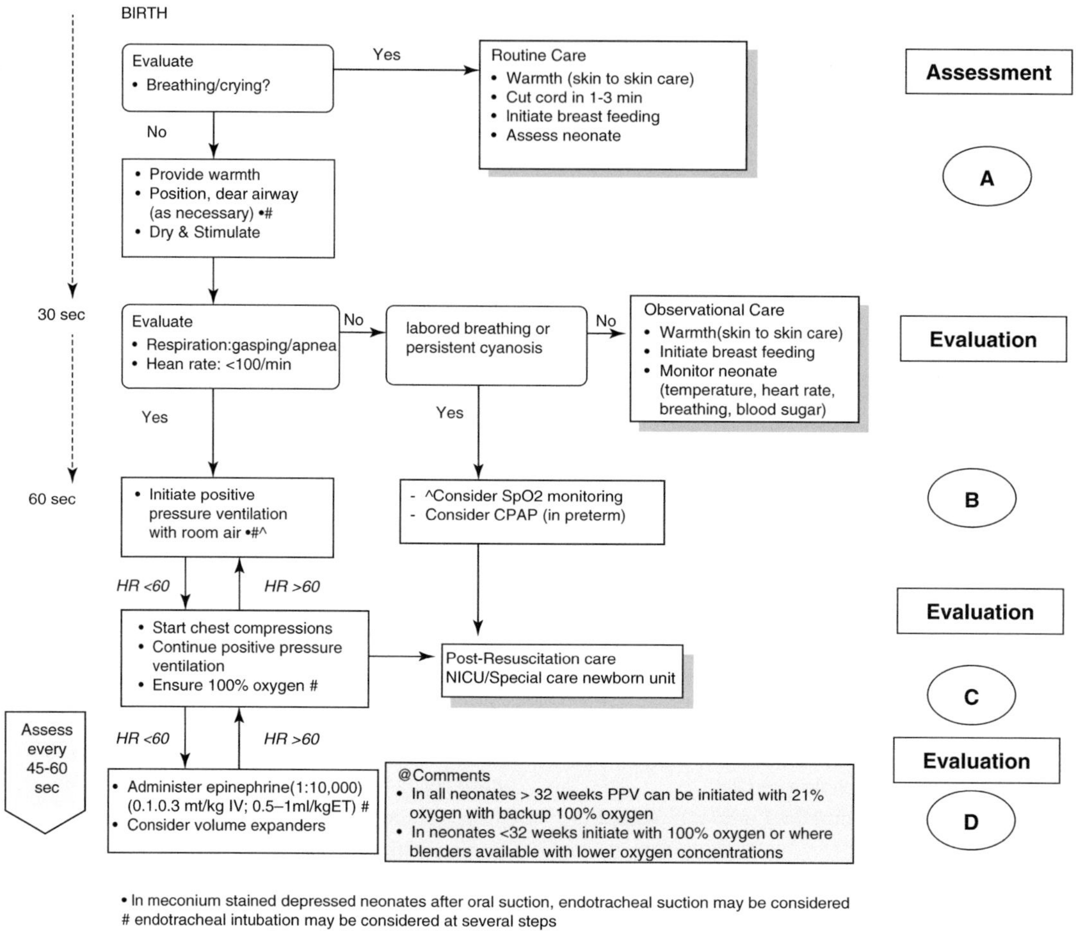


**Fig. 39.1** IAP NRP FGM algorithm for neonatal resuscitation [3]

4. *Dry and stimulate to breath.* To minimize heat loss, the baby should be received in pre-warmed towel. The same can be used to dry him and this should be removed and another fresh pre-warmed towel should be used for continued drying and stimulation. Tactile stimulation can be provided by slapping or flicking soles of the feet or by gentle rubbing the newborn's back, trunk, or extremities.

### Assessment of the Effect of Block A

The next step is to evaluate to determine if further resuscitation actions are indicated. The entire resuscitation process up to this point of initial steps should take no more than 30 s (unless suctioning of meconium from the trachea was required). Evaluate simultaneously for respirations (apnea, gasping, or labored breathing) and heart rate (whether heart rate is greater than or less than 100 bpm [beats per minute]).

*Respirations* – Observe baby for good respiratory efforts. Rate and depth of respiration should increase after a few seconds of tactile stimulation.

*Heart rate* – The heart rate should be more than 100 bpm. The simplest method to determine heart rate is to feel for a pulse at the base of umbilical cord. If you cannot feel a pulse, use stethoscope to auscultate. Counting the number of beats in 6 s and multiplying by 10 provide a quick estimate of the beats per minute.

## Block B (Breathing)

If the baby is apneic, or has gasping respirations, or if the heart rate is below 100 bpm, you should proceed immediately to providing PPV with room air. However, if the baby is breathing and the heart rate is above 100, but the respirations *appear labored or the baby appears persistently cyanotic* administer *continuous positive pressure (CPAP)* with mask. Consider $SpO_2$ monitoring and one should attach an oximeter to determine the need for supplemental oxygen, and it is recommended that the probe be placed on newborns right hand or wrist so as to detect pre-ductal saturation.

### Positive Pressure Ventilation (PPV)

Three devices are available to ventilate newborns to give PPV are self-inflating bag, flow-inflating bag, and T-piece resuscitator [1, 3].

### Concentration of Oxygen During Resuscitation [1]

Meta-analyses showed a decrease in mortality and CNS effects in room air-resuscitated group of neonates. Therefore, it is recommended that:

- In term as well as preterm newborns, resuscitation can be initiated with room air.
- Titrate $O_2$ to achieve $SpO_2$ in target range as described using pulse oximetry for uncompromised babies (the targeted pre-ductal $SpO_2$ at 1 min is 60–65 %, 2 min – 65–70 %, 3 min – 70–75 %, 4 min – 75–80 %, 5 min – 80–85 %, and at 10 min it is 85–95 %).
- Use oxygen blender, if available, to deliver an oxygen concentration between 21 and 100 %.
- If bradycardia (HR <60) after 90 s of resuscitation with lower concentration of $O_2$, increase concentration to 100 % until recovery of normal heart rate is achieved.

### Resuscitation Rate during PPV

Count out loud to help maintain a rate of 40–60 breaths per minute. Say "Breathe" as you squeeze the bag or occlude the PEEP cap of the T-piece resuscitator and release while one says "Two, Three". So the *cadence* is –

Breathe................Two................ Three.............Breathe............Two.......... Three (squeeze) -------------- (release.............) ---------- (squeeze) --------- (release................)

Effective ventilation is defined by the presence of good bilateral breath sounds and chest movement. The most important indicator of successful PPV is the rising heart rate (along with rising saturation if pulse oximetry is functional at this point). If the baby's heart rate and oxygen saturation are not rising and you do not hear bilateral breath sounds or see chest movements, initiate ventilation corrective steps (Table 39.3). One can use the acronym "MR SOPA" to remember the ventilation corrective steps [1, 3].

Signs that PPV has been effective, and indications that PPV may be discontinued, are (a) heart rate rises to over 100 breaths per minute, (b) improvement in oxygen saturation, and (c) onset of spontaneous respirations.

CPAP or supplemental oxygen indications:

- Working hard to breath
- Grunting respiration
- Retractions
- Central cyanosis
- Hypoxemia by oximetry

CPAP can be delivered with a flow-inflating bag or a T-piece resuscitator, but NOT with a self-inflating bag.

**Table 39.3** Ventilation corrective steps

| | | |
|---|---|---|
| M | Mask adjustment – inadequate seal | Mask adjusted to ensure air tight seal |
| R | Reposition airway – inappropriate position | Reposition head to be in "sniffing" position |
| S | Suction mouth and nose – blocked airway | Suction the airway for secretions if present |
| O | Open mouth | Open baby's mouth and lift the jaw forward |
| P | Pressure increase – inadequate pressure | Increase the pressure gradually to achieve the chest rise |
| A | Airway alternative to be considered | Do endotracheal intubation or use laryngeal mask airway |

### Endotracheal Intubation: Indications

- Prolonged PPV required
- Bag and mask ineffective
- If chest compressions required for better coordination
- Tracheal suction required, e.g., MSAF (meconium-stained amniotic fluid)
- Diaphragmatic hernia
- Use of drugs through ET tube

### Evaluation of the Effect of Block B

In almost all cases, with appropriate ventilation technique, heart rate rises above 100 bpm. However, if the heart rate is below 60 bpm, then proceed to block C

## Block C (Circulation)

Circulation is supported by chest compressions. Chest compressions are indicated whenever heart rate is below 60 bpm, despite at least 30 s of effective positive pressure ventilation (PPV). Ensure 100 % oxygen is being given and also endotracheal intubation should be considered at this stage.

### Chest Compressions

- Compress the heart against the spine
- Increase the intrathoracic pressure
- Circulate blood to the vital organs

*Two techniques that are normally used include:*

- *Thumb technique*: In this method both the hands encircle the torso, with thumbs on sternum and fingers supporting back. Thumbs should be flexed at the first joint. Thumb technique is preferred because there is better depth control, provides more consistent pressure, superior in generating peak systolic and coronary arterial perfusion pressure, and is less tiring.
- *2-finger technique*: Tips of the middle finger and either the index finger or ring finger of one hand should be used to compress the sternum, while the other hand is used to support the baby's back.

*Location, depth, and rate of compressions:*

- Compress to depth of one-third AP diameter of chest.
- Compress the lower one-third of the sternum.
- 3:1 compressions to ventilation ratio (90 CC to 30 ventilations, total 120 events in one minute) and the *cadence* is "*One – and – two – and – three – and – breathe – and*"." Do not compress during "Breathe and."

*During chest compressions* ensure that:

- Chest movement is adequate during ventilation.
- Supplemental oxygen is being used.
- Thumbs or fingers remain in contact with the chest at all times.
- Chest compressions and ventilation are well coordinated.

*Adequacy of chest compression*

- Palpate femoral/cord pulsations
- Check HR >30 s of CC

- HR >60 bpm, discontinue CC, continue PPV
- HR <60 bpm, intubate, if not already done for better coordination

Evaluation of the effect of block C – If the heart rate is still below 60, then proceed to block D.

## Block D (Drugs)

One should administer epinephrine as you continue PPV and chest compressions.

- Epinephrine (1:10,000) should be administered intravenously at 0.01–0.03 ml/kg/dose as rapidly as possible.
- While access is being obtained, a higher dose of endotracheal epinephrine may be given but efficacy of this practice has not been evaluated.
- Ineffective response to epinephrine, then one should consider possibility of hypovolemia.

**Evaluation of the Effect of Block D**

If the HR remains below 60 bpm, the actions in block C and block D are continued and repeated. When the HR improves and rises above the 60 bpm, chest compressions are stopped. PPV is continued until the HR is above 100 bpm and baby is breathing. Supplemental oxygen/CPAP can be administered if necessary, based on oxygen saturations measured by pulse oximetry. Care should be taken to avoid allowing the $SpO_2$ to exceed 95 % [1, 3, 5].

## Management in the Presence of Meconium-Stained Amniotic Fluid

### Scenario 1: Meconium Present and Newborn Is Vigorous

If respiratory efforts are strong and muscle tone is good and HR >100 bpm, then use only bulb syringe or large bore catheter to suction the mouth and nose (Fig. 39.2) [3].

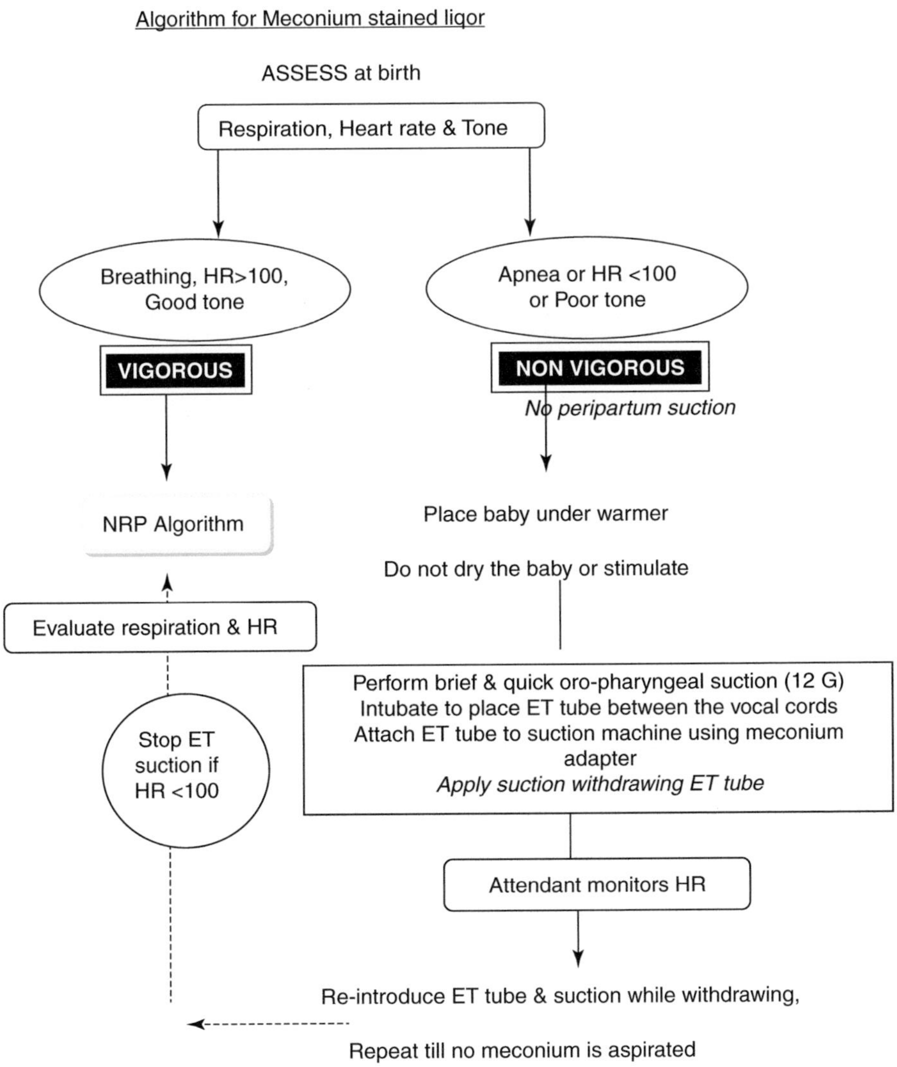


**Fig. 39.2** Algorithm for meconium-stained liquor [3]

## Scenario 2: Meconium Present and Newborn Is not Vigorous

In such a scenario, one needs to do tracheal suction after a brief oropharyngeal suction.

- Administer oxygen and monitor HR.
- Insert laryngoscope and use a 12 or 14 F catheter to clear the mouth and posterior pharynx so that one can visualize the vocal cords.
- Insert endotracheal tube into trachea and then attach it to suction source.
- Apply suction as tube is withdrawn.
- Attendant monitors the heart rate.
- Repeat as necessary until little additional meconium is recovered or until the baby's heart rate indicates further need of resuscitation.

## Post-resuscitation Care

Two levels of post-resuscitation care are routine care and post-resuscitation care [3, 6].

### Observational Care

Observational care is given to babies who required PPV for less than 1 min and it includes providing warmth, initiating breastfeeding, and monitoring newborn for temperature, heart rate, breathing, and color (every 30 s for 2 h).

### Post-resuscitation Care

This is provided to babies who received PPV for more than 1 min or more extensive resuscitation like intubation, chest compression, and are at high risk for deterioration. These neonates are managed in the NICU.

All neonates who required resuscitation must be closely and frequently monitored for potential complications (Table 39.4) [1, 6].

**Table 39.4** Possible complications following resuscitation

| Organ system | Potential complications |
|---|---|
| Brain | Apnea, seizures |
| Lungs | Pulmonary hypertension, pneumonia, pneumothorax, meconium aspiration syndrome |
| Cardiovascular | Hypotension, shock |
| Kidneys | Acute tubular necrosis |
| Gastrointestinal | Necrotizing enterocolitis |
| Metabolic | Hypocalcemia, hypoglycemia |

## Initial Stabilization and Management

Early detection and prompt management of complications prevent further extension of cerebral injury [1, 6].

**Temperature** The temperature should be maintained between 36.5 and 37.5 °C to avoid hypothermia as well as hyperthermia since both are detrimental.

**Airway and Breathing** Patent airway should be maintained with proper positioning and cleaning the secretions. Breathing should be monitored and supported as required.

**Oxygenation** $SpO_2$ should be maintained between 90 and 94 %. Hypoxia and hyperoxia should be avoided.

**IV Fluids and Enteral Feeding** Initiate IV fluids as per day's requirement. Start on enteral feed once the patient is hemodynamically stable and passed meconium and there is no abdominal distention. Start expressed breast milk 30 ml/kg/day and increase daily by 20–30 ml/kg/day or more as the baby tolerates.

**Blood Glucose** Blood glucose should be monitored for at least 48 h. Treat hypoglycemia appropriately with intravenous glucose.

**Blood Pressure** Maintain systemic mean arterial BP at 40 mmHg for term neonate and for preterm neonate; mean BP should be maintained equal to gestational age in weeks as mmHg.

**Seizures** First treat metabolic cause and then consider anticonvulsant therapy.

## Therapeutic Hypothermia

This modality should be tried in neonates more than 36 weeks of gestation with evolving moderate to severe hypoxemic-ischemic encephalopathy and where the expertise and facility for providing therapeutic hypothermia is present. It should be used only strictly following the protocols laid down [1, 3].

## Timing of Cord Clamping

Delayed cord clamping (DCC) for 1 min or more is safe both in preterm and term babies who did not require any resuscitation at birth. However, delayed cord clamping is not recommended in neonates requiring resuscitation. DCC is associated with lesser incidence of intraventricular hemorrhage, higher blood pressure and blood volume, lesser need for blood transfusion, and lesser chance of developing necrotizing enterocolitis. The only disadvantage of DCC being increased chance of developing jaundice and the need for phototherapy.

## Withholding and Discontinuation of Resuscitation

The decision of when to withhold or not to resuscitate is difficult and complex. It will be determined taking into consideration the local neonatal data and ethical issues and a team of the obstetricians, neonatologist, healthcare personnel, and family members should discuss and come to the possible best decision [1, 3].

**Major Criteria to Withhold Resuscitation**

- Anencephaly
- Confirmed gestational age <23 weeks
- Birth weight <400 g
- Confirmed lethal genetic disorder or malformation

**Discontinuation of Resuscitation**

Discontinuation of resuscitation efforts is considered when there is no detectable heart rate after 10 min of complete and adequate resuscitation.

## 2015 American Heart Association Guidelines for Cardiopulmonary Resuscitation

Some of the salient features of the new changes made by AHA 2015 guidelines [2] include:

1. Three assessment questions should be asked at birth in following order:
   Term gestation?
   Good tone?
   Breathing or crying?
2. Delayed cord clamping for >30 s is recommended for non-asphyxiated preterm as well as term babies.
3. New guidelines have reemphasized the need of temperature regulation during neonatal resuscitation. Temperature for non-asphyxiated infants should be maintained between 36.5 and 37.5 °C.
4. Tracheal suction is no longer recommended for non-vigorous baby who is born through meconium-stained amniotic fluid. Appropriate interventions to support ventilation and oxygenation should be instituted at the earliest [2].
5. Use of 3 lead ECG is recommended for assessment of heart rate during resuscitation. The reason for using ECG is because auscultation may not assess heart rate accurately and the

pulse oximeter may underestimate the heart rate.

6. For preterm babies <35 weeks, resuscitation has to be started with low $FiO_2$ concentration, i.e., 21–30 %. $FiO_2$ should be gradually increased to achieve targeted pre-ductal saturations.

**Carry Home Messages**

1. *Always be prepared* to resuscitate.
2. *Provision of warmth* is an essential initial step in resuscitation and helps in normal newborn transition.
3. *Establishing effective ventilation* is the key to nearly all successful neonatal resuscitation.
4. Begin resuscitation of term as well as preterm baby with 21 % oxygen (*room air*).
5. Need of giving oxygen in appropriate concentration should be guided by the pulse oximeter readings. *Pulse oximetry* should be used for evaluation of oxygenation since assessment of color is unreliable.
6. Suctioning following birth should be *reserved for babies who have obvious obstruction* to spontaneous breathing or who require PPV.
7. After clearing the airway as necessary, drying and removing wet linen, repositioning, and stimulating, *evaluate respirations and heart rate* (*not color*).
   (a) If HR is less than 100 bpm, or if newborn is apneic or gasping, begin positive-pressure ventilation.
   (b) If HR is more than 100 bpm and respirations are labored, consider CPAP, especially for preterm newborns.
8. Subsequently, evaluation and decision-making are based on *respirations, HR, and oxygenation* (per pulse oximetry).
9. Using pulse oximetry, whenever possible, supplemental oxygen concentration should be adjusted to achieve the *target values for pre-ductal saturations*.
10. *Chest compressions* are indicated whenever heart rate is *below 60 bpm*, despite at least 30 s of effective positive pressure ventilation.
11. *Epinephrine* is indicated when the *heart rate remains below 60 bpm* after 30 s of effective assisted ventilation (preferably via endotracheal tube) and at least another 45–60 s of coordinated chest compressions and effective ventilation.
12. *Post-resuscitation care and prompt treatment of complications* prevent further cerebral damage and long-term squeal.

## References


1. Kattwinkel J, American Academy of Pediatrics and American Heart Association. Textbook of neonatal resuscitation. 6th ed. New Delhi: Jaypee brothers; 2012. p. 1–236.
2. https://eccguidelines.heart.org/wp-content/themes/eccstaging/dompdf-master/pdffiles/part-13-neonatal-resuscitation.pdf.
3. Soni P. Neonatal resuscitation. In: Pejavar RK, Kulkarni A, editors. Handbook neonatology. 1st ed. Bangalore: Arrow Medical Information Services (Publication of Neonatology Chapter of Indian Academy of Pediatrics); 2013. p. 1–13.
4. Gomella T, Cunningham MD, Eyal FG. Resuscitation of newborn. In: Neonatology: management, procedures, on-call problems, diseases, and drugs. 6th ed. New York: McGraw Hill; 2009. p. 15–22.
5. Ringer S. Resuscitation in delivery. In: Cloherty J, Eichenwald E, Hansen A, Stark A, editors. Manual of neonatal care. 7th ed. Philadelphia: Lippincott Williams & Wilkins/Wolters Kluwer (India); 2012. p. 47–62.
6. Dutta A, Nangia S, Saili A, et al. Post–resuscitation management of an asphyxiated neonate. In: Facility Based Newborn Care (FBNC) training module for Doctors and Nurses. New Delhi: Ministry of health and welfare; 2014. p. 55–8.

MIX
Papier aus verantwortungsvollen Quellen
Paper from responsible sources
FSC® C105338

If you have any concerns about our products,
you can contact us on
**ProductSafety@springernature.com**

In case Publisher is established outside the EU,
the EU authorized representative is:
**Springer Nature Customer Service Center GmbH**
**Europaplatz 3, 69115 Heidelberg, Germany**

Printed by Libri Plureos GmbH
in Hamburg, Germany